a LANGE medical book

Behavioral Medicine

A Guide for Clinical Practice

Fourth Edition

Editors

Mitchell D. Feldman, MD, MPhil, FACP
Professor of Medicine
Associate Vice Provost, Faculty Mentoring
University of California, San Francisco
San Francisco, California

John F. Christensen, PhD
Healthcare Consultant
Pilgrims' Partner Foundation
Corbett, Oregon

Associate editor

Jason M. Satterfield, PhD
Professor of Medicine
University of California, San Francisco
San Francisco, California

New York   Chicago   San Francisco   Athens   London   Madrid
Mexico City   Milan   New Delhi   Singapore   Sydney   Toronto

Behavioral Medicine: A Guide For Clinical Practice, Fourth Edition

1 2 3 4 5 6 7 8 9 0   CTP/CTP   19 18 17 16 15 14

BOOK MHID: 0-07-176770-3
BOOK ISBN: 978-0-07-176770-5

Notice

Medicine is an ever-changing science. As new research and clinical experience broaden our knowledge, changes in treatment and drug therapy are required. The authors and the publisher of this work have checked with sources believed to be reliable in their efforts to provide information that is complete and generally in accord with the standards accepted at the time of publication. However, in view of the possibility of human error or changes in medical sciences, neither the authors nor the publisher nor any other party who has been involved in the preparation or publication of this work warrants that the information contained herein is in every respect accurate or complete, and they disclaim all responsibility for any errors or omissions or for the results obtained from use of the information contained in this work. Readers are encouraged to confirm the information contained herein with other sources. For example and in particular, readers are advised to check the product information sheet included in the package of each drug they plan to administer to be certain that the information contained in this work is accurate and that changes have not been made in the recommended dose or in the contraindications for administration. This recommendation is of particular importance in connection with new or infrequently used drugs.

This book was set in Adobe Garamond Pro by Cenveo® Publisher Services.
The editors were Christine Diedrich and Regina Y. Brown.
The production supervisor was Richard Ruzycka.
Production management was provided by Vastavikta Sharma, Cenveo Publisher Services.
China Translation and Printing Services Limited was printer and binder.

This book is printed on acid-free paper.

McGraw-Hill books are available at special quantity discounts to use as premiums and sales promotions, or for use in corporate training programs. To contact a representative please e-mail us at bulksales@mcgraw-hill.com.

International Edition ISBN 978-1-259-25525-0; MHID 1-259-25525-5. Copyright © 2014. Exclusive rights by McGraw-Hill Education, for manufacture and export. This book cannot be re-exported from the country to which it is consigned by McGraw-Hill Education. The International Edition is not available in North America.

2014007922

Contents

I. THE DOCTOR & PATIENT

II. GLOBAL HEALTH

III. WORKING WITH SPECIFIC POPULATIONS

IV. HEALTH RELATED BEHAVIOR

V. MENTAL & BEHAVIORAL DISORDERS

VI. SPECIAL TOPICS

VII. TEACHING AND ASSESSMENT

Authors

Jonathan Amiel, MD
Columbia University College of Physicians &
    Surgeons
New York State Psychiatric Institute, New York
    Presbyterian Hospital
New York, New York
jma2106@columbia.edu
Chapter 45: Narrative Medicine

Annie Armstrong-Coben, MD
Assistant Clinical Professor of Pediatrics, Associate
    Directory Community Pediatric Training
Columbia University College of Physicians
    and Surgeons
New York, New York
aha2@columbia.edu
Chapter 45: Narrative Medicine

Robert B. Baron, MD, MS
Professor of Medicine, Associate Dean for Graduate
    and Continuing Medical Education
Vice Chief, Division of General Internal Medicine
University of California, San Francisco
San Francisco, California
baron@medicine.ucsf.edu
Chapter 22: Obesity

Kevin Barrows, MD
Medical Director, Osher Center for Integrative
    Medicine
Associate Clinical Professor, Department of Family
    and Community Medicine
University of California, San Francisco
San Francisco, California
barrowsk@ocim.ucsf.edu
Chapter 33: Integrative Medicine

Howard Beckman, MD, FACP, FAACH
Finger Lakes Health Systems Agency, Clinical
    Professor of Medicine and Family Medicine
University of Rochester School of Medicine
    and Dentistry
University Rochester
New York, New York
howardbeckman@flhsa.org
Chapter 4: Difficult Patients/Difficult Situations

Melanie J. Bernitz, MD
Instructor in Clinical Medicine, Department of
    Family Medicine
Columbia University Medical Center
New York, New York
mjb239@columbia.edu
Chapter 45: Narrative Medicine

Thomas Bodenheimer, MD
Professor of Family Medicine and Community
    Medicine
University of California, San Francisco
San Francisco, California
Tbodemheimer@fcm.ucsf.edu
*Chapter 39: Chronic Illness & Patient
    Self-management*

Donald W. Brady, MD FAACH
Associate Dean for Graduate Medical Education
Professor, Department of Medicine
Vanderbilt University
Nashville, Tennessee
donald.w.brady@vanderbilt.edu
*Chapter 17: Lesbian, Gay, Bisexual, & Transgender
    (LGBT) Patients*

David G. Bullard, PhD
Clinical Professor, Departments of Medicine
    and Psychiatry
Consultant, Symptom Management Service, Helen
    Diller Family Comprehensive Cancer Center
    University of California, San Francisco
San Francisco, California
Private Practice of Psychotherapy and Couples
    Therapy
San Francisco, California
dgbullard@yahoo.com
Chapter 32: Sexual Problems

Bethany Calkins, MD, MS
Fellow, Department of Palliative Care
University of Rochester Medical Center
Rochester, New York
Bethany_Arber@URMC.Rochester.edu
Chapter 3: Giving Bad News
*Chapter 40: Palliative Care, Hospice,
    & Care of the Dying*

Lisa Capaldini, MD, MPH
castromedical@aol.com
Chapter 36: HIV/AIDS

Harvey W. Caplan, MD
Former Co-Director of Clinical Training, Human
Sexuality Program
University of California, San Francisco,
San Francisco, California
Private Practice of Psychotherapy and Couples
Therapy
San Francisco, California
hcaplan@ix.netcom.com
Chapter 32: Sexual Problems

Patricia A. Carney, PhD
Professor of Family Medicine and of Public Health
and Preventive Medicine
Oregon Health & Science University
Portland, Oregon
carneyp@ohsu.edu
Chapter 43: Assessment and Evaluation

Rita Charon, MD, PhD
Executive Director and Founder, Program in
Narrative Medicine
Professor of Clinical Medicine, Department of
Medicine
College of Physicians & Surgeons of Columbia
University
New York, New York
Rac5@columbia.edu
Chapter 45: Narrative Medicine

Anna Haseltine Chodos, MD, MPH
Fellow, Division of Geriatrics, Department of
Medicine
University of California, San Francisco
San Francisco, California
anna.chodos@ucsf.edu
Chapter 30: Dementia & Delirium

John F Christensen, MS, PhD
Healthcare Consultant
Pilgrims' Partner Foundation
Corbett Oregon
nagarkot247@gmail.com
Chapter 5: Suggestion & Hypnosis
Chapter 9: Environmental Health and Behavior
Chapter 34: Stress & Disease
Chapter 47: Trainee Well-being
Chapter 25: Depression
Chapter 37: Errors in Medical Practice

David Claman, MD
David.Claman@ucsf.edu
Chapter 31: Sleep Disorders

Steven A. Cole, MD
Professor of Psychiatry, Emeritus
Stony Brook University School of Medicine
stevencolemd@aol.com
Chapter 25: Depression

Ann Cottingham, MAR, MA
Director, Dean's Office of Research in Medical
Education
Indiana University School of Medicine
Indianapolis, Indiana
ancottin@iupui.edu
*Chapter 42: Teaching Strategies, Infrastructures
and Resources*

Thomas Denberg, MD, PhD, FACP
Vice President, Quality and Patient Safety
Atrius Health and Harvard Vanguard Medical
Newton, Massachusetts
tom_denberg@atriushealth.org
Chapter 15: Cross-cultural Communication

Christine Derzko, MD
Associate Professor Obstetrics & Gynecology
and Internal Medicine (Endocrinology)
Faculty of Medicine
University of Toronto, Toronto, Ontario
derzkoc@smh.toronto.on.ca
Chapter 32: Sexual Problems

Mark J. DiCorcia, PhD, OTR
Vice Chair for Education, Department of Obstetrics
and Gynecology
IU School of Medicine
Assistant Professor of Obstetrics and Gynecology
IU School of Medicine
Indianapolis, Indiana
mdicorci@iupui.edu
*Chapter 42: Teaching Strategies, Infrastructures,
and Resources*

M. Robin DiMatteo, PhD
Distinguished Professor of Psychology
University of California, Riverside
California
robin.dimatteo@ucr.edu
Chapter 20: Patient Adherence

Elizabeth Eckstrom, MD, MPH
Associate Professor, Division of General Internal
　Medicine
Oregon Health & Science University
Portland, Oregon
eckstrom@ohsu.edu
Chapter 14: Older Patients

Barry Egener, MD
Medical Director, The Foundation for Medical
　Excellence
Portland, Oregon
Faculty, Legacy Internal Medicine Training Program
Portland, Oregon
BEgener@LHS.ORG
Chapter 2: Empathy

Stuart J. Eisendrath, MD
Professor, Director of the UCSF Depression Center
Department of Psychiatry
University of California, San Francisco
San Francisco, California
stuarte@lppi.ucsf.edu
Chapter 25: Depression
Chapter 28: Somatization

Michael Eisman, MD
mhe49@logical.net
*Chapter 40: Palliative Care, Hospice, & Care of the
　Dying*

Ronald M. Epstein, MD
Professor of Family Medicine, Psychiatry, Oncology
　and Nursing
Director, Center for Communication and Disparities
　Research
University of Rochester Medical Center
Rochester, New York
ronald_epstein@urmc.rochester.edu
Chapter 7: Mindful Practice

Mitchell D. Feldman, MD, MPhil
Professor of Medicine, Associate Vice Provost
Faculty Mentoring
University of California, San Francisco
San Francisco, California
mitchell.feldman@ucsf.edu
Chapter 11: Families
Chapter 15: Cross-cultural Communication
Chapter 25: Depression
Chapter 26: Anxiety
Chapter 36: HIV/AIDS
Chapter 38: Intimate Partner Violence
Chapter 47: Trainee Well-being

Molly Jean Ferguson, MPH
Program Manager, Department of Preventive
　Medicine
Northwestern University, Chicago, Illinois
m-ferguson@northwestern.edu
Chapter 44: Evidence-based Behavioral Practice

Richard M. Frankel, PhD
Professor of Medicine and Geriatrics
Indiana University School of Medicine
Associate Director, Center for Implementing
　Evidence-based Practice
Richard L. Roudebush, Veterans Administration
　Medical Center
Indianapolis, Indiana
rfrankel@iupui.edu
Chapter 46: Professionalism

Lawrence S. Friedman, MD
Professor of Clinical Medicine and Pediatrics
University of California, San Diego School of
　Medicine
San Diego, California
lsfriedman@ucsd.edu
Chapter 13: Adolescents

Julie S. Glickstein, MD
Associate Professor of Clinical Pediatrics
Division of Pediatric Cardiology and Department of
　Pediatrics
Columbia University College of Physicians and
　Surgeons
Columbia University Medical Center
Morgan Stanley Children's Hospital of New York
　Presbyterian
New York, New York
jg2065@columbia.edu
Chapter 45: Narrative Medicine

Matthew J. Gonzales, MD
Assistant Clinical Professor
Division of Hospital Medicine, Department of
　Medicine
University of California, San Francisco
San Francisco, California
Matthew.Gonzales@ucsf.edu
Chapter 35: Pain

Deepthiman Gowda, MD, PhD
Columbia University, College of Physicians
　and Surgeons
New York, New York
dg381@colubia.edu
Chapter 45: Narrative Medicine

Gillian E. Graham, MS
Program in Narrative Medicine
Columbia University College of Physicians
  and Surgeons
New York, New York
geg2120@columbia.edu
Chapter 45: Narrative Medicine

Richard E. Greene, MD, FACP
Assistant Professor, Department of Medicine
New York University School of Medicine
New York, New York
richard.greene@nyumc.org
*Chapter 17: Lesbian, Gay, Bisexual, & Transgender
  (LGBT) Patients*

Damara Gutnick, MD
Assistant Professor of Medicine and Psychiatry
New York University Langone Medical Center
  and Bellevue Hospital
New York City Health and Hospital's Corporation
New York, New York
damaragutnick@gmail.com
Chapter 25: Depression

Frederic W. Hafferty, PhD
Professor of Medical Education, Associate Director
Program in Professionalism and Ethics, Mayo Clinic
Rochester, Minnesota
fredhafferty@mac.com
Chapter 46: Professionalism

Nellie Hermann, MFA
Creative Director, Program in Narrative Medicine
College of Physicians and Surgeons
Columbia University
New York, New York
ngh2101@columbia.edu
Chapter 45: Narrative Medicine

Eric S. Holmboe, MD
Chief Medical officer, American Board of Internal
  Medicine
Adjunct Professor, Yale University School of
  Medicine
Adjunct Professor, Uniformed Services University of
  the Health Sciences
Yale, Connecticut
EHolmboe@ABIM.ORG
*Chapter 41: Behavioral and Social Science
  Competencies for Medical Education*

Thomas S. Inui, ScM, MD, MACP
Director of Research, IU Center for Global Research
Professor of Medicine, IU School of Medicine
Investigator, Regenstrief Institute
Indianapolis, Indiana
tinui@iupui.edu
*Chapter 42: Teaching Strategies, Infrastructures,
  and Resources*

Susan L. Janson, PhD, RN, NP, FAAN
Professor of Nursing and Medicine, Mary Harms/
  Nursing Alumni Endowed Chair
Department of Community Health Systems
University of California, San Francisco
San Francisco, California
susan.janson@nursing.ucsf.edu;susan.janson@ucsf.edu
*Chapter 39: Chronic Illness & Patient
  Self-management*

Bree Johnston, MD, MPH
bree.johnston@ucsf.edu
Chapter 30: Dementia & Delirium

Kavitha Kolappa, MD
kavitha.kolappa@gmail.com
Chapter 8: Global Health and Behavioral Medicine

Patrick T. Lee, MD, DTM&H
Medical Director, Cambridge Primary Care Center
Cambridge Health Alliance Instructor in Medicine
Harvard Medical School
Boston, Massachusetts
ptlee@partners.org
Chapter 8: Global Health and Behavioral Medicine

Mack Lipkin, MD, FACP, FRSM, FAAPP
Professor of Medicine, Director, Section of Primary
  Care
New York University School of Medicine
New York, New York
mack.lipkin@med.nyu.edu
Chapter 1: The Medical Interview

Debra K. Litzelman, MA, MD
Associate Dean, Dean's Office of Research in
  Medical Education
Professor of Medicine, Indiana University School of
  Medicine
Investigator, Regenstrief Institute
Indianapolis, Indiana
dklitzel@iupui.edu
*Chapter 42: Teaching Strategies, Infrastructures,
  and Resources*

Jay S. Luxenberg, MD
Chief Medical Office, On Lok Lifeways
San Francisco, California
Clinical Professor of Medicine, Division of Geriatric
    Medicine
UCSF School of Medicine, San Francisco
San Francisco, California
jay@luxenberg.net
Chapter 14: Older Patients

Elinore F. McCance-Katz MD, PhD
Professor, Department of Psychiatry
University of California, San Francisco
San Francisco, California
Elinore.Mccance-katz@ucsf.edu
Chapter 24: Alcohol & Substance Use

Felise B. Milan, MD
Academic: Albert Einstein College of Medicine
Clinical: Montefiore Medical Center
felise.milan@einstein.yu.edu
Chapter 43: Assessment and Evaluation

Vishnu Mohan, MD
Department of Medical Informatics and Clinical
    Epidemiology
Oregon Health & Science University
Portland, Oregon
mohanv@ohsu.edu
Chapter 1: The Medical Interview
*Chapter 10: Training of International Medical
    Graduates*

Gina Moreno-John, MD, MPH
University of California Medical Center
Department of General Internal Medicine
San Francisco, California
ginam@medicine.ucsf.edu
Chapter 38: Intimate Partner Violence

Diane S. Morse, MD
Assistant Professor of Psychiatry and Medicine
Department of Psychiatry, University of Rochester
    School of Medicine
Rochester, New York
Diane_Morse@urmc.rochester.edu
Chapter 16: Women

Daniel O'Connell, PhD
Training, Coaching and Consultation
Clinical Instructor, University of Washington
Seattle, Washington
danoconn@uw.edu
Chapter 19: Behavior Change

Roberta Oka, PhD, RN, ANP
Associate Chief Nurse for Research
VA Palo Alto HCS
Palo Alto, California
Roberta.oka@va.gov
*Chapter 39: Chronic Illness & Patient
    Self-management*

Steven Z. Pantilat, MD, FAAHPM, SFHM
Alan M. Kates and John M. Burnard Endowed
    Chair in Palliative Care
Director, Palliative Care Program, Division of UCSF
    Hospital Medicine
Department of Medicine, San Francisco
California, San Francisco
stevep@medicine.ucsf.edu
Chapter 35: Pain

Constance M. Park, MD, PhD
Associate Clinical Professor of Medicine
Columbia University, College of Physicians and
    Surgeons
New York, New York
cmp4@columbia.edu
Chapter 45: Narrative Medicine

Steve D. Persell, MD, MPH
Assistant Professor, Division of General Internal
    Medicine
Feinberg School of Medicine, Northwestern
    University
Chicago, Illinois
Spersell@nmff.org
Chapter 44: Evidence-based Behavioral Practice

Timothy E. Quill, MD, FACP, FAAHPM
Professor of Medicine, Psychiatry and Medical
    Humanities
University of Rochester Medical Center
Rochester, New York
timothy_quill@urmc.rochester.edu
Chapter 2: Giving Bad News
*Chapter 40: Palliative Care, Hospice,
    & Care of the Dying*

Michael W. Rabow, MD
Director, Symptom Management Service
Helen Diller Family Comprehensive Cancer Center
Department of Medicine, Professor of Clinical
    Medicine
University of California, San Francisco
San Francisco, California
mrabow@medicine.ucsf.edu
Chapter 35: Pain

Gita Ramamurthy, MD
Assistant Professor, Department of Psychiatry
    and Family Medicine SUNY
Upstate Medical Center
Syracuse, New York
agramam@gmail.com
Chapter 6: Practitioner Well-being

Neda Ratanawongsa, MD, MPH
Assistant Professor, General Internal Medicine
Center for Vulnerable Populations at San Francisco
    General Hospital and Trauma Center
University of California, San Francisco
San Francisco, California
ratanawongsan@medsfgh.ucsf.edu
Chapter 18: Vulnerable Patients

Giuseppe J. Raviola, MD
Instructor Psychiatry and Social Medicine
Department of Psychiatry, Children's Hospital,
    Boston
Department of Global health and Social Medicine,
    Harvard Medical School
Boston, Massachusetts
giuseppe.raviola@childrens.harvard.edu;giuseppe.
    raviola@hms.harvard.edu
Chapter 8: Global Health and Behavioral Medicine

Nancy A. Rigotti, MD
Professor of Medicine, Harvard Medical School
Associate Chief, General Medicine Division
Director, Tobacco Research and Treatment Center
Massachusetts General Hospital
Boston, Massachusetts
nrigotti@partners.org
Chapter 21: Tobacco

Steven J. Romano, MD
Senior Vice President, Medicines Development
    Group, Primary Care, Pfizer, Inc.
New York, New York
steve.romano@pfizer.com
Chapter 23: Eating Disorders

Tracy Ann Rydel, MD
Assistant Clinical Professor, Osher Center for
    Integrative Medicine
Department of Family and Community Medicine
University of California, San Francisco
San Francisco, California
rydelt2@ocim.ucsf.edu
Chapter 33: Integrative Medicine

George W. Saba, PhD
Professor of Clinical Family and Community
    Medicine
University of California, San Francisco
Department of Family and Community Medicine
Associate Program Director, Family and Community
    Medical Residency at San Francisco General
    Hospital
San Francisco, California
gsaba@fcm.ucsf.edu
Chapter 18: Vulnerable Patients

Veronica J. Sanchez, PhD
Department of Psychology
University of California, Riverside
California
vsanc006@ucr.edu
Chapter 20: Patient Adherence

Derek Satre, PhD
Associate Professor, Department of Psychiatry
University of California, San Francisco
San Francisco, California
dereks@lppi.ucsf.edu
Chapter 24: Alcohol & Substance Use

Jason M. Satterfield, PhD
Professor of Medicine
University of California, San Francisco
jsatter@medicine.ucsf.edu
Chapter 26: Anxiety
Chapter 41: Competency-Based Education for
    Behavioral Medicine
Chapter 43: Assessing Learners and Curricula in the
    Behavioral and Social Sciences

Dean Schillinger, MD
UCSF Professor of Medicine in Residence
Chief, Division of General Internal Medicine
San Francisco General Hospital
Director, Health Communication Program
UCSF Center for Vulnerable Populations
Chief, CA Diabetes Program, CA Department of
    Public Health
San Francisco, California
dschillinger@medsfgh.ucsf.edu
Chapter 18: Vulnerable Patients

Jason S. Schneider, MD, FACP
Assistant Professor, Division of General Medicine
Department of Medicine, Emory University School
    of Medicine
Atlanta, Georgia
jsschne@emory.edu
*Chapter 17: Lesbian, Gay, Bisexual, & Transgender
(LGBT) Patients*

Antoinette Schoenthaler, EdD
New York University School of Medicine
New York, New York
Antoinette.schoenthaler@nyumc.org
Chapter 1: The Medical Interview

H. Russell Searight, PhD, MPH
Department of Psychology, Lake Superior State
    University
Sault Ste Marie, Michigan
russellsearight@msn.com
*Chapter 10: Training of International Medical
Graduates*
*Chapter 27: Attention Deficit Hyperactivity
Disorder*

J. Jewel Shim, MD
Associate Clinical Professor of Psychiatry
University of California, San Francisco,
    San Francisco, California
San Francisco, California
jewels@lppi.ucsf.edu
Chapter 28: Somatization

Cheyenne Shinabarger, BS
Department of Psychology
Lake Superior State University
cshinabarger@lssu.edu
*Chapter 27: Attention Deficit Hyperactivity
Disorder*

Clifford Milo Singer, MD
Adjunct Professor, University of Maine
Orono, Maine
Chief, Division of Geriatric Mental Health
    and Neuropsychiatry
The Acadia Hospital and Eastern Main Medical
    Center
Bangor, Maine
CSINGER@EMH.ORG
Chapter 14: Older Patients
Chapter 31: Sleep Disorders

Gregory T. Smith, PhD
Director, Progressive Rehabilitation Associates
Portland, Oregon
Consulting Psychologist, Pain Rehabilitation
    Program
SW Medical Center
Vancouver, Washington
greg@progrehab.com
Chapter 35: Pain

Bonnie Spring, PhD, ABPP
Professor of Preventive Medicine, Psychology
    and Psychiatry, Behavioral Medicine Directory
    & Co-Program Leader for Cancer Prevention
bspring@northwestern.edu
Chapter 44: Evidence-based Behavioral Practice

Jody Steinaur, MD
Associate Professor, Department of Obstetrics
    and Gynecology and Reproductive Sciences
University of California, San Francisco
San Francisco, California
Steinauerj@obgyn.ucsf.edu
Chapter 16: Women

Anthony L. Suchman, MD, FAACH
The Healthcare Consultancy of the McArdle
    Ramerman Center; The University of Rochester
    School of Medicine and Dentistry
Rochester, New York
asuchman@rchcweb.com
Chapter 6: Practitioner Well-being

Howard L. Taras, MD
Professor of Pediatrics
University of California, San Diego
La Jolla, California
htaras@ucsd.edu
Chapter 12: Children

Delphine Taylor, MD
Associate Professor and Clinical medicine
College of Physicians and Surgeons
Division of General Medicine
Columbia University
New York, New York
dst4@mail.lumc.columbia.edu
Chapter 45: Narrative Medicine

Robin Telerant, MD
Geriatric Medicine Fellow
Oregon Health and Science University
Portland, Oregon
telerant@ohsu.edu
Chapter 14: Older Patients

Teresa J. Villela, MD
Professor of Clinical Family and Community
    Medicine
University of California, San Francisco
Department of Family and Community Medicine
Program Director, Family and Community
    Medicine Residency at San Francisco General
    Hospital
San Francisco, California
tvillela@fcm.ucsf.edu
Chapter 18: Vulnerable Patients

Judith Walsh, MD, MPH
Professor of Clinical Medicine
University of California, San Francisco
Women's Health Clinical Research Center
University of California, San Francisco
San Francisco, California
Judith.Walsh@ucsf.edu
Chapter 16: Women

Albert W. Wu, MD, MPH
Professor, Department of Health Policy
    and Management
Johns Hopkins Bloomberg School of Public Health
Department of Medicine, Johns Hopkins School of
    Medicine
Johns Hopkins University
Baltimore, Maryland
awu@jhsph.edu
Chapter 37: Errors in Medical Practice

Kristine Yaffe, MD
Professor Departments of Psychiatry, Neurology,
    and Epidemiology
University of California, San Francisco,
    San Francisco
Veterans Affairs Medical Center
San Francisco, California
kristine.yaffe@ucsf.edu
Chapter 30: Dementia & Delirium

John Q. Young, MD, MPP
Vice Chair for Education
Director, Residency Training
Department of Psychiatry
Hofstra North Shore-LIJ School of Medicine
The Zucker Hillside Hospital
Glen Oaks, New York
jqyoung@lppi.ucsf.edu
Chapter 29: Personality Disorders

Foreword

Caring for patients is challenging work—because people are complicated. Patients seek help not only for acute or chronic medical problems, but they also bring to the clinical encounter their life circumstances, worries, and concerns. Medical problems are rarely only about biomedical issues but are almost always accompanied by problems at work, with family, finances, and a myriad of other life concerns. Physicians and other health professionals need to understand not only the illness but also its impact on the person's life. They must demonstrate a broad understanding of and concern for the patient. As far back as 1925, Dr. Francis Peabody said, "The secret of the care of the patient is in caring for the patient".[1]

While Peabody's adage is still true, we now need to understand a broader variety of behavioral disorders and the best treatments for them. We need to care for increasing numbers of elderly patients and more ethnically diverse populations. We need to tailor our care to a wider variety of patients with more complex needs and with complex problems such as multiple chronic illnesses, palliative care, HIV/AIDS, and other challenging issues such as intimate partner violence.

Behavioral Medicine: A Guide for Clinical Practice, helps practitioners understand the interplay between psychological, physical, social, and cultural issues of patients. It provides practical information about many of the topics listed above and also includes guidance about how to manage common situations. The case illustrations throughout the book are jewels for medical practitioners who need suggestions about how to communicate effectively in challenging situations. For example, the book provides suggestions for ways to coach patients about lifestyle changes or respond to a patient with a somatic symptom disorder.

In addition, the book is useful to those who teach behavioral medicine. It includes topics related to understanding and assessing the competencies of trainees and developing a curriculum in social and behavioral medicine.

One of the significant elements of the book is the recognition that the well-being of physicians and other health professionals is critically important to caring for patients. As a profession we often do not pay enough attention to the feelings of the physicians who can become burned out doing the work they love and, in turn, provide less good care to patients. Chapters on mindful practice and practitioner well-being enhance the book.

It is no surprise that this book is in its fourth edition. With much new content, it provides insight and information not available anywhere else for those who seek to provide comprehensive high-quality care for patients. And it does so in a way that acknowledges patients as people who have problems that often go far beyond the reach of traditional medical care.

Wendy Levinson, MD
Sir John and Lady Eaton Professor and Chair,
Department of Medicine, University of Toronto, Canada

---

[1]Peabody FW. The care of the patient. *JAMA*. 1927;88:877–882.

Preface

Since the publication of the third edition of *Behavioral Medicine: A Guide for Clinical Practice*, there have been considerable advances in medical diagnosis and treatment, as well as changes in the ways in which health care is organized and delivered. The science of genetics has revolutionized the understanding of disease and the design of therapies targeted to specific diseases, and increasingly, to specific individuals. New medications, therapies, and technologies are available for treatment of a variety of behavioral health problems, such as mood and anxiety disorders and substance use. There are new collaborative models of chronic care and patient self-care that increase effectiveness in the treatment of those with chronic illness. The rapid adoption of electronic medical records as the standard in most treatment settings poses new challenges for establishing and maintaining rapport in the clinician–patient relationship. Health care organizations are paying greater attention to the importance of clinician well-being in reducing burnout and error and in maximizing the performance of the organization, including financial outcomes. And the passage of the Affordable Care Act (ACA), with greater emphasis being given to the integration of behavioral health into primary care practice, has the potential to profoundly change how we approach the care of patients with mental and behavioral problems.

This fourth edition addresses these and other new developments in the clinical practice and teaching of behavioral medicine. This edition features extensive revisions of chapters from the previous editions to reflect advances in pharmacotherapy and evidence on the relationship between psychosocial factors and disease.

Recognizing that there is an international context to the practice of behavioral medicine, this fourth edition features a new section on global health. Untreated behavioral and mental illness contributes to the global burden of disease, and there are marked disparities among nations and regions in recognition of these problems and treatment availability. The chapter on global health and behavioral medicine addresses the cultural and economic determinants of these disparities and offers new models for behavioral medicine practice and training to reduce the treatment gaps. Health outcomes globally are also influenced by environmental factors such as climate change, and human behavior is deemed responsible for a growing stress to the earth and its natural functions. The chapter on environment, health, and behavior examines these interrelationships and suggests behavior change models on a societal scale to promote the health of the planet.

The training of physicians and other health professionals has continued to evolve. Greater clarity in defining and assessing competencies, including those in behavioral medicine, have warranted an extensive expansion of the section on teaching and assessment with an emphasis on new approaches to training for behavioral competencies. Among these are more precise descriptions of behavioral competencies, advances in evaluation, novel teaching strategies such as the use of narrative medicine, and evidence-based behavioral practice. Finally, helping trainees in the health professions to find balance in their lives and to develop the life skills for a sustainable career has challenged medical schools and residencies to create curricula and educational experiences to promote well-being. These concepts are addressed in the final chapter of the book.

Although the term "behavioral medicine" is used widely in both medical and social science literature, there is little agreement as to its exact definition. We broadly define it as an interdisciplinary field that aims to integrate the biological and psychosocial perspectives on human behavior and to apply them to the practice of medicine. Our perspective includes a behavioral approach to somatic disease, the mental disorders as they commonly appear in medical practice, issues in the clinician–patient relationship, and other important topics that affect the delivery of medical care, such as motivating behavior change, maximizing adherence to medical treatment, integrative medicine, and care of the dying.

We hope that general internists, hospitalists, family practitioners, pediatricians, nurse practitioners, physician assistants, pharmacists, and other clinicians will find that this book helps them to better understand and care for persons with a wide variety of mental and behavioral problems. For residents and students in health care settings, *Behavioral Medicine: A Guide for Clinical Practice* can function as a valuable resource for understanding the psychosocial dimensions of medicine.

It is our intent that medical educators will find this book to be a clinically relevant text that forms a basis for developing a comprehensive curriculum in behavioral medicine. Training in the core competencies required by the

Accreditation Council for Graduate Medical Education (ACGME) will be enhanced by inclusion of topics covered thoroughly in this book, including clinician–patient communication, professionalism, and cultural competence. For faculty and students who wish to explore a topic in greater depth, the suggestions for further reading and web-based resources provided at the end of each chapter will be helpful.

The principles of behavior change discussed in this book apply not only to individuals, but also to whole societies as they move through the "stages of change" to alter lifestyles that adversely impact the environment and human health. The health and well-being of our personal lives and of the organizations in which we work are intertwined with the health of our planet. Restoring the proper relationship of humans with the earth in a way that promotes sustainability in the whole system is what Thomas Berry has called "the great work" of our generation. Physicians and other health professionals have a vital role to play in this work, for our own health and well-being will only be as good as the health of the planet.

Acknowledgments

This book would not have been possible without the support and mentorship of several people. We are indebted to Stephen J. McPhee, MD, for recognizing the need for such a book almost two decades ago and for continually providing encouragement and advice. Our deep appreciation is offered to Jason Satterfield, PhD, for stepping in as an associate editor for this edition and for organizing the section on teaching and assessment. We thank James Shanahan, Christine Diedrich, Regina Brown, and Laura Libretti at McGraw-Hill for providing expert guidance in the crafting of this fourth edition. We are very grateful to our contributing authors who, despite busy schedules as clinicians and teachers, have been generous and conscientious in going the distance with us.

Countless friends and colleagues at our own institutions, as well as the residents we have been privileged to teach and mentor, have contributed to our own learning and the selection of material for this book. We are especially indebted to our colleagues in the Society of General Internal Medicine and the American Academy on Communication in Healthcare, many of whom have contributed chapters for this book, for being the learning community that has helped us grow professionally.

Jane Kramer and Julie Burns Christensen and our children, Nina and Jonathan Kramer-Feldman and Jake and Hank Christensen, as well as Hank's wife Kerry and Jake's wife Nancy, have continued to be a renewing and cherished presence in our lives. This book would not have been possible without their love and support.

Mitchell D. Feldman, MD, MPhil
John F. Christensen, PhD
San Francisco, California and Corbett, Oregon
June 2014

SECTION I
The Doctor & Patient

The Medical Interview

Mack Lipkin, Jr., MD, Antoinette Schoenthaler, Ed.D. & Vishnu Mohan, MD

INTRODUCTION

The medical interview, the major medium of patient care, is of central importance to practitioners. A successful interview elicits accurate and complete data. It represents a dialogue that determines whether the patient agrees to take a medication, undergo a test, or change a diet. More than 80% of diagnoses are derived from the interview. The doctor–patient interaction is the keystone of patient satisfaction; moreover, interview-related factors impact major outcomes of care, including physiologic responses, symptom resolution, pain control, functional status, propensity to sue in the event of an adverse outcome, and emotional health. The medical interview also influences the quality of care, including malpractice suits and their resolution, the amount of patient disclosure of difficult or stigmatized information, time efficiency, and the elimination of "doorknob" questions as the interview ends.

Clearly, the interview is a major determinant of professional success. Yet, fewer than 10% of medical practitioners have spent time, since medical school, working on their interviewing ability. When asked, most physicians indicate that they have no plan or approach to monitoring, maintaining, or improving this critical skill. Can you imagine a professional musician, athlete, or pilot not practicing? One would question their commitment and competence or potential for remaining successful.

The interview is also key to a practitioner's sense of professional well-being, as it is the factor that most influences satisfaction with each encounter. Physicians with high career dissatisfaction most often attribute this to unsatisfying communication and relationships with patients. Physicians with high job satisfaction have a significant interest in the psychosocial aspects of care, relate effectively with patients, and are able to manage difficult patient situations.

The Ubiquitous Interview

The central role of the interview derives from its epidemiology as well as its "one-on-one" impact. For most physicians, it is more prevalent than any other activity in their work or their lives. The average length of time per ambulatory patient visit for internists, family practitioners, and pediatricians is about 20 minutes, and these groups account for 75% of doctor visits. The average visit time for *all* physicians is 6 minutes, a rate curiously constant in the United States, the United Kingdom, The Netherlands, and elsewhere. Physicians who bring the average down to 6 minutes are moving scarily fast.

Making conservative estimates about how many hours a practitioner will work over a 40-year professional lifetime, a generalist will have around 250,000 patient encounters. Each interview can be the source of satisfaction or frustration, of learning or apathy, of efficiency or wasted effort (Table 1-1), of personal growth and inspiration or dispiriting discouragement. Despite the importance of performing this complex skill expertly, few physicians plan, or even think about, how to improve patient encounters to reach the desirable goals of satisfaction, learning, and efficiency.

Each discipline or special interest, such as psychiatry, occupational health, women's health, or domestic violence support has a specialized set of questions that must be asked of every patient for the interview to be complete and

1

Table 1-1. Gains from improved interviewing techniques.

- Increased efficiency in use of time
- Increased accuracy and completeness of data
- Improved diagnosis
- Fewer tests and procedures
- Increased compliance
- Increased physician satisfaction
- Increased patient satisfaction
- Decreased dissatisfaction
- Increased mutual learning from each encounter

to elicit that patient's particular problems. (If an interviewer were to ask every question recommended by each specialty the interview would take hours.) In most cases, these questionnaires have neither been validated nor shown to be sensitive or specific. Notable exceptions include the CAGE Questionnaire (Table 1-2), which is a highly specific, sensitive, and efficient screening test for alcoholism (see Chapter 24); the two-question depression screen (see Chapter 25); and the one-question domestic violence screen (see Chapter 38).

Rather than the use of a series of over-specific, narrowly focused questions, it is more effective to use a patient-centered approach. First, elicit the patient's complete set of concerns and questions. Then explore the priority, negotiated problem by asking open-to-closed-ended questions to encourage elaboration on the information and elicit the needed data about each concern. Lists of open-ended questions elicit information more efficiently than lists of closed-ended questions. A patient-centered approach ensures that the patient's concerns are understood and accepted—a predictor of increased compliance. Because open-ended questions allow the patient to frame the response, the nature of framing reveals how the patient is processing the issue under discussion information is rarely available from closed-ended questions.

This approach is efficient for several reasons. First, patients usually have a sense of what is relevant and will include key information and data not anticipated by the interviewer. A physician who is thinking of the next question rather than listening to what is being said loses the ability to attend and hear on multiple levels. If the interviewer is talking then the patient is not

Table 1-2. The CAGE Questionnaire.

C: Have you ever tried to **C**ut down on your drinking?
A: Do you feel **A**nnoyed when asked about your drinking?
G: Do you feel **G**uilty about your drinking?
E: Do you ever take an **E**ye opener in the morning?

talking, and so, is not providing data. The physician can always refer to specific items to round out the data once the patient's story is told. If the same format is used for each interview, the variations in responses can be attributed to the patient, thereby providing significant insight.

The evidence favoring a patient-centered approach goes beyond the practical advantages: outcomes of care are also favorable. More complete and higher quality information—with an attendant reduction in procedures and tests—reduces cost, side effects, and complications. Increased patient adherence to diagnostic and therapeutic plans leads to greater clinical efficiency and effectiveness, and patients take a more active role in their own care.

Efficiency & Active Listening

A number of factors enhance interview efficiency, a growing concern, as the corporatization of health care leads doctors and patients to experience care as more rushed. Actual visit lengths have remained constant. However, as knowledge and regulation grow exponentially, tasks to accomplish in a given visit multiply—more diseases and risks to evaluate, more treatments to choose among and explain, and more computer screens and bureaucratic hoops to negotiate. These trends will undoubtedly prove counterproductive: when the visit is jammed with too much to do, psychosocial discussion suffers. This can result in unnecessary testing, patient dissatisfaction, and hazardous or needless procedures and treatments. Challenges to efficiency and effectiveness are exacerbated when behavioral medicine is removed from the medical visit by outsourcing to an external "behavioral management" company. Then both sides compete not to care for the patient, and predictably the relationship and quality of care deteriorate.

Specific techniques enhance cost-effectiveness and efficiency. Open-ended questions allow patients to elaborate on responses, provide additional information, and make interviews shorter. "Active listening" involves listening to what is said on multiple levels—how it is said, what is included and what is left out, how what is said reflects the person's culture, personality, mental status, affect, conscious and unconscious motivation, cognitive style, and so on. Acknowledging or repeating the essence of the information shared, whether clinical or emotional, allows the patient to feel understood and provides an opportunity to correct misperceptions. A skilled active listener acquires data quickly and continuously. Like a jazz musician, an active skilled practitioner creates a harmonious flow in sync with the patient's themes, rhythms, and style to enhance the ability of each to contribute to the complex, shifting improvisation of the interview. The experienced listener gives his or her observations the appropriate weight of clear data, hypotheses, or biases. This creates a complex and textured portrait of the patient that can be used in generating hypotheses, crafting replies, giving information, managing affective responses and nonverbal behaviors, and questioning further.

THE STRUCTURE OF THE INTERVIEW

Recent literature on the medical interview runs to more than 50,000 articles, chapters, and books. Although only a modest portion of these are derived from empirical bases, sufficient work has been done to describe the interview's conceptual framework as having "structure" and "functions." Behavioral observations and detailed, reproducible analyses of interviews have related specific behaviors and skills to both structural elements and functions; performance of these behaviors and skills improves clinical outcomes. The following description of essential structural elements and their associated behaviors or techniques, although comprehensive, is not so exhaustive as to be impractical. Key behaviors are summarized in Table 1-3. One comprehensive model of this approach is shown in Figure 1-1.

Preparing the Physical Environment

Architects and designers believe that form follows function. Similarly, how practitioners organize their physical environment reveals core characteristics of their practice: how they view the importance of the patient's comfort and ease; how they want to be regarded; and how they as practitioners control their own environment. Does the patient have a choice of seating? Do both patient and provider sit at comparable eye level? Is the room accessible, quiet, and private? Optimal environments reduce anxiety and instill calm and a sense of well-being.

Preparing Oneself

Humans can process about seven bits of information simultaneously. Given this limitation, it is advisable to consider how many of these bits are consumed by distractions or trivia in a clinical encounter. The hypnotic concept of focus or the recently accepted psychological concepts of centering or flow apply to the clinical encounter (see Chapter 5). Thoughts about the last or next patient, yesterday's mistake, last night's argument, passion, or movie can affect concentration; information and opportunity are lost. In contrast, a focused practitioner, without external or internal distractions, can expect the interview to be a challenging, fascinating, and unique experience.

Achieving a focused state of mind is personal and related to each situation. Nevertheless, successful centering includes: eliminating outside intrusion by beepers and phone calls, tuning out extraneous sound, eliminating internal distraction and intrusive thoughts by resolving not to work on other matters, letting intrusive thoughts simply pass through your mind for the moment, and controlling distracting reactions within the interview by noting them, considering their origins, and putting them aside.

Such skills do not just happen. We teach our residents self-hypnosis; practitioners are routinely and efficiently able to get to a place of heightened, alert, and energetic focus. Using this skill together with the suggestions in Table 1-4, practitioners can enhance the opportunity for something profound to happen in each patient encounter.

Observing the Patient

A great deal can be learned by thoughtfully observing the patient's behavior and body language both before and during the encounter. Although initial behavioral observations are purely heuristic—used to generate testable hypotheses about the patient—non-verbal behaviors can reveal as much about the patient's state of mind as their verbal behavior. Physicians who are unaware of being influenced by initial reactions and observations in the patient interview may note that when they themselves get on a bus or an airplane, they instantly recognize the person next to whom they would prefer—or not—to sit. Such responses integrate multiple non-verbal cues. Similar input from patients relates to their overall health, vital signs, cardiac and pulmonary compensation, liver function, and more. Observations about grooming, state-of-rest, alertness, and style of presentation reveal the patient's self-confidence, presence of psychosis, depression, or anxiety, as well as the patient's personality style, culture or sub-culture, and important changes from prior visits. The physician may also detect signs of possible alcohol or drug use. Escorting patients from the waiting area, letting them walk slightly ahead into the office, allows the physician to observe gait, how patients use their waiting time, companions, and clues to the relationship with companions. Often, especially with new patients, the very first words spoken by the patient may be epigraphic or may foreshadow the encounter.

Maximizing clinical observation skills starts with the commitment to do so. Developing the habit of systematically retaining and integrating initial observations will provide the physician with important data typically overlooked. Asking pertinent questions about behavioral cues will increase observation speed and comprehensiveness. Practicing in crowds, at rounds or lectures, on the airplane, or at parties will help train oneself to become a more astute observer. It is the physician's equivalent of practicing scales on the piano or taking batting practice.

Table 1-3. Structural elements of the medical interview.

Element	Technique or Behavior
Prepare the environment	Create a private area. Eliminate noise and distractions. Provide comfortable seating at equal eye level. Provide easy physical access.

Prepare oneself	Eliminate distractions and interruptions.
	Focus on:
	   Self-hypnosis
	   Meditation
	   Constructive imaging
	Let intrusive thoughts pass.

Observe the patient	Create a personal list of categories of observation. Practice in a variety of settings. Notice physical signs. Notice patient's presentation and affect. Notice what is said and not said.
Greet the patient	Create a flexible personal opening. Introduce oneself. Check the patient's name and how it is pronounced. Create a positive social setting.
Begin the interview	Explain one's role and purpose. Check patient's expectations. Negotiate about differences in perspective. Be sure expectations are congruent with patient's.

Detect and overcome barriers to communication	Be aware of and look for potential barriers:
	   Language
	   Physical impediments such as deafness, delirium
	   Cultural differences
	   Psychological obstacles such as shame, fear, and paranoia

Survey problems	Develop personal methods to elicit an accounting of problems. Ask "what else" until problems are described.
Negotiate priorities	Ask patient for his or her priorities. State own priorities. Establish mutual interests. Reach agreement on the order of addressing issues.

Develop a narrative thread	Develop personal ways of asking patients to tell their story:
	   When did patient last feel healthy?
	   Describe entire course of illness.
	   Describe recent episode or typical episode.

Establish the life context of the patient	Use first opportunity to inquire about personal and social details. Flesh out developmental history. Learn about patient's support system. Learn about home, work, neighborhood, and safety issues.
Establish a safety net	Memorize complete review of systems. Review issues as appropriate to specific problem.
Present findings and options	Be succinct. Ascertain patient's level of understanding and cognitive style. Ask patient to review and state understanding. Summarize and check. Tape interview and give copy of tape to patient. Ask patient's perspectives.
Negotiate plans	Involve patient actively. Agree on what is feasible. Respect patient's choices whenever possible.
Close the interview	Ask patient to review plans and arrangements. Clarify what patient should do in the interim. Schedule next encounter. Say good-bye.

Begin interview

Prepare
a. Review the patient's chart
b. Assess and prepare the physical environment
  i. Optimize comfort and privacy
  ii. Minimize interruptions and distractions
c. Assess one's own personal issues, values, biases, and assumptions going into the encounter

Open
a. Greet and welcome the patient and family member present
b. Introduce yourself
c. Explain role and orient patient to the flow of the visit
d. Indicate time available and other constraints
e. Identify and minimize barriers to communication
f. Calibrate your language and vocabulary to that of the patient
g. Accommodate patient comfort and privacy

Gather information

I. Survey patient's reasons for the visit
a. Start with open-ended, nonfocused questions
b. Invite patient to tell the story chronologically ("narrative thread")
c. Allow the patient to talk without interrupting
d. Actively listen
e. Encourage completion of the statement of all of patient's concerns through verbal and nonverbal encouragement ("tell me more," the exhaustive "what else?")
f. Summarize what you heard. Check for understanding. Invite more ("anything more?")

II. Determine the patient's chief concern
a. Ask closed-ended questions that are nonleading and one at a time
b. Define the symptom completely

III. Complete the patient's medical database
a. Obtain medical and family history
b. Elicit pertinent psychosocial data
c. Summarize what you heard and how you understand it, check for accuracy

Elicit and understand patient's perspective
a. Ask patient about ideas about illness or problem
b. Ask patient about expectations
c. Explore beliefs, concerns, and expectations
d. Ask about family, community, and religious or spiritual context
e. Acknowledge and respond to patient's concerns, feelings, and nonverbal cues
f. Acknowledge frustrations/challenges/progress (waiting time, uncertainty)

Communicate during the physical examination or procedure
a. Prepare patient
b. Consider commenting on aspects and findings of the physical examination or procedure as it is performed
c. Listen for previously unexpressed data about the patient's illness or concerns

Fundamental skills to maintain during the entire interview

I. Use relationship building skills
a. Allow patient to express self
b. Be attentive and empathic nonverbally
c. Use appropriate language
d. Communicate nonjudgmental, respectful, and supportive attitude
e. Accurately recognize emotion and feelings
f. Use PEARLS Statements (Partnership, Empathy, Apology, Respect, Legitimization, Support) to respond to emotion instead of redirecting or pursuing clinical detail

II. Manage flow
a. Be organized and logical
b. Manage time effectively in the interview

Patient education
a. Use Ask-Tell-Ask approach to giving information meaningfully
  —Ask about knowledge, feelings, emotions, reactions, beliefs and expectations
  —Tell the information clearly and concisely, in small chunks, avoid "doctor babble"
  —Ask repeatedly for patient's understanding
b. Use language patient can understand
c. Use qualitative data accurately to enhance understanding
d. Use aids to enhance understanding (diagrams, models, printed material, community resources)
e. Encourage questions

Negotiate and agree on plan
a. Encourage shared decision making to the extent the patient desires
b. Survey problems and delineate options
c. Elicit patient's understanding, concerns, and preferences
d. Arrive at mutually acceptable solution
e. Check patient's willingness and ability to follow the plan.
f. Identify and enlist resources and supports

End interview

Close
a. Signal closure
b. Inquire about any other issues or concerns
c. Allow opportunity for final disclosures
d. Summarize and verify assessment and plan
e. Clarify future expectations
f. Assure plan for unexpected outcomes and follow up
g. Thank patient—appropriate parting statement

*This model is an expansion of the work of the Kalamazoo Consensus Conference held May 1999 supported by Bayer-Fetzer; in addition other models were consulted directly. These included the Brown Interview Checklist, the Three Function Model, the work of the AAPP Courses Committee-Blue Card. Segue. Calgary-Cambridge Observation Guide, Bayer model, and an extensive review of the literature on communications in medicine completed for the Macy Initiative. This model has been prepared by the Macy Initiative in Health Communication. Please address questions to Regina Janicik (212) 263-2304.

Figure 1-1. The medical interview. *(Developed by the Macy Initiative in Health Communication.)*

Table 1-4. Self-hypnotic suggestions to enhance interview outcomes.

In this encounter I will:
Focus on the patient and his or her concerns
Not hear outside distractors
Let intrusive thoughts pass through unheeded
Connect meaningfully with this person
Learn something new and surprising about him or her
Have a positive encounter
Leave feeling energized
Help the patient grow, change, and heal
Help the patient leave the interview feeling hopeful and committed

Greeting the Patient

The greeting serves to identify each party, to set the social tone, to indicate intentions concerning equality or dominance, and to prevent mistaken identity. It also allows the practitioner to establish an immediate connection with patients, presenting a confident, compassionate professional the patient can trust. It enables the physician to learn how patients assert their own identity and how to pronounce their names. Using a standard greeting—saying virtually the same thing each time—provides data based on the individuality in a patient's response.

Beginning the Interview

The introductory phase of a medical encounter provides an opportunity for both parties to express their understanding of the purpose and condition of the encounter, to check each other's expectations, and to negotiate differences. For example, the patient may expect to be seen by the head of the clinic, but the physician is only a year out of residency. The patient wants relief from back pain and the practitioner is worried about the high blood pressure of the patient that day. The cardiologist expects the consultation to lead to cardiac catheterization, whereas the patient thinks the cardiologist's opinions will be sent to his primary care physician for a decision. Perhaps, the physician planned a 15-minute visit, but the patient feels an hour is needed.

One of the best predictors of the outcome of a dyadic relationship is concordance of expectations; therefore, clarifying and reconciling these is extremely valuable before proceeding to the main part of the interview.

The beginning of the interview, especially with a new patient, sets the interactional tone (although one can always change tone by changing one's behavior). Although many attempt idle social chat, bland social questions may confuse the professional focus or make the patient feel compelled to present a positive tone.

It is useful to consider using a fairly stereotyped beginning, such as "what brings you in to see me today?" (As opposed to ". . . how may I help you" which prejudges the purpose of the interview).

Detecting & Overcoming Barriers to Communication

Many factors that interfere with communication place even more barriers between the doctor and the patient. Sometimes these are tangible barriers: delirium, dementia, deafness, aphasia, intoxication (patient or physician), or ambient noise. Psychological barriers include depression, anxiety, psychosis, paranoia, and distrust. Social barriers often involve language, cultural differences, and fears about immigration status, stigma, cost of the visit, or legal issues. It is essential to detect barriers early in an encounter. Failure to do so not only wastes time but can seriously and, sometimes, dangerously mislead the physician. For example, residents and students often spend an hour or more trying to extract history from a delirious patient, resulting in an hour lost and highly unreliable historical data. In addition, detecting barriers is the first step toward correction, whether by waiting until delirium or intoxication has cleared, finding a professional interpreter or signer, moving to a quiet place, or deferring difficult issues until trust is established.

Surveying Problems

Patients come to medical encounters with multiple problems and, for various reasons, may not lead with the most pressing issue. Physicians typically interrupt very quickly (18–23 seconds on average). It is of vital importance not to jump in at the first important-sounding problem, but instead to elicit all problems. For example, the physician might ask, "What problems are you having?" or "What issues would you like to work on first?" After getting the initial answer or series of answers, the physician can then ask ". . . what else?" until the list of problems is completed and mutual priorities are established.

Negotiating Priorities

Once the physician and the patient clearly understand the full set of problems, the physician should then ask, "Which of these would you like to work on first?" If the physician believes that something else is more important, there should be a negotiation about this difference: "Our time is limited today, and I think your shortness of breath is potentially more dangerous than your back pain. Suppose we deal with that first and, if we have time, go on to your back pain. If not, we'll take that up on your next visit."

Appropriate and understandable resentment results when the physician does not ascertain and acknowledge the patient's priorities. This can lead to treatment adherence problems or failure to return to the office.

Developing a Narrative Thread

Once the physician and the patient have decided which problem has priority, exploration of that problem begins. Note the term "exploration." All too often the approaches are either to jump into a review of systems ("do you have rectal bleeding . . . are your gums bleeding . . . ?") or to elicit the seven cardinal features of the sign or symptom ("where is it, does it radiate, what makes it better or worse . . . ?" and so on). The most efficient method is to explore the problem by asking the patient to tell the story of the problem, as in "Tell me about your rectal bleeding." Although many will begin at an appropriate point and move toward the present, some patients may need guidance to begin when the patient last felt healthy, when the current episode began, or when the patient thinks the problem started. The patient may not appreciate the necessary level of detail and may be too inclusive or superficial. It may be necessary to interrupt to indicate a desire to hear more or less about the problem. Clarifying questions shows the patient what is needed and most patients respond with the appropriate level of detail.

Establishing the Life Context of the Patient

Once the narrative thread is established, the physician can take the opportunity to inquire about specific points. It is important to respond at the patient's first mention of psychosocial matters in order to signal to the patient that such matters are as important as biotechnical ones. Such inquiries help the physician learn in detail about the context in the patient's life—spouse, family, neighborhood, job, and culture. When enough information has been supplied, simply saying, "You were saying . . ." or "What happened next?" returns the patient to the narrative. This approach works because almost everyone knows how to tell a story and remembers key points intrinsically organized by what actually happened.

Creating a Safety Net

Once the problems the patient wishes to discuss have been explored, areas or questions may remain. For these, the physician may choose to ask a series of specific review of systems-type questions. Questions may take the form of the seven dimensions of a complaint, delineated as the location, duration, intensity (use a ten-point scale with zero "no pain at all" and ten "the worst possible pain"), quality, association, radiation, exacerbants, and ameliorants, or a subset of these dimensions. Such final closed-ended questions tie up loose ends and provide the safety of completeness.

Talking During the Physical Examination & Procedures

During the physical examination, there is a tension between the quiet focusing of the senses needed to observe and hear and feel findings and mutually necessary conversation. Practitioners need their senses of smell, sight, touch, and hearing to examine the patient. They need heightened sensory awareness for the encounter. Patients need an explanation of what is being done and what to expect ("this may hurt"), instruction about what to do ("please sit here" . . . "bring up your knees" . . . "hold your breath"), and a check on how they are doing and responding ("does this hurt?"). The examination often stimulates the memory of relevant experiences and problems the patient may have forgotten to mention. Some physicians like to explain what is happening in detail ("I am looking in the back of your eye because it is the one place in the body where blood vessels can be seen"). Others do their review of systems during the physical examination. In general, it is wise to minimize distractions during the physical examination or a procedure by confining talk to the task and the needs of the patient. Explanation of findings can be reserved for the end of the examination.

Presenting Findings & Options

After the history-taking and physical examination have been completed, it is time for the physician and patient to discuss what the problems or probabilities appear to be, related findings, the physician's hypotheses or conclusions, and possible approaches to further diagnostic evaluation and treatment. This should be done in language free of jargon and at a level of abstraction the patient can understand.

Bad news includes any information that will change the patient from their idealized self-image to a lesser one. While telling someone she has diabetes may seem routine to a jaded practitioner, to a patient who has heard tough stories about diabetes, or has a relative who died of it, or is simply a fearful person, it is certainly life-altering and might seem disastrous. It is valuable to foreshadow any bad or potentially upsetting news (see Chapter 3). This prepares the patient to hear and retain the information. It may be useful to suggest the patient bring along a trusted companion (although this flags the likely news as bad). When bad news is a certainty, it is useful to record the explanation and discussion for the patient. These days, a digital recorder in the room allows the doctor to provide a copy of the encounter when it ends. The patient can review it after shock has cleared and share it with family or friends. It has been documented that listening to such recordings produces better patient understanding and improves outcomes like quality of life. It is essential not to underestimate the potential impact of both positive and negative findings on the patient. After presenting each item, the physician should explore the patient's understanding and reactions. The presentation itself should be problem-oriented and systematic—and as simple and succinct as possible. Although the dictum is "be brief," necessary content and empathy should not be sacrificed for brevity.

Negotiating a Plan

Once patients have been factually informed of the diagnosis and prognosis, it is crucial to involve them actively in making choices and in developing diagnostic and therapeutic plans. Such "activation" of patients has been shown to increase their adherence to plans and improve their medical outcome and quality of life.

When the physician and the patient disagree in emphasis or choice, negotiation is necessary. The principles of negotiation can be summarized: find and emphasize areas of mutual agreement (e.g., live as long as possible, retain dignity, and avoid suffering), and avoid the adoption of inflexible positions that lead only to conflict, wherein one side or the other loses. If physicians take time to understand patients' positions and respect concerns, the issues can usually be worked out. For example, it can be agreed upon to do a procedure after a grandchild's graduation or to do non-invasive tests first with hope they will suffice.

Closing the Interview

The closing should include: actively reviewing principal findings, plans, and agreements using a talk back or teach back in which the patient is asked to recall what decisions and recommendations have been made, making arrangements for the next visit and giving patient instructions, making sure outstanding issues have been covered, and saying good-bye. In the future, both the physician and patient may review the physician's notes together.

THE FUNCTIONS OF THE INTERVIEW

The three functions of the interview are the major purposes of the interview. Each is associated with skills and behaviors that inform the process and outcome. The three functions are as follows:

- Gathering information and monitoring progress.
- Developing, maintaining, and, sometimes, concluding the therapeutic relationship.
- Educating the patient and implementing a treatment plan.

These goals are interdependent. For example, patients cannot be expected to reveal personal or humiliating information until they develop trust in their physician. The physician cannot educate a patient effectively without knowing what level of abstraction, language, and literacy to employ; which concepts to use; how to frame things for clarity; and which formulations will interpose barriers to acceptance. Therefore, the three functions must be integrated and pursued in parallel rather than sequentially.

Function 1: Gathering Information & Monitoring Progress

Many physicians consider information gathering to be the principal focus of the interview. The tasks associated with this function include: acquiring knowledge of the patient's current diseases and disorders as well as psychosocial issues and illness behavior, eliciting data relevant to each problem, and generating and testing relevant hypotheses. Useful skills include: use of open-ended questions such as "Tell me about it" and gradually narrowing the queries down to more specific questions, use of minimal encouragers (i.e., "Uh huh" and "Hmmm") to facilitate flow, gentle use of direction to steer without dominating, and use of summarizing and checking ("I think you have said point a, point b, point c; is that right?").

Function 2: Developing & Maintaining the Therapeutic Relationship

The second function of the interview requires defining the nature of the relationship (short- or long-term, consultation, primary care, and disease–episode-oriented). It requires demonstrating professional expertise; communicating interest, respect, empathy, and support; recognizing and resolving relational barriers to communication; and eliciting the patient's perspective. A relationship that engenders trust and safety is pivotal to being able to gather intimate information and actively involve the patient to make lifestyle changes or difficult medical decisions.

The belief that relationships cannot be improved or manipulated has been disproven by empirical psychotherapy literature. It has been shown that the use of appropriate relationship-building skills significantly improves interview outcomes in terms of satisfaction, compliance, data disclosure, quality of life, biological outcomes, and personal growth. These issues are particularly germane in cases involving mental disorders, where skill in managing the patient in a manner compatible with healing is essential.

In general, naming feelings, communicating unconditional positive regard, expressing empathy and understanding, and being emotionally congruent (what you say is actually what you mean and feel) produce the best outcomes. Other skills include reflection, legitimization, partnership, nonverbal skills of touch and eye contact, use of open posture, and avoidance of shame or humiliation (see Chapter 2).

Function 3: Educating the Patient

Patient education and implementation of treatment plans require: an awareness of the patient's level of knowledge, understanding, motivation and cognitive style; a receptive patient who is neither in shock nor disagreement; and the use of plain language that avoids jargon or undue complexity. The tasks associated with this function include: communicating the diagnostic significance of the problems; negotiating and recommending appropriate diagnostic and treatment options, appropriate prevention and lifestyle change recommendations; and enhancing the patient's coping ability by understanding and communicating the psychological and social impacts of the illness. Involving the patient in choices, clarifying uncertainties, and eliciting fears and concerns markedly improve outcomes. Having the patient actively review what has been discussed and decided upon (use of a teach-back or talk-back) is critical to check for understanding and to reinforce memory, thus maximizing the likelihood that the patient can and will do what has been agreed upon (see Chapter 20).

In some cases, the issue is a high-risk health behavior, habit, or addiction such as overeating, smoking, gambling, or medication nonadherence. Two approaches have been demonstrated to be helpful in such situations: (1) the stages of change model and (2) motivational interviewing (see Chapter 19).

A "Stages of Change Model" described by Prochaska and DiClemente involves ascertaining the patient's readiness for change stage and adapting one's interaction to the patient's stage. Stages assess whether patients have begun to think about changing behavior (precontemplative vs. contemplative). If they have, then it is appropriate to move forward with an action plan by setting key milestones such as a quit date for smokers. A plan includes discussion of barriers and how to respond when relapse occurs. Acceptance of the notion that change may involve several cycles that eventually lead to success unloads the weight and shame of the common first failures, reframes them as learning experiences, and may improve the likelihood and stability of eventual success (see Chapter 19).

Motivational interviewing, developed by Miller and Rollnick, is a directive, patient-centered counseling approach designed to motivate people for change by helping them clarify goals, explore perceived barriers to behavior change, and commit to such changes. Motivational interviewing has been used widely for health behavior change in areas such as adherence to behavioral weight control programs, dietary and medication adherence, fruit and vegetable intake, and physical activity. Providing objective feedback about behaviors, acknowledging beliefs, minimizing control, and offering behavioral alternatives have been shown to increase patient self-efficacy and intrinsic motivation to adopt recommended health behaviors. Developed initially for use with addictive behaviors, it uses reflective listening to reframe patients' resistance as self-motivational statements by using such devices as the "readiness ruler," which asks the patient to rate on a scale of 1 to 10 (10 highly and 1 very little) how motivated he or she is to modify behavior. Even if the patient ranks motivation to lose weight at 2, leverage can be gained by asking, "Why wasn't that a 1?" and building on whatever slim reeds of motivation are there. In this way, the approach subtly shifts the physician–patient encounter from confrontation to partnership.

SPECIAL CIRCUMSTANCES & INTERVIEW MODIFICATIONS

Although the preceding principles are applicable to most situations, some circumstances require a modified approach to maximize the usefulness and durability of the interview. Early detection of special situations is crucial, so that appropriate changes in technique can be made. Most special situations require meticulous attention to the particular needs of the patient; for example, with a paranoid or psychotic patient.

Aids to Diagnosing Mental Disorders

There are a variety of tools to diagnose and monitor mental disorders. The simplest aids have relatively high sensitivity (they detect most cases) but lower specificity (they pick up cases that do not meet diagnostic criteria). Screening devices for depression include the Patient Health Questionnaire-9 (PHQ-9), Beck, Zung, and Hamilton scales. The PHQ-9 is a nine-question quantitative scoring method with an abbreviated two-question (PHQ-2) screen. It is useful for depression in primary-care settings (see Chapter 25). Some physicians administer these with the packet of materials to be filled out prior to each initial visit. As with any questionnaire, however, these carry the time-consuming burden to evaluate false positives. The Primary Care Screen for Mental Disorders (PRIME-MD) was developed (with pharmaceutical company support) to screen for common mental disorders. Reasonably sensitive and specific, it is available for telephone use and for computerized administration. However, empathic physicians have two problems with its use: the program asks about feelings but cannot respond and scoring takes several minutes. The role for these screening adjuncts is still evolving.

When the Patient Uses Another Language or Is From Another Culture: Using Interpreters and Eliciting Explanatory Models

Everywhere in the United States, practitioners frequently encounter patients whose first or only language is not English and who adhere to cultural beliefs, which may be divergent from the practitioner's own. As a result, patients' health-related–behaviors are tied more closely to their own health beliefs than to their physician's advice. Kleinman, Leventhal, and others define a patient's health beliefs, or explanatory model, as the conceptual and behavioral framework patients develop to understand the cause of an illness, its likely course, the meaning of specific symptoms, and the implications of these for treatment and recovery. Patient explanatory models tend to be rooted in the experience of their social network, family, ethnicity, and culture, thus reflecting the way people think about their world, themselves, and their health. Physician explanatory models reflect professional ideologies grounded in their medical training (see Chapter 15). For many patients, health beliefs and values intersect with language and acculturation to form a context of experience and expectation discordant from the biomedical model of disease. Patients whose cultural setting is in transition may be confronted with the need to reconcile (or make sense of) the differences between health beliefs that were commonly held in their original culture and the new ones of their current setting. Table 1-5 provides a question set to elicit a patient's health beliefs. Practitioners need to assess patients' salient health beliefs in order to be sure that their teaching, recommendations, and negotiations are not doomed to failure because the patient's cultural beliefs and values suggest that they are contraindicated or irrelevant. Asking about health beliefs enables one to understand them, adjust one's

Table 1-5. Questions for eliciting patient explanatory models for problems or symptoms.

What do you call your problem?
What causes your problem?
Why do you think it started when it did?
How does it work—what is going on in your body?
What kind of treatment do you think would be best for this problem?
How has this problem affected your life?
What frightens or concerns you most about this problem?

From Johnson TM, Hardt E, Kleinman A. Cultural factors in the medical interview. In Lipkin M, Putnam SM, Lazare A., eds. *The medical interview.* New York, Springer-Verlag, 1995, p. 157. By permission.

discussion to reflect and respect the patient's cultural concepts and language, and attain mutual agreement consistent with both patient's and physician's belief systems.

The issues of explanatory model differences virtually always apply when the patient is using another language (akin to the Sapir–Whorf hypothesis which postulates that language inextricably influences and guides the attitudes, cultural beliefs, and views of the user). They are magnified by interpreter variability and bias. In general, use of interpreters introduces the likelihood of errors and misunderstandings. A tight control of interpreter use standards is essential. Where possible, an interpreter should be a professional. Use of a friend or family member raises issues of accuracy and privacy. Remote simultaneous interpretation has the advantages of speed, anonymity, and less adventitious relationship building compared to telephone support or a person in the room. An interpreter in the room should be positioned behind the patient or out of the patient's sight line to keep the focus between doctor and patient. Interpreters should provide literal translation, not rephrase, or become cultural brokers; however, they can be prompted to let you know when a cultural issue is perceived. Principles and standards of interpretation have been defined by the National Council on Interpreting in Health Care (see website below).

Electronic Technology: Gateway or Barrier to Effective Communication?

In today's society, electronic technologies are ubiquitous and becoming increasingly central to daily functions including the medical encounter. With more around the corner, three technologies have already achieved significant presence in the medical encounter: the computer and its associated electronic health record (EHR), the telephone, and electronic communication with patients, such as secure messaging by e-mail. Technologies such as telemedicine and telesurgery may soon allow physicians to practice remotely. Predictably, they evoke conflicting sentiments. Promoters and marketers claim that electronic technology provides greater quality, efficiency, cost-effectiveness and satisfaction. Detractors claim loss of warmth and touch, depersonalization, detraction from patient-centeredness, wasted time, heightened rigidity in practice, and unjustified costs.

The public (i.e., patients), generally likes technology, finds computers easier or safer to "talk" with than practitioners, and accepts technologies as inevitable and related to quality. Physicians may resist most changes and salutatory shifts, such as moving from a paper to an EHR. Consternation is followed by ambivalent acceptance. Practitioners commonly agree that on the one hand, EHR use enhances legibility, completeness, sharing of records, and data organization. On the other hand, it slows the encounter and divides the attention between the patient and computer display. Computers magnify the positive and negative attributes of a physician's communication skills. In general, with a computer in the room, practitioners shift away from patients' psychosocial issues and from patient participation and relationship-building in the medical encounter to a more physician-dominated biomedical information giving, history taking, and attention to computerized note taking. An increase in computer use is also associated with longer medical visits, less dialogue between patient and physician, and lower emotional responsiveness by the physician. How much these impacts alter patient outcomes remains to be proven. So, beware of extravagant claims.

Nevertheless, certain computer-related behaviors seem sensible and can enhance the medical encounter, if utilized properly. First, EHRs can allow physicians to prepare for the visit prior to the patient's entry, saving time during the interview searching for data. Second, with increasing experience (and commitment), physicians can alternate between talking directly to the patient, with good eye contact and open posture, and making explicit breaks to use the EHR for data entry ("I'm sorry, I need to take a minute to . . ."). Third, physicians can use natural breaks in the encounter, such as when the patient is changing or at the end of the visit, for the majority of typing or dictating using voice recognition software. Fourth, physicians can choose to share the screen to enhance collaboration by sharing lab results, providing patient education and showing useful images (where the pathology is, what the procedure will do, dietary portions, etc.). Physicians should avoid typing while the patient is talking, since nonverbal cues will be missed and patients will often interpret too great a focus on the computer as a sign of not caring.

An important, recently completed large scale study (OpenNotes) examined the impact of sharing EHR records with patients. Preliminary findings indicate that such transparency helps patients feel more in charge of their care, promotes increased adherence to treatment plans, reduces content errors, shifts the patient–physician relationship toward greater trust and partnership, and has little adverse impact on the physician's work life. It will take time, however, to understand if and how sharing visit notes affects outcomes and the efficiency of care.

The telephone is not new; it remains a core means of contact between physician and patient, accounting for as much as 25% of interactions. Use of telephones has extended beyond requests for prescription refills and lab results. Phones are now used by practitioners for reminders, monitoring chronic care, delivering manualized treatments, screening, and data transmission from in-home instruments. Cell phones extend access further, including texting and image-sharing capabilities.

Phone answering systems are now emblematic of depersonalization, with patients and physicians frustrated by attempts to reach practitioners behind the unbreachable, automated moat of "please listen to the following options, as they have changed."

Talking with a patient on the phone is rather like looking at a photograph in black and white instead of color. The phone (although it may soon include video) removes the ability to observe nonverbal cues (including lip reading) and forces both parties to listen more, making it possible to hear more. This a-visual quality can be beneficial, especially with patients whose physicality is distracting, but it may be at the expense of nonverbal cues.

While patient acceptance of and satisfaction with e-mail is high, use of e-mail between physicians and patients remains low. Patient barriers include literacy, computer access, language (if discordant), and comfort with writing skills. Physicians resist e-mail out of fear that it will become intrusive, pose a nonreimbursed time sink, be mistaken for real contact in an emergency, enable patients to avoid reimbursable visits, deny the opportunity for verbal interaction and physical examination, and make the physician accountable 24/7 with a permanent written record. However, many of these perceptions are unfounded. The majority of patients sends an average of one e-mail per day and perceives their physician to be more accessible and informed of their individual health-care needs when e-mail is used. More importantly, e-mail messages do not totally eradicate the psychosocial and emotional quality of communication. Patients display higher levels of engagement and attentiveness to detail in their e-mail messages than in actual visits. Most physicians have a tendency to exhibit curtness on e-mail, with a majority of the content focused on information giving. As a consequence, it is easier to forget to match language level with the patient when writing in a medium most often used with peers.

E-mail communication must follow the Health Insurance Portability and Accountability Act (HIPAA) of 1996 guidelines. Patients should be aware of the risks associated with e-mail and informed how confidentiality and privacy will be ensured. Each patient should consent to e-mail use and that consent should be recorded. E-mail should be encrypted. The AMA has published guidelines for e-mail usage.

SUMMARY

The medical interview is the most commonly used diagnostic and therapeutic procedure in medicine. As such it deserves continued attention and skill enhancement throughout a clinician's professional career. The quality of the clinician–patient encounter, patient satisfaction, the accuracy and completeness of data, patient adherence to treatment regimens, health outcomes, and clinician satisfaction are all influenced by a skillful approach to the medical interview. Attention to both the structure and functions of the interview provides a framework for developing mastery in this most central clinical procedure. It also will ensure that the core relationship between physician and patient remains at the center of all advancements in medicine, including the new technologies of electronic communication and information management.

SUGGESTED READINGS

Delbanco T, Walker J, Darer J, et al. OpenNotes: doctors and patients signing on. *Ann Intern Med* 2010;153:121–125.

Delbanco T, Walker J, Bell SK, et al. Inviting patients to read their doctors' notes: a quasi-experimental study and a look ahead. *Ann Intern Med* 2012;157(7):461–470.

Duffy DF, Gordon GH, Whelan G, et al. Assessing competence in communication and interpersonal skills: the Kalamazoo II report. *Acad Med* 2004;79:495–507.

Frankel R, Altschuler A, George S, et al. Effects of exam-room computing on clinician–patient communication: A longitudinal qualitative study. *JGIM* 2005;20:677–682.

Haidet P. Jazz and the art of medicine: improvisation in the medical encounter. *Annals Fam Med* 2007;5:164–169.

Lipkin M, Putnam SM, Lazare A, eds. *The Medical Interview: Clinical Care, Education, and Research*. New York, NY: Springer-Verlag, 1995.

Rao JK, Anderson LA, Inui TS, Frankel RM. Communication interventions make a difference in conversations between physicians and patients. *Med Care* 2007;45:340–349.

Roter DL, Larson S, Sands DZ, et al. Can e-mail messages between patients and physicians be patient-centered? *Health Communication* 2008;23:80–86.

Ventres W, Kooienga S, Marlin R, et al. Clinician style and examination room computers: A video ethnography. *Fam Med* 2005;37:276–281.

Walker J, Leveille S, Ngo L, et al. Inviting patients to read their doctors' notes: patients and doctors look ahead. *Ann Intern Med* 2011;155:891–899.

OTHER RESOURCE

Novack DH, Clark W, Saizow R, et al., eds. *Doc.com: An Interactive Learning Resource for Healthcare Communication*. American Academy on Communication in Healthcare http://www.aachonline.org/. Accessed July 2013.

ORGANIZATIONS AND WEB SITES

American Academy on Communication in Healthcare. www.aachonline.org. Accessed July 2013.

American Medical Association (AMA). Guidelines for Physician-Patient Electronic Communications. http://www.ama-assn.org//ama/pub/physician-resources/medical-ethics/code-medical-ethics/opinion5026.page. Accessed July 2013.

Motivational Interviewing. www.motivationalinterview.org. Accessed July 2013.

National Council on Interpreting in Health Care. http://www.ncihc.org. Accessed July 2013.

Northwest Center for Physician-Patient Communication. The Foundation for Medical Excellence. www.tfme.org. Accessed July 2013.

Empathy

2

Barry Egener, MD

INTRODUCTION

The concept of empathy dates from the early years of this century, when discussions of the topic were restricted to psychotherapists' analyses of their interactions with patients. More recently, the concept has received renewed attention from a wide spectrum of health practitioners and educators. They believe that empathy can positively affect communication with patients and thus lead to improved therapeutic outcomes. Many of the lay public regard empathy as an avenue to the restoration of compassion and humanism to the doctor–patient relationship, which has been increasingly impersonal and threatened by technology and financial pressures. Indeed recent studies have demonstrated that physician empathy increases patient satisfaction and improves clinical outcomes.

The Neurobiology of Empathy

Novel research tools, such as functional MRI scanning, which permit real-time investigation of the brain under experimental conditions, have revealed new insights into the functional neuroanatomy of empathy. The discovery of sensorimotor neurons in the cortex has suggested a mechanism whereby behaviors can trigger an unconscious reciprocal response in an observer. These *mirror neurons* fire when the subject performs a particular task or when the subject simply observes another individual performing the same task. Most of us have had the experience of reflexively smiling when a stranger walking down the street smiles at us. Our motor response often precedes a conscious reflection of what transpired.

This research is preliminary and some of the conclusions speculative. Nevertheless, a model of empathy is emerging in which connections between mirror neurons and other brain structures could facilitate the observed components of empathy. For example, in our example of the stranger-triggered smile, the mirror neuron projections that are downward to the facial muscles and limbic system could provoke the feeling of happiness

concomitant with the motor expression of a smile. These responses are rapid and unconscious. Secondary projections to the more newly evolved cortex provoke awareness of the feeling, thoughts about the social context of the transaction, and decisions about further actions. These are slower, more conscious elements of a complex response.

Empathy as a Clinical Tool

In medical practice, the power of empathy lies in its ability to help us cross, if only for a moment, the divide between clinicians and patients created by their very different circumstances. To briefly bridge that divide and to become simply two humans sharing an experience can help in accomplishing professional diagnostic and therapeutic tasks. We have all experienced the gratitude of patients, isolated by depression or family loss, for our expression of understanding of their sadness.

Succeeding at the greater challenge of putting aside our disagreement with a patient requesting chronic narcotics or perhaps our negative judgment of a patient unable to quit smoking can have proportionally greater rewards. Being willing to imagine what it must be like for these more challenging patients can provide us with insights into what motivates them or what might help them. That is diagnostic information. Communicating that insight may encourage patients to change their behavior, and that is therapeutic. Our disclosure also allows us to check the accuracy of what we think we know about the patient's state. We relinquish nothing of ourselves or our role in that moment; we simply expand our perspective.

Empathy can be defined as an intellectual identification with, or vicarious experiencing of, the feelings, thoughts, or attitudes of another. Thus, there are both cognitive and affective dimensions of empathy. Despite having found neurobiological correlates of both, there remains disagreement about their functional relationship and relative importance. Some have described empathy as a momentary identification with another person in which our human capacity to feel what

Table 2-1. Barriers to discussing emotions.

Doctor
1. Takes too much time
2. Too draining
3. Will lose control of interview
4. Cannot fix patient's distress
5. Not my job
6. Perceived conflicts of interest

Patient
1. Cultural taboo about discussing emotions
2. Preference for interpreting distress in a biomedical model
3. Somatization disorder
4. Desire to meet doctor's expectations
5. Worry about being emotionally overwhelmed
6. Lack of language for emotions

another feels erodes the boundaries of self. If we, in fact, temporarily lose awareness of self, the process might better be termed "sympathy for" or "feeling with" someone else. Remaining aware that we are experiencing empathy prevents total dissolution of ego boundaries and permits a more salutary stance. **Empathy skills** are behaviors that demonstrate empathy. They are among the clinician's most powerful therapeutic tools.

Research suggests that empathy skills can be taught. This chapter will describe how to develop and improve these skills. Research has recently shed light on the frequency of empathic opportunities in clinical practice, on how physicians respond to or neglect these opportunities, and the implications of such choices. Empathic opportunities occur in more than half of surgical and primary care visits, although on average there are more opportunities per visit in primary care than in surgical care. Patients initiate most of the opportunities. Contrary to common belief, surgeons respond empathically at least as frequently as primary care physicians, but both miss opportunities to respond more frequently. Empathic behaviors enhance the effectiveness of care as well as patient satisfaction, and their absence may predispose patients to initiate malpractice suits.

There are numerous barriers to discussing emotions with patients (see Table 2-1), from the impersonal office setting to the disinclination of both physician and patient to address particularly sensitive topics. Nonetheless, appropriate skilled communication can break through these barriers.

OVERCOMING BARRIERS TO EMPATHY

Understanding the feelings, attitudes, and experiences of the patient is the first step toward a more potent therapeutic alliance. Many patients, however, may not be skilled in revealing their feelings to their providers. They need to be made aware that their doctor is interested in their feelings and values them, and that feelings are a legitimate topic for discussion in a medical interview.

Emotions can be difficult for both doctors and patients, and doctors, in particular, may prefer the certainty of science. From the patient's point of view, if difficult emotional issues are manifested as a somatic complaint, denial might be the first reaction to a psychological interpretation of the symptoms. The physician must appreciate and mirror the terms in which a patient will speak about illness. In many cultures, emotions are simply not discussed. In the United States, where the biomedical model of disease predominates over the biopsychosocial model, patients may feel that it is more acceptable to have physical rather than emotional complaints. Because this expectation is often reinforced by their physicians, it is important for physicians to establish a climate conducive to the expression of emotional material and a language useful to that end. Physicians often mention the following barriers to discussing emotions with patients.

1. **It takes too much time.** In a busy practice, concerns about time are legitimate. Given an organized framework, however, it takes only a few minutes to deal effectively with emotion, and the strategies discussed later in this chapter can prove time efficient for the physician. Recent studies suggest that interviews in which physicians respond to emotions may actually be shorter than those in which they do not. An explanation of this finding is that it may be more time consuming to deal with the indirect effects of unaddressed emotions during the rest of the interview. Moreover, it may be useful to distinguish between "acute efficiency" and "chronic efficiency." "Efficiency" should take into consideration not only the duration of a particular visit but also the total amount of time required to address the patient's concerns. Even if it were to take a few extra minutes to address emotions, that time is more than compensated by fewer phone calls and fewer unscheduled visits.

2. **It is too draining.** It is unrealistic to expect all providers to be emotionally available at all times to all their patients. A physician who has been awake all night or is emotionally needy may be justified in putting off a discussion of emotions that should otherwise occur. If the physician chooses to defer, it would be wise to return to the topic at another time. Primary care providers sometimes exert a tremendous amount of energy avoiding emotions in the belief that dealing directly with them will be draining. However, it can be far more efficient to make an emotional connection than to expend so much energy in resisting it.

At times, patients may inadvertently raise issues that are emotionally difficult for their providers. Sometimes the clinician can discuss the difficulty with friends, family, or colleagues; at other times it may be most fruitfully addressed in the physician's own therapy. (A longer discussion of this area is beyond the scope of this chapter, but difficult encounters with patients offer physicians an opportunity for personal growth; see Chapter 4.)

3. **The interview will get out of control.** Although many doctors worry that addressing emotions will cause feelings to escalate, the opposite is often true. Addressing emotions helps diffuse them. Learning a language to handle emotions creates a comfortable distance from the emotions themselves, so that neither the doctor nor the patient becomes overwhelmed.

4. **I cannot fix it for the patient.** Primary care providers are used to "fixing" things. Feelings, however, simply exist, and cannot be "fixed." Patients do not expect their feelings to be eliminated; they just want them to be understood.

5. **It is not my job.** Some doctors believe that their job is to address disease and the psychotherapist's job is to address mental illness. There are several problems with this attitude. Although it is certainly true that collaboration with mental health practitioners is important, at least two-thirds of patients with mental and behavioral problems are cared for mainly by primary care physicians. Physicians who insist on interpreting the physical symptoms of psychiatric disease, such as panic disorder or depression, in purely biomedical terms miss the point—and their patients will not get better. Telling a patient who develops chest pain on the anniversary of his father's death (see "The Therapeutic Language of Empathy") that there is nothing wrong with him will help the patient only briefly. Moreover, many physical illnesses have psychosocial sequelae that must also be addressed.

When a patient keeps returning with the same complaint, unimproved by a physician's interventions, the patient is trying to communicate a message. Physicians are often frustrated by these patients; this frustration can be alleviated and the doctor's satisfaction improved by the progress that comes with addressing the underlying problem.

6. **Perceived conflicts of interest.** Although the more apparent financial conflicts of interest presented by managed care may have diminished in recent years, it is likely that new potential conflicts of interest will continue to arise even as the field upon which these play out changes. Physicians have always needed to balance the needs of the patients in front of them with those of society at large. Research has now demonstrated that patients prefer having their concerns acknowledged and validated rather than the physician blaming an external party for shared constraints. Physicians who feel challenged by patients' questioning their motives are likely to act defensively. The empathy skills offer an alternative that makes the physician a partner again.

THE ROLE OF EMPATHY IN DIAGNOSIS

Feelings that arise in the provider during an encounter may be useful in forming a diagnostic hypothesis about the patient. For example, a doctor who feels burdened, heavy, or "down" during an interview might consider the possibility that the patient is depressed.

All clinicians have had the experience of trying to help a patient with a behavior change, such as weight loss, only to have each suggestion rejected: "I've already tried that, Doc; it doesn't work." The physician's own feelings of frustration and powerlessness in trying to motivate the patient are often mirrored by the patient's sense of frustration and powerlessness in attempting to accomplish the change in behavior. The physician can confirm the hypothesis that the patient is frustrated, as with any other diagnosis, by testing: "I'm feeling frustrated with this problem, and I'm wondering if you're feeling the same way."

Some patients consistently elicit dislike and rejection from their providers. It may seem that the patient is intentionally trying to manipulate the provider into becoming angry. This may in fact be true. When providers become aware of these feelings, they should consider the possibility that their own impulses to punish the patient may be playing into the patient's self-image as deserving of punishment. This pattern may be consistent with a borderline personality disorder (see Chapter 29).

The physician's experience does not invariably reflect the patient's experience. Rather, physicians should notice their own feelings and ask, "Does the way I feel tell me something about the patient or something about myself?" For example, a physician who has recently seen a number of patients seeking drugs begins to feel angry and defensive on noticing that the nurse has recorded "low back pain" as the next patient's chief complaint; these negative feelings indicate more about the physician's recent experiences than they do about the next patient. Feelings are primary data about the person in whom they arise and indirect data about others. The next section clarifies how to test the hypothesis that a patient is feeling a particular emotion and outlines how to respond.

THE THERAPEUTIC LANGUAGE OF EMPATHY

Although empathy is not generally considered a therapeutic tool, discussion of emotional issues can be therapeutic. An empathic relationship is crucial in psychotherapy and enhances the power of all therapeutic relationships. The following sections show how to talk about emotions using specific skills. A premise of this discussion is that biomedical aspects of disease cannot be effectively addressed without considering their emotional consequences. Emotions, whether related to physiologic dysfunction or psychosocial issues, color the discussion in the examining room, and may be so distracting that the patient cannot fully concentrate on other issues until the emotions are addressed.

A clinical scenario helps to illustrate the usefulness of the emotion-handling skills described in this section.

 CASE ILLUSTRATION 1

While you are on call for admissions from the emergency room for patients without a primary care physician, a 45-year-old man is admitted because of concern that his 2-week history of chest pain may represent unstable angina. Although the emergency room physician acknowledges that it is a "soft admission," the patient has a history of elevated lipids, a family history of cardiac disease, and his blood pressure in the emergency room is 180/95. The patient describes a sharp substernal chest pain that occurs at rest, when working in the yard, and while trying to fall asleep at night. He does not smoke or have diabetes. On examination, he appears anxious, his blood pressure on the cardiac floor is 160/90, and he is 5% over ideal body weight. The rest of his examination, laboratory tests, electrocardiogram, and chest X-ray are normal, except for his low-density lipoprotein cholesterol, which is 160 mg/dL.

You greet the patient with outstretched hand:

Doctor: *Good morning, Mr. Swenson, my name is Dr. Bergen. I'll be taking care of you while you're in the hospital.*

Patient: *Well, Doctor, am I having a heart attack?*

Doctor: *You haven't had a heart attack. I can tell from your blood tests and electrocardiograms.*

Patient: *Well is the pain coming from my heart?*

Doctor: *I don't think so.*

Patient: *But you're not sure?*

Doctor: *Nothing in medicine is certain, but your age, the character of your pains, and the fact that antacids help somewhat reassure me that the problem is most likely acid indigestion or muscular pain.*

Patient: *Don't you think we should do more tests to be sure?*

Doctor: *Although you are at low risk for having coronary artery disease, I think it would be prudent to do an exercise stress test as an outpatient just to be sure.*

Patient: *What if I have a heart attack in the meantime? I'm still worried.*

Doctor: *You don't need to be. Besides, you were admitted under "observation status" to make sure you didn't have an unstable cardiac condition, and we have done that. By standard protocols, you fall into the low risk category, and your insurance will not allow you to remain an inpatient for further risk stratification. Don't worry, you'll be all right.*

Patient: *Well, okay, if you say so.*

Despite a diagnosis of non-cardiac chest pain, providing good information, and attempts to reassure the patient, something goes awry in this interaction. The patient still does not seem satisfied. Let us look at the effect empathic skills might have.

The techniques discussed in the following sections are adapted from a three-function model of the medical interview. The goals of the interview are described as gathering medical data, building a relationship with the patient, and educating and motivating the patient (see Chapter 1). The following emotion-handling skills are related to the second function, building relationships with patients (Table 2-2).

REFLECTION

The term reflection refers to naming the emotion the doctor sees and reflecting it back to the patient. Reflection communicates the physician's understanding of the patient's experience. It also has the effect of making the feelings behind the patient's behavior or words explicit, so that they can be dealt with directly.

For example, when a patient greets a doctor who is 20 minutes late with, "My time is as valuable as yours," the doctor might say, "I'm sorry I'm late. You seem pretty angry with me." The patient might then ventilate about the doctor's lateness or his treatment at the hands of doctors. He might even deny his anger, since many patients might view an expression of anger at their physicians as unacceptable.

Table 2-2. The empathic skills.

Skill	Example
Reflection	"You seem upset."
Validation	"I can understand your anger with the callous way you were treated."
Support	"You are doing very well handling your grief."
Partnership	"Perhaps we can work together to make you feel better."
Respect	"You have tremendous compassion for your siblings."

In any case, the doctor has a chance to deal with the emotion directly and then proceed with the interview, rather than trying to work with a patient who is angry and has not had a chance to express his anger.

After reflecting an emotion, the doctor should stop talking and see how the patient responds. Although the patient will usually elaborate, if the physician keeps talking the exploration may be prematurely ended.

Sometimes it is clear that a patient is feeling a strong emotion, but it is not clear what that emotion is. It is perfectly acceptable (and perhaps preferable) to treat the emotion as having a differential diagnosis and test a hypothesis as one would for any other medical entity: "I'm wondering if you're upset," or, more tentatively, "It seems that you're feeling something strongly, but I'm not sure what it is. Can you help me out?"

VALIDATION

Validation informs the patient that you understand the reason for the emotion. This has the effect of normalizing the emotion and making the patient feel less isolated. For example, to a somatizing patient who has been to several doctors to find a cause for her abdominal pain, you might say, "I can understand how frustrating it's been to be no better after seeking so much help." Some physicians are reluctant to validate emotions in difficult patients for fear of adding fuel to the fire. If reflection is the empathy skill that opens Pandora's Box, then validation is the skill that closes it—it is difficult to remain upset with a person who understands how you feel. You do not have to agree with patients to express an understanding of their feelings. For example, to a patient with chronic low back pain who has responded angrily when informed that you will not prescribe narcotics, you might say, "Even though I see it differently, I can understand why you would be angry with me." Although disagreeing with the patient, such a statement allows you to offer support and enhances your chances of continuing a therapeutic relationship. Validation of feelings emphasizes that the patient and doctor are equals in the human condition, although they have different roles in the therapeutic relationship.

SUPPORT

An expression of support tells patients that the physician cares about them and is willing to be present to their emotion. The expression can be verbal or nonverbal. Examples of nonverbal expression are handing the tearful patient a tissue or touching the patient. In judging whether touching a patient will be perceived as supportive, invasive, or inappropriate, the physician should consider such factors as culture, age, gender, sexual orientation, previous experience of abuse, and the presence or absence of psychiatric symptoms, such as paranoia. In general, putting a hand on the patient's hand or arm will not be misinterpreted.

Many physicians prefer taking the lead from the patient by matching the patient's non-verbal behavior.

Some verbal expressions of support are "It's pretty normal to get angry with children when they act out" and "A spouse's death is one of the most difficult life transitions." Again, these responses are not an attempt to suppress, eliminate, or fix the emotion, but rather an offer to help patients, to reassure them that they are not alone with an uncomfortable emotion. These three skills—reflection, validation, and support—are the most important of the emotion-handling skills and will be involved in most of the work physicians do in this area.

PARTNERSHIP

Partnership implies a team approach, in which the patient and doctor work together toward the same goal. Doctors support and are partners with patients in many ways, but in the context of this chapter the word *partnership* makes it explicit that you would like to help the patient with the troubling emotion. An advantage of partnership is that it may help motivate patients to take an active role in their improvement and may lay the foundation for a contract for behavior change. This is consistent with the notion, especially important when illness results from patient behaviors, that physicians facilitate the patient's healing rather than curing disease in the passive patient. The physician's use of the pronouns *we* and *us* expresses partnership, as in "Perhaps we can make a plan to help you feel better" or "Let's figure out a way to help you deal with this difficult diagnosis."

RESPECT

This skill honors the emotional resources within a patient. The doctor might say "You've been through a lot" or "I'm impressed with how well you're holding up under the circumstances."

Physicians may not always know what it would be like to be the patient, but they can acknowledge the patient's experience nonetheless: "I'm not a parent, so I can only imagine what it would be like to lose a child. I can see you're feeling the loss quite deeply." On a happier occasion, she might say "What a joy it must be for you to see your grandchild's birth!"

Although it often makes sense to use reflection or validation first when addressing emotion, these skills can be used in any order, and it may be best to go through the sequence several times at different points in an interview.

 CASE ILLUSTRATION 1 (CONTD.)

Let us return now to the scenario of the 45-year-old man with chest pain to see how that interaction might be improved with a physician who uses

empathic skills. The empathic skills used are listed in parentheses.

Doctor: Good morning, Mr. Swenson, my name is Dr. Bergen. I'll be taking care of you while you're in the hospital.

Patient: Well, Doctor, am I having a heart attack?

Doctor: You're understandably worried. (validation) I can tell from your lab tests and electrocardiogram that you haven't had a heart attack.

Patient: Then why do I have this pain?

Doctor: Our tests don't seem to have reassured you very much. (reflection)

Patient: Wouldn't you still be worried if you thought you were working up to a heart attack?

Doctor: I certainly would be. So you're worried you're going to have a heart attack. (reflection)

Patient: That's what happened to my father. He was raking leaves and just keeled over. I'm the one who found him.

Doctor: That must have been horrible. (support)

Patient: You can't imagine how awful it was. Every time I think of it I get upset. Sometimes it even brings on this chest pain. I've been thinking about him more and more lately, especially when I go to sleep at night. It makes me afraid to fall asleep. I'm afraid I'm not going to wake up.

Doctor: Is there a reason why you've been thinking about him more lately?

Patient: Yeah. I thought I got over his death. But this is the time of year he died. Just raking leaves, which I do every weekend, makes me think of him. Then I get this chest pain and worry about myself. Heart disease runs in families, I don't have to tell you.

Doctor: I'm sorry about your father. (support) It sounds as though there's a pretty strong connection between thinking about your father and the chest pain.

Patient: Yeah. I thought maybe being upset stressed my heart. Do you think maybe this is all in my head?

Doctor: I'm sure you really feel the pain, and I suspect your heart still aches for your father—even if only figuratively. It's pretty hard to lose a father. Now, you know there's a pretty strong connection between the body and the mind, and if you've been worrying about your own health, this could be your way of making sure you take care of yourself. (respect)

Patient: I never thought of it that way. What you say makes a lot of sense, and I think you're probably right. But I still have this nagging worry in the back of my mind.

Doctor: That's understandable. (validation) How about this? Let's work together to reduce whatever risk factors you do have for heart disease to make

sure you don't have a problem down the line. (partnership) Although you are at low risk for having coronary artery disease, I think it would be prudent to do an exercise stress test as an outpatient just to be sure. I'm going to give you my card so that you can call my office to set it up when you get home. Any time in the next few weeks would be fine. And in the meantime, if the pain gets worse or changes in any way, give me a call. Right now you're having some pretty strong feelings about your father, and if that is the source of your chest pain, it may not go away right away. We'll talk more about it when I see you in the office.

Patient: That seems reasonable to me. I appreciate your listening to me.

Doctor: Okay, then, I'll see you in a few weeks. And remember, if the pains get worse or you get new symptoms along with them, call me immediately; don't wait till the next day.

Patient: Thanks, Doc. See you in a few weeks.

Patient satisfaction, as indicated by the patient's responses toward the end of the interview, seems much greater than in the first scenario. Although this scenario is longer than the first, using empathic skills added only approximately 1 minute to the interview, and if that additional minute prevents unnecessary visits by allaying the patient's concerns, the time is well spent. Early in the interview the doctor does very little talking, and what he does say primarily addresses the patient's charged emotional state. He initially resists the patient's invitation to confirm conclusively that this is all in his head, and, instead, allows the patient to continue to explore his feeling state. There is uncertainty at the end of the medical interview, but it seems to be an uncertainty that both the doctor and patient can accept comfortably, with a sense of partnership.

IMPLICATIONS FOR PROFESSIONAL DEVELOPMENT

Suppose the content of what the patient reveals is upsetting, distasteful, or even abhorrent to the physician. In the previous example of the patient with chest pain, suppose that the doctor's mother has just died and his father is scheduled for triple-bypass surgery. The mere contemplation of losing his father is so threatening that the physician withdraws into himself. Psychological defense mechanisms may cause the physician to become distracted from the patient's visit and think about his own concerns.

However, suppose that the patient describes a situation that is emotionally charged, but is so alien to the physician's experience that he cannot empathize. If, for example, a homosexual patient reveals that his partner has become HIV positive, the heterosexual physician may pity (feel sorry *for*) the patient but may be unable to relate to the patient's grief and fears. Or suppose the physician must present certain treatments to a patient that he considers disgusting or repulsive. His own obvious feeling may prevent the patient from making a truly informed decision.

Finding just the right therapeutic stance is essential; it may be partly intuitive and partly learned, and it may vary from patient to patient—or even with the same patient over time—depending on the patient's needs. Opportunities may be lost when the physician is unable to empathize with the patient, or when the loss of ego boundaries makes a therapeutic stance impossible. The most effective physicians are those whose repertoire permits a rapid interplay of objectivity and emotion.

Calibrating responses to patients requires noticing and understanding when clinicians' own emotional issues prevent them from being maximally effective with patients. The first clue may be that a specific patient or type of patient particularly irks a physician. These "irksome patients" are our teachers. They teach us about ourselves. Personal barriers to effectiveness with patients usually originate in the physician's own family of origin. Numerous tools are available to help physicians overcome these barriers: speaking with a trusted colleague, Balint or other support groups, courses that focus specifically on personal awareness, and personal psychotherapy.

On Authenticity

When the language of empathy is new, it can feel foreign and, therefore, phony. Some have likened empathy skills to acting. All new skills, whether in sports, cooking, or the performance arts, are awkward and effortful at first. As one gains experience and tailors these concepts to one's own personal style, empathy skills become part of who we are. If a clinician says something he does not believe, with the goal of manipulating the patient, it is likely to be detected and to backfire. We all have had the feeling of being patronized by service workers trained in customer satisfaction. However, if we express what we imagine the patient is feeling with the goal of strengthening a connection, the patient is likely to detect the authentic intent and forgive any awkwardness in the expression. Returning to the "acting" metaphor, there is a distinction in the performance arts between "surface acting" (acting unconnected to emotions) and "deep acting" (grounded in one's own life experiences or imagination of another's experience). There are both ethical and pragmatic arguments against "faking" empathy. Only the most skilled actors are likely to possess the capacity to match subconscious nonverbal cues with inauthentic verbal expressions.

Non-verbal Expression of Empathy

If one includes voice tone, inflection, cadence, etc., non-verbal communication contains most of the meaning in a conversation. Emotional intelligence includes the capacity to interpret others' emotions, which are less often labeled by patients than expressed in their body language and voice tone. Physicians' expressions of emotion affect patient satisfaction and adherence. Increased physician emotional *expressivity* is correlated with increased patient satisfaction. Conversely, a dominant voice tone has been correlated with the likelihood of being sued.

Nonverbal communication takes place *at the same time* as verbal communication, and, therefore, has the advantage of efficiency—it takes no added time. Simple acts can create the illusion of expanding time. Studies have shown that when a doctor sits down while talking to a patient, the patient in retrospect estimates that the doctor has spent more time in the interaction. Smiling, shaking hands, and nodding as the patient speaks enhance rapport. The electronic medical record, as the paper chart before it, has the potential to impede rapport. Eye contact has been shown to be critical in maintaining a connection with the patient, whereas computer screen gazing has been shown to disrupt it.

Empathy in Medical Training

There is evidence that empathy correlates with the fluctuation of mood state during residency (see Chapter 47, "Trainee Well-Being"). It is remarkable how the fresh enthusiasm and caring of medical students can quickly devolve into the wry cynicism of residents. What accounts for this withdrawal? The usual explanation is that insulating oneself in this way is an act of self-preservation in the face of overwhelming demands. It can be torturous to feel another's pain, and if one's self is already stressed because of long hours and the other exigencies of training, it may be more difficult to sustain an open posture.

The ways in which doctors withdraw depend on both their personalities and their environment. If the culture around the resident tolerates derogatory labels for patients, it can be easy to see patients as *other*, as not sharing some element of humanity with *us*. Even if such labels are not tolerated and caring for patients is a highly preserved value, dark humor may surface as a means of insulation. To take care of others, one must first take care of oneself. Finding the right balance is a major developmental task of the health-care professionals. Perhaps by attending to the well-being of trainees, we will make them better doctors (see Chapter 42). Since empathy directly correlates with well-being in internal medicine residents, it is important that training programs demonstrate that caring for others is valuable.

Experienced physicians can attend to trainees' growth, help them develop effective and healthy working styles, model those styles, and draw attention to the importance of being aware of one's own development. There is a huge contrast between the concept of residency training as nurturing or mentoring and the concept of residency as "trial by fire." And fire, we know, steels metal, making it harder.

Empathy in the Practice of Medicine

What happens after training? For some practitioners, the pressure becomes less, healthy coping styles develop, and the caring physician reemerges. Far too many, however, are casualties of the training process. Physicians' compulsive personality styles are susceptible to a pattern of delayed gratification. Constantly nurturing others, physicians may have no time left for themselves. Relationships with family and friends may atrophy. The most effective physicians may be those who attend to their own needs as well as those of their patients, who understand their own unique struggles, so that these struggles—by making physicians aware of their own humanity—can enhance, rather than detract from, their relationships with patients.

Because the culture of an institution strongly influences the practice of medicine within its purview, physicians who practice together have a unique opportunity to enhance each other's empathic skills. Patient-care conferences can incorporate psychosocial issues into the discussions of difficult cases. Reviewing videotaped interviews with difficult patients is a powerful tool that allows physicians to examine their own contributions to the difficulty of such interactions.

Regular videotaped conferences, in which physicians take turns presenting cases, allow them to feel at ease in front of the camera, demonstrate collaboration and mutual support, and reinforce the importance and value of empathy to the group. Balint groups or other types of support groups, which may include non-physician office staff, can help health practitioners cope with collegial interactions or family relationships that have become stressed by practice. Such groups also show that a psychosocial perspective can benefit both physicians and their patients.

Understanding the interaction between illness and emotion helps us become more effective clinicians. Familiarity and practice with the skills in this chapter can make us more comfortable discussing this interaction with our patients. Becoming aware of our own personal response to patients promotes personal growth as well. The emotional demands of the medical profession can be enriching or impoverishing. Using the skills of empathy, we may become more satisfied and effective clinicians, and at the same time, our patients also may become more satisfied and healthy.

SUGGESTED READINGS

Blatt B, et al. Does perspective-taking increase patient satisfaction in medical encounters? *Acad Med* 2010;85:1445–1452.

Cohen-Cole S, Bird J. Building rapport and responding to the patient's emotions (relationship skills). In Cohen-Cole S, ed. *The Medical Interview: The Three Function Approach.* St. Louis, MO: Mosby Year Book, 1991.

Colliver JA, et al. Reports of the decline of empathy during medical education are greatly exaggerated: a reexamination of the research. *Acad Med* 2010;85:588–593.

Decety J. Dissecting the neural mechanisms mediating empathy. *Emotion Review* 2011;3:92–108.

Halpern J. What is clinical empathy? *J Gen Intern Med* 2003;18:670–674.

Hojat M, et al. Physicians' empathy and clinical outcomes for diabetic patients. *Acad Med* 2011;86:359–364.

Jordan JV. Empathy and self boundaries. In *A Developmental Perspective.* Wellesley, MA: Wellesley College Press, No. 16, 1984.

Novack DH, Suchman AL, Clark W, et al. Calibrating the physician: personal awareness and effective patient care. *JAMA* 1997;278:502–509.

Roter D, Frankel R, Hall J, Sluyter D. The expression of emotions through nonverbal behavior in medical visits. *JGIM* 2006;21:S28–S34.

Shanafelt TD, West C, Zhao X, et al. Relationship between increased personal well-being and enhanced empathy among internal medicine residents. *JGIM* 2005;20:559–564.

Spiro H. What is empathy and can it be taught? *Ann Intern Med* 1992;116:843–846.

Suchman AL, Markakis K, Beckman HB, et al. A model of empathic communication in the medical interview. *JAMA* 1997;277:678–682.

Wilmer HA. The doctor-patient relationship and the issues of pity, sympathy, and empathy. *Br J Med Psychol* 1968;41:243–248.

Zinn W. The empathic physician. *Arch Intern Med* 1993;153:306–312.

OTHER RESOURCE

Egener B. Responding to strong emotions. Web-based Learning Module in *Doc.com: An Interactive Learning Resource for Healthcare Communication.* American Academy on Communication in Healthcare (www.aachonline.org). Accessed January, 2014.

WEB SITES

American Academy on Communication in Healthcare Web site. www.aachonline.org. Accessed January 2014.

The Foundation for Medical Excellence. www.tfme.org. Accessed January 2014.

Giving Bad News

Bethany Calkins, MD, MS & Timothy E. Quill, MD, FACP, FAAHPM

INTRODUCTION

With the passage of time, attitudes about how much information is to be divulged to patients about their medical conditions have evolved. In *Decorum*, Hippocrates wrote, ". . . conceal most things from the patient while you are attending him. Give orders with cheerfulness and serenity, turning attention away from what is being done to him [because] a forecast of what is to come can cause a turn for the worse." In 1847, when the American Medical Association (AMA) published their First Code of Medical Ethics they agreed stating that "The life of a sick person can be shortened not only by the acts, but also by the words or manner of a physician. It is, therefore, a sacred duty to guard himself carefully in this respect, and to avoid all things which have a tendency to discourage the patient and depress his spirits."

There has been a dramatic change in attitudes and practice patterns in this regard among physicians. In 1961, 90% of physicians preferred not to share a cancer diagnosis with their patients. In 1990, the data showed an upward trend in disclosure with 97% of surveyed physicians telling patients about their unfavorable diagnosis. This could be partly due to the improvement in treatment regimens for chronic diseases, such as cancer and AIDS, over time; with these advances, it has become easier for physicians to give bad news to patients while simultaneously offering the hope for effective treatment necessary to sustain them through their illness. However, along with treatments come treatment failures, recurrence of disease and what may be irreversible side effects of those treatments, requiring physicians to explore these less favorable scenarios with patients. Unfortunately, the literature has shown that most doctors receive little or no training in communicating bad news to patients, and even those who do it regularly are unsure of their ability to do it effectively.

COMMUNICATING BAD NEWS

Bad news is defined in the literature as "any information which adversely and seriously affects an individual's view of his or her future." Objectively, bad news can be a serious condition, particularly cancer, but could also include other fatal or serious diagnoses, the death of a loved one, treatment failures, or transitions in care (i.e., to hospice). It is important to remember that bad news is a subjective experience that depends on the patient's expectations and understanding of the situation. It is hard to know how news will affect a person without this personal knowledge, but effective communication can help a patient to better understand and move forward with the information tailored to their particular clinical situation.

Common sense dictates that there are better and worse ways to offer bad news to patients. This type of conversation is delicate and challenging and has implications for both the provider and the recipient, yet most physicians are not trained in the art of this kind of communication. In one survey, only 5% of oncologists said that they learned to give bad news through a formal teaching program; most had either learned by sitting in on other clinicians giving bad news or had no formal teaching at all. Others learn by doing or by relying on their intuition and prior experience in breaking bad news to patients. However, research shows that communication skills do not improve with experience alone (see Chapter 1). Cultural and ethnic variables further complicate the process and will be discussed further toward the end of this chapter.

THE IMPORTANCE OF THE BAD NEWS DISCUSSION

Optimal communication in relaying bad news leads to better outcomes for both the physician and the patient. As providers feel more comfortable with their communication skills, they report less job stress, higher levels of personal accomplishment, higher levels of confidence, and less emotional stress and burnout. Patients will often feel encouraged to participate in difficult decision making when they are connecting with their physician, which can result in higher quality medical decision making.

Good, open communication encourages trusting relationships to develop between doctor and patient, and patients report better outcomes, better satisfaction, improved understanding of their condition, and better adherence to treatment plans. Significant decreases in rates of litigation occur when patients feel that they were involved in a conversation that they felt was clear, honest, and empathic.

When communication surrounding the bad news discussion goes poorly, it can negatively affect the patient's view of humanity; of the medical field, in general; and of their particular medical-care providers. Patients may see a poorly run conversation as a breach of the patient–physician partnership, which ultimately could affect their compliance with the treatment plan, level of hopefulness, and subsequent psychological adjustment to their disease. When the patient's quality of life suffers, so could their health outcomes. There have been many studies to show that the inability of oncologists to deliver bad news effectively leads to short courses of futile, unnecessary chemotherapy being administered at the end of life.

The delivery of bad news is a complex interaction. Providers need to arrange the verbal component of actually giving the bad news, while simultaneously eliciting and responding to the patient's emotions, dealing with the stress created by patients' expectations for cure, involving patients in decision making, involving as many family members as are present, and all while trying to provide them with hope in the face of a potentially bleak situation. With such an emotionally charged environment, the opportunity for miscommunication is enormous. Given all of the issues surrounding breaking bad news to patients, it quickly becomes evident why learning communication as a skill is important for everyone involved.

Patient-centered communication is an approach in which attention is placed on using verbal and nonverbal behaviors to establish partnerships with patients. Physicians should help create and maintain patient-centered communication by clarifying with patients, in advance, how much information they would like to know before discussing it with them. Using the six-step approach described below—initially created by Dr. Robert Buckman and others—to establish patient-centered goals can smooth the progress in transitions of care.

SPIKES: A PROTOCOL FOR THE DELIVERY OF UNFAVORABLE NEWS

Buckman created a six-step protocol for giving unfavorable information to patients. In a review of the literature on Breaking Bad News published in the Journal of American Medical Association, most authors agree that following the SPIKES framework reduces stress on the patients receiving the bad news as well as the physicians charged with delivering the bad news (Table 3-1).

Physicians may have several goals on entering a discussion in which they plan to divulge bad news to a patient: they may wish to gather information from the patient in terms of what they know already of their illness as well as how much they want to know; to provide information to the patient that is clear and within the boundaries of what they desire; to support the patient by responding to emotional needs that arise during the conversation; and to develop a treatment strategy with the help of the patient. These are no small goals, but the SPIKES protocol can assist professionals in realizing them.

Step 1 of the six-step SPIKES protocol (**Set** up the interview) involves advanced preparation for the discussion and choosing an appropriate physical setting in which it will occur. Mentally rehearse what you will tell patients and anticipate what they may ask or how they may react. Remember that although the conversation that is ahead will be challenging to hear for everyone, it will be important to communicate the information clearly and succinctly to begin preparing patients to plan their future. Consider where the conversation will happen. The space chosen for this purpose should be private, quiet, comfortable, and convenient for everyone involved. Identify the key players that should be

Table 3-1. The SPIKES protocol for delivering bad news.

Set up the interview	Advanced preparation, pay attention to the physical setting: sit down, make eye contact, avoid interruptions, and invite patient to ask family to stay
Assess patient's **Perception**	"Tell me how you are doing." "What do you understand about what's happened so far?"
Obtain the patient's **Invitation**	"Is it okay to speak freely about the information that I have here?" "Is there anything that you wouldn't want to know?"
Give **Knowledge** and **Information** to the patient	"I'm afraid that I have bad news for you." "The biopsy confirmed cancer."
Address the patient's **Emotions** with empathic responses	"I wish I had better news for you." "I can see that you're upset. Tell me more about what you're feeling."
Set goals	Summarize the conversation and make a plan to go forward

present, this includes family or friends whom the patient identifies as being close supports, as well as practical additions to the team, such as nurses, interpreters, social workers, and consultants who know the patient well. Having a supportive colleague present during the discussion may also potentially bolster the comfort level of the provider when the news is particularly bad. In a hospital, the physical setting adds another level of complexity to an already difficult discussion. Finding a space to have a private conversation where the patient can comfortably attend—while maintaining the peaceful, supportive environment required to openly discuss sensitive information—often proves difficult. Seeking out empty family rooms or offices in advance can be helpful. In the outpatient setting, the physical space may not be as much of a problem as the time constraints. It is recommended in this step of the SPIKES protocol to set aside a large amount of time where one does not feel pressured to truncate the conversation in favor of other responsibilities. Many experienced clinicians find that time set aside at the end of a patient-care session is most convenient for this discussion. If possible, providers should hand off their pagers to another colleague and ask staff to hold telephone calls or other interruptions until the conclusion of the bad news discussion.

In addition to the optimal physical setting, physicians should prepare for the conversation by finding out the medical information necessary to answer any anticipated questions. Talking to consultants about specific diagnoses or test results in advance will help when formulating the treatment plan with the patient.

Something else to consider before escorting the patient into the conversation is who should be present and who should be delivering the bad news. There is no single right answer, but the healthcare provider who knows the patient best is the right person in most cases. The use of an interdisciplinary team helps in preventing discrepancies in information presented to the patient, and potentially aids in identification of patient needs. Nurses can also be helpful in acting as a supportive liaison between patients and physicians. Social workers can provide essential services such as talking with patients on how best to communicate with doctors, setting up interpreters, and arranging meetings with key people.

When entering into a discussion, in which sensitive information will be divulged, be mindful of body language and non-verbal cues that could be sending additional information to patients. In addition, be vigilant about identifying what information the patient's body language is providing to you. Sitting down lets the patient know that there is no rush and making eye contact (though sometimes uncomfortable) assists in strengthening rapport between patient and provider.

In **Step 2** of the SPIKES protocol (**Perception**), the goal is to assess the patient's perception of what has thus far occurred to bring everyone together. Introduce yourself

and state your role, and invite everyone else in the room to introduce themselves and state their reason for being there. This is a good time to acknowledge any time constraints that you might have. For example, "I have thirty minutes to meet with you before my next meeting." Start then by stating the goals of the meeting, such as, "I asked you here today to discuss Mr. Green's recent test results and how this affects the plan for the future." An excellent rule of thumb at this point of the conversation is "before you tell, ask." Find out what the patient and family know and what they want to know. Some patients may choose less-than-full disclosure in regard to their medical conditions, and you cannot know without asking. Some cultures protect their members from bad news by relaying this information to family instead of the patient; these issues must be explored early in the interview to ensure that this is truly the desire of both the patient and the family. Cultural differences in medical care and in discussing bad news are explored in more detail later in this chapter.

Once it is determined that everyone in the room wants to participate in the ensuing discussion, invite the patient to speak freely about their understanding of their experience thus far. Studies have shown that satisfaction in family meetings increases as the proportion of family talktime goes up. Attempt to minimize interruptions and actively listen to what patients and families describe. Invite them to participate freely in the information exchange and to dictate how much information is divulged at this initial meeting. Active listening ensures that nothing is left out of the conversation simply due to over-estimating what the patient and family already know. Step 2, when patients are invited to express what they already know, is a great time also to correct any misinformation that the family or the patient may harbor. It is also a good time to assess whether the patient or their support group are engaging in any sort of denial about their condition. As examples, wishful thinking, unrealistic expectations of treatment or omitting important details of medical care might surface during this time of the interview.

The purpose of **Step 3** of the protocol (**Invitation**) is to obtain the patient's invitation to the clinician to talk further about what he or she knows about the patient's condition. Ideally, one would have previously asked the patient when ordering a test that might result in serious news how they would want to receive bad news if the need should arise. Do they want to tell their family on their own? Or would they prefer to let everyone hear together and be able to ask questions of the provider as the news is divulged? When asking the patient for an invitation to speak, ask also if it is okay to speak freely in front of family in the room. Most patients indicate during research studies that they want as much information as possible about their illness, though they may not express their full desire to providers (and they may not retain the details of what has been shared if they have a strong emotional response to the news).

Step 4 (**Knowledge**) is the actual process of giving information to the patient. If the news is bad, many clinicians are advised starting with a "warning shot;" this may lessen the shock that follows disclosure and may facilitate processing of the information to follow. The warning shot may be prepared earlier in the process as well. For example, it can be provided when the office calls a patient to set up an appointment, as in: "Is there anyone that you'd want to bring with you to this appointment? I'm afraid we have some serious things to discuss." The separation in time between the warning shot and the actual disclosure may ease the patient into the coping process.

Once the patient has been told that it is not good news, follow the "Ask, tell, ask" procedure. In Step 3, the patient was asked how much information they wanted to know. Use Step 4 to actually tell them that information in small quantities. Reevaluate the patient's verbal and non-verbal cues throughout the discussion and ask if it is okay to proceed with the conversation. Use non-technical words, but be sure to use words that will allow the patient to clearly understand what you are telling them when they are ready. For example, instead of telling a patient that there is an "invasive mass" in their liver, one might say, "There is a large cancer in your liver" (not a "tumor"). Instead of "metastasized," use "spread." Instead of "dyspnea," say "shortness of breath." Excessive bluntness must be avoided ("There is nothing we can do to treat this cancer") to keep patient's feeling engaged in the conversation and to avoid inciting a feeling of isolation and anger—but one should try to gage what additional information is given by soliciting what additional questions the patient and family may have.

A good rule of thumb along the lines of "ask, tell, ask" is to give at most three pieces of information at a time before checking for understanding. Repeat information as much as is necessary for the patient and their family. Asking the patient to summarize periodically what you have shared with them thus far can be helpful in checking to see if information is being received.

Most importantly, help the patient and family find hope. If the hope is no longer in the form of a cure, assist the patient in changing the therapeutic goal or the "hope object." Hope objects will be addressed in more detail later in this chapter. Sometimes patients may have to deal with strong negative emotions (see next section) after hearing bad news before they are able to see hope. But just because there is no treatment for their cancer, one can potentially be hopeful for a good quality of life moving forward or for other important personal or family outcomes.

Step 5 in the SPIKES protocol (**Emotions**) is to respond humanistically to the patient's emotions. Most people find this to be the most difficult part of giving bad news. Although one can hypothesize how a patient might react to life-altering news, the range of emotions is endless. Following your disclosure, wait for the patient to react. Begin by acknowledging and if possible naming the emotion ("I see that you're sad, Mr. Green."). It is helpful also to identify the reason for the emotion. "I imagine that you feel this way because you were hopeful that the treatment was going to work." Legitimize the emotions that you have identified ("Most anyone hearing such news would feel [sad, angry . . .]"). Rather than trying prematurely to reassure, try exploring the emotion so you fully understand it ("Tell me about the most difficult part . . ."). Let the patient know that you have connected their emotion to the feeling behind it with a statement to reflect your understanding. "I would probably feel the same way if I were you." It is important to allow the patient sufficient time to express their fears and emotions. Listen carefully and do not interrupt. Allowing patients to talk freely about what they are experiencing and feeling will improve how you both feel about the value of the conversation.

An approach to responding to patient emotion.

Acknowledge that emotion is being expressed	"I can see that this is upsetting to you."
Legitimatize the normalcy of the emotion	"Anyone receiving this news would be devastated."
Explore more about what is behind the emotion	"Tell me more about that . . ."
Empathize with the emotion if you genuinely feel it	"I can imagine that this feels disappointing."
Explore strengths	"In past circumstances, what has helped?"

Empathy is defined as being able to personally imagine what the patient is feeling and experiencing. (see Chapter 2). Empathy can be a very powerful tool in building trust and relationships with patients if done correctly; empathic statements made by the physician are associated with increased family satisfaction. However, if an empathic response is done without sincerity or when a patient is not ready to accept another's compassion, it can end up being harmful to a therapeutic relationship. For instance, if a patient is silent at the conclusion of the divulgence of bad news, they are not clearly expressing any emotion to the physician. In this case, it is helpful to explore what the patient is thinking and feeling prior to offering an empathic response. Sometimes the feelings of the provider can provide a clue as to how the patient is feeling, but this is not always accurate. If a physician is feeling anxious while anticipating a response from a patient after having given bad news, this may represent the physician's own response and not necessarily a guide to how the patient is feeling (countertransference).

Addressing a patient's emotions during the conversation may help mitigate anxiety in both provider and patient, prevent depression later in the course of the illness, and improve overall satisfaction with the interaction. Patients report less distress when they feel that their physician detected and addressed their concerns. Although identifying and responding to emotional cues requires focus, experience, and time, clinical interactions may actually take longer when emotional cues are missed.

Physicians often want to respond empathically to a patient's visual cues and feelings, though sometimes physicians may also be experiencing feelings such as hopelessness and perhaps guilt at not having detected the disease earlier. Providers may fear that responding empathically may be construed as evidence of inadequacy, mistakes, or failure. Before expressing empathy, clinicians should try to be sure that they are responding to the patient's feelings and not their own. Clinicians' feelings and reactions are important, but unless they relate directly to the patient's experience, they should be explored in other settings with trusted colleagues.

When giving bad news to a patient or family, generally avoid apologizing unless you have clearly made a mistake that you are ready to acknowledge. Apologies can be mistaken for admissions of guilt or of error on the part of the clinician. Though we may feel like we need to apologize for being the bearer of bad news, apologies can be problematic to physicians for many reasons. Patients may confuse an apology as an expression of pity or can change the emphasis of the conversation from the feelings of the patient to the feelings of the physician. "I'm sorry" may also limit further exploration of the patient's feelings. A good surrogate expression for "I'm sorry" as proposed by Quill is an "I wish" statement. "I wish I had better news for you" allows the physician to walk in the patient's shoes while acknowledging that the news is unlikely to change.

Compassion can take many forms. For instance, empathy can be shown by giving recommendations in light of what the physician knows of the patient's beliefs, goals, fears, and medical situation. For example, "From what I know about your ideals, Mr. Green, I would recommend switching to a hospice plan of care. This will allow for you to have the best possible quality of life for whatever time you have left."

Factors that improve attentiveness to and empathy for the patient during this difficult discussion include older age, female gender, and personal experience on the part of the physician. One study illustrated that physicians who had personally experienced life-threatening illness were more attentive to the emotional needs of the patient than those who had not. The same study concluded that older physicians give more emotional support to patients than their younger counterparts. Female physicians spend more time giving bad news to patients than male physicians.

Step 6, the final step of the SPIKES protocol (**Set goals**), is to summarize the conversation and to engage with the patient in creating a clear plan for the future. This step is essential in decreasing a patient's anxiety and level of uncertainty. At this point into the conversation, the patient has heard a lot of information that affects them very personally. Ask, first, if the patient and family are ready for a discussion about the plan. If they are not, briefly review the conversation to that point and ask for further questions about what has been said. Most likely at this point patients will be eager to plan for and discuss the next step. Present the possible treatment options in small bits and elicit patients' values and preferences as it relates to the possible treatment options. Clearly state each option and make a recommendation based on your medical expertise and experience as well as your knowledge of the patient's values as to which one you think would work best. Work together to come up with a decision; shared decision making with the patient relieves some pressure for the physician should the treatment not be completely successful. Referring patients to support groups within the community has also shown some benefits in those with terminal illnesses. There has been some evidence to suggest that patients who share experiences with supportive physicians and a group of peers with similar experiences have improved quality of life, experience less pain, and cope more effectively with terminal illnesses than those who do not attend support groups.

Some providers might consider briefly writing down the diagnosis and possible treatment plans for the patient to look up when they feel ready. In some studies, physicians audio-recorded these consultations, so that patients could take them home; however, reliving this experience may contribute to poorer mood and increasing rates of depression for patients. Schedule a follow-up appointment with you and other appropriate consultant(s) for the patient before he or she leaves your office. They may not feel up to completing these tasks while they are processing their bad news.

Patients are not likely to ask about prognosis during this initial discussion. In one survey of over 30 patients newly diagnosed with cancer, only 1 patient asked for a specific prognosis. Studies have shown that patients value qualitative estimates of prognosis far more than quantitative assessments. Doctors consistently overestimate survival in terminally ill patients, especially those who have a short life expectancy. Patients may vary in their desire for prognosis disclosure over the course of their illness as well; at their first visit, they may be more interested in information about their disease and possible course of treatment, with curiosity regarding prognosis revealed at later visits. If a patient desires some information at the time of the initial discussion, provide an average range of survival with caveats that they may lie also outside of that range in either direction. *"The average person with your condition will live (3-6) months. Some will live longer, and we will do our best to try to have you be in that group, but also some may live shorter, so you should get prepared just in case."* Clinicians need to be aware if they tend to be optimists or pessimists in their prognostication, but the inclusion of the possibility of being outside the expected range helps compensate for that to some degree.

It has been generally agreed upon by clinicians and researchers in this area that the SPIKES protocol assists both patients and physicians in breaking bad news. Most guidelines are based on expert opinion with little evidence about the best method for breaking bad news. Remember that all guidelines recommend tailoring the interview to the patient, and that each discussion will be different, depending on differences between patients. Not every conversation surrounding unfavorable information will require all six steps, but when it does, the steps of the SPIKES protocol should generally be done in sequence.

STRESS ON THE PROVIDER: BEFORE AND AFTER DIFFICULT CONVERSATIONS

Research and anecdotal information remind us that patients do not often remember most of the initial bad news discussion once the diagnosis is spoken. The divulgence of bad news is a stressful conversation for both providers and patients, but patients still need and want information regarding their disease. Although some stress may be adaptive, stress that is experienced at too high a level or as uncontrollable can have negative effects on the recipient. The emotional response of the patient depends on a number of factors, such as age, familial obligations, and levels of psychosocial support; for example, a 35-year-old father of young children might respond differently to the news of a new lung cancer than would a 96-year-old great-grandfather (but there are exceptions to every rule).

The doctor–patient relationship comes with expectations from both parties. The bad news discussion, when done well, is a good opportunity to strengthen this relationship. Earlier, we discussed shared decision making as a way to mitigate pressure on the physician when deciding on a treatment plan. This model of decision making is the norm in Western culture, but not in all cultures. For this reason, it is important for providers to assess early on how much of a role patients desire in their care. Some patients may want the physician's guidance, while others may only want the medical facts, so

that they can then make up their own mind. A multicultural approach to the bad news discussion is addressed in more detail later in this chapter (also see Chapter 15).

The reaction of the provider to the bad news is just as important as the patient's reaction to the difficult discussion. Due to the nature of the relationship between physicians and patients, physicians receive the bad news in advance of the patient. Breaking bad news to patients is stressful and psychologically difficult. There are multiple stressors on those charged with delivering the bad news; challenges include being honest without destroying hope, not knowing what the patient's emotional reaction will be, how to deal with the variety of reactions that might result, and how to deal with one's own feelings and reactions that may be very different from the patient and family. All of these variables create anxiety for the physician, even before the patient knows that anything is wrong. A lack of experience in delivering bad news may also contribute to the stress and anxiety present in the provider before giving the patient the news. This level of stress and anxiety sometimes dissipates quickly after divulging the information to the patient, but other times when the patient and/or family have a strong negative emotional reaction, the clinician's feelings may intensify.

When the physician is stressed, the possibility of avoiding the bad news discussion exists. Also, the physician may convey unwarranted optimism during the actual conversation. Talking with colleagues and getting support from coworkers prior to speaking with the patient can be helpful in difficult cases. Providers must be aware of their personal beliefs about illness, death, and dying prior to sitting down with the patient, to ensure that they are not inadvertently pressuring patients to respond in a certain way. As an example, a provider who recently lost a family member to breast cancer after forgoing chemotherapy treatments may push harder for their patient with breast cancer to take this treatment. During the conversation, be alert for emotions that you are projecting onto the patient and for emotions that the patient may be projecting onto you. Discussing strong emotional reactions on either side of the relationship with a trusted colleague may help in sorting out these issues and allow clinicians to care for themselves as well as their patients.

Those charged with the task of bearing bad news often experience high levels of stress, anxiety, and fear of negative evaluation. There may be a reluctance to deliver bad news, known as the "mum effect" which may result in the physician holding onto the bad news for a prolonged time prior to contacting the patient. How much stress a physician experiences prior to sharing the news is exacerbated when the physician is inexperienced, when the patient is young, and when there are limited prospects for successful treatment. Physicians may feel uncertain about how the patient will react or how they will manage the patient's emotions. They may fear destroying the patient's hope. Alternatively, physicians may feel embarrassed that they gave too much hope earlier in the process or may feel inadequate in the face of disease that is uncontrollable. All of these emotions factor into how a physician handles the news prior to getting it to the affected patient and can put up barriers to actually having the bad news discussion. Talking with trusted colleagues and members of multidisciplinary teams can help sort out these complex issues, which is critical to both self-care and patient care.

HOPE AS AN IMPORTANT PART OF THE BAD NEWS DISCUSSION

Hope becomes an important part of the patient's new life after hearing the news of a serious illness. As part of the healing process from the time of diagnosis, hopes will continuously change in the eyes of the patient as their disease evolves. Early in the discussion, clinicians may have to explore and empathize with elements of hopelessness, as when the expectations for a cure or for effective disease-directed treatments are no longer realistic. After exploring and empathizing with the loss of hope in the form it had been, the discussion should eventually evolve to refocus, reframe, or find hope again. For the patient with an imminently terminal disease, the hope now is no longer for a cure, but it can be shifted by the patient or the physician to alternatives, such as hope for a comfortable future or hope for the best-possible quality of life. Reframing hope can be an important role for the physician in a discussion involving the divulgence of bad news.

Physicians must walk along a critical path that balances optimism and honesty; patients need enough information to make the decisions that are of value to them, but truthfulness is just as important. However, evidence shows that regardless of the nature of information divulged or the amount of truthfulness as perceived by the patient, patients place more importance on the attitude of the physician and the manner in which the physician gives the news.

In searching for hope, it is helpful to identify that there are two kinds of hope, *specific* and *generalized*. With this knowledge, it becomes possible for providers to help distressed patients find hope even when the chance of a good outcome, in terms of longevity, is small. *Specific hope* is the state of desiring a specific possible event or future state of affairs, called the hope object. For something to qualify as a hope object, it must be possible, though it need not be probable. An example of specific hope is the hope for a cure of a patient's specific disease. Specific hope varies among two dimensions, desire (whose strength varies on a scale between lukewarm and intense) and the perceived likelihood of the event occurring (which varies on a scale

between uncertain and nearly certain). The patient's desire for their specific hope and the perceived likelihood of that specific hope occurring are independent of each other.

Generalized hope is a sense that there is some future beneficial, but uncertain, development that is not linked to a particular object, and is broad in scope, in other words, a sense of "open-endedness". Faith, which is distinct from hope, is a belief that life always has meaning, even with its unavoidable loss and suffering. By using two distinct types of hope, physicians can help despairing patients find hope even when the chance of a good outcome is small.

Hope should always be sought with patients, but one must also be truthful. It may sometimes seem hopeless to both patient and physician during a conversation about bad news; in these difficult cases, continuing to honestly explore feelings of hopelessness may eventually help in finding new avenues of hope. Sometimes patients will initially put all their hope in an experimental treatment that is statistically unlikely to be effective. After ensuring informed consent, it is useful to move forward with supporting treatment and "hope for the best," but at the same time, the clinician might offer the patient and family to "prepare for the worst," so that the developmental issues of preparation for death are not necessarily avoided. These two strategies, hoping for the best and preparing for the worst, need not be mutually exclusive. Hoping, while simultaneously preparing, minimizes the weakness of each strategy on its own.

When patients and physicians discuss serious illness only in terms of hope, physicians are potentially missing opportunities to improve upon pain and symptom management, discuss the patient's fears and concerns, and to grow the patient–physician relationship. By expanding the conversation to include both hoping for the best while preparing for the worst, physicians can now help address needs surrounding symptom management, spiritual, and psychosocial issues. Patients who rely only on hope may not be aware of their limited life expectancy and may go forward with costly, difficult treatments that are unlikely to work. Physicians who focus the relationship on hope alone may feel as if they are being dishonest with the patient, and may withdraw from the relationship as the patient becomes more sick.

THE EVOLUTION OF HOPE AND WORKING THROUGH GRIEF

Hope often initially focuses on outcomes that are strongly desired and reflect individuals' varying beliefs, values, and sense of possibility. The main focus of hope can develop and change over time as the disease progresses. At the start of a serious illness, most people will have an implicit hope for cure of their disease and continued life. As the prognosis changes, patients often need to be helped to modify the focus of their hope toward sustaining their quality of life or perhaps having important conversations with family members about "unfinished business." These transitions are initially not only filled with loss and grief but also potentially open up new avenues for hope. Physicians can help patients find hope by offering specific alternate foci that might be adopted when and if they are ready. Near the end of a terminal illness, patients may find hope in the doctor's ability to control symptoms and minimize discomfort. Using "I wish" statements at a time when giving bad news helps to redefine an unrealistic hope as a wish, thereby allowing for empathy without false hope.

Patients normally experience the onset of a life-threatening illness in an evolving state, starting with the idea that something is wrong, then absorbing the diagnosis, adapting to the disease, and, finally, changing their lives to live with the disease. The moment when the clinician is giving the bad news is usually the moment when the reality of the bad news dawns on the patient and stress peaks. After receiving the bad news, patients enter a period of attempted accommodation to changed life circumstances. This may end in denial, acceptance, or anger. Acceptance is usually the optimal outcome for patients. Those who reach acceptance have integrated the illness and the limitations that it imposes by establishing new priorities, shifting the focus of hope and finding a renewed sense of purpose. This grief work may take a very long time and some patients may never complete it. Often, patients will find a period of "middle knowledge," where they vacillate between continued adjustments and life's losses while preparing for death. It is important for clinicians to support the evolution of new kinds of hope as well as the preparation for death over time.

Patients and families are not the only people affected emotionally during the discussion of a bad news. Physicians, too, are often left with feelings of sadness, grief, incompetence, or anger after having to divulge bad news to patients, with whom they may or may not have had a longstanding relationship. These emotions should not be ignored. Allow time for self-reflection and seek out responses from those professionals who experienced it with you, including trainees. Identify the feelings that you have and talk them over with a colleague. Try keeping a journal to elaborate on the experience for the immediate relief of strong feelings and for your future development as a clinician (see Chapter 6).

THE ROLE OF CULTURE IN THE BAD NEWS DISCUSSION

Before giving bad news to patients, physicians must seek out the type of information that the patient and family would like. In some cultures, disclosure of truth

Table 3-2. Ways to explore cultural beliefs in discussing bad news.

What do you think might be going on? What do you call the problem?
What do you think has caused the problem?
What do you think will happen with this illness?
What do you fear most with this illness?
Would you want to handle the information and decision making, or should that be done by someone else in the family?

Source: Back and Curtis, *West J Med,* 2002; 176: 177–180.

is believed to cause bad outcomes, and nondisclosure can be protective and benevolent. Asking the patient and family what their culture dictates in terms of information sharing and decision making prior to giving bad news can strengthen the relationship between provider and patient. As an example, pose this question: "If we had to discuss a serious illness, how would you like me to handle this news?" Using open-ended questions to explore cultural differences before the actual disclosure can be helpful in outlining boundaries for clinicians (Table 3-2). Western culture puts a high value on truth-telling and a scientific explanation of disease; however, other cultures may value different degrees of truth-telling and prefer family-centered styles of decision making over patient-centered decision making. Clinicians can ask patients if they would personally want to hear bad news and handle the decision making should something serious arise, or if they would prefer delivering the news to family members. Understanding the patient's reasoning in advance can help circumvent conflict between patient/family and the health care team should they desire serious bad news information to be withheld from the patient. Having this sort of information about the patient in advance will help to keep the patient–physician relationship intact when unfavorable news does have to be discussed.

In western culture, patient autonomy and informed consent have created ethical and legal obligations to provide patients with as much information as they want about their illness and treatment. Nondisclosure is unethical unless there is clarity that the patient is deferring decision making, in which case enforcing full disclosure to the patient would be unethical. Hypothetical discussions before the news is actually available can go a long way to avoiding such conflicts. Bad news cannot be unilaterally withheld, but patients can clearly "choose" not to hear it. Communicating bad news must be done sensitively and with high regard given to the patient's readiness to hear and understand the discussion.

If the communication of bad news does not go well, misunderstandings can ensue, causing increased conflict between providers and patients and families, which has been shown to lead to poor quality decision making. Before sitting down with a patient, attempt to identify whatever cultural biases might be present on both sides of the conversation. Recognize also that although some patients may come from a similar cultural background, culture-based preferences vary within groups, and should, therefore, never be assumed. Patients may also have beliefs that vary considerably from their cultural heritage. In terms of decision making, Europeans generally mimic Americans, in desire, for more information and a stress on patient autonomy. Asians and Eastern Europeans may prefer family to be the decision makers while in general. African Americans tend to prefer family to be heavily involved in the end-of-life decision making.

Anytime there is a language barrier in the patient–physician interaction, interpreters should be used to allow the patient to ask questions of the provider and to fully understand the extent of the conversation. The use of family members as interpreters is discouraged, as they frequently misinterpret or omit words either for essential in the comfort of themselves or the patient. Children of patients, as an example, frequently leave out words relating to bodily functions. Interpreters who are trained to work in a medical setting are essential in enhancing communication with patients, particularly when the subject matter entails sensitive issues, such as delivery of bad news. Medical interpreters are trained to translate exactly what the provider and patient have said, but also may be used to gain insight into sensitive cultural issues that may help them to better understand the patient's context.

SUGGESTED READINGS

Baile WF, Buckman R, Lenzi R, Glober G. SPIKES: A six-step protocol for delivering bad news: Application to the patient with cancer. *The Oncologist* 2000;5:302–311.

Casarett DJ, Quill TE. "I'm Not Ready for Hospice": Strategies for timely and effective hospice discussions. *Ann Intern Med* 2007;146:443–449.

Barclay JS, Blackhall LJ, Tulsky JA. Communication strategies and cultural issues in the delivery of bad news. *J Palliat Med* 2007;10:958–977.

Quill TE, Holloway RG, Stevens Shaw M, et al. Primer for palliative care. 5th Edition. *American Association of Hospice and Palliative Medicine.* 2010;[vol 1]:102–119.

Ptacek JT, Eberhardt TL. Breaking bad news: A review of the literature. *JAMA* 1996;276:496–502.

Ambuel B, Weissman D. *Fast Facts and Concepts #6. Delivering Bad News part 1.* http://www.eperc.mcw.edu/fastFact/ff_06.htm. Accessed January 2014.

Back AL, Curtis JR. Cultural issues in breaking bad news. *West J Med* 2002;176;177–180.

Ambuel B. *Fast Facts and Concepts #29. Responding to Patient Emotion.* http://www.eperc.mcw.edu/fastFact/ff_29.htm. Accessed August 2011.

Weissman DE, Quill TE, Arnold RM. *Fast Facts and Concepts #224. Responding to Emotion in Family Meetings.* http://www.eperc.mcw.edu/fastFact/FF_224.htm. Accessed October 2011.

Quill TE, Arnold RM, Plass F. "I Wish Things Were Different": Expressing wishes in response to loss, futility and unrealistic hopes. *Ann Int Med* 2001;135:551–555.

Back AL, Arnold RM, Quill TE. Hope for the best, and prepare for the worst. *Ann of Int Med* 2003;138:439–443.

Glare P, Virik K, Jones M, et al. A systematic review of physicians' survival predictions in terminally ill cancer patients. *BMJ* 2003;327:195.

Whitney JN, McCullough LB, Fruge E, McGuire AL, Volk RJ. Beyond breaking bad news: The roles of hope and hopefulness. *Cancer* 2008;113(2):442–445.

Difficult Patients/Difficult Situations 4

Mitchell D. Feldman, MD, M.Phil, FACP; Howard Beckman, MD, FACP, FAACH;
& John F. Christensen, PhD

INTRODUCTION

Whenever and wherever health professionals congregate, it does not take long for them to bring up the topic of difficult patients. Patients and families we experience as difficult often increase the frustration and decrease our satisfaction with work. They make it difficult to deliver the person-centered care that is at the heart of high-quality, satisfying, and effective health care. Why, we ask, would someone come to the office, emergency department, or hospital and harass, abuse, demean, or lie to us?

Fortunately, most difficult interactions are both diagnosable and repairable. Apart from the rare patient who seems determined to be difficult, most problematic situations are created by unsatisfactory communication between practitioners and patients or by personal issues the practitioner or patient unknowingly bring into the visit. Such issues can mirror similar problems within the practitioner's own world and provoke negative reactions to an inherent or overt aspect of the patient's physical condition, sexual orientation, personality, or lifestyle.

At times, practitioners consider patients difficult based on their similarity to family members or others with whom they have had a close relationship or interpersonal problems. For example, a physician whose uncle used anger to control her may now have problems with an older male patient who responds angrily when she refuses to prescribe an antibiotic for an upper respiratory infection. Another common situation is the practitioner who is unusually intolerant of patients who will not stop smoking. This practitioner may well have had a close relative whom he or she could not convince to stop smoking, who later died from lung cancer. Developing the self-awareness to separate one's own past experiences and relationships from the current clinical interaction can significantly moderate one's aversive response and reduce difficult interactions. The key to dealing with such situations is to carefully examine how visits are progressing while monitoring one's own responses to the patient and the interaction. Greater self-awareness about their own feelings, experiences, and beliefs can help practitioners approach the clinical interaction with more self-reflection and less judgment and frustration. The case illustrations that follow focus on some of the more common challenging patients and situations that practitioners will encounter, and offer specific approaches to dealing with them. Table 4-1 summarizes some general guidelines for working with difficult patients. Table 4-2 recommends practical strategies for approaching specific situations.

THE ANGRY PATIENT

 CASE ILLUSTRATION 1

Dr. Swanson enters the room to see her fourth of the 12 patients scheduled for her Thursday morning session. Her patient, Ms. B., a 35-year-old social worker, is sitting with arms crossed, refusing to make eye contact. Dr. Swanson greets the patient by asking, "Ms. B., how are you?" She responds, "I've been waiting 35 minutes! This is no way to run an office." The doctor, who is emotionally drained after spending the last 50 minutes talking with a patient about breast cancer, wonders why she's chosen medicine as a career. She follows up by saying, "I apologize for being late. Besides that, are there other things that are upsetting you?"

Ms. B. replies, "You said that when I went to the Emergency Room last week with back pain, you would call and tell them I was coming. When I got there, no one knew why I was there or anything about my medical history. It was very embarrassing."

Table 4-1. General guidelines for working with difficult patients.

- Seek broader possibilities for the patient's emotion or problems
- Respond directly to the patient's emotions
- Solicit the patient's perspective on why there is a problem
- Avoid being defensive
- Seek to discover a common goal for the visit

Diagnosis

It is generally easy to recognize an angry patient. Even without the explicit expression of anger, harsh non-verbal communication, such as rigid posturing, piercing stare, a refusal to shake hands, gritting the teeth, and confrontational or occasionally abusive language, provide unmistakable evidence. More subtle behaviors that may indicate anger include refusing to answer questions; failing to make eye contact; or constructing non-verbal barriers to communication, such as crossed arms, turning away from the provider, or increasing the physical distance between them.

All too often, practitioners assume that the patient is angry with *them*, and, as a result, feel blamed for something they must have done or forgotten to do.

Table 4-3. Possible causes of patient anger.

- Difficulty in getting to the office
- Problems with the office staff
- Anger toward the illness from which the person suffers
- Anger at the cost of health care
- Problems with consultants to whom the practitioner referred the patient
- Unanticipated problems from a procedure or medication recommended by the practitioner
- Previous unsupportive or condescending treatment by a physician
- Absent or miscommunication between members of the healthcare team
- Other significant news or problems unrelated to medical service, such as work- or family-related conflicts

Although that certainly is one possibility, other important reasons must be considered as the cause for a patient's or family member's anger. These include, but are not limited to, those listed in Table 4-3.

Psychological Mechanisms

Many patients come to rely on the special relationship they develop with their medical practitioners. When successful, these relationships are anchored in trust and safety.

Table 4-2. Tips for approaching difficult situations or patient behaviors.

Situation	Recommended Techniques
Angry patients	Elicit the patient's reason for being angry: *You seem angry; tell me more about it.* Empathize with the patient's experience: *I can understand why you would be angry.* Solicit the patient's perspective: *What can we do to improve the situation?* If appropriate, apologize: *I'm sorry you had to wait so long.*
Silent patients	Point out the problem: *You're being very quiet.* Elicit the patient's reason for silence: *Why are you being so quiet?* Explain the need for collaboration: *For me to help you, I really need you to talk to me more about your problem.* Respond to cues of hearing impairment or language barriers: *Are you having trouble hearing or understanding me?*
Demanding patients	Take a step back from the demand: *You seem adamant about the MRI. Why do you think it's so important?* Solicit the goal of the demand: *Is there a particular problem you think the MRI will help us diagnose?* Acknowledge emotions unexpressed at the time of the demand: *It must be very frustrating that your back still hurts.* Solicit the patient's perspective: *What do you think is causing your problem?* *In what way had you hoped I could help you?*

It is, therefore, quite common for patients to share emotions they would never consider revealing or discussing with others. Patients want to have their concerns evaluated with compassion and interest. Any perception that their concerns are not taken seriously or are viewed as mundane, may be considered a violation of their trust and result in their feeling violated, vulnerable, and angry.

Patients have lofty expectations of practitioners. They expect timely service, relevant and up-to-date information about evaluations and treatments offered, and advice on how to cope with their illness. From their point of view, interactions that fall short can result in feelings of shame and rejection. The resulting humiliation can easily turn to anger.

From the practitioner's point of view, the patient's expression of anger may trigger feelings as diverse as guilt at having failed the patient, or feeling insulted by the patient's disrespectful behavior. As a result, practitioners may become defensive. This expresses itself as a reciprocal anger, a withdrawal from the relationship, or a denial of the practitioner's own behavior that may have prompted the anger in the first place. The difficulties are magnified if the expression of anger is or has been problematic in the practitioner's own family. After recognizing the contributions of one's own experiences, openly exploring a patient's anger can help create a more honest relationship, define the problem more explicitly, and facilitate an accurate and timely response.

Management

In most anger situations, evaluation and understanding should begin the therapeutic process. Responding calmly without judgment or projection with "You seem angry" tests whether the practitioner has correctly identified the emotion of the patient. (At times, it may be more effective and less threatening for patients to label the behavior with a less powerful emotion, for example, "You seem upset"). Failing to confront anger informs the patient that the practitioner is impervious to or unsettled by anger, discourages any meaningful sharing of feelings, and ensures eliciting superficial information. However, constructively acknowledging and working with the anger is both efficient and medically appropriate.

Although many patients in this situation respond with, "You bet I'm angry," some deny their anger. Nonetheless, their body language or tone of voice betrays the denial. In this case, the practitioner can address the denial: "Maybe 'angry' is too strong a word. It seems to me that you're upset by something; if you'd like to tell me about it, I might be able to help." This invitation to explain offers patients the opportunity explicitly to express their feelings. As a result, the practitioner develops a more complete understanding of the patient's point of view, and both can reach a deeper agreement on the nature and magnitude of the problem. At this point in the encounter there is usually a reduction in the patient's anger, relief on the part of the practitioner, and the restoration of a positive collaboration that facilitates a solution to the identified problem. Understanding the particular cause of the anger will help manage the problem in the future.

CASE ILLUSTRATION 1 (CONTD.)

The doctor apologizes, saying that the office had gotten busy and that she had simply forgotten to make the call. She explains that to prevent problems like that in the future, the staff decided at a recent meeting to put up a "follow-up" board so that process errors could be reduced. Ms. B. feels better understood, accepts the apology, and ends by saying, "I hope this doesn't happen again; I have enough stress at work as it is." Remembering the same patient's earlier complaint about waiting 35 minutes in the office to be seen, the doctor says, "I should have asked the receptionist to tell you that I was running late—I'm sorry about that. We're really trying hard to make sure that we communicate more effectively with our patients and our consultants." The whole exchange takes 50 seconds—time that is certainly well spent.

Patient Education

It is important for patients to understand that it is not only permissible but also important for them and their families to express their feelings. Encouraging the expression of anger helps to identify unresolved conflicts that can interfere with providing appropriate care. Encouraging patients and their families to express concerns or disappointments actually offers the practitioner an opportunity to become more effective by identifying and then removing significant barriers to effective, honest collaboration. Encouraging the hospital, emergency department, or office staff to use this approach can do the same.

Summary

Too often we assume that angry patients are angry with us. Sometimes this is so, but often there are much more complex reasons for the anger. The patient's reasons must be sought directly before mistakenly projecting our own beliefs onto the patient. By working hard to avoid being defensive, practitioners can acknowledge and then constructively resolve the cause of the anger. Confronted with such a responsive approach, most angry people are satisfied and resume an effective collaborative relationship with their practitioner.

THE SILENT PATIENT

CASE ILLUSTRATION 2

Dr. Cren begins his afternoon office hours with Mr. K., a 47-year-old man who has recently relocated to the area. On entering the room, Mr. K. fails to make eye contact and fiddles with a piece of paper folded over many times. In response to "Good afternoon; I'm Dr. Cren," Mr. K. quietly says, "Good afternoon." When asked what problems he is having, Mr. K. answers, "I've been really tired." After waiting a few seconds, the patient is asked to tell him more. Mr. K. responds, "I don't know what to say."

In response to "You seem quiet," Mr. K. responds, "Today is 3 months since my favorite aunt died." When Dr. Cren says, "I'm sorry to hear that; would you like to reschedule the visit?" The patient thanks him for the offer, adding that he's concerned about the fatigue and would like to talk about it. With that, the patient becomes more animated and discusses his fatigue. It is subsequently diagnosed as being related to depression.

Diagnosis

Silent patients offer little verbally, but there are a number of important non-verbal cues that deserve attention. The patient may seem withdrawn, as indicated by sitting a greater distance from the physician than usual, failing to make eye contact, seeming distracted, or not acknowledging the physician's attempts at interaction. Alternatively, the patient may seem anxious, evidenced by nervous or repetitive habits such as nail-biting, pacing, or folding and refolding papers. Finally, the patient may exhibit signs of sadness like deep sighs, red eyes, or tears. Some of the more common etiologies of silence in patient visits are provided in Table 4-4.

Table 4-4. Possible causes of silence in patients.

Cause	Discussion
Adverse reaction to prescription medication (e.g., sedation)	Check for overdose or drug interactions
Alcohol or other drug intoxication	Screen with CAGE Questionnaire and elicit history of substance abuse
Alzheimer or other dementia	Age dependent; although some dementias strike as early as the mid-forties, most occur in the 65+ age group. Silence is usually a sign of advanced disease associated with withdrawal from the environment
Anger	The patient is feeling wronged or slighted and is trying to elicit an emotional reaction (see Table 4-3)
Cultural or language barrier	Ask whether the patient can understand; use an interpreter or bilingual staff member, if available
Depression, dysthymia, or adjustment disorder with depressed mood	Name the feelings; request elaboration
Distraction secondary to depression	Associated with drawn features, sad affect, and lack of eye contact
Fear of being told that serious disease is causing the presenting problem	State clearly that, regardless of the outcome, the practitioner will be there to help
Fear of physician authority	Family background, other experience with domineering authority figures may have demanded submissiveness; a gentle demeanor, reassurance, and an explicit request for collaboration can help win the patient's confidence
Hearing impairment	Use the whisper test
Passive or shy personality	Change to a more direct, closed-ended pattern of questions; encourage descriptions and elaboration
Preoccupation with auditory or visual hallucinations	Request additional information from family or attendant
Quiet person	Usually responds to encouragement, offers to elaborate
Stroke, transient ischemic attack (TIA), mass lesion	Conduct thorough neurologic examination for focal findings.

Psychological Mechanisms

In many families, authority figures may demand "silence unless spoken to." This may be transferred to the practitioner–patient relationship. This deference may also extend to interactions in which differences in gender or social class exist. A history of humiliation or perceived mistreatment in previous medical relationships may also contribute to withdrawn silent behavior.

When patients feel that they have a serious or potentially life-threatening illness, silence may represent denial and serve as a protective function. For example, a woman can avoid confronting her fears about having breast cancer if she does not mention feeling a breast lump while in the shower. Silence may be a sign of a passive personality or, in some cultures, may be consistent with an appropriate way to communicate with doctors. These individuals want the interviewer to take control and direct the flow. Silence may also indicate a depressed mood, an adverse effect from a medication, or another medical condition that interferes with the patient's ability to communicate. Those struggling with depression or dysthymia may find it difficult to express their concerns or even find the energy to initiate conversation.

Management

When confronted with a silent patient, exploring the behavior is usually best begun by reflecting, "You seem very quiet." This offers the patient the opportunity to acknowledge the behavior and share the reason for it. Providing time for a response may encourage a tentative, frightened, or passive patient to begin speaking. When a patient seems passive, it is appropriate to explain the need for the patient to collaborate in the visit: "In order for me to help you, I really need you to tell me about what you are experiencing in more detail." If the patient seems distracted, it is fair to ask, "Are you hearing voices or seeing things you think might not be real?" If the patient appears angry, commenting on that would be appropriate. Particularly with older patients, if the patient responds with "What?" the most likely diagnosis may be hearing impairment, and the practitioner needs only to speak louder. One of the most common complaints by older patients is that their practitioners do not speak as clearly or as loudly as needed.

Patient Education

By explaining that silence may create additional barriers to effective care, practitioners can invite patients to be more involved in evaluation and treatment decisions. Emphasizing the importance of this involvement underscores the value of their taking an active role in decision making. It also discourages the patient from making the practitioner solely, and inappropriately, responsible for evaluation or treatment plans.

Summary

There are many reasons for a patient's silence during the visit. Openly acknowledging it and then asking for an explanation offers patients the chance to express a feeling, an extenuating circumstance, fear of an outcome, or fear of the practitioner. Further questioning can also result in the diagnosis of an anatomic cause, like an acoustic neuroma, or a psychiatric condition. Testing a hypothesis too early runs the risk of insulting patients and worsening the relationship.

Silent patients may be particularly challenging for practitioners who value the social and interpersonal aspects of their work. Learning respectfully to encourage more verbal collaboration is usually beneficial and rewarding. As with anger, the reason for struggling with silent patients may be that they remind us of others from our previous or personal experiences. These reminders can evoke strong negative responses. For example, a practitioner easily frustrated by silent patients may be reminded of a parent who died and did not reveal that he was having exertional chest pain. Recognizing the sources of these intense personal responses can be most helpful in assisting practitioners to focus on the patients and avoid unproductive replays of unsettling past experiences.

THE DEMANDING PATIENT

 CASE ILLUSTRATION 3

Dr. Hartwick is seeing her fifth patient of the afternoon. Mr. G. is a 48-year-old bricklayer, who is being seen for chronic back pain. In the initial visit, after excluding conditions suggestive of an underlying cancer or spinal cord injury, Doctor H. prescribed limited activity, exercise as tolerated, nonsteroidal anti-inflammatory medications, and a heating pad. Two weeks later, Mr. G. returns, and when asked how things have gone in the last 2 weeks, responds, "I'm no better. I've checked into a web-based back pain chat room and everyone agreed I should have a prescription for some stronger medicine like opioids." The doctor leans back in her chair, anticipating a frustrating encounter.

Diagnosis

Patients often make various requests or demands in the course of their visit for things such as diagnostic tests, referrals to specialists, and for specific treatments. These demands are often tied to dissatisfaction with the recommended evaluation, treatment concern about the accuracy of the diagnosis, or a failure to solicit important aspects of the history. A recommended test or treatment, however, may trigger a memory of a family member or friend's similar and unpleasant experience. The consequence is that the patient projects an undesirable outcome on the recommended plan.

Sometimes the reason for an unexpected demand involves secondary gain, such as workers' compensation, a disability claim or lawsuit, or seeking psychoactive medication. Another possibility is that the patient has found something on the Internet, talked to a friend, or read something in the press. The patient may be concerned that the practitioner is withholding a more expensive test or treatment to limit cost. Finally, it may be that the patient is frustrated with the lack of relief because additional testing or treatment is actually indicated. By listening carefully to a patient's concerns, the practitioner may rethink the diagnosis and/or seek alternatives to the current treatment plan.

Patients who are isolated from family and friends during times of illness may begin to doubt that the practitioner is sufficiently interested in their problem to ensure the best possible outcome. If the distrust grows, the patient may feel increasingly responsible and seek alternative sources of care. The patient may become fearful and demanding. If secondary gains are associated with the illness, however, the patient may demand testing to demonstrate greater levels of disability or to prove that the problem is sufficiently severe. This is especially true in pain syndromes for which testing is generally unrevealing and treatment not satisfactory.

Practitioners often experience feelings of rejection, distrust, blame, or humiliation in response to demanding patients, leading them to become defensive. By doing so prematurely, the clinician loses the opportunity to explore the patient's subtle reasons for the demands. For example, casual asides; postural shifts in response to a topic; and expressions of fear, agitation, and grief are often ignored. Possible reasons for demanding additional interventions are listed in Table 4-5.

Management

Rather than responding to the presumed cause, the first step in evaluating or reevaluating the demand is to identify the patient's affect.

 CASE ILLUSTRATION 3 (CONTD.)

Because Mr. G. seems frustrated, the practitioner reflects the feeling: "You seem frustrated." The patient responds, "I am frustrated. My father had a similar condition, and 2 years later they found he had a herniated disk which was successfully treated surgically. I don't want to wait that long to find out what I have."

In response to the practitioner's comment about frustration, the patient usually confirms or denies it. If the patient responds affirmatively (e.g., "I am angry, frustrated, sad, nervous"), the practitioner would ask, "Why are you . . ." This permits the patient to explain and share the experience behind the emotion. Often, this prompts an interaction between practitioner and patient that provides important information. In Mr. G.'s case, a better understanding of what prompted the request for more pain medication helps to determine to what extent education, a redescription of the results of evaluation or treatment, another examination, or questions about possible secondary gain might be most appropriate. As all aspects of a demand are explored, an appropriate response can usually be constructed.

When this approach is less successful, more probing questions may be useful. One is to ask patients what they think is causing their problem; often patients do not offer their opinions without being asked. Given the opportunity, patients frequently say that after an evaluation they were told the test results were all negative, but they believe that the cause of the problem was not

Table 4-5. Possible reasons for demanding additional interventions.

Feeling	Discussion
Anger	The patient is feeling wronged or is reexperiencing a previous bad outcome (see Table 4-3)
Fear	The patient may be afraid that the illness is terminal, serious, horrible, disfiguring, and so on, if not attacked quickly
Frustration	The patient may feel that no—or insufficient—progress has been made
Personal responsibility for health outcome	Previous experience may have convinced the patient that physicians are not trustworthy, competent, or interested
Doubt	The patient may wonder if economic reasons are driving decision making or if the practitioner is skilled enough or up-to-date with the current evaluation and treatment technologies

addressed. This point cannot be stressed enough: To provide meaningful reassurance, the patient's feelings about what caused the symptom must be elicited and confronted.

Another useful question is: "How had you hoped I could help you?" This gives the patient the opportunity to express dissatisfaction with the extent of evaluation, treatment, or commitment by the practitioner; it often lightens the practitioner's burden, since the patient's request may be significantly less difficult than what the practitioner anticipated. A typical example might be the arthritic patient who complains bitterly about the pain in his hip. When the physician asks, "How had you hoped I could help you?" the patient responds, "I'd like a prescription for a cane." The physician had anticipated a request for additional imaging and narcotics.

Primary care practitioners often find it challenging when patients make requests for opioid pain medication. In response to Mr. G's request for opiates to treat his back pain, the doctor should *acknowledge* the patient's experience of pain and his hope for relief, *reflect* her understanding of the patient's request, and express concern and *explain* that it is not the standard of care to prescribe narcotics for chronic back pain. In addition, the doctor can reframe pain as an "ability." For example, "It's clear that your ability to feel pain is intact. This is important, since pain is an alarm that is wired into us to call our attention to something that may need fixing. In your case, given the history of your pain and the medical workup, it's clear that there is no medical procedure that will make a difference. Nevertheless the alarm is continuing to go off." It may be helpful to use a metaphor to describe the adaptive nature of pain, for example, "It is like a car alarm designed to signal something to attend to. In the case of chronic pain it is like a car alarm set too sensitively. Rather than removing it, we need to reset the sensitivity of the alarm."

The doctor may give a rationale for why she is not in favor of using narcotics for chronic pain: "It will make the alarm more sensitive." "It can lead to sluggish thinking and interfere with your ability to do your job." "It can lead to addiction." In the common case where patients give a history of previous prescriptions of narcotics by physicians and that they helped, the doctor may want to comment on how the standard of care in medicine has changed with new knowledge about pain and about narcotics. "Our understanding of how pain functions and the nature of narcotic medications has changed the standard of care, which is not to use these medications for the kind of chronic pain you are experiencing." It is advisable to avoid personalizing the nonuse of narcotics as your preference. Rather refer to it as "the standard of care in this clinic." Finally, suggest that there are a variety of safe pharmacological and nonpharmacological options for managing chronic pain. Instill curiosity, but do not

elaborate too soon. "You may not be ready just yet to discuss these with me, but when you are, I'd like you to contact the clinic and set up an appointment so we can discuss the alternatives. I'm confident they can make a difference for you." (This communicates nonabandonment of the patient, even though the patient will not be receiving the desired narcotic medication.)

CASE ILLUSTRATION 3 (CONTD.)

Dr. Harwick ends the visit with Mr. G by saying: "What I would like to do is continue our present course of treatment, since in 90% of cases the symptoms you describe resolve within several weeks. If at the end of that time you're still having these symptoms, we can consider further evaluation with imaging studies and a different approach to reducing your pain. I appreciate your suggestions and I will continue to work with you until you feel better."

When practitioners believe that the demand is related to secondary gain (e.g., a desire to remain away from work for an extended period), they can gently confront the patient and offer a plan that provides ample time for recovery.

Patient Education

Patients respond to instruction when they believe it will be helpful in solving their problems. Until there is an agreement on the need for education by practitioner and patient, however, the patient might perceive education as the practitioner's way to control the visit. The patient's usual response in such an encounter is either to tune out the information or to construct mental barriers to implementing the recommendation. However, once the patient's concerns have been successfully addressed and a partnership formed, the patient often asks for and benefits from information supporting the practitioner's point of view.

Summary

Exploring the reasons for a patient's demands in a nonjudgmental manner allows most demands to be understood and addressed. Knowing the cause of the demand, a plan that is mutually agreeable can then be negotiated. If such a negotiation is not possible, the patient should be informed of realistic limits to what the practitioner can offer. The patient can then decide whether he or she is willing to accept the practitioner's boundaries or should seek alternative services.

THE "YES, BUT ..." PATIENT

 CASE ILLUSTRATION 4

Mrs. M. is a 58-year-old woman being followed for obesity and poorly controlled high blood pressure. Her doctor is frustrated because his continued attempts to get Mrs. M. to lose weight have been unsuccessful. As a result, he is pessimistic about their ability to work together to treat her hypertension, which he feels is a clear risk to her health. When the doctor notes that Mrs. M.'s blood pressure is still elevated, he asks whether she is still taking her medication.

She responds, "Oh, I'm sorry, doctor; I ran out of my medicine 3 days ago and didn't want to bother you for a refill." Later in the visit the doctor asks, "Did you join that exercise program you said you would last time?" Mrs. M. replies, "I've been so busy. I'll do it next week." The doctor pulls back in his chair, thinking to himself, "This will never go anywhere."

He leans forward and says, "Mrs. M., your actions tell me I'm pushing you to do something you don't want to do. I'm concerned about your weight; what are your thoughts on this?" Mrs. M.'s eyes moisten and she responds, "I want to lose weight, but I can't do it. I've tried for years, and it's so frustrating." The practitioner nods and says, "Let's hold off on the weight control for now. How about taking one thing at a time and focusing on your blood pressure?"

Diagnosis

When problems are being discussed, this type of patient's non-verbal behavior is usually engaged and active: leaning forward, bright affect, and dynamic gestures. As recommendations for evaluation and treatment are made, however, the patient typically becomes withdrawn, eye contact diminishes, and language becomes significantly less animated. Verbally, during the discussion of evaluation and treatment, the patient becomes quiet, volunteers little, and characteristically offers no solutions to problems. In fact, as the practitioner makes recommendations, the patient often responds with the classic, "I'd like to do that but . . . ."

Frequently, this behavior indicates a passive–aggressive personality (see Chapter 29). The practitioner initially feels encouraged to offer the patient suggestions, who then invariably rejects the offer or agrees to the plan but does not carry it out.

However, there are other possibilities that are often not explored. Probably most important is that the practitioner's plan has not taken the patient's perspective

into account and is, therefore, unrealistic or economically or logistically impossible. Another consideration is that the patient comes from a highly controlling family and is attempting to follow the recommendations but for psychosocial reasons is unable to.

Finally, the patient's previous experiences with practitioners may have been so hierarchical and paternalistic that the thought of disagreeing or negotiating a position does not come to mind, even when the suggested approach is not acceptable.

Psychological Mechanisms

Passive–aggressive behavior may emerge when patients do not feel capable of asserting themselves directly. They may position themselves so that others feel they want to, or must, save them. The practitioner's attempt to solve the problem is invariably followed by the patient's frustrating failure to collaborate. The patient successfully transfers responsibly for his or her problem to the practitioner and then rejects each solution offered. Continued failure results in repeated visits, offering the patient continuing attention while increasing the practitioner's frustration.

Some patients who are unable to fully collaborate may have been emotionally, verbally, or physically abused or may have had family or other personal experiences that taught unquestioning submission to authority.

Most people who enter the healing professions have a desire to be helpful. Passive–aggressive patients' solicitations for practitioners to save them can be seductive, luring practitioners into believing that these patients will singularly benefit from their expertise. The extent to which practitioners use a patient's recovery to validate their competence or professional value may determine how frustrated and angry they will become when treatment is unsuccessful. Rather than focusing initially on outcomes, the practitioner is better served answering the questions "Am I encouraging patients to take a more active role in their care?" and "Am I giving patients the chance to say why they're not using the treatments I thought we agreed on?"

Management

It is important to clearly communicate that to get better the patient must take responsibility for his or her own health. To help differentiate patients who are dependent from those who cannot participate because of a definable medical or personality disorder, the practitioner can say, "I'm frustrated with how things are going. Let's start again and see if what I see as a problem is really a problem for you."

The next step is to ask what he or she thinks would be helpful in solving the problem. One can ask, "Do you really think you can do this?" If the question is asked in a supportive fashion, most patients who initially agreed to fulfill an unrealistic plan (perhaps to please the practitioner), respond more honestly, acknowledging that they are unable to do so. Again, if asked respectfully, patients will share their reasons. Once this is done, the practitioner can encourage collaboration by saying, "Let's explore what we *can* do to solve this problem together. As we discuss options, it will really help if you tell me what's possible for you and what's not."

If the patient displays passive–aggressive behavior, the practitioner can seek agreement on the nature of the problem and then make very specific contracts for what the patient will do. They can be as direct as, "So, until our next visit, you will remain abstinent from alcohol," or "Between now and our next visit, you'll keep a diary and record when, and under what conditions, your headaches occur." The practitioner's support and enthusiasm can be directly tied to the degree to which both parties carry out the contract. In this way, the practitioner can promote patient autonomy and offer support, without taking full responsibility for the patient's behavior.

Over time, patients learn to respond to the support offered and begin to take a more active role in their care. Of course, there is always the risk that a passive–aggressive individual attempting to control the relationship will choose to seek another practitioner who can be more easily manipulated.

Patient Education

Patients who are unfamiliar with a collaborative model can be given specific information about the practitioner's understanding and particular style of collaborating. Explicit requests for patients' opinions about collaboration can be extremely useful. Over time, given the opportunity to state opinions and formulate plans, most people find such an approach satisfying, engaging, and motivating. Indeed, there is convincing evidence that patients taught to be more assertive improve their health outcomes, such as lowering blood pressure and controlling diabetes.

Educating patients who exhibit passive–aggressive behavior about such behavior can begin a process of introspection and self-awareness. Encouraging patients to explore the origins of these behaviors and consider a therapeutic relationship that facilitates the process can be rewarding for both patient and practitioner. Descriptions of behavior that hit home can provoke emotional responses in patients, but penetrating long-held psychological defenses can spur growth. The practitioner might say, for example, "You say your mother was overbearing and controlling and withheld praise. Isn't that what your children are telling you?" In most instances, the benefits outweigh the risks.

🖼️ **CASE ILLUSTRATION 4 (CONTD.)**

Mrs. M. agrees to take her medication and to return for a blood pressure check in 2 weeks. The practitioner gives her a card so that she can record her own blood pressure when she checks it at the drug store or the mall.

Summary

Setting limits and providing explicit feedback can teach patients to collaborate more effectively. Being aware of "yes, but" patterns can help promote a strategy of shared responsibility and prevent the ultimately unhelpful rescuing behaviors that interfere with successful treatment.

Appreciative Inquiry and Difficult Patients

Appreciative inquiry can be applied to our work with difficult patients. It allows us to shift the focus away from the sense of frustration that often accompanies these interactions to recognize and appreciate our successes. One technique is to write a brief narrative of a patient with whom you had initially a difficult interaction, but with whom your relationship became positive over time. As you reflect on the case, keep in mind the following questions to identify the factor or factors that helped transform that initially difficult relationship into one where you felt successful.

- What did you say or do that contributed to moving beyond the difficulty?
- What did the patient contribute to changing your relationship in a positive direction?
- What was it about the environment or circumstances of your encounter that improved the situation or your relationship?
- What changes did you make in your internal appraisal or perception of this patient that made a difference?
- What will you do differently the next time?

INDICATIONS FOR REFERRAL

Indications for referral include inability to make a diagnosis, an objective assessment that the patient is not benefiting from evaluation or treatment, or the practitioner's feeling of being threatened or in danger. Outside assistance and advice is always required when an inability to work with a patient impairs the provision of effective care. Since negative feelings often relate to a

DIFFICULT PATIENTS/DIFFICULT SITUATIONS / **39**

practitioner's previous family and life experiences, a patient who is difficult for one physician is often not difficult for another.

Once the decision to refer is made, framing the referral in a positive way is particularly valuable. One strategy is to acknowledge the need for assistance in managing difficult situations or problems. The dialogue might take the following form:

> **Doctor:** Mrs. S., for the last 2 months I've been trying to figure out how to help make your headaches better. I think it would help me if you were evaluated by a psychologist; I might be able to get a better handle on what else I could do to assist you in improving the problem.
>
> **Mrs. S.:** Are you saying that I'm imagining this? Do you think it's all in my head?
>
> **Doctor:** No, not at all. But nothing we've tried has stopped your headaches. It often helps me to have another person listen to the story and maybe find a new direction to take. Dr. F. has helped me with a number of people in the past, and I'm hopeful she can help us also.
>
> **Mrs. S.:** What do I have to do? I really do want these headaches to end.
>
> **Doctor:** Great. In addition to the referral, I'll schedule you for two visits with me over the next 12 weeks to see how things are going and see what else I can do.

Proposing a positive outcome from the referral can be remarkably useful. In addition, scheduling a visit for the person to return after the referral reassures the patient that the referring physician is truly seeking assistance rather than simply "dumping" the problem on someone else.

Learning to understand the patient's perspective, negotiating for realistic evaluation and treatment plans, and being aware of and responsive to verbal and non-verbal evidence that a recommendation was misunderstood or rejected creates a collaboration that can be satisfying for both participants. Underused skills such as soliciting the patient's attribution for a problem, offering praise and support, listening carefully to the patient's description of a problem, and explicitly confronting problematic or confusing behavior inform the patient that a serious attempt is underway to understand and successfully manage the patient's concerns. To the extent practitioners become more self-aware and address their feelings, they become more effective.

Finally, in the last few years, there has been increasing recognition of the role the work environment plays in a physician's effectiveness. As we ask practitioners to be more aware of their feelings and influences, manage the complexities of chronic and life-threatening illnesses, and recognize both verbal and nonverbal clues to overlying psychosocial components of disease, the medical establishment has a responsibility to create caring, responsive practice settings that nurture practitioners as we ask them to nurture patients.

SUGGESTED READINGS

Beach MC, Inui T. Relationship-centered care: a constructive reframing. *J Gen Intern Med* 2006;21:S3–S8.

Lazare A. Shame and humiliation in the medical encounter. *Arch Intern Med* 1987;147:1653–1658.

Levinson W, Gorawara-Bhat R, Lamb J. A study of patient clues and physician responses in primary care and surgical settings. *JAMA* 2000;284:1021–1027.

Quill TE. Partnerships in patient care: a contractual approach. *Ann Intern Med* 1983;98:228–234.

Safran DG, Miller W, Beckman H. Organizational dimensions of relationship-centered care: theory, evidence and practice. *J Gen Intern Med* 2006;21:S9–S15.

Suchman AL, Markakis K, Beckman HB, et al. A model of empathic communication in the medical interview. *JAMA* 1997; 277:678–682.

Suggestion & Hypnosis

John F. Christensen, PhD

Photo by Hank Christensen (www.hankchristensen.com)

INTRODUCTION

The history of hypnosis as a healing art dates back millennia. Its modern expression as a medical treatment emerged in the eighteenth century, with proponents such as Franz Anton Mesmer, an Austrian physician who practiced in Vienna and Paris in the late 1700s. Mesmer, from whose name the term "mesmerize" was derived, believed that illness was caused by an imbalance of magnetic fluids in the body, which could be corrected by the "personal magnetism" of the hypnotist. Discredited in 1784 by a French royal commission appointed to investigate Mesmer's techniques and chaired by Benjamin Franklin, hypnosis has since regained respectability. Franklin himself wrote an opinion that the patient's beliefs could influence bodily effects. The Scottish surgeon James Braid in 1843 coined the term "hypnosis," from the Greek word for "sleep," and espoused its use as a medical treatment. In the 1930s, Clark Hull and his student Milton Erickson conducted early research on hypnosis. Erickson went on to become a pivotal practitioner, researcher, and teacher of a generation of hypnotherapists. In the 1950s, the British and American Medical Associations recommended incorporating hypnosis into the medical curriculum. The American Psychological Association in 1960 endorsed hypnosis as a branch of psychology. In 1995, the US National Institutes of Health issued a consensus statement with evidence supporting the use of hypnosis for the alleviation of chronic pain.

Hypnosis appears to be a special manifestation of the mind–body system's ability to process information by transforming it from a semantic to a somatic modality. Its therapeutic effectiveness is supported by both research and clinical experience. Today, hypnosis is widely used to treat a variety of conditions—pain, airway restriction, gastrointestinal disorders, skin lesions, burns, and anxiety—as well as to prepare patients for surgical procedures and to facilitate behavior change (such as smoking cessation or weight loss).

Trance and suggestion occur naturally throughout human experience and are a function of how the mind works. Becoming absorbed in a novel and being unaware of surrounding sounds, or daydreaming while driving and not remembering the last few miles, are common experiences that illustrate the ubiquitous nature of trance. Responding to subliminal messages in advertising by purchasing a product represents a familiar reaction to suggestions made in a carefully crafted trance. These common experiences of trance and suggestion also occur with patients in health care.

This chapter will describe the therapeutic use of suggestion within the context of the patient's naturally occurring trance states and in the course of clinician–patient discourse. This application can be used routinely by clinicians in all patient encounters. We will also describe the role of therapeutic hypnosis, usually provided by a specialist trained in this procedure, in treating a variety of medical conditions.

DEFINITIONS

Derived from a Greek word meaning "sleep," hypnosis is, in fact, a therapeutic procedure that requires active cooperation on the part of the patient. The following definitions, used in this chapter, describe the states and processes involved:

Trance: A state of focused attention, in which a person becomes uncritically absorbed in some phenomenon and defocused on other aspects of reality. Trance states can be positive or negative.

Suggestion: A communication that occurs in trance, with special power to elicit a particular attentional, emotional, cognitive, or behavioral sequence of events.

Hypnosis: A communicative interaction that elicits a trance in which other-than-conscious processes effect therapeutic changes in the subject's mind–body system. Hypnosis can be either other- or self-induced.

Induction: The process by which a trance is initiated. This can occur naturally or as the first phase of hypnosis.

Utilization: The therapeutic use of trance to achieve desired outcomes and the phase of hypnosis following induction in which this occurs.

TRANCE & SUGGESTION IN THE MEDICAL ENCOUNTER

Both patient and clinician may undergo a mutual trance induction that, depending on the self-awareness of the participants, can leave either more susceptible to suggestion by the other. This state is neither pathological nor unwarranted, but part of the natural pattern of human

awareness in this environment. Generally, because of the power imbalance inherent in help-seeking situations, the patient is more vulnerable to suggestion. Being cognizant of trance and suggestion can give clinicians greater flexibility and influence in leading their patients to more positive outcomes.

Many patients waiting in an examining room are in a trance that has developed through a series of events that started with the onset of the symptom. The patient's awareness of this symptom then leads to an internal search for meaning. Prior beliefs, personal experience, or prompting of family or friends may lead the patient to attribute a particular meaning to the symptom. This attribution constitutes the initial suggestion, perhaps solidifying into a concern, "I wonder if that can be something serious." This preoccupation, in turn, increases awareness of the sensation and further restricts the patient's attentional field. Increased absorption in the symptom and decreased awareness of other sensations are the essence of the trance.

The decision to see the doctor further deepens the trance, and this process continues as the patient, waiting first in the doctor's office and then in the examining room, rehearses how to describe the symptom and discuss it with the doctor. As noted earlier, this process of trance induction around a symptom is not pathological, but is part of the natural unfolding of awareness surrounding a medical visit.

By the time the physician enters the examining room, the patient is in a trance and consequently susceptible to suggestion. Whatever the clinician says or does not say in the course of the interview can, because of the power generated by the patient's suggestibility, further develop the patient's trance, shift its focus, augment or diminish the patient's somatic awareness, and influence ongoing patient emotions, cognitions, and behaviors surrounding the symptom.

The clinician is also susceptible to trance. Patients can sometimes unwittingly induce a trance in the clinician through a combination of verbal and non-verbal techniques such as the initial verbalization of the problem, hand gestures, grimacing, and changes in voice tone and tempo. All these contribute to focusing the attention of the clinician on the problem or on what hurts. This narrowing of the physician's focus (even while a differential diagnosis is being developed) may preclude other internal images, such as the future good health of the patient or a positive doctor–patient relationship, that could otherwise give rise to helpful discussions. A too-rapid response by the clinician results in premature closure on the nature of the patient's problem and solidifies the clinician's initial trance. However, attending to and eliciting the whole story from the patient (see Chapters 1 and 2) keeps that focus fluid. Sometimes patients induce a recurrent negative trance in the provider, leading to antagonism or aversion for the patient or to feelings of powerlessness in the face of the patient's problem (Chapter 4).

 CASE ILLUSTRATION

A 55-year-old single woman was being followed by her primary care physician for chronic chest pain after a thoracotomy. The pain led the patient to withdraw from social activities. Her complaints, which continued for several months, appeared inconsistent with the progress of healing around the surgical wound. Various pain-management strategies that the physician proposed, including physical therapy, acetaminophen, and an antide-pressant, had little effect on the complaints. Both patient and doctor became frustrated, with the patient feeling that nothing new was being done for her pain and the physician feeling powerless to alleviate the patient's suffering.

Eventually, seeing this patient's name on the appointment schedule would produce a sinking feeling and tightness in the physician's stomach, and his breathing would become shallow. As he walked into the examining room and observed the patient's slumped posture and grim facial expression, he could predict how the discussion would go:

Doctor: How have you been doing since our last visit?
Patient: (*pointing to her chest, and responding with slow speech and long latencies*) This pain really has hold of me, and I can't escape it.
Doctor: (*anticipating a negative answer*) Did you try any of the exercises the physical therapist recommended?
Patient: (*grimacing, shifting position, looking down and then back at doctor*) I've tried that before, and it only makes the pain worse. (*eyes filling with tears*) Can't you do something for me?

This case illustrates several components of trance in both patient and doctor. The patient's recurring chest pain induces a trance in which her attention becomes narrowly focused on her suffering and disability. Anticipation of a visit to her doctor further restricts her focus, and her rehearsal of how she can convince the doctor of how bad it really is further heightens the trance. She has learned to associate the image of her doctor's face and the sound of his voice with frustrating discussions about the intractable nature of her pain. Her continued presence at these appointments corresponds with a belief that the power to alleviate her suffering lies outside of herself. If only this doctor knew everything there

was to know about her pain, he would be able to help. This expectation keeps her in a suggestible state.

The doctor, too, has shifted into a negative trance by the time he enters the examining room. The induction begins as he anticipates seeing the patient and continues as his accompanying somatic responses shift him from his habitual openness to the field of possibilities to absorption in his own powerlessness to effect change. His trance is deepened by the patient's non-verbal and verbal communications about her continuing pain. The doctor becomes more vulnerable to suggestion, and the patient's plea to do something for her creates the expectation in him that he must. This expectation, in the face of the patient's persistent pain, deepens his sense of powerlessness.

Therapeutic Uses of Trance & Suggestion in the Medical Encounter

The clinician can use the patient's trance to make specific suggestions that enhance therapeutic outcomes. The language used in medical encounters can lead to unintended patient beliefs and behaviors that influence both illness and healing. For example, the prediction of continued problems for a patient with a weak knee—"You'll probably always be bothered by some pain in that joint"—in the first postsurgical visit has an enhanced power to influence negatively the patient's future awareness of and belief in the knee's integrity. The warning becomes a self-fulfilling prophecy as the patient unwittingly guards the knee and develops a compensatory gait. A positive suggestion—"Whatever residual discomfort you feel, in time you will notice more freedom of motion and activity"—can create expectations that are more likely to enhance healing and the resumption of activity.

A more subtle strategy is the use of positive images and avoidance of negative modifiers. Consider the following statement to a patient after surgery:

Doctor: Your ankle ought to hurt less in a few weeks.

The unconscious mind tends to delete negative modifiers, in this case "less." The embedded suggestion becomes: "Ankle . . . hurt . . . in a few weeks." A positive suggestion would be:

Doctor: You will notice much more comfort within a few weeks.

Because the primary words of the sentence are positive, the suggestion might be incorporated as:

Doctor: You will notice . . . comfort . . . within a few weeks.

In the context of discussing sleep hygiene with an insomniac patient, the well-intended suggestion, "When you go to bed, try not to worry about staying awake," might contain several unintended messages leading to disturbed sleep. The word "try" connotes effort; it becomes associated with "bed;" the negative modifier "not" is deleted by the unconscious mind, leaving the additional message to "worry about staying awake." The suggestion could be positively restated:

> **Doctor:** After you get into bed, you can enjoy a few minutes of deep relaxation before falling soundly asleep.

Clinicians can also use temporal clauses to embed suggestions that lead to positive patient expectations. For example, linking pain with expectations for healing can be accomplished by the following statement:

> **Doctor:** When you first experience postoperative pain, it is important to realize that the healing has already begun.

Predicting positive change that precedes the patient's awareness of it can build positive expectations—even if the discomfort continues. For example, the physician might predict the course of recovery as a patient responds to antidepressant medication:

> **Doctor:** Your spouse and others close to you will notice the changes in you long before you begin to feel better.

The implied suggestion is that you will begin to feel better, and when you do, positive changes will already have occurred.

The clinician can also reframe uncomfortable side effects of some medications as an indicator of their potency, thus enhancing the placebo effect. In prescribing an antidepressant, a physician could disclose the anticipated side effects:

> **Doctor:** If you notice this kind of discomfort as you begin to adjust to the medication, keep in mind that this is a potent drug that has the capability of achieving the results we want.

The message contains two positive associations with the side effects: adjustment to the medication and movement toward the desired outcome.

The clinician who appreciates the trance-like nature of the medical encounter can use the patient's openness to suggestion not only to present positive suggestions and avoid those that are negative but also to promote healing. This is true for both the clinician's own trance and that of the patient.

Shifting from a Negative Trance to a Positive Trance

Clinicians have several options to shift a dysfunctional trance in a more open direction.

CHANGING BODY POSITION

This works directly with the somatic configuration that maintains a trance state. A depressed patient may have a frozen, slumped posture, downcast eyes, and shallow breathing. This frozen posture amplifies negative images and self-statements and inhibits any focus on possibilities for change. The physician can comment on this posture and suggest modifications, such as raising the eyes while walking outside to observe cloud formations, birds, or airplanes, and shifting breathing to the abdomen. The clinician might also suggest that the patient occasionally put on some music and dance—even alone—at home. Clinicians, too, can use a shift of physical position to break an unwanted trance in themselves. A physician who feels ineffectual in the face of an inordinately blaming or demanding patient and reacts physically with chest tightness and throat constriction can stand up, say "Excuse me while I adjust the light," walk to the window, adjust the blinds or shade, move the chair to a slightly different location, and then sit down. During this activity, the physician can shift breathing to the abdomen and prepare to open a new line of discourse with the patient:

> **Doctor:** It's quite obvious how frustrated you are with the way things are going. Let's refocus for a moment on our goals and how things will look for you then.

CONFUSION

Confusion can be helpful in breaking a pattern that locks patient and clinician into repeatedly acting out a script whose negative outcome both can predict. The following caricature illustrates a common script:

> **Patient:** Fix me.
> **Doctor:** Try this.
> **Patient:** That won't work.
> **Doctor:** What do you think will work?
> **Patient:** I don't know. You're the doctor.

When the clinician becomes aware of such a circular pattern, it is helpful to ask "What is the patient anticipating I will say or do next?" If at this point the clinician can do something unpredictable, the result will be temporary confusion, which can be used to shift the patient's trance in a more resourceful direction. The unpredictable action might be the "Columbo technique" (named for the television detective). In this technique, the physician suddenly and dramatically remembers some minor personal problem (e.g., forgetting a spouse's birthday gift), asks the patient's forgiveness for the distraction, and requests the patient's aid (e.g., in suggesting a store to purchase the gift). The momentary confusion that ensues (whether or not the patient is able to offer any help) breaks the previous trance and allows the formation of a new one. This temporary role reversal is only one example of the use of unpredictable behavior to induce confusion and interrupt the pattern, thus allowing greater rapport and more effective communication.

MINING FOR GOLD

This phrase refers to a technique that shifts the focus of discussion away from distress and toward an exploration of the patient's resources. Useful at any time, this strategy is especially helpful when the tone of meetings with the patient is persistently hopeless, when the patient appears to legitimize the visit by focusing exclusively on somatic complaints, or when the patient's continuing complaints make the clinician feel ineffective or frustrated. In "mining for gold," the physician may inquire about things the patient is proud of—past successes, hobbies, travels, relationships, and obstacles overcome. The clinician observes when the patient becomes animated or otherwise shifts out of the negative trance and notes the topic in the chart, returning to this topic briefly in subsequent sessions. Sometimes the change in the patient's state leads to a change in behavior, emotions, or outlook that had been precluded by the "what's wrong with me" trance. Similarly, the clinician's feeling about the patient may change; renewed interest and curiosity about the patient's personal resources may transform a previously difficult relationship.

ELICITING TARGET STATES

Here the clinician engages the patient in thinking and talking about a future well-state, asking the patient to describe what things will be like when the medical problem is resolved or no longer interferes with the patient's life. It is important that the patient be able not only to name the target state ("I want to feel good again" or "I want to be free of pain") but also generate visual, auditory, and kinesthetic images of activities associated with that state. This discussion helps physician and patient establish criteria for knowing when the problem is resolved; it also engages the patient in imagining a future well-state unrelated to and incompatible with present suffering. This trance shift may be accompanied by positive physiologic changes and increased animation and hope.

 CASE ILLUSTRATION (CONTD.)

In the case of the woman with post-thoracotomy pain, the physician tried using the technique of eliciting a target state to alter the patient's trance.

Patient: (*grimacing*) I feel trapped. I never imagined it would hurt this bad.
Doctor: How do you imagine it will be when you've completely recovered from your surgery?
Patient: Well, I hope I'll feel better.
Doctor: Well, let's think about what that would be like for you. Once you're feeling better, what do you see yourself doing differently?
Patient: Fly fishing.
Doctor: (*smiles; eyebrows raised, voice more animated*) You like to fish? (*the doctor enjoys fly fishing and has shifted automatically into a state of high interest*)
Patient: (*looks at doctor, smiles*) I used to enjoy being out on the river in my waders, fishing for steelhead and Chinook salmon.

The doctor and patient proceeded to discuss various rivers they had fished. The patient had momentarily shifted her mental imagery and her kinesthetic state away from the pain trance toward future health. This created a context in which she could construct a full sensory image of that future well-state that was incompatible with the pain behaviors she had displayed. In addition, her image of the doctor, previously associated exclusively with her pain awareness, became, in subsequent visits, associated with images of recovery and hope. The doctor's impression of the patient also changed, so that he looked forward to their meetings instead of dreading them.

MEDICAL APPLICATIONS OF HYPNOSIS

Hypnosis can be an effective therapeutic option for a variety of problems. The neurophysiologic processes by which hypnosis can effect change in such a wide range of complaints are still a subject of exploration. One current theory uses information processing as a heuristic model, with the body, brain, cells, and organs regarded as an information-processing system. In the brain, semantic information (encoded in language) is transduced into molecular information, which uses neurochemical and neurohormonal channels to cause changes in diverse organ systems.

Recent brain imaging studies, employing PET and MRI, have shown that the hypnotic state is related to a widespread set of cortical areas involving the occipital, parietal, precentral, premotor, and ventrolateral prefrontal and anterior cingulate cortices. The antinociceptive effects of hypnosis correlated with activity in the mid-cingulate cortex.

In deciding whether to use hypnotic procedures with patients (or to refer them to a hypnotherapist), it is important to consider patients' beliefs about hypnosis, their openness to other therapeutic modalities, and their locus of control. Some religious groups (e.g., Jehovah's Witnesses) forbid use of hypnosis, and some patients may fear that they will surrender control to a powerful "other," who can then control their minds. Brief education by the physician about the nature of hypnosis and its usefulness as a tool to help patients increase control over their symptoms may correct these beliefs. If the patients are not convinced, they are probably not good candidates for hypnosis.

Furthermore, some patients may resist hypnosis because they infer that the physician thinks the problem "is all in their head." For such patients, anything other than a biomedical intervention may be viewed with suspicion. Assuring them that hypnosis is simply part of a comprehensive medical management of their problem may increase their openness.

Locus of control—internal or external—is also a significant factor. Patients with an internal locus of control believe that they can influence many of life's rewards or punishments, and they may be better candidates for hypnosis than those with an external locus of control. This latter group may respond better to biofeedback, which relies on equipment that is external to the patient.

In the following brief descriptions of clinical situations, hypnosis can be considered as an adjunctive or, in some cases, primary treatment.

Relaxation & Stress Management

One of the physiologic effects of therapeutic hypnosis is stimulation of the parasympathetic nervous system (see Chapter 34, Figure 34-2). Several stress-related conditions have been attributed to hyperstimulation of the sympathetic nervous system, which is modulated by the parasympathetic nervous system in a dynamic interrelationship. Sympathetic activation can be part of the fight-or-flight response to perceived threats. Given the plethora of real or perceived threats in today's world, stress-related illnesses may be a common presentation of patients' habitual levels of sympathetic arousal (see Chapter 34). Sympathetic responses include tachycardia, muscle tension, adrenaline release, pupil dilation, inhibited intestinal mobility, shortness of breath, and sweating. This autonomic activation is downregulated during hypnosis, and with parasympathetic stimulation the individual becomes relaxed, leading to energy restoration, conservation, and renewal.

Anxiety

Hypnosis can be quite effective as a primary or adjunctive treatment for anxiety. Patients with an internal locus of control will find self-hypnosis an especially satisfying alternative to anxiolytic medication. When introducing this as an alternative treatment, the physician can say:

> **Doctor:** You have a powerful pharmacy in your brain that can produce significant healing effects. Through hypnosis you can learn to mobilize that pharmacy and let it work cooperatively with the other approaches we use.

The clinician can devote 15–20 minutes to inducing a trance, during which the patient is led to form a full sensory recall of an experience in which he or she felt deeply relaxed. In this process, it is important that clinicians avoid imposing their own images of relaxation, instead facilitating the patient's exploration by means of non-specific suggestions. These suggestions can lead the patient through each sensory modality (e.g., vision) and submodality (e.g., color, brightness, and quality of reflected light) to allow the patient to become absorbed in a full sensory representation of an actual experience associated with relaxation. If the session is audio recorded, patients can take the recording home for daily practice, thereby learning to self-induce trances and regulate their own levels of autonomic nervous system arousal. The extra time taken for the hypnotic induction can often be compensated by a decrease in time spent on phone calls from anxious patients, since the audio recording allows the patient to access the clinician's voice and suggestions whenever needed.

Pain Management

Because cortical elaboration of nociception is a component of pain, hypnosis can be used to shift the focus of attention away from pain sensations. In some surgical or dental procedures, hypnosis can be used as an adjunct to, or instead of, anesthesia. In addition, patients with chronic pain can be taught to relax the muscles they tense around areas of pain as part of their "guarding" or bracing efforts. This hypnotic relaxation reduces the component of the pain that is due to muscle contraction. Patients with migraine headaches can be taught to dilate blood vessels in their hands and feet through hand- and foot-warming imagery—sitting in front of a campfire, for example. In the early prodromal stage of migraine, this procedure can sometimes reverse the progress of the headache, possibly by increasing peripheral vasodilation and allowing relaxation of blood vessels in the head. Temporomandibular disorders, pain from repetitive strain injuries, and tension headaches have also been treated effectively with hypnosis. For pain relief during childbirth, a meta-analysis showed that hypnosis reduces analgesia requirements in labor. In one study, older female patients with osteoarthritis experienced significant increase in their health-related quality of life following a 12-week treatment using guided imagery with relaxation. Brain imaging studies have suggested that in hypnosis-induced analgesia prefrontal and anterior cingulate cortices form important structures in a descending pathway that modulates incoming nociceptive input.

Hospice & Palliative Care

Hypnosis has been used adjunctively with other therapies to help patients with chronic and terminal illnesses. Relaxation, overcoming insomnia, relief from pain and dyspnea, and enhancing relationships with relatives and other support persons are some of the benefits of this modality in the hospice setting.

Cancer

There is evidence that hypnosis is effective in alleviating the chronic pain associated with cancer. In addition, hypnosis can control symptoms such as nausea, anticipatory emesis, and learned food aversion; it is also helpful in managing anxiety and other emotions associated with cancer. Hypnosis may also be effective in reducing hot flashes in breast cancer survivors.

Skin Problems

Certain dermatological conditions, such as warts and alopecia, have been treated successfully with hypnosis. While in trance, patients are given the suggestion to experience tingling or flushing in the affected area. Warts may respond to these suggestions by shrinking in size or—in some cases—disappearing. Burns have also responded to hypnotherapeutic suggestion, both in lessening the degree of the burn and in controlling pain. Other dermatoses for which therapeutic hypnosis may be helpful are acne, atopic dermatitis, herpes simplex, hyperhidrosis, pruritus, psoriasis, and rosacea.

Immune System Function

Hypnosis has been used successfully to treat genital herpes, both in reducing the number of flare-ups and in decreasing the duration of flare-ups. Hypnosis has been shown to decrease blood levels of herpes simplex virus and to increase T-cell effectiveness, NK-cell activity, secretory immunoglobulin A (IgA), and neutrophil adherence. A meta-analysis has shown that hypnosis can reliably alter immune system function. Hypnosis incorporating immune suggestions showed a positive influence on total salivary IgA concentration and neutrophil adherence, along with a modest suppression of intermediate-type hypersensitivity erythema. These effects were mediated through relaxation. Some studies have shown differential delayed skin sensitivity reactions on the right and left arm of subjects depending on which arm was suggested under hypnosis to show no changes.

Respiratory Problems

Patients with asthma have been taught to use self-hypnosis to expand airways and minimize stress-induced attacks, as well as reduce anticipatory anxiety about having an attack. Some patients are able to decrease their bronchodilator use with daily self-hypnosis. Weaning patients off a ventilator in the intensive care unit has been facilitated by the use of hypnosis.

Hypertension

Hypnosis for relaxation can be a useful adjunct to other therapies for hypertension. Individual hypnosis treatments for eight sessions was shown to reduce mild essential hypertension immediately posttreatment and at one-year follow-up.

Gastrointestinal Problems

Problems such as irritable bowel syndrome (IBS), are amenable to adjunctive treatment with hypnosis. The primary approach is to reduce anxiety, induce relaxation, incorporate abdominal breathing, and suggest warmth in the abdomen and proper functioning in the bowels. Preoperative suggestions have been used successfully to promote an early return of gastrointestinal motility following intraabdominal surgery, leading to shorter hospital stays.

Sleep Problems

Sleep-onset insomnia—associated with anxiety, obsessive worrying, or sympathetic arousal conditioned to the cue of getting into bed—can be treated with hypnotherapy. By making an audio recording of an induction in which the patient is led into a relaxed state and invited to form positive associations with lying in bed before falling asleep, the clinician can give the patient a new nightly ritual that will enhance relaxation. A relaxing trance can also help the patient return to sleep more quickly after waking up.

Pediatrics

Pediatricians and family physicians skilled in hypnosis find it a useful adjunct in the treatment of children. Children are often amenable to the use of imagination and story-telling as trance induction techniques. Some of the conditions that respond well to primary or adjunctive use of hypnosis include nocturnal enuresis, night terrors, functional abdominal pain, surgical and other office procedures, chronic dyspnea, and symptoms related to cystic fibrosis. Hypnosis was shown to be effective in reducing distress and the duration of an invasive diagnostic test in children with urinary tract abnormalities. In a review of studies on psychological interventions to reduce needle-related procedural pain in children, hypnosis showed the most promise in reducing self-reported pain.

Pregnancy

Hypnosis has been used successfully to reduce symptoms of hyperemesis gravidarum. Habitual aborters have been helped to relieve anticipatory anxiety and lessen the psychogenic risks of spontaneous abortion when organic etiologies have been ruled out.

Preparing for Surgical and Other Difficult Procedures

Patient expectations appear to play a role in the degree of pain and distress felt with surgery and procedures such as colonoscopy. Hypnosis has been used to anesthetize patients who are allergic to anesthetic drugs and to decrease the use of postoperative pain medication. Usually hypnotic anesthesia requires a deep level of trance, which calls for advanced skill on the part of the hypnotist along with the patient's ability to be hypnotized. Using the naturally occurring trance of patients anticipating surgery, physicians can make simple suggestions to enhance surgical wound healing and reduce postoperative pain. Referring to pain as "discomfort" or an "unusual sensation," the physician can offer the patient a statement such as:

Doctor: No matter what you've been thinking about the time after surgery, you'll be pleasantly surprised at how little discomfort you have.

Presurgical hypnosis can also decrease disorientation and confusion following surgery.

Habit Change

For patients in the preparation/determination or action stage of readiness to stop smoking or to change eating behavior (Chapter 19), hypnosis can be a useful ally. The ritual pattern of patient behavior around smoking can be viewed as a trance phenomenon. There is an automatic, other-than-conscious sequence of kinesthetic (tactile, visceral, emotional, and postural) awareness and behavior usually set in motion by contextual cues (e.g., finishing a meal, drinking coffee or alcohol, and talking on the telephone). Hypnosis can be described to patients in the preparation/determination stage as a useful tool "to help you come out of the smoker's trance and into a more satisfying, health-promoting trance." The clinician can call patients' attention to the automatic behavioral sequence while taking a smoking history (Table 5-1). Asking patients to describe in detail which hand they use to pick up the cigarette pack, take the cigarette out of the pack, hold the lighter or strike the match, and so on, will call their attention to the automatic, trance-like nature of their

Table 5-1. Hypnotic smoking-cessation interview.

The following questions are designed not only to gather information about the patient's smoking behavior and its parameters but also to raise the patient's awareness about behaviors that are usually automatic and unconscious. The interview presupposes that the patient has already expressed a desire to stop smoking.

- Have you ever quit smoking before? How long were you successful at curtailing your smoking? What allowed you to succeed at not smoking for that long?
- What other habits have you overcome? How have you done that?
- What brand of tobacco have you been using?
- What motivates you to continue smoking?
- Where do you have your first cigarette of the day?
- Where do you have your second cigarette?
- What is the sequence of activities that precede the first cigarette of the day?
- Describe the different situations in which you are likely to smoke.
- Describe the mood or emotional state that usually precedes smoking.
- Describe the urge to smoke in detail.
- Describe how you light a cigarette (if the response is vague, offer the following prompts):
  - Which hand do you use to reach for the pack?
  - Which hand do you use to pull the cigarette out of the pack?
  - Which hand do you use to put it in your mouth?
  - Which hand do you use to light it?
  - Which hand do you use to continue smoking?
- Will you describe in detail all of the reasons that you can think of for not taking a first puff after you have stopped smoking?
- How long will you have to stop before you realize that you are permanently free of smoking?
- How will you tell people that you have stopped smoking?

behavior. After inducing a hypnotic trance, the clinician can suggest that patients visualize in slow motion the entire sequence prior to lighting each cigarette. When the previously automatic behavior is raised to the level of awareness, patients are able to break the previous pattern and approach each episode of smoking with increased deliberation. Once patients are in the action stage of cessation, the parasympathetic effects of self-hypnosis can be used as an alternative stress-reducing activity.

Hypnosis, when combined with cognitive-behavioral therapy, has been shown to be effective in promoting weight loss.

SELF-HYPNOSIS

With proper training, patients who respond well to hypnotic trances can learn to self-induce hypnosis to achieve both relaxation and specific therapeutic effects. A useful transition to confidence in self-hypnosis is the patient's regular use of a recorded hypnotic induction made by the clinician (primary care provider or referral specialist) in the office, thereby extending the clinician's presence into the patient's milieu. As the patient gains experience going into a therapeutic trance by listening to the tape, the clinician can teach the patient one of several self-induction protocols, such as the one shown in Table 5-2 (this can also serve as a handout). Some patients are able to develop their skill at self-hypnosis and retain it as a life-long health resource.

Table 5-2. Eyeroll technique for self-hypnosis.

1. Find a relaxed, quiet place to sit or lie down.
2. Open yourself to a few minutes of inner renewal and refreshment.
3. Use a one-two-three count:
   One: Roll your eyes up to the top of your head.
   Two: Slowly close your eyelids over raised eyes. Inhale deeply.
   Three: Slowly exhale while you relax your eyes.
4. Continue breathing in a relaxed way from your abdomen.
5. Imagine yourself in some pleasant scene or experience for a few minutes.
6. Imagine the sights, sounds, feelings, and smells.
7. While imagining this scene, focus on the desired outcome of this trance (relaxation, pain reduction, etc).
8. To alert yourself, use a three-two-one-zero count:
   Three: Tell yourself, "I'm ready to be alert."
   Two: Roll your eyes up under your closed eyelids.
   One: Slowly open your eyes and make a fist.
   Zero: Relax your eyes and your hand. Enjoy reorienting yourself to your surroundings.

One use of a self-induced trance is to enhance one's inner awareness or state of mind by accessing somatic memories of positive resource states. This can be useful for either patient or clinician when preparing for a stressful encounter. The method (Table 5-3) is based on the observation that various sensory cues (e.g., music or smell) can trigger associated memories of feeling states. By choosing a desired resource state, constructing a full sensory memory in which that state was felt, then anchoring that feeling state to a tactile cue, the desired state can be reactivated in the new situation. Clinicians might find this especially helpful in shifting toward a positive trance before a patient encounter.

REFERRAL FOR TREATMENT WITH HYPNOSIS

The various medical applications of hypnosis described in the above sections require one or more sessions with a trained hypnotherapist. Skilled hypnotherapists spend time with patients prior to hypnosis discussing their understanding and expectations of the hypnotic experience and addressing their anxieties and misconceptions. The aim is to establish rapport and raise positive expectations in the patient's mind. When this preliminary discussion is completed, the clinician proceeds to the induction of a trance, using one of several approaches. (The specifics of these inductions are too numerous and complex to be discussed in detail in this chapter, and special training is required to use them appropriately and with flexibility to the patient's responses.) Once the patient exhibits signs of a trance, the clinician proceeds to the utilization of that trance for the specific benefit desired. This involves offering suggestions for the patient to imagine changes in somatic sensations, emotions, or future behaviors. The clinician then concludes by alerting and reorienting the patient to the external surroundings. After the procedure, the hypnotherapist can discuss the patient's subjective experiences and answer questions.

As noted earlier, some clinicians become trained in hypnosis (see final section) so they can integrate this treatment into their medical practices. Others may choose to refer patients to a specialist (psychiatrist, psychologist, clinical social worker, or psychiatric nurse practitioner) trained in hypnosis and familiar with its medical applications. To maximize the therapeutic outcome, it is essential that the referring practitioner communicate with the specialist—before the visit—about the nature of the medical problem, the desired clinical outcome, and the patient's expectations about treatment. It is also important to prepare the patient by explaining the nature of therapeutic hypnosis and by

Table 5-3. Developing resourceful states with self-hypnosis.

This technique is useful when you anticipate a stressful situation where you would like to access a positive internal resource that is already a part of you. It is founded on the reality that you have already experienced all the inner states you need to be effective in the anticipated situation. These inner states are part of the body's kinesthetic memory and the files containing them can be cross-referenced with your mental representation of the new event. This is a reprogramming technique that allows you to rapidly activate the desired kinesthetic state.

1. Allow yourself to become quiet, breathe from your abdomen, close your eyes.
2. Build a full sensory image (visual, auditory, and kinesthetic) of the stressful situation you expect to encounter. Notice your emotional and physical response.
3. Now break your physical state by changing positions. Become quiet again.
4. Think about the kind of internal resource (attitude, feeling state, and level of energy) you would like to have available to you in the stressful situation. Examples would be "confidence," "calmness," or "compassion."
5. Once you have decided on the resource state you want to access, search in your memory for an experience or situation in which you felt that resource to be strong in you. This remembered experience may have nothing to do with the stressful situation you are anticipating and may be from a totally different sphere of your life.
6. Build a full sensory image of the positive experience in which you felt that resource (visual, auditory, and kinesthetic). Allow the resourceful feeling to grow in you as you recall that experience.
7. When the resourceful feeling becomes strong in you, **anchor** it by touching together your right thumb and little finger. (An anchor is any stimulus that can serve as a cue for that resource state—it may be a word you say internally, a melody, a fragrance. The tactile anchor is useful, since it is very portable.)
8. Break your emotional state by changing positions. Now test the anchor you developed by touching your thumb and finger together. Notice what feelings emerge.
9. If you wish to add additional resources to the same anchor to be used in the anticipated situation, repeat steps 4–7 for each additional resource.
10. Now again fantasize the stressful situation. Imagine yourself stepping across a threshold into that scene. As you step across the threshold, activate the anchor and carry the resources you developed with you into the encounter.

explaining that its intent is to increase the patient's control over symptoms and their impact.

SUMMARY

Hypnosis has a long tradition as a healing art and as adjunctive treatment for many medical conditions and primary or preferred treatment for some conditions. Clinicians can refer patients for hypnotherapeutic treatment to licensed psychologists, clinical social workers, nurse practitioners, or physicians who have formal training in hypnosis through an accredited organization such as the American Society of Clinical Hypnosis or the Milton Erickson Foundation. Whether or not formally trained in hypnosis, the astute clinician can utilize the naturally occurring trance states frequently found in patients in the medical setting, including the primary care encounter and presurgical consultations, to reduce fear through the reframing of symptoms manifest in common presentations such as chronic nonmalignant pain or anxiety disorders. In these naturalistic trances, careful attention to language is paramount in using suggestion. Avoiding the unwitting use of negative suggestions and maximizing positive expectations for a future experience of healthy functioning can mobilize mind–body healing potentials inherent in the patient.

TRAINING IN HYPNOSIS

Clinicians who are interested in developing their own skills in hypnosis are encouraged to receive formal training from an accredited training program or receive supervision from a licensed health professional with formal training in hypnosis. Several of the organizations listed here provide accredited training:

- The American Society of Clinical Hypnosis (ASCH) http://www.asch.net (Accessed July 2013).
- The Society of Psychological Hypnosis http://psychologicalhypnosis.com/ (Accessed July 2013).
- The Milton H. Erickson Foundation http://www.erickson-foundation.org (Accessed July 2013).
- Society for Clinical and Experimental Hypnosis http://www.sceh.us/ (Accessed July 2013).
- Societies of Hypnosis http://www.societiesofhypnosis.com/ (Accessed July 2013).
- International Society of Hypnosis http://www.ish-hypnosis.org/ (Accessed July 2013).

SUGGESTED READINGS

Christensen JF, Levinson W, Grinder M. Applications of neuro-linguistic programming to medicine. *J Gen Intern Med* 1990;5:522.

Faymonville ME, et al. Functional neuroanatomy of the hypnotic state. *J Physiol* 2006;99:463–469.

Gonsalkorale WM, Whorwell PJ. Hypnotherapy in the treatment of irritable bowel syndrome. *Eur J Gastroenterol Hepatol* 2005;17:15–20.

Kupers R, et al. The cognitive modulation of pain: hypnosis- and placebo-induced analgesia. *Prog Brain Res* 2005;150:251–269.

Levinson W. Reflections: mining for gold. *J Gen Intern Med* 1993;8:172.

Miller GE, Cohen S. Psychological interventions and the immune system: a meta-analytic review and critique. *Health Psychol* 2001;20:47.

Pittler MH, Ernst E. Complementary therapies for reducing body weight: a systematic review. *Int J Obes* 2005;29:1030–1038.

Rossi EL. *The Psychobiology of Gene Expression: Neuroscience and Neurogenesis in Hypnosis and the Healing Arts.* Norton, 2002.

Smith CA, et al. Complementary and alternative therapies for pain management in labour. Cochrane Database of Systematic Reviews 2006.

Uman LS, et al. Psychological interventions for needle-related procedural pain and distress in children and adolescents. Cochrane Database of Systematic Reviews 2006.

Practitioner Well-being

Anthony L. Suchman, MD, MA, FAACH & Gita Ramamurthy, MD

INTRODUCTION

CASE ILLUSTRATION

Don, a 38-year-old primary care physician, sighs as he sees Mrs. D.'s name as a last-minute addition to his patient list. It is mid-afternoon on Friday, and he had blocked out the last hour of the day to attend his son's final softball game of the season. "Of all the days for one of her 'crying headaches,'" Don mutters to himself, "why today?"

Don's skill in handling patients with somatoform problems is respected throughout the health center. Since he assumed responsibility for Mrs. D.'s care, her emergency-department visits have fallen by 90%, and she has even taken a part-time job. Don has almost always been able to help her through these spells by sitting with her, holding her hands, and letting her talk.

When he was growing up, Don was always a leader. In the Boy Scouts, his college newspaper, student service projects in medical school, he was always the one who could organize everyone and get things done. People came to depend on him for that, and while he never showed it outwardly, his capacity to hold responsibility was a source of pride. "Hey, Don!" The greeting comes from Grace, one of Don's partners, breezing toward the door with briefcase in hand. "What a great afternoon! My last patient just canceled . . . I'm going to go home, pour myself a glass of white wine, sit out on the deck, and catch up on some journals. Hope you have a great weekend!"

The door opens, the door closes, and frustration, sadness, loneliness, and anger come together as Don watches Grace leave.

Primary care practice can be both an enriching source of personal growth and meaning and an unmerciful and depleting taskmaster. It provides us with access to a broad range of human experience—an intimate view of the characters and stories of a thousand novels—and an opportunity to have our very presence matter to others. At the same time, it makes constant demands and surrounds us with perpetual uncertainty; it relentlessly confronts us with our limitations of time, energy, knowledge, and compassion. It is a job that is never done; at best, problems are stabilized until something else goes wrong.

The balance each of us strikes between our own enrichment and depletion is critical to our own physical, emotional, and spiritual health and to our ability to care for others. All too often, however, we lose sight of this balance. We become so outwardly focused, attending to clinical problem solving, that we do not tend to our own renewal. This lack of balance is not surprising, our education has taught us much more about how to care for others than how to care for ourselves. The socialization processes of medical school and residency have cultivated a variety of unrealistic self-expectations and attitudes, especially concerning control and self-sufficiency.

Over time, this imbalance can produce a vague but increasing sense of demoralization, in which the joy of work is lost and patients seem increasingly annoying and adversarial. Work becomes the means to some other end—skiing trips or a vacation house—rather than meaningful in its own right. When the root causes of this dissatisfaction are invisible to us, we blame external sources such as the government, insurance companies, or lawyers. Although there are many legitimate complaints about restrictions and bureaucracy, the most fundamental determinants of satisfaction and well-being are not external but rather are found within.

In this chapter, we will examine important values, attitudes, and skills that affect our well-being. We will also consider the subtle but powerful effect of our work environment and personal practices that can keep us healthy.

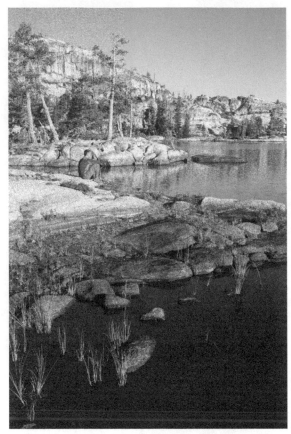

Photo by Hank Christensen (www.hankchristensen.com)

BASIC NEEDS OF PRACTITIONERS

The foundation of our well-being is the acknowledgment that we are human, that we have needs and limits, and that to keep on giving we must know and have reliable access to those things that sustain and revitalize us. Unfortunately, the notion that clinicians have needs has been put off-limits by traditional professional ideals. An excessively narrow interpretation of the scientific model calls on us to be detached and objective observers, leaving no room for our own subjective experience. We are also exposed early, and often, to the ideal of the clinician who is selfless, invulnerable, and omnipotent.

In actuality, each of us has a variety of needs, both universal and neurotic, that cannot fail to assert themselves. Our health and well-being depend upon the degree to which we are aware of and attend to them consciously and purposefully.

Among our most fundamental needs are those for human connection, meaning, and self-transcendence—experiencing ourselves as part of something larger than we are. Clinical work is particularly rich with opportunity for human contact and appreciation. Many studies have shown the patient–clinician relationship to be the single most important factor contributing to physician satisfaction (mirroring its central importance to patients). When we are working under excessive pressure or in situations for which we are not adequately prepared, however, clinical work can interfere with the satisfaction of these needs resulting in depersonalization and alienation from and hostility toward our patients.

Clinical work can also threaten the fulfillment of transpersonal needs through family and community life. Family and career often compete intensely for time and attention, too often to the detriment of the former. Moreover, we sometimes have difficulty shedding the white coat—leaving our professional caretaking role and expressing the spontaneity and vulnerability necessary for intimacy. As tensions build at home, putting more time into work can provide a short-term escape. In the long term, however, avoidance of difficult relationship problems leads to alienation and potentially to the breakdown of crucial personal support systems.

In addition to our universal needs for connection and meaning, we also have very individual neurotic needs—born of pain and conflict—that are intimately related to our medical work. These needs influence both our motivation to go into medicine in the first place and the way we practice. Out of a need to feel loved or appreciated, we often find ourselves in the role of overfunctioning caretakers, and our difficulty saying "no" quickly leads to over commitment. Feelings of impotence engendered by childhood experiences of illness—our own or those of a close friend or relative—may be relieved through our work with patients, but the wishful fantasy of controlling disease is constantly challenged by reality. Voyeuristic desires, fear of death, and the fulfillment of parental expectations are other factors, conscious or unconscious, that can motivate our careers.

These darker, neurotic needs are no less legitimate than those less hidden; they, too, are a normal part of life. When these needs operate outside our awareness, however, they can drive us to work excessively, assume unrealistic degrees of responsibility, and otherwise distort our work lives, thereby causing us to suffer. If we invest ourselves in unrealistic solutions that must inevitably fail, we risk chronic anxiety, substance abuse, and even suicide. Through various processes of self-exploration (such as psychotherapy, peer support groups, or mindfulness workshops) we can become more aware of these needs that underlie our work and find healthier ways to satisfy them. We ignore them at our own peril.

PERSONAL PHILOSOPHY

Another important but under-recognized determinant of our well-being is our personal philosophy—the deeply held beliefs and values that address the most fundamental questions of our lives: the meaning and purpose of life, death, joy, and suffering; why things happen the way they do; the nature of our relationship to other people and to the world; and the nature of our goals and responsibilities as human beings. Our personal philosophies define our expectations of ourselves and other people. They guide the way we perceive and respond to our world and help us identify our place in it. They define the framework by which we imbue things in our lives with meaning, joy, or pain and by which we determine what seems right and what seems wrong.

Developing a personal philosophy tends to be a subliminal process—a gradual internalization of attitudes and values from family, culture, education, and life experience. This process makes it possible for us to be entirely unaware of our core beliefs as an ideology; we may take them so completely for granted that they just seem to be part of the way things are. If we do not understand how these beliefs filter our perceptions and shape our behaviors, then we are unable to subject them to critical reflection and to decide which parts work well for us and which parts need to be changed.

The Control Model

An aspect of personal philosophy with special importance to clinical practice is our attitude toward control. Through the influence of Western culture in general and medical culture in particular, we often perceive being in control (of diseases, patients, and the health care team) to be the ideal state (Table 6-1). We use specific intellectual tools for gathering and applying knowledge: *reductionism*—"Sickle cell anemia is attributable to the substitution of a single nucleotide;" *linear causality*— "*A* causes *B*;" and *generalization*— "Asthma responds to bronchodilators." All have a distinctly controlling, outcome-oriented focus, that is, to manipulate *A* so as to control *B*. Although this approach has led to important technological advances, it also has important adverse consequences.

The control model creates unrealistic expectations that limit our opportunities to feel successful. Consider,

for instance, how our expectations of good control in caring for a diabetic patient allow us to feel successful only when the blood sugar is tightly regulated. The patient's blood sugar, however, is influenced by many factors over which we have no control, the patient's own behavior being foremost among them. We become angry at the patient whose noncompliance stands in the way of our success. If success for us is defined only in terms of controlling disease, we are precluded from feeling successful in many, if not most, situations. Accepting responsibility for outcomes over which we have little or no control is highly stressful and leads us to feel helpless, anxious, and angry.

Our quest for control also creates distance and detachment in the patient–clinician relationship, which, as we have already seen, is an important factor in professional satisfaction. A strong orientation toward control leads to hierarchic relationships. This, coupled with the reductionism and labeling inherent in medical thinking, turns patients into objects, and we find ourselves working more with *things*—organs, diseases, medications, and tests—than with people. We, too, become depersonalized in this process, leaving no room for our own subjective experience.

The Relational Model

An alternative philosophy that avoids many of these problems emphasizes relatedness rather than control. This model does not reject the insights of reductionism, but rather builds on them by adding an appreciation of context and relationship. Therefore, although *A* may seem to cause *B*, there are also other mediating factors and bidirectional interactions (*A* and *B* influence each other). For example, the tubercle bacillus causes tuberculosis, but not everyone who is exposed to this bacterium becomes ill; environmental and socioeconomic factors also contribute to the process. The illness, in turn, affects those contextual factors; no portion of the system exists in isolation.

In the relational model, we seek to be with and to understand the patient in a number of dimensions simultaneously—biological, experiential, functional, and

Table 6-1. A comparison of control- and relationship-based personal philosophies.

Attribute	Control	Relational (I–Thou)*
Phenomenon of interest	Thing-in-itself	Thing-in-context
Epistemologic strategy	Reductionist; linear causality	Emergent; systems model
Clinician's stance	Detached observer	Participant observer
Information deemed relevant	Objective data only	Subjective and objective data
Model for patient–clinician relationship	Hierarchy	Partnership
Focus of attention	Outcome-oriented	Process-oriented

*Terms are from Martin Buber. *I and Thou*. New York: Scribner, 1970.

spiritual. As we come to understand patients' experiences, we may or may not identify opportunities to recommend strategies or undertake treatments to ameliorate their suffering. We are mindful that patients are ultimately responsible for their own lives; they may or may not accept our suggestions. In some cases, we may have no suggestions or treatment to offer, but we can still find success in offering, in the words of Arthur Kleinman, "empathic witnessing," honoring the patient's need for connection—a healing intervention in its own right.

This relational model helps us avoid unrealistic expectations of ourselves. It offers us the opportunity to feel successful in situations, such as untreatable illness or a patient's refusal to accept our good advice that would seem like failures under the control model. The relational model also leads us to more effective action. In contrast to the control model, which attends exclusively to outcomes, this model calls for explicit attention to process, to the quality of communication, and to the values enacted in the way we work together. Paradoxically, it is by letting go of outcomes and focusing more on making the process as good as possible that we achieve the best outcomes. The relational model also gives us more room to look outside ourselves for guidance and solutions—and to admit our own limitations or powerlessness.

Whereas the control model creates barriers between clinicians and patients, the relational model keeps us closer to the experience of both our patients and ourselves, thereby increasing the opportunities for our work to be meaningful and decreasing the potential for frustration, alienation, and burnout.

SKILLS

There are a number of skills that can make the difference between depletion and thriving in practice.

Time Management

These skills are essential both within the office visit and in arranging work schedules. For example, negotiating an agenda at the start of each visit focuses attention on the issues that are most important to the patient and the clinician, minimizes time spent on unnecessary tasks, and drastically reduces the frequency with which new topics emerge late in the visit ("Oh, by the way, Doc, I've got this chest pain . . .") that lay waste to office schedules. Informing patients at the outset how long their visits will last and reminding them a few minutes before ending allow them to share responsibility for using time effectively. On a more global level, time-management skills can help preserve the balance among work, family, community, and recreation that is so important to life satisfaction. Keeping time logs for several days can help us discover whether we are apportioning our time in accordance with our personal goals and priorities. Time logs can also point out time wasters in daily work habits and help us devise more efficient office procedures.

Communication

Given the important contribution of the patient–clinician relationship as a source of meaning, the communication and relationship skills described elsewhere in this book become critical tools for well-being as well as for good patient care. Learning to *be with* the patient requires broadening the goal of the interview from making a diagnosis to understanding the story of the patient's illness as a lived experience. We need to understand the meaning of the illness to the patient—why this disease in this particular patient at this particular time, how it is affecting the patient's function, and what role it might be playing in the patient's life. Thus, we need skills for eliciting deeper levels of patients' stories and responding to their emotions. As we become more able to do this, it becomes apparent that there are no longer routine or uninteresting cases—each patient is unique. The patient's personhood enriches our own.

Coaching & Negotiation

Sharing responsibility more effectively and more realistically with patients requires both coaching and negotiation skills. Specifically, we must know how to facilitate patients in articulating their own values, goals, and opinions, including their feedback about their medical care. We must be willing to relinquish our traditional—and burdensome—role of unquestioned authority and adopt instead a more flexible stance, trying to combine synergistically our own knowledge of medicine with patients' knowledge of themselves and the patterns, problems, and balances of their daily lives. We must learn to see patients' increasing capacity for gathering information and making their own decisions as a valuable resource and a sign of our success rather than as a challenge to our competence and authority. Knowing how and when to set firm boundaries without being judgmental and how to discuss communication and relationship problems openly can help resolve impasses with many seemingly difficult patients, making their care less frustrating and more rewarding. We also need to know how to recognize when we are over-functioning, hooked by unrealistic hopes or expectations of control, and to respectfully, but clearly, give responsibility back to the patient.

Self-Reflection & Self-Care

We need to be able to reflect on our own feelings and actions, to acknowledge our vulnerabilities and needs, to seek and courageously follow our sense of calling, and to act in support of our own health. Rather than judging and shutting out such feelings as anger, attraction, or insecurity that inevitably arise in us, we can learn to accept them with self-compassion, to manage them appropriately, and to harvest from them insights about ourselves and our patients. Through solitary reflection and honest conversation with trusted colleagues (informally or in more organized formats such as Balint groups, workshops, executive coaching, or psychotherapy) we can attend more closely to what our hearts are telling us about the state of our lives. Shedding the mask of omnipotence and invincibility and recognizing our vulnerabilities are essential for working amidst uncertainty and coping with mistakes. And finally, we can thoughtfully examine our lifestyle choices, starting with our work hours. Simplifying our material needs to reduce financial pressures can give us more time for exercise, healthy eating, social interaction, pursuing diverse interests, and whatever else it is that truly gives us joy and meaning.

Collective Self-Care

Over the past 10–15 years the attention given to clinician well-being has grown enormously. Early pioneers such as the Foundation for Medical Excellence and the Institute for the Study of Health and Illness have been joined by larger mainstream organizations such as the American Medical Association (AMA), Canadian Medical Association (CMA), and American Hospital Association in offering programs and resources. There is now a biennial international conference on physician well-being sponsored by the AMA, CMA, and British Medical Association. Nearly all hospitals and many medical societies in the United States and Canada offer wellness programs of some sort and excellent online resources are available.

These programs may be effective not only by virtue of the education they offer but also because they convene healing communities. Most practitioners experience high levels of isolation, even when they work as part of busy group practices. They seldom talk about their patients in any depth with colleagues and almost never talk about their own responses and struggles. Participants in a program on mindfulness and communication valued the connection and validation that came from honest conversations with peers ("I'm not the only one") as much as the new skills and insights that they gained. The most effective self-care may be that which we pursue in concert with others.

HEALTHY WORK ENVIRONMENTS

Our workplaces have an important effect on our well-being. The local culture of the institutions in which we work—be they hospitals, individual practices, or medical communities—subtly reinforces values through both formal educational processes and everyday policies and practices. The local culture can determine whether we feel able to disclose uncertainty and vulnerability to one another or feel constrained always to maintain the iron man façade; whether we act and negotiate collegially or retreat into always protecting our "turfs" against other disciplines; whether we can discuss mistakes and ask for help or be forced to work in perpetual isolation; whether we receive encouragement and respect for setting reasonable limits on our workload so we can be present in our families or feel shamed for being "lazy."

Surveys from both industry and academia have identified common characteristics of organizations with greater employee well-being. Organizational cultures that promote employee trust, engagement, and thriving are characterized by collaborative decision making, ethical behavior toward employees and customers, mutual respect between members, growth, and learning toward increasing competence, and a reasonable work–life balance. In contrast, organizations that ignore employee input, are riddled with political favoritism, and tolerate rudeness appear to breed employee apathy, cynicism, and burnout. Employee trust and engagement—i.e., commitment to the organization—correlate positively not only with the well-being but also with the organizations' financial and operational success. Studies of hospital work environments have yielded similar results.

Creating environments that support relationship-centered care is a large topic; a few general principles must suffice for this discussion:

- As clinicians, we tend to treat patients in the same way that we ourselves are treated within our institutions. Core values such as respect, partnership, honesty, and accountability must be explicitly articulated and embodied in institutional policies and procedures. Clinicians and administrators alike may need to learn new communication and relationship skills, and redesign processes for making decisions and maintaining accountability.

- The principle of reciprocity governs much of human interaction. Mutually helpful behavior and camaraderie creates a virtuous cycle in which employees thrive and succeed. Reciprocity can also tear an organization apart. A few acts of unchecked incivility can spiral into widespread acrimony. Incivility at work has been linked to a lack of job satisfaction, decreased organizational commitment, and impaired job performance. Organizations can foster civility through hiring policies that specifically screen for interpersonal skills, team-development activities, and codes of conduct with meaningful (and respectful) accountability. Respecting values and attending to the quality of process must be embraced as the most effective means to high-quality outcomes at the organizational level, just as at the clinical level. This requires a departure from traditional, hierarchical approaches of top-down decision making and control of the work process.

- Clinicians in the "front lines" providing patient care, but not in leadership positions, may feel helpless to change a dysfunctional organization. The feeling of helplessness reflects the false belief that only the leaders are responsible for organizational culture. *Leaders co-create an organizational culture with followers.* If leaders are unable or unwilling to promote teamwork, clinicians need not passively react by fragmenting into insular, self-serving cliques. Instead, clinicians can choose to reach out across specialties and disciplines to promote a culture of mutual respect and accountability. Offering appreciation and "going the extra mile" for colleagues, particularly from other disciplines, can begin a virtuous cycle of civility. Physicians unhappy with an organizational culture can work on "being the change" they seek. Finding like-minded colleagues can create a mutually supportive group that catalyzes creation of a better culture.

- We can replace the current culture of rugged individualism with a culture of teamwork, accountability, and mutual support. Support groups for all staff, including physicians, may encourage self-awareness, increase sensitivity to patients' concerns, and diminish the isolation and depersonalization that both characterize and accelerate burnout. We can be vigilant to ways in which the local culture reinforces work addiction and inhibits collaboration and work to improve it.

In this time of concern about health care costs and patient safety, clinicians, administrators, patients, and families need to work together in partnership to redesign our medical institutions, making them more respectful and humane, more collaborative in terms of care, and more responsive to the needs of the people they serve and the people who work within them. Clinical outcomes, financial performance, patient satisfaction, and staff satisfaction have all been associated with factors that create healthy work environments for health care providers; thus, institutions have a direct stake in maintaining the well-being of their clinicians and staff.

CONCLUSIONS

Whether the rigors of clinical work become sources of meaning or exhaustion depends on a number of factors. We must be able to know and address mindfully the personal needs that affect our work. Fulfilling our needs for connection and meaning is particularly sustaining.

Unrealistic expectations of control interfere with connection and confront us with an ongoing specter of inadequacy and failure. Instead, we need a more mature perspective of balance, acceptance, and relation. We need skills for working with uncertainty, sharing responsibility, and promoting relationship. We need personal disciplines of reflection and self-care, supported by participation in a healing community of peers. We must become more attentive to the values expressed subliminally but powerfully in our work environments and begin to make necessary changes so that these environments call forth the best and healthiest of what we have to offer, both as professionals and as human beings. These approaches can help us to appreciate fully the privilege of caring for patients and to realize our best potential for personal fulfillment and growth.

SUGGESTED READINGS

American Hospital Association. Long-range Policy Committee, John W. Bluford III, chair. A Call to Action: Creating a Culture of Health. Chicago: American Hospital Association, January 2011.

Krasner MS, Epstein RM, Quill TE, et al. A continuing education program in mindful communication: Effects on primary care physician burnout, empathy and attitudes. *JAMA* 2009; 302:1284–1293.

Safran DG, Miller W, Beckman H. Organizational dimensions of relationship-centered care. Theory, evidence, and practice. *J Gen Intern Med* 2006; 21:S9–S15.

Spreitzer G, Porath C. Creating sustainable performance. *Harvard Bus Rev* 2012;90:92–99.

Suchman AL, Matthews DA. What makes the patient-doctor relationship therapeutic? Exploring the connexional dimension of medical care. *Ann Intern Med* 1988;108:125–130.

Vaillant G: Some psychologic vulnerabilities of physicians. *N Engl J Med* 1972;287:372.

WEB SITES

American Medical Association Physician Health page. http://www.ama-assn.org/ama/pub/physician-resources/physician-health.page. Accessed September 2012.

Canadian Medical Association Centre for Physician Health and Well-Being. http://www.cma.ca/living/centrephysicianhealthwellbeing. Accessed September 2012.

Center for Positive Organizational Scholarship. http://www.centerforpos.org/. Accessed September 2012.

Institute for the Study of Health and Illness: Finding Meaning Discussion Groups. http://www.ishiprograms.org/programs/all-healthcare-professionals/. Accessed September 2012.

Relationship Centered Health Care. http://www.rchcweb.com/. Accessed September 2012.

The Foundation for Medical Excellence. www.tfme.org. Accessed September 2012.

Mindful Practice

Ronald Epstein, MD

CASE ILLUSTRATION 1

Jeffrey Borzak, a patient I knew well, seemed to be recovering from coronary artery bypass surgery. On rounds, I sensed that there was something that was wrong, but I could not put my finger on it. In retrospect, his color was not quite right—he was grayish-pale, his blood pressure was too easily controlled, he was even hypotensive on one occasion, and he seemed more depressed than usual. He reported no chest pain or shortness of breath, and had no pedal edema, elevated jugular venous pressure, or other abnormalities on his physical examination. But still I did not feel comfortable, and although there were no "red flags," I ordered an echocardiogram which showed a new area of ischemia. An angiogram showed that one of the grafts had occluded. After angioplasty, Mr. Borzak looked and felt better, and he again required his usual antihypertensive medications.

CASE ILLUSTRATION 2

Elizabeth Grady recently came to be a patient in our practice. The practice, despite having long waits for appointments, was recently reopened to new patients to boost productivity. Mrs. Grady left her previous physician's practice because of a disagreement over seeking care in the emergency room rather than in the office for her out-of-control diabetes. Her blood sugar has never been below 400, and often was in excess of 600 mg/dL. Despite claiming to be on a diet, her weight kept increasing, and now she weighed nearly 500 lb. At the first visit, an irate sister accompanied her demanding that the patient be hospitalized immediately. On the second visit, Mrs. Grady was so anxious that she could not sit in the examination room; she was pacing in the waiting room until her appointment, and then indicated that she was in a rush to leave even though the appointment was on time. She no-showed for the subsequent appointment, and is now returning for her third appointment.

Excellent patient care requires not only the knowledge and skills to diagnose and treat disease but also the ability to form therapeutic relationships with patients and their families, recognize and respond to emotionally demanding situations, make decisions under uncertainty, and deal with technical failures and errors. These capabilities require that clinicians have self-awareness to distinguish their values and feelings from those of their patients, recognize faulty reasoning early in the diagnostic thinking process, be attentive to when a technical procedure is not going as it should, recognize the need to gather more data, and be able to incorporate disconfirming data into an evolving assessment of the patient. Often, there is no tool or instrument that can help physicians with these situations on a moment-to-moment basis other than their own cognitive and emotional resources.

Mindful practice refers to a clinician's capacity for reflection, self-monitoring and self-awareness during an actual clinical practice in order to practice with clarity, insight, expertise, and compassion. Clinicians generally value the principles of mindful practice—attentive observation, critical curiosity, presence, and capacity to see a familiar situation with new eyes ("beginner's mind"). Yet, during training and practice, clinicians spend little time "sharpening the saw"—developing, refining, and calibrating their own capacity for self-understanding as they think and feel their way through the complex demands of clinical practice. For psychotherapists, athletes, and musicians, self-calibration and self-awareness are considered fundamental to excellence and are often explicit aspects of training. Yet, for clinicians, there is often the assumption that knowledge and technical expertise are sufficient, when on reflection most clinicians value "adaptive expertise" and cultivating habits of mind that allow them to self-calibrate and reflect continuously during everyday work. This chapter will suggest why mindful practice is important and indicate ways in which it can be cultivated.

Mindful practice is fundamental to excellent patient care. It means being attentive, on purpose, to one's own thoughts and feelings during everyday clinical practice and educational activities. Mindfulness implies a nonjudgmental stance in which the practitioner can observe not only the patient's situation but also his or her own reactions to it. A mindful practitioner can see a situation from several angles at the same time. Mindful practice implies curiosity rather than premature closure and presence rather than detachment. Mindfulness is especially helpful when dealing with difficult relationships with patients and families, challenging clinical situations, and in recognizing the need for self-care. Furthermore, recent research among students, residents, and practicing clinicians suggests that mindfulness is associated with better communication, better quality of technical (e.g., fewer errors) and interpersonal (e.g., empathy) care, and greater clinician well-being (e.g., lower burnout).

In contrast, mindless practice involves self-deception, often with the illusion of competence. Blind certainty, ignoring of disconfirming data, and arrogance without self-examination or reflection dooms us to "seeing things not as they are, but as we are." An example of mindlessness is the common practice of reporting findings that were not actually observed, because "they must be true."

Mindfulness is especially important in the diagnosis and treatment of mental disorders because there are few anchors other than the clinician's own judgment to assess the severity or pervasiveness of anxiety, depression, or psychosis in a particular patient. However, mindfulness also applies to other cognitive and technical aspects of health care. Self-monitoring and mindfulness are equally essential to expertise in other domains of medicine as they are to primary care or behavioral medicine. For example, hepatobiliary surgeon Carol-Anne Moulton eloquently describes ways in which expert surgeons remain "attentive in automaticity." They work quickly, yet recognize aberrant and problematic situations, and slow down accordingly, thus switching from automatic to deliberative thinking. In this chapter, I will explore several aspects of mindful practice and some ways of recognizing and practicing mindfulness in clinical settings.

Fushimi Inari Shrine, Kyoto, Japan. Photograph by Mitchell D. Feldman, MD, MPhil

MINDFULNESS & CLINICAL CARE

Mindful practice depends on the ability to be aware in the moment. The champion tennis player is being mindful when he or she is not only attentive to the ball but also to his or her state of balance, expectations for what will happen next, physical sensations such as pain or discomfort, and level of anxiety. All of these factors can affect performance and can be modified by specific attention to them. Like tennis players, physicians' lapses in awareness and concentration can have dire consequences. For physicians, these lapses directly affect the patient's welfare. The result of lapses may include avoidance, overreactions, poor decisions, misjudgments, and miscommunications that affect survival and quality of life for the patient. Thus, physicians have a moral obligation to their patients and themselves to be as aware, present, and observant as possible.

By cultivating the ability to be attentive to the unexpected, mindful practice can improve the quality of care and help prevent errors. Case Illustration 1 presents some observations that led to a change in care resulting in an improved outcome. Being aware in the moment and receptive to new information—especially information that is unexpected, unwanted, or upsetting—can help the clinician be more attentive to patients' needs and, thus, be more likely to meet them. The clinician's job in Case 1 would have seemed easier, at least in the short run, if he had ignored his intuitions.

Mindful practice involves allowing awareness of our own areas of ignorance, as well as our areas of expertise. Yet many clinicians are not as aware as they should be of the accuracy of their first impressions and tacit judgments. Clinicians, whether beginners or experts, often are aware of things before they are named, categorized, or organized into a coherent diagnosis. For example, the unusual gait of a patient walking toward the chair in the examining room may be the first clue to a neurodegenerative disorder, and such first impressions can often be quite accurate. Educators, psychologists, and cognitive scientists have called these automatic nonconscious mental processes "unconscious competence," the "unthought known," or "preattentive processing."

Conversely, the capacity for inattentiveness and self-deception can be impressive. The same capacity for automatic nonconscious processing can backfire if unexamined biases and preconceived ideas dominate clinical reasoning without some capacity for deliberation. Thus, the goal might be to be attentive in automaticity. A patient of mine, hospitalized with urinary infection, was suspected of having adrenal insufficiency because of hyperpigmented skin. He was later noted to only have hyperpigmented forearms and face, whereas the rest of the body was pale. Yet, the residents and attending physicians continued to evaluate the possibility of adrenal insufficiency in spite of being made aware of the faulty observation. A classic article on curiosity in clinical education reported a story about a patient who was presented on rounds as "below knee amputation (BKA) times 2"; clearly no one had noticed that he actually had two legs, and, through several hospital admissions, did not correct the mistranscribed "diabetic keto-acidosis (DKA)." Although these examples are dramatic, similar misperceptions are perpetuated with regard to patient personality or psychological states. For example, one study showed that patients asking for antidepressant medications tend to receive them regardless of whether they fulfill diagnostic criteria for depression. Patients who are labeled "difficult," "uncooperative," or "demanding" (such as Mrs. Grady, Case Illustration 2) seem to be stuck with such labels for life, and disconfirming data tend to be ignored. Furthermore, the "difficult patient" is approached as if the difficulty is only the patient's, rather than considering that the physician's expectations and attitudes may also contribute to the difficulties.

Mindfulness means being simultaneously attentive to external data as well as to internal data—the clinician's own thoughts, feelings, and inner states. Negative thoughts about a patient might promote a pejorative label ("somatizer"); negative feelings might provoke anger or disgust; and negative inner states might induce boredom or hostility. Positive feelings also present difficulties. Sexual attraction toward a patient obviously can be problematic, but so can an unusually keen interest in a patient's illness. As a medical student, I was assigned a patient with hairy-cell leukemia, a disease whose genetic basis was just being uncovered. Although she was considered an "exciting" and "fascinating" case, I was disappointed, when meeting her, that she was a sad, weak, pale woman dying of cancer, hardly matching my excitement and that of my colleagues.

Mindfulness of thoughts allows clinicians to follow intuitions while also accommodating for biases and cognitive traps in the process of making clinical decisions. Awareness of feelings is particularly useful in diagnosing mental disorders; clinicians tend to feel "down" when in the presence of a depressed patient, or confused in the presence of patients with subtle delusions and mild dementia. Awareness of their own fatigue can help clinicians recognize when their cognitive, attentional, or technical capacities are not at their best; the fatigued resident in the emergency room late at night might then get corroboration for an important finding on physical examination (such as the degree of nuchal rigidity in a febrile child) from a trusted colleague.

Mindfulness improves learning. Trainees who are more aware of the difference between what they believe and their actual performance can make adjustments and improvements. Key features of mindful learning are the ability to see novelty in familiar situations and the ability to consider facts provisional and contextual. Studies show that mindfulness and self-awareness training can improve reasoning and communication skills.

Mindfulness can be a corrective for those who otherwise might believe that they are expert and are surprised when that notion is challenged by an outside observer or objective test. Other types of professionals—not only medical personnel—also can suffer from the illusion of competence. Musicians know the delusion of the "practice-room virtuoso"—an illusion which is often shattered when the performer is put in front of a discerning audience. Clinicians, however, usually practice unobserved, so the opportunities for external validation and learning are much scarcer than for the musician—and the stakes are much higher than a wrong note.

Mindful practice involves cultivating the ability to monitor and modulate one's own emotional reactivity. Faced with emotionally challenging situations, humans often overreact by blaming (oneself, another clinician, or patient) or becoming overinvolved. Others may underreact by avoiding, minimizing, or distancing. In contrast, mindful practitioners can observe their own reactions, and thus have choices about the way they might respond that enhances quality of care and quality of healing relationships. Clinicians thus respond with empathy based on an understanding of the patient's experience rather than making assumptions about the patient leading to further alienation (see Chapter 2). This same awareness can inform the small ethical decisions that clinicians make during everyday practice—such as which patient's phone call to return first, or whether to acquiesce to a patient's slightly unreasonable demand.

Finally, mindfulness involves monitoring the clinician's own needs. Self-awareness can directly enhance clinicians' own well-being by helping them feel more in touch and in tune with themselves. Self-awareness can also motivate the clinician to seek needed help and support. Mindful self-care can lead to greater well-being and job satisfaction; clinicians who report greater job satisfaction and well-being tend to express empathy more readily, report making fewer errors, and have patients who report greater satisfaction. The self-reinforcing process of self-care and well-being can contribute to productivity and reduce burnout and attrition (see Chapter 6).

CULTIVATING MINDFULNESS IN ONESELF & TRAINEES

Although it is self-evident that self-awareness is a necessary ingredient in developing and maintaining clinical expertise, achieving a state of moment-to-moment self-awareness in a chaotic and busy health care environment is not straightforward. For several years, a variety of training venues in medicine, psychology, and other disciplines have offered small group settings for trainees and practitioners to present difficult situations for group discussion, with the intent that the resulting insights then might inform future clinical practice. These sessions have been associated with improvement in communication skills and satisfaction with clinical practice. One program (Krasner et al., 2009) reported the results of an intensive course in "mindful communication," which included a variety of self-awareness and body-awareness exercises, narratives about meaningful clinical experiences, appreciative interviews, didactic material, and discussion. Participating physicians not only reported lower burnout and lower psychological distress but also greater empathy and psychosocial orientation in care. Some small group formats are listed in Table 7-1, each with a particular focus but with the common thread of providing both support and insight.

Domains that are amenable to training include:

• Clinicians' habits (meditation, body awareness, exercise, interactions with others, and so on).

• Clinicians' beliefs and attitudes (health beliefs, beliefs about human behavior and relationships, attitudes toward patient autonomy or psychosocial aspects of care, family, cultural influences, and so on).

• Clinicians' feelings and emotions (joy, fulfillment, vigor, attraction, anger, frustration, conflict, setting boundaries, and so on).

• Challenging clinical situations (difficult decisions, sharing bad news, facing mistakes, apologizing to patients, dying patients, demanding or "difficult" patients, conflict within the health care team, and so on).

• Clinician self-care (impairment, balance between home and work, burnout, healthy approaches to stress, finding meaning in work, and so on).

Other educational strategies can enhance the capacity for reflection and mindfulness. Reviewing video-recordings of patient sessions are surprising and instructive, whether reviewed individually or with a tutor. Learning contracts or agreements can focus learning on areas of deficiency, including becoming more self-aware. Peer evaluations of work habits and interpersonal attributes with medical students can foster greater awareness of how students function on the clinical team and interact with their colleagues and patients. Keeping a journal not only promotes reflection on one's actions but also appears to be therapeutic in itself, offering a venue for self-expression so needed by busy and overwhelmed clinicians.

However, these individual and small group activities may not necessarily translate the insights gained into the moment-to-moment drama of clinical practice. Mindful practice refers not only to reflection on one's actions but goes one step further by emphasizing habits of mind during actual practice. Mindful practice refers not only to the social and emotional domains of practice but also to the cognitive processes of data gathering and making decisions as well as the technical skills employed during physical examinations, surgery, and procedures. Following are some general suggestions on how to enhance mindfulness in practice, for oneself and for trainees:

Table 7-1. Group learning experiences that promote mindful practice.

Type of Group	Description	Qualifications of Facilitator
Mindfulness-based stress reduction courses	Promote attentive awareness through meditation, yoga and discussion	Mindfulness training
Support groups	Promote balance between the human and technical aspects of health care by sharing difficult and challenging situations	Training in psychotherapy or group facilitation
Balint groups	Recognizing that the clinician is a "drug" (a therapeutic agent), groups aim to improve clinician effectiveness by examining thoughts and feelings that may interfere with care	Training through the International Balint Society
Family of origin groups	By drawing genograms (family trees), participants learn about influences family and culture have on their values and attitudes	Family therapy training
Personal awareness groups	Unstructured experience focused on individual needs of participants, these groups examine personal issues that affect a broad array of aspects of being a clinician	American Academy of Communication in Healthcare offers training courses
Literature in medicine groups	Using published written works or writings of group members, participants explore the human dimensions of health care	Narrative medicine training
Challenging case conferences	Using videotapes or critical incident reports, participants explore the moment-to-moment actions they took during a clinical encounter	Facilitation training

- *Priming.* This involves creating the expectation for mindfulness. By observing what they do during clinical practice, clinicians can be more present, curious, and attentive. Sometimes, it is as simple as pausing and taking a breath before entering the patient's room or taking time to look at the patient rather than at the chart or screen. Clinicians use these techniques to bring themselves into the present, and then can be invited to pay attention to how those techniques enhance their capabilities as clinicians and to expand their ways of applying those or similar techniques to other aspects of their practice. Trainees can be expected to pay attention not only to the patient but also to their own thoughts and emotions during the clinical encounter. These thoughts and emotions are fodder for discussion following an encounter, whether it occurs in hospital or in outpatient settings. Writing narratives about these experiences can help practitioners recognize their own mental states and learn to be aware of how they contribute to creating a coherent patient story while eliciting what often seems like fragmented information from the patient.

- *Availability.* Just as clinicians can make themselves psychologically and physically available to their patients, teachers should carve out time and space in which they are available to observe and discuss students' progress toward greater self-awareness, whether in a small group setting or individually.

- *Asking reflective questions.* Reflective questions explore the inner landscape; only clinicians themselves can answer them. They are designed not to elicit facts or answers but rather to foster reflection in the moment. Teachers can ask reflective questions, but more importantly, clinicians themselves can adopt a habit of self-questioning. Examples of reflective questions are shown in Table 7-2. The internal dialogue that they foster can contribute to mindful practice.

- *Active engagement.* When in learning situations, mindful practice can and should be observed directly. Students' reports of what they said and did during a clinical encounter are biased by their own values, expectations, and anxiety; thus the presence of a tutor or observer has no substitute. Imagine if in music instruction or tennis lessons, the student simply reported on his or her progress and difficulties, giving a narrative account of how the piece of music or tennis match went. Ludicrous as it sounds, we often do exactly that in medical education.

- *Thinking out loud.* When facing a challenging clinical situation it can be useful to describe one's observations, impressions, or clinical reasoning to a colleague or tutor, or to put them down on paper in the form of a written narrative. Similarly, experienced clinicians can think out loud in the presence of learners to demonstrate how recognizing one's own ignorance, biases, and predispositions can lead to more deliberative responses rather than mindless reactions. These methods help clinicians hear the story or rationale as if it were told by a third person, allowing them to examine their own thinking processes and emotional reactions,

Table 7-2. Reflective questions.

- "What am I assuming about this patient that might not be true?"
- "If there were data that I neglected or ignored, what might it be?"
- "What about my prior experience with this patient (or with other patients) is influencing my thinking and reasoning process?"
- "What surprised me about this patient? How did that surprise affect my clinical actions?"
- "What would a trusted colleague say about the way I am managing this patient?"
- "What outcomes am I expecting from this clinical situation? Are those expectations reasonable?"
- "How do I know when I have gathered enough data?"

---

identify what might be missing in their perception of the situation, and correct faulty logic. These methods can allow for reflection that cannot be accomplished simply by moving forward with problem solving.

- *Practice.* Medicine, like music and tennis, must be practiced; the same is true of mindfulness. There is both formal and informal practice. Formal practice includes mindfulness exercises, such as meditation, yoga, movement exercises, and body awareness exercises. Equally important are informal practices that can be incorporated into daily work, and may be unobserved by others.

Most important is the practice of stillness. Even momentary stillness during a busy day can open the mind, allow for new possibilities, and allow greater self-awareness. The stillness may be short informal practices—a momentary pause before seeing the next patient, or a "huddle" before commencing a surgical operation. Touching the doorknob before going into an examination room, a clinician might develop a habit of stopping momentarily, taking a breath, being aware of potentially distracting thoughts, feelings and preconceptions, allowing him or her to set aside what has just occurred and be more attentive to the next patient. Longer episodes of stillness might include formal meditation exercises or other contemplative activities. A daily meditation practice can provide a powerful means for learning how to be centered, observant, and attentive. Meditation involves watching one's thoughts, feelings, and bodily sensations (such as breathing) without necessarily trying to change them. By learning to evoke similar states of attentiveness, even briefly, during clinical practice, the clinician can learn to approach new situations with a lowered reactivity and to tolerate ambiguity. Meditation can be an entirely secular activity and need not have religious or spiritual overtones.

For clinicians and educators, "mantras" for daily practice can be cultivated. Clinicians might use the "it might not be so" mantra when facing a new patient or new diagnosis; the clinician develops a habit of trying to see the situation from another angle that might question an emerging hypothesis. "Unexpecting" is a practice of becoming aware of one's own expectations or eliciting those of a learner, and then actively imagining another outcome (the "it might not happen that way" mantra). The goal of using these techniques is not to adopt a different, contrasting perspective; rather their purpose is to debias one's

Gardens at Tofukuji Temple, Kyoto, Japan. Photograph by Mitchell D. Feldman, MD, MPhil

thinking, recalibrate feelings, and train the mind to consider two or more perspectives at the same time.

- *Praxis.* Clinical skill is not truly learned and known until it is used. Increasing expertise is associated with the development of habits that become second nature. At that point, an expert clinician may not be able to describe easily exactly why he or she is making each decision, because many of the early steps in the decision process may have become automatic or tacit. Just as a habitual approach to history taking or physical examination becomes second nature, mindfulness training should have as its goal developing habits of reflection, self-questioning, and awareness in the moment during clinical practice.

- *Assessment and confirmation.* As is true for any newly acquired skill, some kind of assessment and confirmation of achievement are important for learning and reinforcement. Facilitated self-assessment, assessment by peers, and feedback from supervising clinicians are important to identify markers of and barriers to practicing mindfully. A supervisor might evaluate, for example, the degree to which the learner was able to articulate his or her reactions to a particular patient. Patients and peers can assess presence and attentiveness.

CONCLUSIONS

Mindful practice is a process and a goal, not a static state of mind. Even the most accomplished practitioners cannot claim to be mindful all the time. Efforts toward becoming more attentive, curious, and present, and approaching familiar situations with a "beginner's mind," can lead clinicians to be better listeners and diagnosticians, and to critique their own technical skills more objectively. Many medical schools and some residency programs offer training in mindfulness and self-awareness, in recognition that these approaches help in the process of professional development, reduce burnout, and improve communication. Resources for mindfulness and self-awareness training are also available through organizations such as the Center for Mindfulness at the University of Massachusetts (www.umassmed.edu/cfm/index.aspx) and the American Academy on Communication in Healthcare (www.aachonline.org), the Northwest Center for Physician Well Being (www.tfme.org), and the Mindful Practice Programs

at the University of Rochester (www.mindfulpractice.urmc.edu). Research using functional magnetic resonance imaging (MRI) scanning, cognitive testing, and other techniques is only beginning to uncover reasons why mindful practice improves performance, compassion, and well-being in a variety of professional activities.

SUGGESTED READINGS

Balint E, Norell JS. *Six Minutes for the Patient: Interaction in General Practice Consultation.* London: Tavistock Publications, 1973.

Beach MC, Roter D, Korthuis PT, et al. A multicenter study of physician mindfulness and health care quality. *Annals of Family Medicine* 2013;11(5):421–428.

Beckman HB, Wendland M, Mooney C, et al. The impact of a program in mindful communication on primary care physicians. *Academic Medicine* 2012;87(6):1–5.

Epstein RM. Mindful practice. *JAMA* 1999;282:833–839.

Epstein RM. Just being. *West J Med* 2001;174:63–65.

Epstein RM, Krasner MS. Physician resilience: what it means, why it matters, and how to promote it. *Academic Medicine* 2013;88(3):301–303.

Grepmair L, Mitterlehner F, Loew T, et al. Promoting mindfulness in psychotherapists in training influences the treatment results of their patients: a randomized, double-blind, controlled study. *Psychother Psychosom* 2007;76: 332–338.

Krasner MS, Epstein RM, Beckman H, et al. Association of an educational program in mindful communication with burnout, empathy, and attitudes among primary care physicians. *JAMA* 2009;302(12):1284–1293.

Novack DH, Suchman AL, Clark W, et al. Calibrating the physician. Personal awareness and effective patient care. *JAMA* 1997;278:502–509.

Sibinga EMS, Wu AW. Clinician mindfulness and patient safety. *JAMA* 2010;304:2532–2533.

Smith RC, Dorsey AM, Lyles JS, et al. Teaching self-awareness enhances learning about patient-centered interviewing. *Acad Med* 1999;74:1242–1248.

WEB SITES

Center for Mindfulness at the University of Massachusetts. www.umassmed.edu/cfm/index.aspx. Accessed July 2013.

Mindful Practice Programs, University of Rochester School of Medicine and Dentistry. www.mindfulpractice.urmc.edu Accessed January, 2014.

Northwest Center for Physician Well Being www.tfme.org. Accessed July 2013.

SECTION II
Global Health

Global Health and Behavioral Medicine

Patrick T. Lee, MD, DTM&H; Kavitha Kolappa, MD; & Giuseppe J. Raviola, MD

INTRODUCTION

Global health and behavioral medicine intersect in two important ways. First, mental, neurological, and substance use (MNS) disorders affect every community in the world. We relate to MNS disorders at a local level, where they are embedded in our customs, culture, and context. MNS disorders also exert global influence, through their massive burden of disease, the human and economic costs of treated and untreated illness, and their secondary (often less visible) effects on the outcomes of other health conditions.

Second, the integration of behavioral, social, and biomedical sciences can improve health care globally. Adapting interdisciplinary lessons to tackle local problems may result in more effective, efficient, and responsive health care delivery. Similarly, understanding the interdependence of social determinants, health, and development may inform enlightened approaches to promoting health and empowering communities.

An interdisciplinary approach also has important implications for health worker training. Health workers in all settings should be trained to treat and prevent behavioral, social, and biological problems. They should be taught communication, leadership, and team membership skills. Burnout among health workers begins during training and leads to a range of dysfunctional behaviors. While learning to care for others, health workers should also be taught to care for themselves.

The intersection of global health and behavioral medicine is a complex and rapidly evolving area. With the goal of offering students a concise entry point into the relevant issues, we have organized this chapter into four sections:

1. The global treatment gap.
2. The need for new models of care.
3. The importance of context.
4. Health worker training and support.

THE GLOBAL TREATMENT GAP

The Problem

To appreciate the global treatment gap, we must first understand the level of need. One in four people will suffer from a mental illness in their lifetime. Major depression is the third largest contributor to the overall global disease burden and is expected to be the number one contributor by 2030. The World Health Organization (WHO) estimates that nearly 850,000 people commit suicide annually. Eighty percent of these suicides are in low- and middle-income countries. As a group, MNS disorders (including conditions such as depression, substance abuse, schizophrenia, dementia, and epilepsy) account for 14% of the overall global disease burden. According to a recent report by the World Economic Forum, the direct and indirect costs of mental illnesses totaled 2.6 trillion dollars in 2010 alone. By 2030, the cumulative costs are expected to exceed 15 trillion dollars. Underlying these staggering financial costs is a flood of measured and unmeasured human suffering.

Despite the enormous need, MNS disorders have received scant attention globally. Why is this the case? The following section presents a brief gap analysis, charting a cascade of inadequate global response from policy, to funding, to treatment.

Policy Gap

At each governance level (international, national, state/province, and local), policies influence funding priorities, timelines, and targets. It is not only health policies but also economic, trade, agricultural, educational, and environmental policies that matter. This is because health in general, and mental health in particular, is closely linked to the conditions in which people are born, grow, live, work, and age, which these policies shape. For the purposes of this gap analysis, we will focus on the prioritization of mental health in international and national health policies.

At the international level, significant strides have been made in recent years with the creation of the Mental Health Gap Action Programme (a series of evidence-based care protocols for MNS disorders), the Mental Health Atlas Project (more accurately mapping the global burden of disease for MNS disorders), and the Movement for Global Mental Health (a global advocacy group). Setbacks have also been common, with mental health too often marginalized or ignored in the international policy arena.

BOX 8-1. THE WORLD HEALTH ORGANIZATION (WHO) ON MENTAL HEALTH

The adoption of a mental health programme must be regarded as a truly historic step taken by the Assembly to bring this new field of medicine into the area of inter-governmental action. The programme . . . will do much for the implementation of one of the W.H.O.'s fundamental principles – namely, that without mental health there can be no true physical health.

–Dr. Brock Chisholm, MD,
psychiatrist and first Director General of the WHO

Since its inception in 1948, the WHO has engaged at the international health policy level in both mental and physical health. Dr. Brock Chisholm, a psychiatrist and the first Director-General of the WHO, helped articulate the WHO's holistic definition of health as "a state of complete physical, mental, and social well-being and not merely the absence of disease or infirmity."* Over half a century later, the 2005 WHO Ministerial Conference in Denmark continued to advocate for an integrated approach, aptly coining the phrase, "No Health Without Mental Health.†

---

*Outline for a Study Group on World Health and the Survival of the Human Race. Material drawn from articles and speeches by Brock Chisholm. Geneva: World Health Organization; 1954. Available from: http://whqlibdoc.who.int/hist/.../ChisholmBrock_1953_Compilation. pdf. Accessed December 6, 2012."
†WHO Mental health: facing the challenges, building solutions. Report from the WHO European Ministerial Conference. Copenhagen, Denmark: WHO Regional Office for Europe, 2005.

 CASE ILLUSTRATION 1

In the months leading up to the 2011 United Nations General Assembly Special Session (UNGASS) on Noncommunicable Diseases (NCDs), MNS disorders became an issue of considerable debate. Notably, the 2000 WHO Global Strategy for the Prevention and Control of NCDs made no mention of MNS disorders. In 2008, MNS disorders only made it into a footnote in the WHO Action Plan on NCDs. In May of 2010, the UN passed a resolution calling for the UNGASS on NCDs, and the subsequent modalities resolution in December 2010 called for six regional consultations on NCDs.

Although MNS disorders had not featured prominently in discussions up until that point, the WHO Regional Office of Africa consultation in Brazzaville in April of 2011 revealed that MNS disorders, hemoglobinopathies, and injuries were major priorities for the region. Weeks later, African nations and India pushed for the inclusion of MNS disorders and garnered their inclusion in the preamble of the Moscow Declaration, which was approved during the Global Ministerial Conference on Healthy Lifestyles and NCDs.

NEW DELHI: India achieved a major success on the global platform by pushing for inclusion of mental health in the list of non-communicable diseases. India fought alone to get mental disorders included in the non-communicable diseases (NCDs) list at the just-concluded first Ministerial Conference on Healthy Lifestyles and Non-communicable Disease Control in Moscow.

–Excerpt from *The Hindu* May 5, 2011

Unfortunately, MNS disorders were excluded from the list of priority conditions in the 2011 UNGASS on NCDs final summary report and recommendations. Time will tell whether the momentum created by the Global South's advocacy push for MNS disorders in 2011 will yield tangible results. Following the UNGASS on NCDs, advocacy groups resolved at the 2011 World Mental Health Day to push for a stand-alone UNGASS on MNS disorders.

At the national level, many countries lack mental health policies (which services should be covered, for whom, and at what cost), plans (how these services should be implemented and evaluated), and legislation (to protect the rights of people who are mentally ill). Global disparities exist. Less than 40% of African countries have a mental health policy, compared with more than 70% of European countries. More than 70% of African countries do not have a national mental health plan, compared to more than 80% of European countries who have one. Globally less than 40% of countries have specific mental health legislation. The absence of mental health legislation (or their enforcement) encourages human rights abuses, which have been widely reported and described as a "failure of humanity."

Funding Gap

The policy gaps described above lead to critical funding gaps. Compared to the burden of disease and economic loss they cause, the amount of health care spending targeted to MNS disorders is remarkably low. Again, global disparities exist. While high-income countries spend, on average, 5% of their health budgets on mental health, low-income countries spend around 0.5%. As a result, high-income countries spend 2.6 million dollars on psychiatric medications per 100,000 people each year, while low-income countries spend only 1700 dollars per 100,000 people each year. This funding stream is simply insufficient to build or sustain the necessary people, tools, infrastructure, or services needed to provide effective care for the one out of every four people worldwide who will suffer from MNS disorders in their lifetime.

Increased funding for mental health is needed at national and international levels. Whereas a multilateral,

international funding mechanism exists for the prevention and treatment of HIV/AIDS, tuberculosis, and malaria, no such mechanism exists for noncommunicable diseases, including MNS disorders. The Grand Challenges in Global Mental Health, a joint-initiative between the US National Institute of Mental Health, Global Alliance for Chronic Disease, and other institutions seeking to fund mental health research, represents a step in the right direction.

Treatment Gap

Policy and funding gaps bear significant responsibility for the massive global treatment gap. Approximately 85% of people with MNS disorders worldwide do not receive appropriate care. Major deficits and global disparities exist in the workforce, essential medicines, and services necessary to provide effective mental health care.

There are insufficient numbers of mental health workers at all levels. These disparities are particularly pronounced in poorer countries. For example, Africa has 0.05 psychiatrists, 0.04 psychologists, and 0.61 mental health nurses per 100,000 people. Staffing levels in the United States and Europe are two to three orders of magnitude higher. New models of mental health care may be able to make better use of (and perhaps expand) the limited mental health workforce, as we discuss later. Nevertheless, the severe shortage of providers, resulting from the withering policy and funding environment, represents a major barrier to delivering safe, effective, community-centered mental health care to all who need it. Figure 8-1 shows the uneven distribution of mental health professionals globally per 100,000 population.

Similar absolute and relative disparities exist in essential medicines for MNS disorders. For example, the antipsychotic section of the WHO Essential Medicines List (EML) has not been modified since 1977. The antipsychotics currently included in the EML (chlorpromazine, fluphenazine, and haloperidol) are significantly more toxic than newer, equally efficacious agents such as risperidone. Worse still, even the outdated medicines included in the EML are often unavailable in low- and middle-income countries. A survey conducted by the WHO in 40 developing nations found that the mean availability of antidepressant medicines was 45.1% in private sector pharmacies and 27.8% in public sector pharmacies. Similar results were found for antiepileptic medicines. Though a full discussion is beyond the scope of this chapter, it bears mentioning that international policies (and the complex factors that determine them) directly shape instruments such as the EML, which profoundly influence the scope of available care in poorer countries. Millions of people live with unnecessary disability, resulting in massive economic loss and, in some cases, conflict and humanitarian crises.

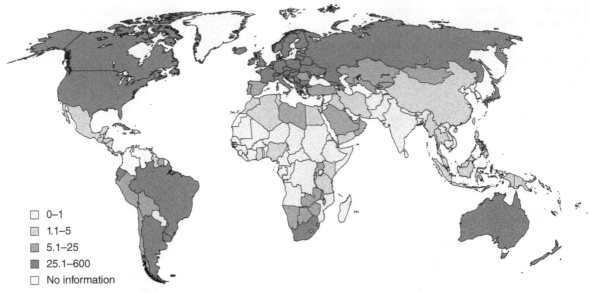

Figure 8-1. Human resources for mental health per 100,000 population. (Redrawn from WHO Health Atlas.)

Legend:
- 0–1
- 1.1–5
- 5.1–25
- 25.1–600
- No information

In summary, one in four people suffer from MNS disorders in their lifetime; 85% of these are unable to access appropriate care; and trillions of dollars are lost as a result each year. The causes are complex but knowable. Gaps at the policy level result in insufficient funding which translates into the extreme global shortage of mental health care.

THE NEED FOR NEW MODELS OF CARE

The Problem

In most of the world, mental health care consists of episodic treatments delivered by psychiatrists in specialized, often locked, facilities. This prevailing model is problematic for four reasons. First, it is too expensive. Teams of mid-level providers and community health workers can be deployed in less time and for a fraction of the cost of training and supporting a single psychiatrist. Second, it fails to achieve sufficient coverage. Even if we assume areas near specialized facilities have access to optimal mental health care (a debatable point), such concentration of resources leaves many areas too far away to maintain longitudinal care. This exacerbates the third problem, which is the overemphasis on treatment at the expense of prevention. The root causes of mental ill health are social as well as biological. If we focus only on the terrible cases that present to the psychiatric hospital, we will miss the forest for the trees. Finally, such treatment models promote stigma and fear surrounding the treatment of mental disorders. This is a particularly sensitive issue in countries where there has been a history of colonialism or violations of human rights by government authorities.

 CASE ILLUSTRATION 2

Decades of civil war and authoritarian rule had ruined Liberia's economy and destroyed its health system. Liberia's people had suffered enormously. In some areas of the country, an estimated 90% of women had been raped, half of the population had fled the country or been internally displaced, and less than 20% of the population had a paying job. In 2008, a nationwide survey documented a massive burden of mental disorders. Forty percent of Liberian adults had major depression, 44% suffered from post-traumatic stress disorder, and 10% were actively suicidal. In contrast to the overwhelming need, Liberia had only a single psychiatrist, one psychiatric nurse, and one psychiatric facility located in its capital city.

The Liberian government recognized the importance of mental health for the overall health, development, and security of the nation. Several policy steps were taken. Mental health was included as one of six priority areas in the 2007 National Health Policy. Following this, Liberia formulated a National Mental Health Policy and a Basic Package of Mental Health Services (both notable achievements for a poor, postconflict country). However, the actual implementation of these policies was constrained by weak physical infrastructure, overwhelmed health services, the absence of trained health workers, and limited financial resources.

In 2011, a disputed presidential election in neighboring Ivory Coast led to genocide-level violence. Over 180,000 Ivorian refugees fled into Liberia, carrying with them the trauma of recent violence and displacement from their homes. The Ivorian refugee crisis triggered a modest influx of international personnel and resources, creating a window of opportunity to strengthen Liberia's fledgling mental health services.

Best Practice

How should mental health services be delivered? This remains an area of significant controversy and, at present, insufficient research. Nevertheless, five elements of best practice emerge from the current literature:

1. Collaborative care.
2. Packages of care.
3. Integration into primary care.
4. Quality improvement.
5. Direct action on the social determinants of health.

The following sections briefly describe each of these best practice elements. For students interested in reading further, we suggest several key references at the end of the chapter.

1. COLLABORATIVE CARE

Collaborative care is team-based care facilitated by smart systems. Complex care pathways are boiled down to discrete tasks that may be shared across different members of the team. These team members may include community health workers, health coaches, social workers, psychologists, nurse care managers, nurse practitioners, physician assistants, primary care physicians, and/or psychiatrists. In the most enlightened models, patients, families, and communities are viewed as active team members with specific and outcome-relevant expertise and knowledge.

Protocols provide decision support (i.e., what to do when, when to ask for help, and when to refer), thereby enabling each team member safely and efficiently to perform tasks that might otherwise be outside their usual scope of practice. Smart tools further support this work. These tools range from paper-based population registries (e.g., lists of patients and active issues that facilitate coordination of care) to smartphone-based decision support and data entry applications.

A strong body of evidence indicates that collaborative care models are as or more effective than other ways of delivering mental health care. In addition to demonstrable efficacy, team-based care has the advantages of lower cost, increased coverage, and better resilience in cases of staff turnover.

2. PACKAGES OF CARE

The term "packages of care" refers to evidence-based bundles of interventions for specific MNS disorders. In

Table 8-1. Packages of care for depression.

Low Resourced Settings	High Resourced Settings
Routine screening for detection	High-risk or routine screening with confirmation of diagnosis by skilled clinician
Psychoeducation	Psychoeducation
Generic antidepressants	Choice of antidepressants
Problem-solving	Choice of brief psychological treatments
	Electroconvulsive therapy

doi:10.1371/journal.pmed.1000159.t003

Source: Patel et al., Packages of care for depression in low- and middle-income countries. PLoS Medicine 2009.

settings where the need is great and resources are limited (the case for MNS disorders in most of the world), difficult decisions need to be taken regarding what treatments should be provided. A series of papers published in *PLoS Medicine* reviewed the evidence and proposed such packages of care. Table 8-1 is excerpted from one of these papers. It summarizes two evidence-based packages of care for depression, appropriate for low- and high-resourced settings.

3. INTEGRATION INTO PRIMARY CARE

There are three compelling reasons for integrating mental health services into primary care. First, such integration locates services closer to people's homes, thereby improving access and reducing costs associated with seeking specialist care in distant locations. Second, it minimizes stigma and discrimination while reducing the risk of human rights violations that may occur in psychiatric hospitals. And third, it generates good health outcomes at reasonable costs. Notably, such integration is not without its pitfalls. Collaborative planning, effective task-sharing among multidisciplinary team members, and adaptation to local context are important adjuncts to care integration. In its 2008 report, *Integrating Mental Health Care into Primary Care: A Global Perspective*, the WHO reviewed the evidence for integration of mental health services into primary care and presented ten best practice case studies from countries around the world. The Case Illustration 3 and Table 8-2 (summary of key messages) are excerpted from the WHO report.

 CASE ILLUSTRATION 3

Juan from Chile has suffered from schizophrenia his entire adult life. Before integrated services for mental health in primary care were introduced, his condition

Table 8-2. Key messages from who report, integrating mental health into primary care: a global perspective.

Key messages of this report
1. Mental disorders affect hundreds of millions of people and, if left untreated, create an enormous toll of suffering, disability and economic loss.
2. Despite the potential to successfully treat mental disorders, only a small minority of those in need receive even the most basic treatment.
3. Integrating mental health services into primary care is the most viable way of closing the treatment gap and ensuring that people get the mental health care they need.
4. Primary care for mental health is affordable, and investments can bring important benefits.
5. Certain skills and competencies are required to effectively assess, diagnose, treat, support and refer people with mental disorders; it is essential that primary care workers are adequately prepared and supported in their mental health work.
6. There is no single best practice model that can be followed by all countries. Rather, successes have been achieved through sensible local application of broad principles.
7. Integration is most successful when mental health is incorporated into health policy and legislative frameworks and supported by senior leadership, adequate resources, and ongoing governance.
8. To be fully effective and efficient, primary care for mental health must be coordinated with a network of services at different levels of care and complemented by broader health system development.
9. Numerous low- and middle-income countries have successfully made the transition to integrated primary care for mental health.
10. Mental health is central to the values and principles of the Alma Ata Declaration; holistic care will never be achieved until mental health is integrated into primary care.

Source: WHO (2008) Integrating mental health into primary care: A global perspective. Geneva: World Health Organization and World Organization of Family Doctors (Wonca).

was poorly managed and he was shuffled repeatedly in and out of a psychiatric hospital, where he endured and witnessed numerous human rights abuses. This part of his story is unfortunately all too familiar. However with the advent of primary care services for mental health in his community, Juan's condition became well-managed and he was able to be reintegrated with his family. He hasn't been back to the psychiatric hospital for four years now.

Excerpted from: WHO (2008) Integrating mental health into primary care: a global perspective. Geneva: World Health Organization and World Organization of Family Doctors (Wonca).

4. QUALITY IMPROVEMENT

Quality improvement is the disciplined use of performance data to improve processes, systems, and outcomes. Various approaches exist. All share a focus on clearly defined goals, methods to link actions to outcomes, and steps to translate new lessons into better processes and systems. As distinct from research, which emphasizes methodological rigor at the expense of real world relevance, quality improvement takes a more pragmatic approach. Like the instrumentation of a plane, it provides continuous feedback on airspeed and altitude, enabling safe landings under difficult conditions. In multiple areas of health care, quality improvement has saved many lives at reasonable cost.

The application of quality improvement to mental health care, however, is in its infancy. The Institute for Healthcare Improvement's *Breakthrough Series for Depression* demonstrated early success in the implementation and maintenance of quality improvement for depression treatment in the US primary care settings. Partners In Health and the Millennium Villages Project have begun to embed performance feedback systems into their community-based mental health programs in Haiti and Nigeria. Though the principles are sound, the evidence connecting quality improvement practices to measureable health outcomes is still forthcoming.

This should not deter the disciplined use of performance data to drive better outcomes in mental health care. Rather, we would suggest all health professional students (and indeed, all health professionals) learn the fundamentals of quality improvement and seek to apply the core principles in their daily practice. One note of caution: quality improvement processes, like all tools, are only as useful as the context and skill with which they are applied. Of particular relevance to global health and behavioral medicine, health students and professionals should marry the discipline of performance improvement to a nuanced understanding of local context (see **The Importance of Context** section).

5. DIRECT ACTION ON THE SOCIAL DETERMINANTS OF HEALTH

Mental, neurological, and substance use disorders and social determinants (i.e., the conditions in which people

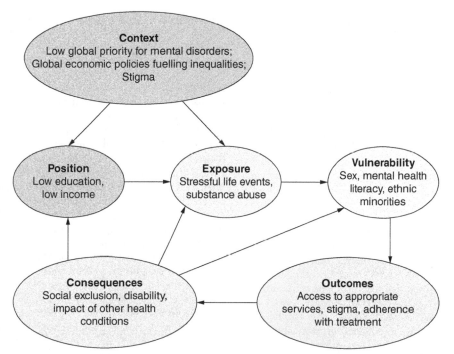

Figure 8-2. Vicious cycle of social determinants and mental disorders. *Source:* Patel V, Lund C, Heatherill S, et al. Mental disorders: equity and social determinants. In Blas E, Sivasankara Kurup A., eds. *Equity, Social Determinants, and Public Health Programmes.* Geneva: World Health Organization, 2010.

are born, grow, live, work, and age) are closely linked. On the one hand, the incidence of MNS disorders goes up with every step down in the social gradient. The poorest populations in every society have the highest rates of depression and alcoholism, for example. On the other hand, MNS disorders and social determinants actually drive one another in a vicious cycle, as summarized in Figure 8-2.

Given the complex range of social determinants that drive MNS disorders, traditional models of facility-based care seem ill prepared to address the root causes of disease (e.g., poverty, stigma, and local context). Rather, an approach that integrates clinical medicine with public health, community empowerment, and direct action on poverty and stigma is needed. Such an approach tends to reorient the usual workforce pyramid. Instead of the most highly trained providers at the top, it is the team members who are closest to the community that are best able to earn trust, understand the local context, and coordinate care in a patient- and community-centered way.

THE IMPORTANCE OF CONTEXT

The Problem

Context is important for four main reasons. First, the history of global health and behavioral medicine is littered with examples of good (and sometimes not so good) intentions gone awry. A nuanced and locally informed understanding of context can reduce the likelihood of unintended harm.

Second, context influences perception and stigma. The origins and effects of mental health programs—what, when, where, how, why, and with whom they are implemented—can dramatically alter their local acceptability, their cultural meaning, and their eventual impact.

Third, the root causes of mental ill health are social as well as biological. Each situation is unique: prisons are different from war zones and urban slums, and no two slums are the same. Effective action on the social determinants must necessarily be tailored to local context. Similarly, MNS disorders present and respond differently in different settings. Diagnostic and therapeutic strategies must account for these local variations, while forging past the inaction that sometimes results from such uncertainty.

Fourth, intersecting with all of the above problems, is the issue of trust. Given the complex and sometimes troubled history of global health and behavioral medicine, strategies to build and strengthen trust between communities and care providers must be grounded in a shared understanding about what truly matters, how best to partner, and how to determine the priorities and metrics for success.

For students interested in reading further about how to consider the issue of context, we recommend Arthur

Kleinman's four social theories for global health, referenced at the end of the chapter.

Complexities in Global Health and Behavioral Medicine

Behavioral medicine is complicated by a number of historical tensions that persist to the present day. For example, diagnostic systems for MNS disorders (the International Classification of Diseases, developed by the WHO, and the Diagnostic and Statistical Manual of Mental Disorders, produced by the American Psychiatric Association) are not fully supported by scientific evidence, and may to some degree reflect Euro-American concepts of illness. Additional tensions that undermine consensus on how to provide mental health services in different contexts include: spiritual (supernatural or religious) and scientific (natural or biological) approaches to understanding etiology and causation; strength- ("resilience") and illness-based interpretations of human distress in adversity; traditional and biomedical approaches to treatment; and community- and clinic-based approaches to service delivery.

Additional layers of complexity arise from the relationship of behavioral medicine to historical precedents. Specifically, psychiatry has at times been used as an instrument of political or government control. This occurred, for example, in Nazi Germany, Communist Russia, apartheid South Africa, and in a number of developing countries during the colonial period. The legacy of these kinds of practices continues to affect the perception of mental health professionals, and compounds the already strong cultural predisposition to stigmatize MNS disorders and mental health services.

A third area of complexity is the relationship of behavioral medicine to humanitarian emergencies (both "natural" and "man-made" disasters). On the one hand, these complex emergencies have created opportunities to engage the international community in strengthening mental health services in developing countries. On the other hand, humanitarian mental health responses in low-resource settings have been characterized by difficulties in coordinating the efforts of international agencies, nongovernmental organizations (NGOs), and other groups and individuals with the priorities of governments and local communities. International humanitarian response mechanisms have often contributed to a lack of local agency in decision making. These challenges underline the importance of framing humanitarian mental health efforts within a pragmatic, do-no-harm, human rights-based approach that prioritizes the engagement of local leaders and experts across disciplines (see Box 8-2).

BOX 8-2. INTERNATIONAL HUMANITARIAN RESPONSE MECHANISMS

The United Nations (UN) Office for the Coordination of Humanitarian Affairs (OCHA) was created in 1998 to assist governments in mobilizing international assistance when the scale of a disaster exceeds national capacity. The Inter-Agency Standing Committee (IASC), created in 1992 by the UN, has served as an inter-agency forum for coordination, policy development, and decision-making involving key UN and non-UN humanitarian partners. In 2007, the IASC developed a set of guidelines for mental health and psychosocial response in complex emergencies, which now serves as a point of reference for organizations responding to disasters. These guidelines are based on a set of core principles: human rights and equity; local participation; doing no harm and avoiding unintentional harm; building on available resources and capacities; developing support systems that integrate into wider systems (e.g., existing community support mechanisms, formal/nonformal school systems, general health services, general mental health services, social services, etc.); and developing a layered system of complementary supports that concurrently meets the needs of different groups.

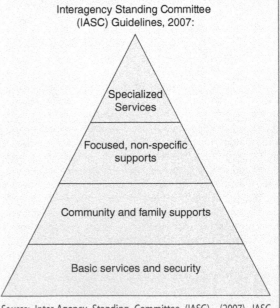

Interagency Standing Committee (IASC) Guidelines, 2007:

- Specialized Services
- Focused, non-specific supports
- Community and family supports
- Basic services and security

Source: Inter-Agency Standing Committee (IASC) (2007). IASC Guidelines on Mental Health and Psychosocial Support in Emergency Settings. Geneva: IASC.

CASE ILLUSTRATION 4

In January 2010, a major earthquake struck Haiti, crumbling the city of Port-au-Prince and causing massive casualties. Partners In Health (PIH), an international health care organization with 25 years of experience in health care delivery and program implementation in Haiti, was among the first responders to the disaster. At the time of the earthquake, PIH was operating 11 hospitals in partnership with the Haitian Ministry of Health (MOH) and had a staff of approximately 5000 Haitian providers, including 2500 community health workers.

Partners In Health chose to take a long-term view of the problem, recognizing that building mental health systems of care in the context of the disaster would require an integrated, evidence-based, and multisectoral approach. In the weeks following the disaster, immediate linkages were made with the Haitian MOH. Partners In Health also met biweekly with UN and other NGOs interested in post-earthquake mental health services. Initial needs assessments were completed. A proposal was developed for a model of community-based mental health services that could be piloted within the PIH health care system, with the potential to be scaled across the country in partnership with the Haitian MOH.

The empowerment of Haitians to meet locally identified mental health needs was viewed as a critical component for long-term programmatic success. Partners In Health hired additional staff, expanding its team from three Haitian psychologists to 17, and from 20 social workers to 50. Approximately 18 months after the earthquake, PIH staff had provided 20,000 individual services for mental health needs. All of these services were linked to a system of social and economic support on the one hand, and advanced medical care on the other. A qualitative study of local beliefs and perceived needs resulted in the creation of locally valid screening tools for use by community health workers. A stepped care model for mental health services—including treatment algorithms, training curricula, and evaluation tools—was being developed.

Informed by decades of collaborative care with local Haitians and the Haitian MOH, PIH was able to respond to a complex humanitarian disaster from a position of trust, resilience, and deep familiarity with local context. This response addressed urgent needs, strengthened local capacity, and positioned mental health services within a continuum of care spanning basic needs, common MNS disorders, and more complex conditions.

Assessing Local Context

Given the importance of context in designing effective, community-centered mental health services, how then do we approach the task of assessing local context? The elements of this assessment include: qualitative and quantitative assessment of needs, prioritization of needs, and identification of available resources. We will expand briefly on qualitative assessment.

The first question should be: how are MNS disorders understood, described, and addressed locally? Iterative experience and ongoing assessment may be needed to plumb the depths of this critical question. As the local context comes into view, ethnographic or similar qualitative analysis should be used to adapt and modify treatments based on international standards of best practice. The adaptation of generalizable knowledge to local context is a routine, not exotic, challenge captured by the oft-described goal of linking evidence-based practice with practice-based evidence. The purpose is to enable caregivers to use proven treatments in ways that make local sense, and to leverage local understandings and resources to be more effective.

Structured interview guides can facilitate such qualitative assessment. The guides can be designed to understand the nature and impact of mental and emotional conditions, as well as how people seek, or would seek, care for these conditions. Community members, local leaders, health workers, and potential community partners (such as religious leaders or traditional healers) should be asked specifically about the local acceptability of carrying out certain care and treatment functions. These functions include case finding and diagnosis, patient education and engagement, use of appropriate medications, use of specific psychosocial interventions, use of community-based support systems, systematic follow-up and outcomes monitoring, expert consultation and supervision, and referral rules.

The use of qualitative methods in health care implementation is an emerging area of best practice and can be performed with varying degrees of rigor. But as a general rule it should be repeated iteratively and include a set of participatory queries that inform the understanding of MNS disorders and the use and acceptability of mental health services. For students interested in reading further on the assessment and adaptation of mental health services to local context, we recommend the framework described by Belkin et al. for implementing and delivering community mental health care.

HEALTH WORKER TRAINING AND SUPPORT

The need for more robust training in the social and behavioral sciences for all health professionals has been well recognized. The final section of this book, *Teaching*

Behavioral Medicine in Medical Settings, offers a fuller discussion of the nature and potential solutions to this problem. In this section, we wish to briefly emphasize three points relevant to global health and behavioral medicine.

First, new skills are needed. These include an understanding of the global treatment gap, the need for new models of care, and the importance of context, as described above. In order for such skills to be incorporated into training systems, they will need to be aligned with locally relevant terminology, qualification schemes, and practice patterns. For US physician training, for example, this means linking skills to professional competencies, evaluating performance in licensing and certification exams, and considering the set of metrics and incentives that will continue to foster these skills when trainees enter professional practice.

Second, a new ethos may be needed. Communication, leadership, and team membership skills have all been emphasized in recent calls for medical education reform. These skills are linked to cohesive team dynamics and effective care coordination across multiple providers and health systems. Based on our experience in global health practice, we would suggest an additional ethos that may integrate this set of skills and foster the development of collaborative behaviors, namely, the ethos of "accompaniment."

Accompaniment refers to the long-term commitment to do "whatever it takes" to improve another person's health and dignity. In practice, accompaniment translates the belief in health as a human right into pragmatic and results-oriented service. Because it is grounded in mutual respect and long-term commitment, accompaniment often helps to bridge distrust, stigma, and other social distances. This ethos carries over into the organization of teams and systems. The commitment to equity and justice creates a culture of transparency, shared accountability, and horizontal collaboration among leaders, frontline workers, patients, families, and communities. In our experience, accompaniment often unlocks the "purpose motive" for both international and local health workers, amplifying the impact of team members who are motivated by intrinsic (i.e., core values and shared commitments) rather than extrinsic (i.e., rewards and punishment) factors.

Third, self-care is essential to prevent burnout and promote resilience (see Chapters 6 & 47). The loss of empathy during health professional training, as well as the development of dysfunctional behaviors during and after training, has been well documented. Several educational initiatives, such as the *Healer's Art* curriculum created by Rachel Remen and the curricular reform at Indiana University School of Medicine, have attempted to address these issues. However, these initiatives tend to cluster earlier in the training pathway, whereas burnout and dysfunctional behaviors continue to accumulate at the graduate medical education and professional levels. In particular, the complexity of practicing behavioral medicine in a global context (including the tendency of those who do "whatever it takes" to subsume personal needs) requires health workers with a high degree of resilience and self-awareness. New programs and professional norms will be needed to safeguard hope and empathy throughout training, and prepare health workers to harness the power of shared values and commitments in themselves and others in their professional practice.

CONCLUSIONS

This chapter has considered the rationale for integrating the study of global health and behavioral medicine, the magnitude and causes of the global treatment gap for MNS disorders, five elements of best practice for new models of mental health care, the importance of local context and how to assess it, and the need for new skills, an ethos of accompaniment, and better self-care in health worker training.

We have aimed for breadth, envisioning a concise introduction for a primarily US or European medical student audience. The depth of coverage has necessarily been limited. We hope readers will find the chapter useful, and that at least several students will be stimulated to read further and perhaps contribute to global health and behavioral medicine in their professional careers.

SUGGESTED READINGS

Becker AE, Kleinman A. Mental health and the global agenda. *N Engl J Med* 2013;369:66–73.

Belkin G, Unützer J, Kessler R, et al. Scaling up for the "Bottom Billion": "5×5" implementation of community mental health care in low-income regions. *Psychiatric Services* 2011;62:1494–1502.

Bloom, DE, Cafiero, ET, Jané-Llopis, E, et al. (2011). The global economic burden of non-communicable diseases. Geneva: World Economic Forum.

Collins, et al. Grand Challenges in global mental health. *Nature* 2011;475:27–30.

Gilbody S, Bower P, Fletcher J, et al. Collaborative care for depression—a cumulative meta-analysis and review of longer-term outcomes. *Arch Intern Med* 2006;166:2314–2321.

Kleinman A. Four social theories for global health. *Lancet* 2010;375(9725):1518–1519.

Kohn R, Saxena S, Levav I, Saraceno B. The treatment gap in mental health care. *Bull World Health Organ* 2004;82:858–866.

Mathers CD, Loncar D. Projections of global mortality and burden of disease from 2002 to 2030. *PLoS Med* 2006;3:e442. doi:10.1371/journal.pmed.0030442.

Patel V, Lund C, Heatherill S, et al. Mental disorders: equity and social determinants. In Blas E, Sivasankara Kurup A, eds. *Equity, Social Determinants, and Public Health Programmes.* Geneva: World Health Organization 2010.

Patel V, Saxena S. Transforming lives, enhancing communities–innovations in global mental health. *N Engl J Med* 2014. doi: 10.1056/NEJMp1315214.

Patel V, Thornicroft G. Packages of care for mental, neurological, and substance use disorders in low- and middle-income countries. *PLoS Med* 2009;6(10):e1000160. doi:10.1371/journal.pmed.1000160.

WHO. Integrating mental health into primary care: a global perspective. Geneva: World Health Organization and World Organization of Family Doctors (Wonca). 2008.

World Health Organization. Closing the gap in a generation: health equity through action on the social determinants of health. WHO Commission on Social Determinants of Health. 2008.

WEB SITES

"Project Atlas: Resources for Mental Health." World Health Organization website. Accessible online at http://www.who.int/mental_health/evidence/atlas/en/. Accessed July 2013.

World Health Organization (2008) Mental Health Gap Action Programme (mhGAP): scaling up care for mental, neurological and substance abuse disorders. Geneva: WHO, Available: http://www.who.int/mental_health/mhgap/evidence/en/. Accessed July 2013.

Environment, Health, and Behavior

John F. Christensen, PhD

If you want to learn about the health of a population, look at the air they breathe, the water they drink, and the places where they live.

Hippocrates, Fifth century BCE

Photo by Hank Christensen (www.hankchristensen.com)

INTRODUCTION

This chapter looks beyond the individual patient and clinician to the behaviors of human populations and their impact on the environment, which itself exerts a profound influence on human health and illness. We will discuss opportunities and strategies for modifying those behaviors—on the individual and societal scale—that affect human health and well-being.

The attention of health professionals to environmental factors is warranted by developments in our scientific understanding of three interrelated domains: (1) the impact of environmental degradation and enhancement on human health; (2) the impact of human behavior on the environment; and (3) the effectiveness of initiatives to modify human behavior on a population scale. This chapter will review each of these domains and conclude with suggestions for clinicians to draw upon this information in the care of patients and to become engaged in the process of societal behavior change for the well-being of the planet.

EFFECTS OF ENVIRONMENTAL DEGRADATION ON HUMAN HEALTH

As Hippocrates observed millennia ago, the quality of the biosphere that supports us has a marked impact on our health. Disease burdens due to environmental degradation include altered fertility rates, challenges to the health of newborns, disorders of human development, malnutrition, vector patterns of infectious diseases, skin cancers due to ultraviolet radiation exposure, respiratory disorders, and obesity. Understanding connections between environmental change and these kinds of health problems has increased as agencies such as the World Health Organization (WHO), US National Institutes of Health (NIH), US Centers for Disease Control (CDC), Institute of Medicine (IOM), and others have compiled research on the environment–health connection. A few of these connections are summarized here.

Air Pollution

The WHO estimates there are 3 million deaths worldwide each year from air pollutants—3 times the number of traffic fatalities. Over an 18-year period increased

death rates from dementias such as Alzheimer and Parkinson have been linked to a rise in the concentration of pesticides, industrial effluents, car exhaust, and other pollutants in the environment. Sulfur dioxide, produced by combustion of fossil fuels, has been shown to induce acute bronchoconstriction in asthmatics. Particulate air pollution has been implicated in respiratory ailments and in derangement of heart rate variability, a risk factor for cardiac events. Carbon monoxide (CO), primarily emitted from internal combustion engines in motor vehicles, has serious health effects in high concentrations leading to carbon monoxide poisoning. More frequently, however, lower-level exposures to CO may increase platelet activity and coagulation, leading to increased risks of thromboembolism. A global meta-analysis found an association between air pollution and heart failure hospitalization or death, particularly with increases in carbon monoxide, sulfur dioxide, and nitrogen dioxide. In Northern China, where the government's Huai River policy has provided free winter heating with coal, total suspended particulates (TSPs) air pollution has been associated with a lower life expectancy of 5.5 years, compared with populations in the south. A meta-analysis of 17 population cohorts in Europe found a significant association between particulate matter concentrations and lung cancer.

Degraded Water Quality and Availability

The quality of water can be associated with human disease in several ways. Bacterial pathogens, including *salmonella, Shigella, Escherichia coli,* and *Vibrio cholerae*— all of which cause diarrheal disease, can be spread by

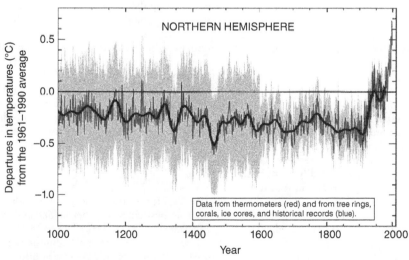

Figure 9-1. Northern Hemisphere temperature changes over last millennium. (The curve of temperature changes takes on a "hockey stick" appearance, with accelerated warming since the Industrial Revolution resembling the blade of the stick.) (Intergovernmental Panel on Climate Change [IPCC].)

water, particularly in developing countries with inadequate water treatment. Water quality is also compromised by various toxic chemicals that accumulate in ground and surface water from runoff and industrial discharge. Examples are nitrates, pesticides, the gasoline additive methyl tert-butyl ether (MTBE), radon, arsenic, lead, and the by-products of disinfectants. These toxins have been associated with a variety of health problems, including various forms of cancer, decreased intelligence quotient (IQ) and behavioral problems in infants and children, adult hypertension, and neurotoxicity.

Water availability per capita is shrinking worldwide. The total amount of freshwater available for human use worldwide is about 0.007 of all the water on earth. Currently, humans use about half of this amount. In many underdeveloped parts of the world, millions of humans live in "hydrological poverty," in which water for direct human consumption through drinking and indirect consumption through grain production is becoming increasingly scarce. In these areas, water for drinking and irrigation is over-pumped beyond the recharge rate of underground aquifers. Resource wars, in which arable land is contested in civil wars, such as that occurring in the Darfur region of Sudan, are increasing in frequency due to diminished water availability for irrigation.

Malnourishment

Of the 7.2 billion comprising the earth's human population, over 4 billion are prone to malnourishment of some form. Hunger afflicts 1.2 billion; another 2 billion suffer from micronutrient deficiency. Most of these people live in the preindustrial or developing world. At the other end of the malnourishment spectrum, 1.2 billion people, primarily in the developed world, suffer from over-consumption of food with its associated problems of obesity, cardiovascular disease, and type 2 diabetes.

Climate Change

There is a preponderance of evidence from various domains of scientific measurement that the earth's climate is warming at an alarming rate that exceeds the normal background fluctuation of temperature. Global temperatures have been rising steadily for nearly 40 years; 9 out of the 10 warmest years on record have occurred since 2001; and the global combined land and ocean surface temperature for 2010 was tied with 2005 as the warmest years on record, at 0.62°C above the twentieth century average. Figure 9-1 shows the increase in the Northern Hemisphere temperature over the last thousand years.

The major driver of this global warming is the accumulation of "greenhouse" gases—primarily carbon dioxide, methane, and nitrous oxide—which reached their highest concentrations over the last millennium during the 1990s. These greenhouse gases allow radiant energy from the sun to be absorbed by water vapor, clouds, and aerosols, and then trap the reflected infrared radiation, absorbing and reemitting it to further warm the lower atmosphere and the earth's surface (see Figure 9-2).

Current estimates are that the earth's warming is accelerating, and climate models predict that the average surface temperature will rise by 2.4 to 6.4°C by the year 2100.

The *direct effects* of climate change on human health include heat-related illnesses and deaths; the impacts of increased floods and droughts (often followed by malnutrition due to loss of cropland); the spread of infectious diseases to wider geographical ranges, both in latitude and altitude as mosquito-borne illnesses such as West Nile virus, tick-borne illnesses such as Lyme disease, and rodent-borne illnesses such as hantavirus follow the warming trends; a longer seasonal duration of biogenic allergens; cardiorespiratory problems due to increased ground-level ozone concentrations; increase in water-related diseases as water scarcity leads to freshwater contamination; algal blooms with associated cholera outbreaks; increased outbreaks of cryptosporidiosis due to heavy rainfall; and the threat to human health and well-being by the more violent storms associated with warming.

The *indirect health effects* include water scarcity, with the number of people living in water-scarce countries expected to rise six-fold from 470 million to 3 billion between 1990 and 2025; nutrition deficits driven by a drop in crop yields combined with increased demand due to population growth and higher levels of consumption as affluence promotes shifting to a meat-based diet; undernutrition (indicated by stunting and underweight in children under 5 years) due to lowered crop yields; decreased nutritional content of grains due to increased atmospheric CO_2 concentrations; and finally population displacement—with associated immune system challenges, infectious diseases, housing and sanitation challenges, lack of safe drinking water, malnutrition, violence, and post-traumatic stress disorder (PTSD).

Environmental Toxins

The leaching into groundwater of industrial chemicals such as pesticides and herbicides and into the air of substances such as dioxin due to incineration of medical waste has led to an accumulation of persistent organic pollutants (POPs) in the human body. Almost all humans have residues of these chemicals in their tissues, and there is increased concern among public health officials that these levels could reach thresholds

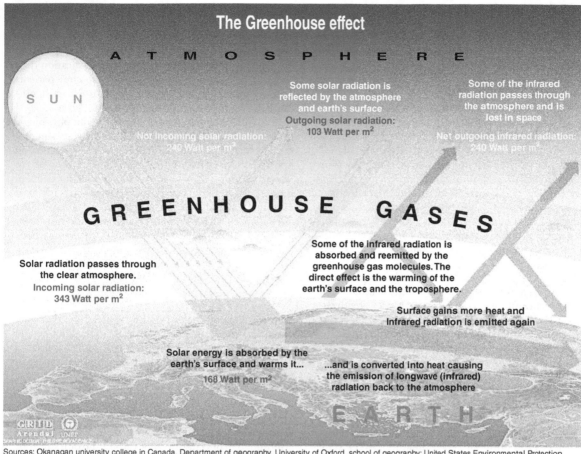

Figure 9-2. The greenhouse effect on earth's atmosphere. (Greenhouse gases, which include water vapor (H_2O), ozone (O_3), carbon dioxide (CO_2), methane (CH_4), and nitrous oxide (N_2O), are able to absorb and reemit infrared radiation, while not blocking visible light. The greenhouse effect occurs when solar radiation is absorbed by the earth's surface, converted into heat, and subsequently emitted into the atmosphere as infrared radiation. Some of this infrared radiation escapes into outer space; however, some is absorbed and reemitted back toward the earth's surface by greenhouse gases. These returning waves of infrared radiation warm the troposphere and the earth's surface once again.) (Intergovernmental Panel on Climate Change [IPCC].)

harmful to human health. The emerging toxicological field of endocrine disruption focuses on the influence of POPs in imitating or blocking the actions of hormones, possibly leading to a variety of reproductive and neurodevelopmental disorders.

Built Environment

The ways in which cities grow to accommodate increased population may be contributing to worsening human health. The "built environment" refers to the impacts of urban sprawl, traffic congestion, and the associated sedentary lifestyle of the population as people spend more time in cars and in gridlock driving to work or shopping. The US CDC estimates that urban sprawl due to lack of adequate land use planning is associated with increases in obesity, cardiovascular disease, and type 2 diabetes.

POSITIVE HEALTH EFFECTS OF NATURE

Engagement with nature has a positive influence on human health. The biologist E.O. Wilson proposed in his *biophilia hypothesis* that humans have an innate inclination to affiliate with other forms of life. There is a growing awareness of the restorative benefits of spending time in nature—including physical, mental, and spiritual renewal.

Different theories have been advanced about what constitutes the restorative effects of nature. *Attention restoration theory* suggestions that the effort required for focused attention, especially in complex urban environments, requires inhibition of competing demands for attention, often leading to "directed attention fatigue." The restorative benefits of nature involve recovery from this attentional fatigue through the experience of *being away* (having a distance from routine mental tasks), *fascination* (involving interest-driven attention), *extent* (being in a coherently ordered environment of substantial scope), and *compatibility* (the demands and supports posed by the environment match the individual's inclinations).

A theory of *psychological stress recovery* proposes that particular qualities and contents of the natural scene facilitate this recovery—moderate depth, moderate complexity, the presence of a focal point, gross structural qualities, and natural contents (e.g., vegetation and water). These features of the natural scene evoke positive emotions, sustain nonvigilant attention, restrict negative thoughts, and facilitate reduction of sympathetic arousal. From an evolutionary perspective, humans are biologically prepared to respond positively to environmental features that signal possibilities of survival.

There is growing evidence supporting the restorative and health-promoting influence of nature. Several studies have shown that children who have access to green environments with trees and other vegetation have an increased ability to focus and concentrate. Children with attention deficit hyperactivity disorder (ADHD) have shown improvement in symptoms when they are in contact with nature. A study of childhood asthma and the number of street trees in neighborhoods in New York City found that an increase of tree density of one standard deviation was associated with a lower prevalence of asthma. Neighborhood greenery has also been associated with lower body mass index (BMI) in children, indicating the value of urban planning for greenspaces as a means of addressing childhood obesity.

A number of studies have shown positive impacts of natural environments on cognitive performance and attentional enhancement in adults. Recovering breast cancer patients who participated in nature-based restorative activities showed better coping ability and attentional performance than those who did not. College students whose dormitory windows had views of nature functioned more effectively on daily tasks requiring directed attention than those with views of buildings. These studies lend support to the attention restoration theory of how nature influences human performance.

There is also evidence supporting the role of engagement with nature in psychological stress recovery. Hospital inpatients recovering from cholecystectomy whose rooms had views of trees had a shorter length of hospitalization and lower need for pain medication than patients with views of buildings. Bronchoscopy patients exposed to images and sounds of nature had significantly better pain control than those who did not.

The influence of natural environments on physiologic parameters related to stress and illness suggests some of the pathways mediating the positive impacts of nature on human health. Studies in Japan on *shinrin-yoku*, or "forest bathing trips" have shown significant effects of time spent walking in forest settings on enhanced immune function, including increase in natural killer cell activity; decreased levels of adrenalin and noradrenalin; and increased activation of the parasympathetic nervous system.

IMPACT OF HUMAN BEHAVIOR ON THE ENVIRONMENT

Figure 9-3 shows the growth of the earth's human population over the last two millennia. The doubling of this population since 1950 to its current 7.2 billion in 2013 has led to a cumulative and negative impact of human alteration of the environment.

The consensus of the scientific community as expressed in the 2007 Intergovernmental Panel on Climate Change (IPCC) report is that the earth is warming due to human activity. The dramatic rise in atmospheric concentrations of carbon dioxide since the Industrial Revolution—especially due to carbon emissions from automobiles, coal power plants, and other industrial sources—coupled with a destruction of natural carbon sinks due to deforestation, especially the loss of tropical rainforest, is correlated with the increased

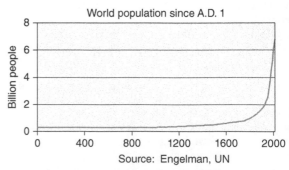

Figure 9-3. Growth in the earth's human population over the last two millennia. (The acceleration of population growth over the last century assumes a "hockeystick" curve, similar to Figure 9-1 for northern hemisphere warming.)

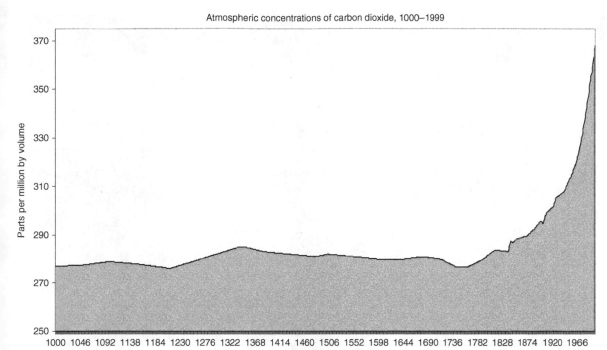

Atmospheric concentrations of carbon dioxide, 1000–1999

Compiled by worldwatch institute

Figure 9-4. Increase in atmospheric concentrations of carbon dioxide over the last millennium. (The accelerated increase in CO_2 since the Industrial Revolution assumes the familiar "hockey stick" curve, as in Figures 9-1 and 9-3.) (Compiled by Worldwatch Institute.)

warming trend noted over the same period (see Figure 9-4). For the first time in geological history, the behavior of a single species is now altering on a global scale the sustaining fabric of all life.

Global disparities in consumption of energy—for transportation, heat, lighting, food production, and industrial output—can be seen dramatically in photos of the earth at night from the international space station (Figure 9-5). The relatively dark contours of continents such as South America and Africa in the Southern Hemisphere contrast sharply with the brilliantly lit cities and megalopolises of the United States and Western Europe.

The United States, leading the world in carbon emissions per capita, released over 17.2 tons per person in 2011, compared with the European Union (EU) (7.3 tons), China (6.6 tons), and India (1.8 tons). Yet automobile use continues to rise, and with the annual economic growth rate of China (about 10.4% per year from 1990 to 2010) and India (about 6.4% per year in the same time period), their enormous populations (together exceeding 2 billion) threaten to overwhelm the carrying capacity of the earth's atmosphere with carbon emissions. Already China's total CO_2 emissions are the highest (27% of the world's total), compared with the United States (18%), the EU (13%), and India (5%).

In addition to its influence on global warming, human behavior is responsible for the failure to limit population globally, thus magnifying geometrically the "human footprint" on the earth. That footprint is distributed unevenly among the nations, with the United States showing an overall environmental deficit of −8.2 (the amount of hectares per capita by which human use exceeds the available land capacity), while the Indian subcontinent shows a surplus of 0.8 ha. Currently the global environmental deficit due to the human footprint is −0.9 ha per capita (see Figure 9-6).

Human behavior is implicated in all of the environmental threats to human behavior mentioned above. Poor or absent land use planning; waste of water and the over-pumping of underground aquifers below their recharge rate; deforestation; over-fishing of the seas; indiscriminate discharge of pollutants into air, ground, and water; over-cultivating and mismanaging the soil; and over-consumption of material goods whose manufacture and disposal further degrades the environment—all are behaviors that in the aggregate alter the fabric that sustains life and supports human health.

Behavioral medicine, especially as practiced in the individual clinician–patient encounter, traditionally targets the behaviors, emotions, and relationships of patients and clinicians in the amelioration of disease in the individual

Earth at Night
More information available at:
http://antwrp.gsfc.nasa.gov/apod/ap020810.html

Figure 9-5. Composite picture of earth at night from international space station. (Density of nighttime lighting is a good proxy for unequal distribution of greenhouse gas emissions.) (Earth at Night Credit: C. Mayhew & R. Simmon [NASA/GSFC], NOAA/ NGDC, DMSP Digital Archive.)

patient. In the context of the environment–health connection, however, behavioral medicine focuses more broadly on the behavior of populations, while maintaining the individual patient encounter at its core.

CHANGING POPULATION BEHAVIOR IN RELATION TO THE ENVIRONMENT

How can health care clinicians influence behavior change at the population level? There is a growing awareness that several approaches have either demonstrated effectiveness or hold promise for exerting a meaningful influence, if professionals organize to take action.

Leading by Example

Individual clinicians can adopt environmentally friendly practices by the way their offices and clinics are furnished. The use of low-watt fluorescent light bulbs and

low flow toilets, and the purchase of products from vendors known to use environmentally sensitive practices demonstrate to patients that their clinician is committed to sustainability. In their personal lives as well, health professionals can lead the way in the choices they make by using mass transportation and lower-carbon-emission vehicles, owning energy-efficient homes and appliances, using renewable sources of energy, being mindful of consumer patterns that favor environmentally friendly products, and dealing responsibly with waste.

Patient Education

Mentioning the link, where appropriate, between patients' illnesses and environmental factors that are the result of human behavior can plant the seed for behavior change. For example, mentioning the link between exposure to diesel exhaust and asthma, or between

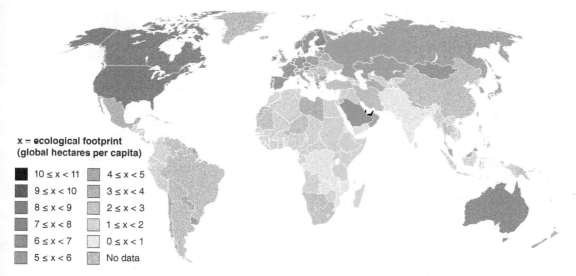

x = ecological footprint (global hectares per capita)

- $10 \leq x < 11$
- $9 \leq x < 10$
- $8 \leq x < 9$
- $7 \leq x < 8$
- $6 \leq x < 7$
- $5 \leq x < 6$
- $4 \leq x < 5$
- $3 \leq x < 4$
- $2 \leq x < 3$
- $1 \leq x < 2$
- $0 \leq x < 1$
- No data

Figure 9-6. World map of countries by ecological footprint in 2007. (Map based on data from 2007 published by Global Footprint Network in 2010. Data is given as global hectares per capita. The world-average ecological footprint in 2007 was 2.7 global hectares per person. With a world-average biocapacity of 1.8 global hectares per person, this leads to an ecological deficit of 0.9 global hectares per person. If a country does not have enough ecological resources within its own territory, then there is a local ecological deficit and it is called an ecological debtor country. Otherwise, it has an ecological remainder and it is called an ecological creditor country.)

pesticide overuse and endocrine disruption, can in the aggregate begin to educate a community, using teachable moments related to individual health care. The Pediatric Environmental Health Toolkit developed by Physicians for Social Responsibility (PSR) and endorsed by the American Academy of Pediatrics (http://www.psr.org/site/PageServer?pagename=pediatric_toolkit) to assist pediatricians in educating parents about POPs is one example. Another example is *Healthy Aging and the Environment: a Pocket Guide*, a resource developed by the Collaborative on Health and the Environment (http://www.healthandenvironment.org/). Having literature available in the waiting room linking environmental factors with human health may provide a context for further clinician–patient dialogue on this issue.

Community-based Social Marketing

This population-based intervention targets a specific behavior, such as reducing residential water use in summer months, that if practiced by the majority of a community can have a beneficial effect on resource use. Community-based social marketing employs a variety of channels to get a message out to a community about the rationale and method of making a specific change. Among these are newspaper articles, radio and TV spots, direct mailings to households, door-to-door canvassing by volunteers, gaining commitment from individuals,

and making the desired behavior more convenient. The behavior change strategy is usually pilot tested on a small scale, then outcomes are measured and evaluated, and once tested, the strategy is implemented. Using this methodology, an entire suburb of Toronto was persuaded to restrict lawn watering to odd or even days linked to street addresses.

Community Education

Health professionals can offer community education lectures through their hospital systems, civic clubs, community associations, schools, and churches. Resources such as the Worldwatch Institute, Earth Policy Institute, Collaborative on Health and the Environment, CDC, PSR, and others have web sites and databases from which presentations can be easily assembled. Letters to the editor and op-ed submissions to local newspapers are other ways of informing communities about the link between the environment and health, as well as about behaviors that can mitigate deleterious health impacts.

Land Use Planning

Decisions made at the neighborhood, municipality, state, and national levels about the built environment and the protection and promotion of natural areas have relevance for human health and well-being. Health professionals can play an informative role with land use planning bodies, providing testimony about the importance of wilderness areas, parks, and open spaces in promoting human health.

Public Policy Advocacy

Professional associations at the local, state, and national level are potent vehicles for public policy advocacy. Clinicians who are interested and informed about environmental issues and their health effects can organize interest groups and public policy advocacy teams within their organizations. They can also work with the governance structure of their organizations to endorse policy positions both to influence public opinion and to lobby local, state, and federal government for legislation and regulations to promote environmentally friendly practices. Examples are the number of municipalities and local governments that have passed ordinances ratifying the Kyoto accords on limiting greenhouse emissions. The states of California, Oregon, and Washington have established laws and regulations to reduce greenhouse emissions from automobiles. Health professionals have played important roles in these efforts.

The Clean Air Act of 1970 is an example of a public policy success involving regulation of industrial pollution in the United States. With support from the medical community, the Clean Air Act provided a broad regulatory framework for air pollution standards. It set ambient air emission standards, including acceptable levels for particulate matter, ozone, carbon monoxide, nitrogen dioxide, sulfur dioxide, and lead. The law required the US Environmental Protection Agency to use scientific evidence relating air quality to public health in setting standards. Over the last 40 years this has led to a progressive national reduction of these air pollutants. Even in the first year after the law went into effect, there was a sharp reduction in total suspended particulates of air pollution and infant mortality, with a 1% decline in TSPs resulting in a 0.5% decline in the infant mortality rate.

The Precautionary Principle

Many professional associations have adopted versions of this principle, which states: "When an activity raises threats of harm to the environment or human health, precautionary measures should be taken even if some cause and effect relationships are not fully established scientifically." When applied to a phenomenon such as global warming, this principle states that the probable connection between human behavior and planetary warming, coupled with the probable and irreversible health consequences to humanity and other species if preventive action is not taken, creates a moral imperative for governments and human society to act now to reduce greenhouse gases, even before all the scientific causality is established. Health professional associations have played a role in getting this principle adopted by municipal and local governments.

Changing the Corporate Behavior of Health Care Organizations

Health professionals affiliated with medical centers and other health care organizations can influence these organizations to alter practices that have an impact on the environment. Examples are the use of "green" building design to make new facilities more energy efficient and utilize materials that leave a lower environmental footprint, environmentally preferable purchasing of supplies, healthy food options for patients and staff, safe disposal of medical waste, and recycling of materials produced by the healthcare enterprise.

CONCLUSIONS

These are but some of the ways in which clinicians and health professionals can influence the behavior of populations, corporations, and governments. The principles of behavior change (see Chapter 19) may be applicable not only to individuals but whole societies, as they move through stages of readiness to alter lifestyles that strain the earth's carrying capacity. In the aggregate these behavior changes can reduce the human footprint on the earth.

Finally, the health and well-being of our personal lives and of the organizations within which we work is embedded within the health of our planet. Being mindful of the factors that promote environmental and planetary health can give us insights into the sustainability of our lives and careers in medicine. Land use planners, when determining where human population growth in a region should be allowed to occur, employ the following equation: $C - L = M$ (*Capacity – Load = Margin*). Here, *capacity* refers to the carrying capacity of the land, which includes available water, natural resources, transportation corridors, and the ability of the land to absorb the wastes of human activity. *Load* refers to the impact or "ecological footprint" of that human activity upon the land. When the carrying capacity of the natural environment is greater than the additional load of human activity, then there will be a *positive margin* and population growth is *sustainable*. Conversely, when the load exceeds the capacity of the land, then there is a *negative margin* and growth is *unsustainable*.

This same equation, $C - L = M$, can be applied to our own lives and the organizations within which we work. When our capacity as persons is chronically overloaded by work, family, and other commitments, then we are in a negative margin state, which is a way of defining *burnout*. At this point our lives as human beings are unsustainable. It is as if we are drawing off the principal of our resources rather than living off the interest. Conversely, when our capacity routinely exceeds the load we assume, then we are in a positive margin state, and our lives are sustainable.

We must awaken to the full context of our lives on this planet, that we are that part of the earth that has become conscious of itself. Restoring the proper relationship of humans with the earth in a way that promotes sustainability in the whole system is what Thomas Berry has called "the great work" of our generation. Physicians and other health professionals have a vital role to play in this work, for our own health will only be as good as the health of the planet.

SUGGESTED READINGS

Berry T. *The Great Work*. New York: Bell Tower,1999.

Chen Y, Ebenstein A, Greenstone M, Li H. Evidence on the impact of sustained exposure to air pollution on life expectancy from China's Huai River policy. *PNAS* 2013;110:12936–12941 www.pnas.org/cgi/doi/10.1073/pnas.1300018110

Epstein PR. Climate change and human health. *N Engl J Med* 2005;353:1433–1436.

Epstein PR, Ferber D. *Changing Planet, Changing Health*. University of California Press, 2011.

Hansen J, Sato M, Ruedy R. Perception of climate change. *PNAS* 2012;109:E2415–E2423 www.pnas.org/cgi/doi/10.1073/pnas.1205276109

Haines A, Patz JA. Health effects of climate change. *JAMA* 2004;291:99–103.

Lopez R. Urban sprawl and risk for being overweight or obese. *Am J Public Health* 2004;94:1574–1579.

McCally M (ed.). *Life Support: the Environment and Human Health*. MIT Press, 2002.

McKenzie-Mohr D, Smith W. *Fostering Sustainable Behavior: an Introduction to Community-based Social Marketing*. New Society Publishers, 1999.

Myers N, Stein J, Schettler T, et al. *Environmental threats to healthy aging*. Greater Boston Physicians for Social Responsibility and Science and Environmental Health Network, 2008. (http://www.agehealthy.org/pdf/GBPSRSEHN_HealthyAging1017.pdf) Accessed January 2012.

Raaschou-Nielsen O, Andersen ZJ, Beelen R, et al. Air pollution and lung cancer incidence in 17 European cohorts: prospective analyses from the European Study of Cohorts for Air Pollution Effects (ESCAPE). *The Lancet Oncology* 2013;14:813–822.

Samet JM. The Clean Air Act and health—a clearer view from 2011. *N Engl J Med* 2011;365:198–201.

Shah ASV, Langrish JP, Nair H, et al. Global association of air pollution and heart failure: a systematic review and meta-analysis. *The Lancet* 2013;382:1039–1048 http://dx.doi.org/10.1016/S0140-6736 (13)60898-3

Vitousek PM, et al. Human domination of earth's ecosystems. *Science* 1997;277:494–499.

Weart SR. *The Discovery of Global Warming*. Harvard University Press, 2003.

WEB SITES

350.org (an online grassroots movement dedicated to reducing CO_2 concentrations in the atmosphere from its current 392 parts per million to below 350 ppm) www.350.org. Accessed July 2013.

Centers for Disease Control articles on the built environment and health http://www.cdc.gov/healthyplaces/articles.htm. Accessed July 2013.

The Collaborative on Health and the Environment (CHE) http://www.healthandenvironment.org/. Accessed July 2013.

Healthy Aging and the Environment: a Pocket Guide available for download. http://www.healthandenvironment.org/initiatives/healthy_aging/training_materials#report Accessed January 2014.

Earth Policy Institute http://www.earth-policy.org. Accessed July 2013.

Intergovernmental Panel on Climate Change (IPCC) http://www.ipcc.ch/. Accessed July 2013.

Physicians for Social Responsibility http://www.psr.org/. Accessed July 2013.

PSR Environmental Health Toolkit for pediatricians http://www.psr.org/site/PageServer?pagename=pediatric_toolkit. Accessed July 2013.

The Worldwatch Institute http://www.worldwatch.org/ Accessed July 2013.

Training of International Medical Graduates

10

H. Russell Searight, PhD, MPH; Jennifer Gafford, PhD; & Vishnu Mohan, MD

INTRODUCTION

This chapter will review issues involved in the training and education of international medical graduates (IMGs), including differing views of psychiatric conditions and treatment; differences in educational experiences; clinical issues involving interactions with patients and nonphysician staff; technology and documentation; psychosocial issues; and medical ethics. General suggestions are offered regarding possible modifications to residency education to address the special needs of these trainees. As in any discussion of cross-cultural differences, the tremendous variability in the backgrounds of IMGs must be acknowledged. Generalizations will always be qualified and may not reflect the experience of all IMGs.

CASE ILLUSTRATION 1

The primarily U.S.-trained family medicine residency faculty meets one last time to review candidates before submitting their final rank order list to the National Resident Matching Program (NRMP). With few exceptions, the rank order begins with the U.S. medical graduates (USMGs) and ends with IMGs, who comprise two-thirds of the total list. Visa issues further complicate the selection process. "She is a strong applicant, but her visa status is likely to cause some administrative difficulties." Thoughtful, sensitive discussions sort out which applicants, particularly among the IMGs, appear genuinely interested in family medicine; which applicants are more familiar with the U.S. medical system; which applicants might effectively relate to and communicate with this residency's low-income, urban population; and which applicants might appreciate and attend to psychosocial issues in patient care. One faculty member comments, "The ranking process was more straightforward when we considered only USMGs." Another adds,

"So was residency education!" A third retorts, "Don't forget, some of our strongest residents have been IMGs!"

GROWING NUMBER OF IMGS IN US RESIDENCY PROGRAMS

International medical graduates are filling an increasing proportion of openings in US primary care specialties. Match results from 2013 indicate that 13% of postgraduate year (PGY)1 family medicine residents were non-US citizen IMGs with comparable figures of 27% for internal medicine and 11% of pediatrics. The percentage of IMGs entering internal medicine residencies has remained fairly constant over the past several years while percentages of non-US citizen IMGs entering family medicine and pediatric residencies has declined slightly. In 2013, the top three countries for IMGs' medical education were India, the Philippines, and Mexico. At present, about 30% of practicing physicians in primary care specialties come from outside the United States. A similar pattern exists for Canada, Britain, and Australia. For example, in Britain, one-third of all practicing physicians are IMGs. As noted above, in the United States, IMGs are well represented in primary care specialties (family medicine, internal medicine, and pediatrics) and it is estimated that they will soon represent 35% of the primary care physician workforce. International Medical Graduates currently provide a disproportionate share of health care in medically underserved areas.

As noted by geographic data, a high proportion of US and Canadian noncitizen physicians come from less developed countries that are poor in resources. In addition to the differences in educational content and pedagogy, many IMGs come from cultures in which norms differ from the United States regarding communication style, male–female relationships, and views of children and the elderly. Given this increased internationalization of medical residents, assumptions about prior medical training, based on US-educated physicians, are likely to be inaccurate.

PRIOR TRAINING IN THE BIOPSYCHOSOCIAL MODEL

In the United States, the biopsychosocial model has strongly influenced primary care and community medicine. While the diverse backgrounds of IMGs are valuable in caring for a multiethnic and increasingly diverse US population, the extent to which IMGs have been trained in the biopsychosocial model differs tremendously depending on the country in which the resident was trained. For instance, with a few exceptions, such as Canada, England, Australia, South Africa, and the Netherlands, applied behavioral science and psychology is much better developed in the United States than elsewhere in the world. One recent study examined whether differences in medical training affected IMGs' recognition of late-life depression in standardized vignettes of older patients. Among 178 primary care physicians and 321 psychiatrists, IMGs were significantly less likely than the US medical graduates (USMGs) to make the correct diagnosis of depression or recommend treatment with a first-line antidepressant. The authors proposed that the decreased diagnosis and treatment of late-life depression by IMGs may be attributable to decreased familiarity with depressive symptoms due to different training or cultural paradigms of depression.

A biopsychosocial framework also implicitly underlies sexual medicine and pain management, topics also largely absent in non-Western medical school curricula. In the case of sexual medicine, cultural factors associated with prohibitions regarding premarital sex, sexual orientation, and sexual activity in later life may make it less likely that IMGs will broach these topics with patients. This reluctance is likely to extend to assessing and treating medication-induced sexual dysfunction. With respect to pain management, a recent report found that only 5 out of 300 medical schools in India included pain management and/or palliative care in their curricula.

Our experiences in family medicine residency training are consistent with these observations. As our programs matched greater numbers of IMGs, physician faculty increasingly commented that many of these residents did not appear to appreciate the psychological and social components of primary care. For example, without prompting and even with direct modeling, an IMG resident might interview a 17-year-old pregnant patient without inquiring about the patient's feelings about the pregnancy; the father of the child; parental/family support; whether and how she plans to continue her education; and the availability of other social supports.

Moreover, comments by the IMGs with whom we worked suggested that many of the common mental health conditions seen in the United States were not commonly diagnosed or treated in their home countries. These comments are supported by cross-cultural research. For example, in Japan major depressive disorder, as defined in the Diagnostic and Statistical Manual of Mental Disorders, 5th Edition (DSM-V), is only currently gaining acceptance. Historically, *Utsobyo* was the term for clinically significant depression; however, this condition is severe and involved debilitating psychotic symptoms requiring inpatient care. A related condition, *Yuutsu*, a melancholic state having moral connotations, was often prized in Japanese culture. *Kokoro no kaze*, the Western construct of depression, is beginning to gain acceptance as a "cold of the soul."

Many IMGs that we trained viewed attention deficit hyperactivity disorder (ADHD), as misbehavior rather than a medical condition requiring medication. These differences in practice appeared to stem both from differences in previous training (i.e., limited education in behavioral medicine) as well as acculturation factors (i.e., the way mental health was conceptualized in the resident's home country).

DIFFERENCES IN EDUCATIONAL EXPERIENCES PRIOR TO US RESIDENCY TRAINING

While medical schools vary widely internationally, residents from non-Western countries describe vastly different educational experiences than the typical US graduate. First, in many Asian countries, entrance into medical school occurs directly after completion of high school. While there are some 6-year medical school programs in the United States that take students at a similar point in their educational career, most students in the United States earn a bachelor's degree before applying to medical school. While meeting medical school requirements in the sciences, many US medical school applicants major in fields such as English literature, history, psychology, foreign language, or even art history. In contrast, in those countries in which students enter medical school at 17 years of age, a direct career trajectory heavily loaded with education in the biological sciences precludes broadening the student's scope of knowledge and intellectual exploration in the humanities.

Approaches to teaching and evaluation of students' knowledge also frequently differ by country. In many international schools, rote memorization of information from textbooks and lectures is the principle learning style. In the United States, there is more emphasis on the application of medical knowledge and on small group learning experiences such as "problem-based learning" (PBL), rather than pure memorization of information. The current US medical school emphasis on evidence-based medicine (EBM), combined with PBL, encourages critical analysis of knowledge and its applicability to a given context rather than retention of facts. The interactional style of many US educators, often including games requiring learner participation (e.g., "Pharmacotherapy Jeopardy"), is a new experience for many IMGs. Ironically, however, the United States relies heavily on multiple-choice exams to evaluate medical students, residents (in training exams), and practicing physicians (board exams)—thereby reinforcing the memorization of facts. Outside of the United States, essay and oral exams are more commonly used to assess medical students' knowledge. In addition, Objective Structured Clinical Examinations (OSCEs) featuring role playing by standardized patients are not widely used outside of the United States, Canada, and Western Europe. In many developing countries, rather than being observed by faculty, it is assumed that directly observing faculty mentors' interactions with patients will provide adequate training to medical students. In these societies, the relationship component of the clinical encounter is often minimized.

International medical graduates frequently come from societies in which there is a rigid hierarchy between students and teachers. International graduates often demonstrate much greater deference toward faculty than their US-trained counterparts. An ongoing Canadian study concluded that an IMGs' medical school experience is characterized by ". . . an authoritarian didactic professor in large group settings." In these countries, two-way exchanges of ideas are also very rare—a learner openly questioning a faculty member would be considered impolite, if not disrespectful. These differences are particularly evident when learners are asked to evaluate their teachers. The US-trained residents and students have considerable experience evaluating faculty; student evaluations are commonly used for promotion and tenure decisions in undergraduate colleges and universities. International Medical Graduates often indicate that they are very uncomfortable evaluating their US faculty and consider it inappropriate.

This reticence to speak up in the presence of authority often extends to rounds and precepting interactions, frequently leading the US-trained faculty member to conclude erroneously that the IMG has a deficient knowledge base. While limited, available patient outcome data suggest otherwise. Norcini and colleagues examined a large pool of patients with congestive heart failure and/or myocardial infarction. The US-licensed IMGs had significantly lower mortality rates compared with patients cared for by the American-educated or the US-citizen IMGs. However, the IMG's knowledge may not be evident in precepting encounters. Rather than providing to preceptors the presenting problem, evaluation results, diagnosis, and plan as USMGs are trained to do, some IMG's may provide only the patient evaluation findings, and not offer problem lists, diagnoses, or treatment recommendations. This reticence is often mistaken for a deficient knowledge base by the US-trained faculty. International Medical Graduates from some cultures may perceive that offering this concluding information without specific prompting from the supervising physician is "showing off" and a sign of disrespect for a faculty member. In many Asian countries, teachers are held in very high esteem and a learner who "knows too much" would be seen as offending a supervising clinician. Even when presenting diagnoses and treatment recommendations, this information may be tentatively communicated out of respect. Similarly, when desiring assistance with a patient, the IMG resident may not make a direct request but expect that the omniscient faculty member will recognize their difficulties and spontaneously provide the necessary help.

CLINICAL ISSUES

Patient Care & Physician–Patient Interaction

Many IMGs come from third-world countries and have a wealth of experience with diseases that their US counterparts rarely see. For example, early childhood death due to diarrhea and parasitic diseases are relatively uncommon in the United States compared with the developing world. The physician–patient relationship also differs across cultures. Many IMGs come from countries in which a paternalistic style of medical practice still predominates. Under the basic tenets of informed consent, patients have a right to know what is wrong with them, what treatments are being recommended, the risks and benefits of the treatment(s), and alternatives—including no treatment. The ultimate decision maker is the patient with the physician acting more as an expert facilitator. This model is in stark contrast to the approach in India described by a family medicine resident from that country:

> In India, the doctor is God-like. "The doctor cured me, saved my life, my God." Whatever the doctor says, that's enough. . . . Patients don't ask questions, they don't doubt. That wouldn't be taken very nicely. "I am the physician. If you are coming to me, my rule goes."

Similar to the authority-based instructional style characteristic of medical schools in many developing countries, IMGs are often accustomed to respectful, deferential patients. Coming from this background, IMGs are likely to be disoriented and perhaps insulted by American patients coming to them requesting specific tests or medications that they have seen on television and the Internet, or that have been recommended by friends. Because much of primary care in the United States emphasizes chronic disease management rather than treatment of acute illness, patient adherence has become a particularly challenging issue. Some IMGs were brought up in systems that have little respect for patients who do not take their antihypertensive medications or follow their diabetic regimen. The concept of having a repertoire of communication skills for enhancing patient adherence is new to IMGs trained in a country where physician authority, power, and control are unquestioned. The idea of a difficult patient, requiring specialized interpersonal management skills, may not have been viewed as part of the physician's responsibility. Models such as the transtheoretical approach in which patient adherence is conceptualized by stages of change (e.g., precontemplation, contemplation, preparation, and action) are unlikely to be part of the IMG's knowledge base. Health behavior change requires active listening, negotiation, setting initially small goals, and providing social support for the patient (see Chapter 19). These skills are unlikely to be taught outside the United States, nor are health behavior models that provide a conceptual framework for counseling these patients.

Even if the IMG begins practice with an appreciation of the American patient as a consumer, there are still concrete challenges, such as language barriers. Often IMGs who have spoken English much of their lives still find conversations with US patients challenging:

> My first day in clinic in the U.S., I couldn't understand most of my patients. My entire education has been in English but these patients could have been from Mars.

Particularly those IMGs who have learned English as a second language find it confusing that their patients do not speak "proper" English. American English is strongly impacted by regional and ethnic factors influencing word choice, idioms, intonation, and emphasis. Similarly, US patients may be unfamiliar with the accent and terminology (some of which includes British words) of IMGs who acquired much of their English outside the United States. Finally, social psychologists suggest that 90% of communication is nonverbal. As anthropologists and international businessmen have noted, gestures and other physical styles of communication are culture bound. For example, the shaking of the head from side-to-side, while meaning "no" to most Westerners is often an expression of agreement among persons from India.

Interactions with the Nonphysician Staff

US medical care is multidisciplinary. International Medical Graduates need to learn to work with and respect social workers, pharmacists, nurses, care managers, nurse practitioners, physicians' assistants, physical therapists, and other professions who are all involved in the care of patients. These teams often have a horizontal rather than hierarchical power configuration. Physicians frequently manage patients as a member of a complex team, and though in many cases they coordinate care, in other instances (e.g., hospice care), nonphysician providers take the lead in many aspects of patient care. As one IMG said: "I can't believe the number of people who tell me how to do things their way—and I'm the one who went to medical school."

In many countries, the interdisciplinary nature of health care is not as well developed, if recognized at all. Physicians are the lead decision makers, and their orders are obeyed unquestioningly. Additionally, in countries with social and economic distinctions, ancillary workers are typically from different social strata than physicians. In US outpatient settings, the easy familiarity existing between staff, including calling physicians by their first names, is often seen as disrespectful and overly familiar by those trained in a more formal, hierarchical system.

Medical Ethics

Many IMGs come from societies where physician paternalism is still the rule. In countries in which physician paternalism predominates, ethical principles such as autonomous informed consent are often not culturally normative. Ethical dilemmas can be evaluated from the perspective of four principles: autonomy, benevolence, nonmaleficence (do no harm), and justice. Over the past 50 years, US health care has deemphasized beneficence and increasingly valued autonomy as a preeminent principle. Changes in disclosing a cancer diagnosis to patients clearly illustrate this historical shift. In 1961, 90% of American oncologists indicated that they would not disclose a cancer diagnosis to a patient. Twenty years later, this pattern had been reversed, in that oncologists routinely informed patients of their condition. The US emphasis on autonomy, which takes the form of giving patients choices about how to treat their condition (e.g., "You could take any of these three medicines; which one would you like to try?"), is likely to be disorienting to IMGs from countries where the physician remains an unchallenged authority.

For a number of years, the first author routinely polled groups of internal medicine residents (comprised of approximately 75% IMGs) about whether physicians in their home countries routinely disclosed serious or terminal conditions to patients. Many, if not most, residents from India, Pakistan, and Eastern Europe responded "no." Cross-cultural research suggests that beneficence typically guides nondisclosure. In these societies, it is seen as cruel to inflict emotional distress on an already ill person through such a disclosure. In Jain and Krieger's study of IMGs' communication strategies, a third year resident expressed distress about American medicine's standard of honesty:

> *The one thing I don't like about the American system is that you are telling the patient face-to-face that he is going to die . . . You are telling a dying patient that he only has a few weeks or months left. . . . [if I was the patient] I wouldn't want to know that.*

In societies in which patients are not informed of their diagnosis, the locus of decision making is likely to differ from the US norm. Family members, often within a network that includes the physician, make medical decisions for the patient. In Pakistan, where family decision making is common, the physician may become adopted into the family and addressed as "parent," "aunt," "uncle," or "sibling."

This collectivist value may conflict with US laws and ethics emphasizing individual autonomy. International Medical Graduates from traditional societies, particularly when treating a patient in the United States from their own ethnic background, may feel caught between the legal requirements for disclosure and their own culture's ethics about proper physician conduct.

Technology

Many IMGs are from countries with far less access to sophisticated laboratory and radiologic testing or choices for pharmacotherapy. As a result, they are often particularly skilled in obtaining maximum information from the history and physical examination, since other data sources are limited. The educational system in many international medical schools rewards acumen in physical exam skills, which is heavily emphasized in evaluating the competence of medical students and residents. The routine of ordering multiple tests is initially surprising to many IMGs: "When I first started my training in the US, I was stunned by the number of tests that we ordered. I wish I had the luxury of ordering an echocardiogram for every heart murmur or a CT scan for every head injury back home!"

The influence of technology has spread to the medical record, commonly used pharmaceutical reference sources, and treatment guidelines—all of which are increasingly digitized in the United States. Personal digital assistants (PDAs) and electronic medical records further challenge physicians trained in systems with significantly less technology.

Meghani and Vijay noted that many IMGs had rarely or never prescribed opioid analgesics. This lack of experience often reflects the limited availability of these drugs in their home countries. For example, the amount of fentanyl available to one person in the United States is the same quantity available to 2323 individuals in the Philippines.

Documentation & Litigation

Depending on their training, IMGs have varying degrees of exposure to medical documentation formats common in the United States. While some are aware of the Subjective, Objective, Assessment, and Plan (SOAP) format, others, once exposed to this approach, cannot understand its significance. The vast majority indicate that the amount of detail required in patient notes far exceeds customary practice in their home countries. Additionally, the presence of third parties "looking over the physician's shoulder" at the chart notes creates some anxiety. One IMG resident observed: "Documentation is a huge issue here. Not just documenting in a professional way, but in a legal way. Every word is important."

Malpractice litigation is a relatively new concept in many developing countries. Concerns such as patient abandonment, negligence, and the dictum "if it isn't written in the chart, it didn't happen," are new to many IMGs. Some report frequently being worried that they have "missed something" in a patient's care that could lead to a lawsuit.

PSYCHOSOCIAL & MENTAL HEALTH ISSUES

IMGs' Views of Psychiatric Conditions

International medical graduates often have different views of psychiatric conditions compared to US-trained residents and faculty. In a qualitative study investigating the behavioral science training of IMG residents prior to coming to the United States, the majority of respondents commented that rates of mental disorders appeared to be higher in the United States than in their home countries. International Medical Graduate residents will sometimes attribute these higher rates to differences in the US social structure—such as the widespread use of nursing homes, elders without visitors in the hospital, and mothers raising several children alone—as the primary reasons there is more depression in the United States. These residents perceive family support to be stronger in their home countries, buffering against mental illness. The well-established finding by the World Health Organization of better outcomes for persons diagnosed with schizophrenia in less-developed versus more-westernized countries provides some indirect support for these observations.

International medical graduates also tend to perceive strong religious faith as a valuable coping skill.

These residents suggest that Americans often become "depressed" in response to chronic or daily struggles, in contrast with their international counterparts who may be more likely to accept their fate and avoid converting emotional distress into a medical condition:

> It is a religious society (India), so if there is a difficult life event, people accept it and move on . . . The strong belief in God means that if something bad happens, that's because of God.

Other cultures share with the United States the belief that psychiatric mental disorders are a form of illness, but the perceived causes of mental illness may differ. For example, in Karachi, Pakistan, Qidwai and Azam found that 30% of primary care patients believed that psychiatric illness was caused by supernatural powers and spirits. These patients commonly sought treatment from a Hakim (12%), spiritual healer (12%), and family support (2.5%).

The stigma of mental illness also affects how these issues are addressed by IMG residents in primary care. In many cultures, mental health issues are viewed as shameful and taboo: "You practically never do this . . . [in my country] . . . psychiatry is for the mad man." Due to their own culturally based misgivings about mental health issues, many residents fear they will offend patients and therefore avoid such questioning.

Views of Mental Health Treatment

Not surprisingly, many IMGs report minimal exposure to behavioral medicine prior to residency education in the United States. Many cultures view anxiety and milder mood disorders as variations on normal functioning rather than as illnesses. In these societies, the prototype of a psychiatric condition is a severe illness such as psychotic depression, bipolar I disorder or schizophrenia. Clinical training often involves observerships or walking rounds in institutions for patients manifesting debilitating psychiatric conditions. One resident from India reported:

> I had minimal training or no training in anxiety and depression. I was in a mental hospital and I had one month. It was in my fourth year. We had lectures for two weeks and two weeks in an institution. We looked at locked-up people all the time. We did not interview patients; we just walked through. It was like looking at specimens.

Even in countries in which primary care physicians inquire about and treat psychiatric symptoms, there may be little diagnostic specificity. For example, one IMG from Bosnia stated:

> Mental health does not look the same there as it does here. In my country, our people are simply "nervous." All psychiatric problems, depression, posttraumatic stress disorder, everything, it is just "nervous." . . . People in my country, they come to the office and say they are nervous, so we just give them some benzodiazepines.

The sociopolitical history in IMGs' home countries may influence how they approach mental disorders. Family physicians in Russia revealed a reluctance to refer for mental health care, in part due to a history, in which psychology and psychiatry were used by the State to control political dissidents. In the Stalinist era it was said, "No person, no problem." Diagnoses such as schizophrenia meant that there was "no person," and the "patient" could be locked up indefinitely in a mental hospital, which was little different than a prison. (This practice has recently been resurrected in Russia by the Putin government.) People became afraid of psychiatrists. As one of the interviewees said, "The fear of that kind of specialist is probably somewhere in the genetic code."

Family Life

International medical graduates, particularly from East Asian countries and the Philippines, are startled by many aspects of US family life, including single-parent families, cohabiting relationships, and serial monogamy. Before beginning residency, IMGs obtain their knowledge about the U.S. families from several sources, including television "talk" shows as well as from listening to the discussions of the personal lives of office staff in settings where they were completing observerships.

Usually, IMGs are stunned by the permissive parenting practices in the United States and the childhood behavior problems that they believe result from this approach. Many find it odd that conditions like childhood ADHD, not commonly diagnosed in their home countries, are so common in the United States. As one resident from Eastern Europe said:

> Parents in this country, they let the kids do whatever they want . . . ADHD is not diagnosed in my country— it's simply a matter of discipline. Here it seems to calm down parents and teachers when you give the kids medicine.

International medical graduates tend to view parental discipline, even when physically harsh, as important for preventing oppositional and disrespectful behavior among children. The notion of child physical abuse is new to many IMGs. They are surprised that the state becomes involved when parents physically discipline their children. Child protective services' power to remove children from their parents' custody is very troubling to many of these residents. What is considered abusive in the United States may be seen as responsible parenting that builds character in their home countries. A resident from India noted that the children of strict parents do very well in school and college. In addition to influencing the clinical context, many IMGs have children of their own that they are raising in a new country with different parenting practices. They may themselves be experiencing conflicts regarding appropriate discipline.

Sexual Behavior

Early sexual experiences are particularly troubling to IMGs raised in traditional societies governed by strong religious and collectivist values. Sciolla and colleagues suggest that IMGs raised in many non-Western cultures may view sexuality as intensely private or even shameful. Premarital sex, while occurring, is a taboo subject.

Our observations of IMG residents suggest two common patient management styles. One approach is to avoid discussing sexuality with adolescents seen in the office. Preceptors often need to remind residents repeatedly to raise these issues (see Chapter 32). Even then, residents often appear uncomfortable with the topic—speaking awkwardly while looking at the floor rather than the patient. The other approach is to accept that the West is a sexually permissive society. The resident may address sexuality in a matter-of-fact, almost business-like manner. For example, an IMG seeing a 14-year-old girl who recently had her first sexual intercourse approached the patient in much the same way as an adult. A Pap smear and pelvic examinations were conducted, and customary guidance about pregnancy, contraception, and safe sex provided. There was no discussion about the circumstances under which the girl had intercourse (e.g., was it coerced?), the age of the partner, or the patient's perspective on the experience. Despite research evidence that early sexual activity is associated with sexual abuse history, smoking cigarettes, and using marijuana, the resident raised none of these issues until some of them were suggested by the behavioral scientist observing the encounter.

Nonmarital cohabitation is also a unique experience for many IMGs. In one instance, a resident from the Asia-Pacific region was seeing a hospitalized patient with injuries reportedly sustained through an assault by her boyfriend. The supervising physician had urged the resident to address the issue with the patient and provide her with resources for victims of domestic violence (see Chapter 38). The IMG was confused and didn't follow through at first. When asked about her reluctance, she responded: "It's not domestic violence. They are just boyfriend and girlfriend; they're dating. Each of them has their own house." The resident was surprised to learn that adult "boyfriends" and "girlfriends" often live together, and domestic violence can indeed occur in these situations.

The increased nuclearization and isolation of generations among the US kinship networks is troubling for IMGs from non-Western cultures, where extended families are common. To those from East Asia, for example, domestic violence in their home country was not a dyadic event with a perpetrator and a victim, but a situation in which the wife's family members would rightfully intrude into the marriage to protect her. The family should handle this problem rather than the medical–legal system:

> Back home, if I hit my wife, they would not take that to the doctor. There is family support. Women are abused here, and they often do not want to do anything about it. Back home, women are hit and their dad says: "Come home." Here, women get put out on the street.

Caring for geriatric patients in institutional settings contributes to a view of American families as isolated and cut-off from their extended kinship network. Residents from societies that care for aging family members at home have difficulty comprehending the practice of placing senior family members in impersonal nursing homes: "Nursing homes do not exist in India—because no son or daughter would ever lose the honor of caring for his or her elders, especially a parent." Similarly, hospitalized patients receiving no visitors—even when family members live nearby—are troubling to IMGs. One resident commented that he could now understand why he saw so many depressed patients here in the United States compared with his home country: "Back home families are crucial. Here, people are left alone. You have a chance to get depressed much more here."

Challenges In Learning Behavioral Science

At a fundamental level, many IMGs are challenged by the inclusion of psychiatry and psychosocial aspects of the patient's life as a significant component of Western medical practice. Coming from societies where diagnosis of mental health problems was often less common and those syndromes that were diagnosed were typically severe, many resident IMGs initially feel inadequate to diagnose and treat these conditions. Early in residency, some IMGs respond by referring nearly all depressed and anxious patients to psychiatrists. It is important that preceptors establish early in training that diagnosis and treatment of common mood and anxiety disorders, dementias, childhood behavior and adjustment problems, as well as sexual dysfunction, are expected competencies. Unless the case is complicated and beyond the scope of a nonspecialist (e.g., schizophrenia), the resident should learn to manage the patient.

Diagnostic interviewing for mental health conditions is particularly challenging for IMGs. After taking the United States Medical Licensing Exam (USMLE), most IMGs are familiar with the Diagnostic and Statistical Manual of Mental Disorders (DSM) system and the use of explicit criteria for diagnosis. It may be difficult for them, however, to convert these dimensions to conversational questions. Often the questions tend to be verbatim recitations of the DSM criteria and have a stilted quality that confuses the patient (e.g., "Are you having feelings of worthlessness or inappropriate guilt?" Or "Do you have chronic feelings of emptiness?"). IMGs often recognize that they do not know how to ask about these types of symptoms and consequently omit them. This reluctance may be particularly pronounced for questions about self-harm, suicide, abuse, and illegal acts. One IMG resident describes his experience of learning how to ask sensitive questions:

First, you are very uncomfortable, then you feel better and better . . . how to ask questions, how to ask about suicide. For me, that was very embarrassing. I was surprised people responded normally to these questions. "How will this influence her relationship with me?"

Another IMG said:

In my country, if I asked a woman with a child if she was married, she'd get mad at me.

During their behavioral science training, we have noticed unspoken discomfort when IMG residents are asked to interview, for example, a 14-year-old unwed mother, an openly lesbian couple, or divorced parents—each present with their new spouse. The resident who has done quite well interviewing other patients with psychosocial issues often seems at a loss about how to proceed with these family configurations. After sensing that they are uncomfortable asking the patient(s) further questions, the behavioral science faculty member will take over the interview for awhile. Later in the interview, we typically try to turn it back over to the resident who often at this point appears less confused and can follow the faculty member's lead. After the encounter, when asked about their reaction and reason for not continuing the interview, a common response is something like:

I know these relationships exist in America, but I have never seen them face-to-face. I don't know what to say to these people.

RECOMMENDATIONS FOR IMPROVING THE EDUCATION & TRAINING OF INTERNATIONAL MEDICAL GRADUATES

General Suggestions

More recently, several programs of educational research and training recommendations for IMGs have emerged. The ECFMG has produced a series of brief video physician–patient vignettes addressing confidentiality, patient requests for specific therapies based on Internet information, interaction with pediatric patients and adolescents, customer service, child abuse, informed consent, and working with nursing staff.

A consistent theme arising in recent research on IMGs is their experience of being "second class citizens." Having been educationally and often professionally successful in their home countries, proving oneself in a new country and health care system is frustrating and onerous. This issue is particularly sensitive for those IMGs who had practiced independently in their home countries and now are having to undergo re-training. Alienation, loneliness, and anger are common emotional reactions to these challenges. Some residents have shared their fear that they may be unsuccessful in the long sought-after US residency program and be required to return to their home countries. Fears of revealing any knowledge deficiencies may prevent IMGs from directly asking for appropriate faculty assistance. When providing clinical supervision to IMGs, educators should maintain awareness of these underlying dynamics.

International medical graduates would benefit from early acclimatization. Instead of the typical July 1 start date, it would be helpful if some preparatory experiences could begin at least 8–12 weeks before the formal residency year begins. English immersion, and when possible including information on common US medical abbreviations as well as idiomatic English experiences, would be helpful for IMGs with uneven abilities in written and/or spoken English. For those residents who learned English late in life and whose accent is a barrier to understanding, there are specialists in accent reduction who can be quite helpful. There are CD-ROMs and other resources for learning specialized medical terminology.

Other areas that could become part of a preresidency curriculum include medical documentation, the mechanics of ordering lab work and radiographic studies, writing prescriptions, and how to use a PDA. An overview of the US health care system including legal, ethical, and insurance issues would also be valuable. Basic medical interviewing skills can be taught through use of videotapes, simulated patients and role-plays. One resource that may be helpful is the *Doc.com* interactive web-based curriculum on clinician–patient communication, produced by the American Academy on Communication in Healthcare (see "Other Resources" at the end of chapter). The general "style" that a primary care physician uses when relating to patients, however, is difficult to reduce to a set of skills. IMGs might benefit from shadowing faculty or seasoned primary care physicians as they see patients.

The individualist–collectivist distinction that plays a significant role in ethics and determining moral responsibilities should be discussed explicitly in the context of ethical decision making, end-of-life care, and other relevant areas in medicine. For both US-trained physicians as well as IMGs, an open exploration of these issues, including their cultural and religious background, would allow all physicians to be more sensitive with a broader cultural array of patients.

When IMG residents are having apparent difficulty meeting performance criteria, faculty should consider both cultural and language issues. As anyone who has learned a second language knows, people can appear to understand even if they are only picking up bits and pieces of what is being said. The deference that IMGs show toward faculty may be misinterpreted as a lack of assertiveness, an absence of independent thinking, inadequate knowledge base, or poor motivation. Before drawing conclusions, it would be helpful to have several supportive, noncritical conversations with these residents to better understand their background. During observation of clinical interactions with patients, we noted that an IMG from Pakistan never sat down during any of four to five encounters. In our discussion afterward, the resident indicated that she knew that sitting was the correct thing to do in terms of carrying out an effective interview, but thought it would be disrespectful to sit while the supervisor was present. If we had not clarified this point, we would have "graded" her interview skills as less than optimal.

Suggestions For Teaching Psychiatry & Psychosocial Medicine

Psychosocial content should be introduced early in the first year of residency. To address educational and training needs in behavioral science, a formal block rotation can be scheduled during the resident's first year. At our program, we added a first-year rotation in addition to the second-year rotation that had been in place for many years. The first-year behavioral science rotation focused more on effective interview skills and several common psychiatric conditions, while the second-year block focuses exclusively on diagnosing and treating mental disorders.

To help residents with wording questions about psychiatric symptoms, we heeded their advice and developed a series of "cheat sheets." Specifically, we made up a series of laminated cards (they easily fit into a lab coat) with helpful questions to elicit symptoms for many common psychiatric disorders. These became very popular among residents.

Faculty should be aware that patients with diverse backgrounds, customs, and family configurations are likely to be somewhat disconcerting to the IMG resident. In an individual discussion with a resident, the faculty member may want to begin by asking questions such as, "How often have you had the experience of . . . interviewing an openly gay male, a teenager being raised by foster parents, or a patient who requests a specific test that you don't think is indicated? Would physicians see patients or situations like these in your home country? Why do you think it's different here?" The faculty member should demonstrate genuine interest in the resident's experiences, respect, and intellectual curiosity during this exchange. These conversations can be useful learning experiences for both parties. Next, the clinical instructor should provide some focused information on the topic (e.g., "In the inner city, up to 50% of children are being raised by grandparents. Research shows that raising grandchildren has a negative effect on the grandparents' health compared to grandparents not raising grandchildren." Or, "About a third of the US children are born to unmarried women. What is your reaction to that norm?")

We typically do joint patient interviews with residents as part of their behavioral science training. This allows observational learning of the faculty's unspoken acceptance of patients and a way of responding to them "like anyone else." In discussing these issues with IMGs, faculty should appreciate the extent to which patterns of family organization, views of the physician role, and so forth, are culturally relative. For example, many Westerners who automatically accept the norm of "companionate marriage"—a product of an extended friendship, dating relationship, and often a period of cohabitation—may be disturbed by the East Asian custom of arranged marriage. However, the teacher's genuine, noncritical interest in the background of arranged marriages often creates a climate in which the IMG is receptive to learning about the US relationship variations.

As many seasoned clinical faculty know, patients can be great teachers. IMGs who have been successful in understanding the US patients in a cultural context approach these patients with respect, intellectual curiosity, concern, and a genuine desire to learn. While obtaining pertinent historical and symptomatic information, these physicians can also encourage patients to "tell their story," and in so doing provide meaning and satisfaction for both doctor and patient.

SUGGESTED READINGS

Guey-Chi Chen P, Nunez-Smith M, Bernheim SM, et al. Professional experiences of international medical graduates practicing primary care in the United States. *J Gen Intern Med* 2010;25:947–953.

Huijskens EGW, Hooshiaran A, Scherpbier A, et al. Barriers and facilitating factors in the professional careers of international medical graduates. *Med Ed* 2010;44:795–804.

Jain P, Krieger JL. Moving beyond the language barrier: The communication strategies used by international medical graduates in intercultural medical encounters. *Patient Educ Couns* 2011;84:98–104.

Meghani SH, Rajput V. The need for practice socialization of international medical graduates—An exemplar from pain medicine. *Acad Med* 2011;86:571–574.

Norcini JJ, Boulet JR, Dauphinee WD, Opalek A, Krantz ID, Anderson ST. Evaluating the quality of care provided by graduates of international medical schools. *Health Affairs* 2010;29:1461–1468.

Sciolla A, Ziajko LA, Salguero ML. Sexual health competence of international medical graduate psychiatric residents in the United States. *Acad Psychiatr* 2010;34:351–368.

Searight HR, Gafford J. Cultural diversity at the end of life: issues and guidelines for family physicians. *Am Fam Physician* 2005;71:515–522.

Searight HR, Gafford J. Behavioral science education and the international medical graduate. *Acad Med* 2006;81:164–170.

OTHER RESOURCES

Novack DH, Clark W, Saizow R, et al., eds. *Doc.com: An Interactive Learning Resource for Healthcare Communication.* American Academy on Communication in Healthcare Web site. http://aachonline.org. Accessed October 2011.

WEB SITES

Educational Commission for Foreign Medical Graduates. http://www.ecfmg.org/. Accessed April, 2013.

International medical graduates in American medicine: Contemporary challenges and opportunities. American Medical Association, 2010. http://www.ama-assn.org/resources/doc/img/img-workforce-paper.pdf. Accessed April 2013.

A longitudinal cross-sequential study of the professional integration of international medical graduates (IMGs): From application to licensure. An interim report, April, 2011 Co-investigators: Claudio Violato, David Watt, Deidre Lake Website: www.m-cap.ca/pdf/IMGStudyInterimReport_Apr2011.pdf. Accessed April 2013.

SECTION III
Working with Specific Populations

Families

Mitchell D. Feldman, MD, MPhil & Steven R. Hahn, MD

INTRODUCTION

Our experience of health, illness, and health care, as patients and as practitioners, occurs in a social context. The "family" is at the heart of that context. Making the patient's social context an explicit part of medical care affects every step of the clinical process, from basic assumptions about who the patient is to the conceptual framework for the database, theories of causality, and the implementation of treatment. Consider the following vignettes:

1. Despite wondering whether she could have done something more for Joe, the doctor is gratified and reassured by the family's overwhelming thanks for the "wonderful care" she provided for the past 10 years, and in particular during the time preceding the patient's death. The family is grateful for her help in family discussions about end-of-life care.

2. Eric is a 40-year-old man with diabetes who has extraordinary difficulty following a reasonable diet. His partner has been unwilling to change his expectations about their meal plans and he has been unable to negotiate a change with him.

3. Mary, 50 years old and previously without complaints, presents with headaches that have been ongoing for 2 months. She is afraid she has a tumor or "something bad." A brief discussion about her family reveals that her 60-year-old husband has been depressed and forgetful for at least 6 months. Two months ago he got lost on his way home from the hardware store. After her doctor listens to her story, she agrees that she too is depressed and very concerned about her husband. She is upset that he has

refused to see a doctor. She accepts her doctor's offer to help her get him evaluated, but she is still worried that her headache is something bad.

4. Eva, who is 27 years old, has multiple somatic complaints and panic disorder. She was raised by her grandmother after her mother died, and when her grandmother died 4 years later, by an aunt 20 years her elder. She and her aunt became very close, "almost like sisters, we did everything together." After completing college she returned to live with her aunt, who had recently begun the first serious relationship of her life. Eva does not understand why her aunt needs a boyfriend, and reports that her panic attacks often interrupt her aunt's plans to spend time alone with her fiancé.

In every case, the family context is critical to understanding the situation. In the case of Joe, the doctor has attended to both patient and family and the family is a partner in care and grief. Family function has become a significant barrier to critical self-care for Eric. Mary is having a psychophysiologic reaction to family stress. Eva is a vulnerable young woman whose panic disorders are not only partially a response to her aunt's perceived abandonment but also a high-cost and inadequate "solution."

All health care providers have an intuitive understanding about "the family" and how families work and develop. However, lack of clinically useful tools for making the family an explicit part of care may prevent successful application of this knowledge. Caring for the patient in the context of the family goes beyond involving some families in the management of care. Two case illustrations are presented throughout the chapter that will illustrate the conceptual foundation and basic skills of family assessment and intervention.

THE FAMILY AS THE CONTEXT OF ILLNESS

The family is the primary social context of experience, including that of health and illness. The individual's awareness and perception of health and disease are shaped by the family, as are decisions about whether, how, and from whom to seek help. Use of health care services and acceptance of and adherence to medical treatments are all influenced by the family.

Reciprocal Relationships

There is a reciprocal relationship between healthy family systems and the physical and mental health of its members. Physical symptoms and illness can significantly influence the family's emotional state and behavior, often causing dysfunction in family relationships; and dysfunction in the family system can generate stress and lead to physical illness. Dysfunctional family systems can incorporate a physical illness and symptoms into the family's behavioral patterns, thereby reinforcing the sick role for one or more members and sustaining or exacerbating illness and symptoms. In these "somatizing" families, the presence and persistence of the symptom or illness cannot be understood without examining its meaning in the context of the family.

What Is a Family?

Our understanding of family is based on our experience with our own family and experiences with the families of others. The variety of groups that make up a family is enormous: two-parent nuclear families, single-parent families, foster parents with children from different biological families, families of divorcees blended through remarriage, families with gay or lesbian couples as parents, and married or cohabiting couples without any children. In some cultures, the "family" may be other members of the clan who are not related by blood or marriage. Isolated elderly individuals may think of their home health attendants as family, and for other solitary individuals the only family they may know is their pets.

All of these groups can be experienced as families. They share similarities in the structure of the relationships between their members and the role that the family group plays for the individuals and for the society in which the group exists. So, rather than define the family in terms of its members, we describe it as a *system having certain functional roles*.

The Role of the Family

Family relationships are described more by their roles than by the labels traditionally applied to individuals.

Table 11-1. The role of the family: a partial list.

- Reproduction
- Supervision of children
- Food, shelter, and clothing
- Emotional support
- Education: technical, social, and moral
- Religious training
- Health care—nursing
- Financial support
- Entertainment and recreation

For example, in one family an elderly woman may obtain companionship and emotional support from a home health attendant, a friend at the local senior citizen's center, and a daughter, whereas a woman in another family may find these needs met by her marital partner. In one society, the primary education and socialization of children may be accomplished in the household of the child's parent(s) and in community schools. In another, parent collective or unrelated individuals may accomplish these educational tasks, and play a more prominent, family-like role in children's lives. Hence, for health care practitioners, the patient's family context must be understood as the individuals in the social system, who are involved in the roles and tasks that are of central importance to the patient (Table 11-1).

The Family as a System

Families as systems are characterized by:

1. External and internal boundaries;
2. An internal hierarchy;
3. Self-regulation through feedback;
4. Change with time, specifically family life cycle changes.

The qualities of these four system characteristics in a particular family help shape the family's internal milieu and functioning.

BOUNDARIES

The family is partially separated from the outside world by a set of behaviors and norms that are embedded in specific cultural systems. Family boundaries are created by norms that determine who interacts with whom, in what way, and around what activities. For example, teaching children "not to talk to strangers" creates a boundary around the family. Different parts of the family system (i.e., subsystems), such as "the parents" and "the children," or each "individual," are separated from one another by boundaries. Internal boundaries work in the same way: children who speak back to a parent may be told that they "don't know their place"; they have crossed a boundary that defines their role. Healthy boundaries balance the individual identity of family subsystems with the openness required for interaction and communication across boundaries.

INTERNAL HIERARCHY

Subsystems of the family relate to one another hierarchically: parents have authority over the children, the older children over the younger children, and so on. A healthy hierarchy is clear and flexible enough to evolve with the needs of the family, and localizes power and control in those who are the most competent. Hierarchies may become dysfunctional for a number of reasons; for example, when they are unable to adapt to change, when the allocation of power or authority is not consistent with the location of expertise or competence in the family, or when the lines of authority are blurred and effective decisions cannot be made.

SELF-REGULATION THROUGH FEEDBACK

Relationships within the boundaries of the family system and its subsystems are regulated by "feedback." All behaviors in the family set a series of actions in motion that in turn influence the original actor.

Feedback maintains the integrity of the family system as a unit, establishes and maintains hierarchies, and regulates the function of boundaries in accordance with the individual family's norms and style. This tendency toward maintaining "homeostasis" is critical. All family systems must learn to balance the desire for stability with the inevitable need to evolve and change.

CHANGE AND THE FAMILY LIFE CYCLE

The family must continually adapt as its members evolve both biologically and socially (Table 11-2). For example, the family with young children must protect them within the boundaries of the family (or that of specific delegates, such as the schools). Adolescents need to achieve a degree of independence and the ability to function without immediate adult supervision. To facilitate this, the family must develop new norms of behavior and relax the boundary between the child and the world and redraw the boundaries between parent and child (e.g., provide more areas of autonomy and privacy). Each stage of the family life cycle presents new challenges, and healthy families are able to modify their hierarchic relationships and boundaries. Families whose

Table 11-2. The family life cycle.

Life Cycle Stage	Dominant Theme	Transitional Task
The single young adult	Separating from family of origin	Differentiation from family of origin Developing intimate relationships with peers Establishing career and financial independence
Forming a committed relationship	Commitment to a new family	Formation of a committed relationship Forming and changing relationships with both families of origin
The family with young children	Adjusting to new family members	Adjusting the relationship to make time and space for children Negotiating parenting responsibilities Adjusting relationships with extended families to incorporate parenting and grandparenting
The family with adolescents	Increasing flexibility of boundaries to allow for children's independence	Adjusting boundaries to allow children to move in and out of the family more freely Attending to midlife relationship and career issues Adjusting to aging parent's needs and role
Launching children	Accepting exits and entries into the system	Adjusting committed relationship to absence of children in the household Adjusting relationships with children to their independence and adult status Including new in-laws and becoming grandparents Adjusting to aging or dying parents' needs and role
The family later in life	Adjusting to age and new roles	Maintaining functional status, developing new social and familial roles Supporting central role of middle generation Integrating the elderly into family life Dealing with loss of parents, spouse, peers; life review and integration

Source: Adapted, with permission, from Carter CA, McGoldrick M, eds. *The Family Life Cycle: A Framework for Family Therapy.* New York, NY: Gardner Press, 1980.

boundaries, hierarchies, and self-regulatory feedback are dysfunctional have difficulties at each transition.

HEALTH AND ILLNESS IN FAMILIES: THE "SICK ROLE"

Behavior in social settings can be understood in terms of "roles" that are shaped by shared expectations, rules, and beliefs. All roles have prerequisites, obligations, and benefits or dispensations. One such role is the "sick role," which is temporarily and conditionally granted to individuals when they have an illness perceived to be beyond their control, seek professional help and adhere to treatment, and accept the social stigma associated with being sick. Individuals in the sick role are exempt from many of their usual obligations and entitled to special attention and resources. The sick role therefore has a profound effect on relationships within the family.

The exemption from obligations that is part of the sick role is critical to recovery from illness and adaptation to disability. The obligations and stigmatization of the sick role are important to protect others from abuse. Physicians play a critical role in establishing the legitimacy of the sick role by certifying the prerequisite illness or disability, and attesting to adequate adherence to treatment. Because the sick role has such a profound effect on the family of the sick individual, physicians' obligate role in establishing the sick role makes them a powerful actor in the patient's family system, and makes the family system an intrinsic part of the doctor–patient relationship, whether the physician is aware of these ramifications or not.

The Doctor–Patient–Family Relationship & the Compensatory Alliance

A positive relationship with an active and concerned family can be one of the physician's most powerful tools and rewarding clinical experiences. In these circumstances, working with the family seems quite natural and the complexities of the doctor–patient–family relationship are not apparent. On the other hand, when significant family problems exist, the doctor–patient relationship can become entangled in the family system's dysfunction.

When one or more members have assumed the sick role in response to family problems, the task of providing appropriate care for the patient may be subverted and subsumed by family dysfunction. Some families can achieve internal stability and meet the needs of their members only when one or more individuals are perceived as being sick.

The physician's role in determining that the patient is entitled to the special prerogatives and dispensations of the "sick role" makes the physician a central and powerful member of these family systems. The authority to prescribe changes in role function for the patient further involves the physician in the life of the entire family. In effect, the physician and patient develop an alliance that compensates for the dysfunction and deficit at home. Hahn, Feiner, and Bellin have termed this a *compensatory alliance.*

When the physician is unaware of underlying family dysfunction, the compensatory alliance can become dysfunctional and contribute to somatization and noncompliance, and support the ultimately inadequate coping mechanism afforded by the sick role.

PATIENT CARE IN THE CONTEXT OF THE FAMILY: FAMILY ASSESMENT & INTERVENTION FOR PRIMARY CARE

General Considerations

Treating the patient in the context of the family requires a practical method that can be learned and used by health care providers in real world practice and training. The large number of tasks that occupy the provider places limits on the complexity of and time available for family assessment and intervention. A family assessment and intervention method must be focused, time efficient, and consistent with the general scope of care.

All patients should receive a "basic" family assessment that allows the doctor to understand how the family milieu will influence the basic tasks of care, and that identifies family problems requiring intervention (Table 11-3). Basic family assessment consists of two

Table 11-3. Goals of basic family assessment and intervention.

- Understand the pattern of family involvement with the patient's medical problems.
- Communicate with other family members about the management of patient's medical problems.
- Recognize the presence of problem behaviors (e.g., alcohol or drug abuse, somatization, domestic violence, physician experience of the patient as "difficult") and family dysfunction affecting the patient's medical problems or functional status, which require further assessment and intervention.
- Assess the family's behavioral and emotional response to the patient's problems, and provide emotional support to the patient and family.
- Provide counseling to enhance the family's emotional and functional adaptation to the patient's medical problems.
- Perform a preliminary assessment of the doctor–patient–family relationship and recognize a "dysfunctional compensatory alliance" when present or developing.
- Refer the patient or family for further assessment and intervention, or obtain a family systems consultation.
- Understand the triangular relationships and repetitive patterns of interaction among members of the family system, including the development of a "dysfunctional compensatory alliance" in the doctor–patient–family triangle.

processes: (1) conducting a genogram-based interview and identifying the relevant family life cycle stages, and (2) screening for family problems that are associated with family life cycle stage tasks, or the patient's medical problems. A subset of patients with problems rooted in serious family dysfunction will then require the four-step family intervention described below.

Treating the patient in the context of the family does not necessarily mean bringing the family into the examining room and in adult medicine usually does not. Family assessment and intervention can be accomplished by meeting exclusively with the patient, though meeting with other family members is very often desirable, sometimes necessary, and almost always enhances the care. Using a family systems orientation without meeting directly with other family members requires the ability to explore the life of the family and bring the family into the room through the patient's narrative.

The genogram-based interview, described below, is a powerful technique for accomplishing this goal. However, the task of understanding the patient's family system in this way can be complicated by the fact that patients often give a distorted and incomplete presentation of family life. Such distortion may be conscious, unknowing, or some of both. Therefore, clinicians need to learn to infer what is going on at home—to "see the family over the patient's shoulder"—by imagining how members of the patient's family might be reacting or behaving in ways that the patient does not understand or would not report.

BASIC FAMILY ASSESSMENT: CONDUCTING A GENOGRAM-BASED INTERVIEW, IDENTIFYING FAMILY LIFE CYCLE STAGE ISSUES, & SCREENING FOR PROBLEMS

 CASE ILLUSTRATION 1

Ariana is a 40-year-old Italian-American woman with multiple somatic complaints. She has complained of chronic diarrhea, dyspepsia, and "asthma" but has had a thorough normal gastrointestinal (GI) and pulmonary evaluation. She has made multiple visits to her primary provider and to an urgent care clinic, has been hospitalized two times, and has been seen in several subspecialty clinics. She has made an average of 15 visits per year for the past several years.

Constructing a Genogram

The first step to treating the patient in the context of the family is to create a picture of the family by conducting a "genogram-based interview." A genogram is a graphic representation of the members of a family. It uses the iconography of the genetic pedigree (Figures 11-1 and 11-2) and can be used to record data ranging from family medical history to life events and employment, as well as family issues. The overall objective of the genogram interview is to help the patient tell the family's story.

CONDUCTING A GENOGRAM INTERVIEW

Begin with a blank page, or a designated section of the patient's chart. Place the genogram where the patient can see it and draw a family tree with the patient's help. Note important dates such as marriages, divorces, and deaths, and the general location of individuals in other households. Family systems data can be recorded using lines to enclose household boundaries, double lines between individuals to indicate strong relationships or coalitions, jagged lines to indicate conflict, and triple lines to indicate dysfunctional over-involvement. At subsequent visits take a brief look at the genogram to recall the patient's family context, and expand or alter the genogram as the family changes or new issues arise.

FOCUSING THE GENOGRAM

The type of information explored, the number of generations, and the level of detail included in the genogram depend on an initial sense of the importance of family issues. A detailed, comprehensive genogram interview going back more than one generation can be a powerful clinical tool but is too complex for everyday practice. The genogram must be "focused" on the most clinically useful information while providing the foundation for treating the patient in the context of the family. As with most clinical databases, it is harder to know what can safely be excluded than it is to include the entire range of family-oriented data. However, skillful parsimony is acquired with experience, and efficiency is produced by following three principles:

1. Engage patients and encourage active participation—they will take you to the heart of the story.
2. Focus the interview on family life cycle tasks and issues—they are almost always the focal point of stress and dysfunction.
3. Draw and examine the genogram—a picture is worth thousand words (e.g., picture a single mother, six children, parents, and siblings in another country; three different fathers in various places; and a new boyfriend).

Begin with the core members of the family, that is, household members, parents, children, and past and present partners and spouses. Identify the family life cycle stage of the patient's family from the ages, relationships, and household composition of the nucleus of the patient's family. As described below, the family life

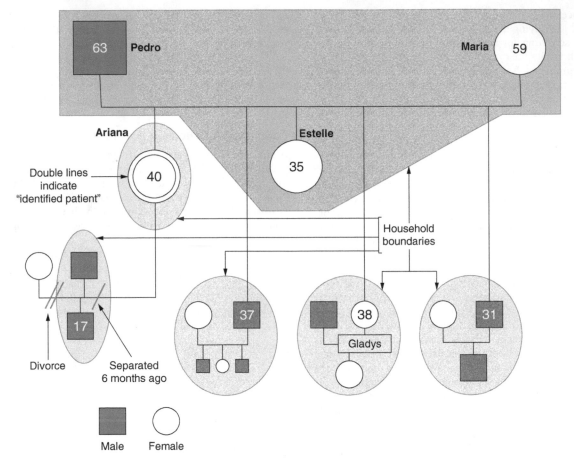

Figure 11-1. Genogram showing household composition and key family members in Ariana's family (Case Illustration 1).

cycle stage will almost always predict the locus of stress, challenge, or conflict in the patient's family system.

Inquire about the family's responses to any known or presenting problems, and to issues identified using the family life cycle screening questions described later. If no significant major problems or dysfunctions are identified, stop the focused genogram interview when you understand the family well enough to take the family into consideration in addressing the patient's medical and other problems. If significant family problems are discovered, continue with the four-step family intervention described later.

Figure 11-1 shows the skeleton of the genogram for Case Illustration 1. The amount of information you gather about each individual and the family should be guided by the evolution of your hypotheses about family function as you go along. When major family issues emerge from the shape of the genogram or the patient's narrative, exploration of family relationships and history can be very focused. If the nature of family issues is

initially obscure, but you suspect something important is going on, expand the genogram to include more peripheral family members and examine individual relationships more completely.

In general, it is useful to obtain brief descriptions of family members and important relationships, the history of major life events, immigrations, and comings and goings from the household(s). Record important information on the genogram as the interview progresses to create a picture of the family. Remember, the greatest efficiency in the genogram interview comes from the patient's active participation.

Identifying the Family Life Cycle Stage & Predicting Stress & Conflict

FAMILY LIFE CYCLE STAGE ASSESSMENT

Determining the life cycle stage of the family is the first task of a genogram assessment. The stages of the life

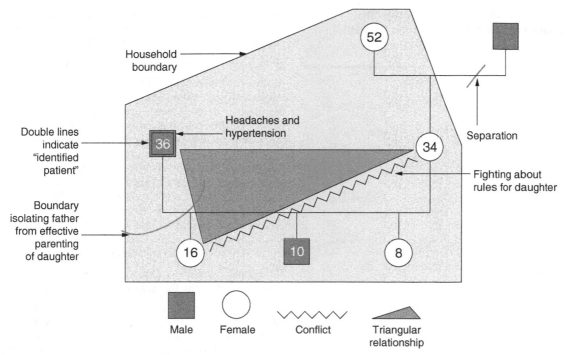

Figure 11-2. Genogram of the family in Case Illustration 2.

cycle are a road map for exploring the important issues in the life of a patient and family.

The family life cycle consists of six stages (Table 11-2). Each stage is grounded in biologically driven and socially and culturally shaped patterns of individual development. The cycle usually "begins" with the separation of the individual from the family of origin (stage 1), followed by the formation of a new family (stage 2), the raising and "launching" of children into the world (stages 3, 4, and 5), and the family later in life (stage 6). Each of these stages is dominated by a theme and principal task. Each task requires two to four major changes in family structure and function. More often than not, family problems revolve around difficulty with one or more of the developmental tasks of the family's life cycle stage. Of course, the family life cycle is grounded in a specific sociopolitical and cultural context that helps to determine and shape the themes and tasks of each stage.

THE FAMILY LIFE CYCLE: ROLES AND GENERATIONS

With each stage of the family life cycle individuals acquire new roles: for example, from single adult to husband or wife *and simultaneously* to son or daughter-in-law. Note these roles as you and the patient scan the genogram. A directed open-ended question to screen for problems in each role is an efficient way of exploring the patient's relationships: "What's it like being a grandmother of six? Joe's wife? The daughter of a 95 year old?" If the patient is suitably activated, the whole story may come out after the first inquiry: "Being a grandmother is great, it's being a mother-in-law that I can't stand!"

THE LIFE CYCLE AND PATTERNS OF PARENTING

In probing for life cycle problems, be sensitive to the influence of culture, ethnicity, and social class on norms and expected patterns. Pay particular attention to the structure of the parental subsystem: the adaptational strategies of families with one parent, one "working" and one "child care" parent, two working parents, families with extended-family parenting, blended families, and so on have differences that can be anticipated.

CASE ILLUSTRATION 1: DISCUSSION

Ariana (see Figure 11-1) is in the first stage of the family life cycle, an unattached young adult, in her case between families. Her divorce from her husband suggests difficulty forming a new family and moving on to the second stage of the family life cycle. It is noteworthy that the patient's sister Estelle is still at home and having difficulty with the first phase of the life cycle.

Screening for Family Function

After drawing the genogram and determining the life cycle stage of the family, the next step is to screen for

Table 11-4. Presentations and problems associated with family dysfunction that should trigger screening for family dysfunction.

- Noncompliance with self-care regimens
- Alcohol or substance abuse
- Mental disorders, especially psychotic, mood, and anxiety disorders
- Unexplained medical symptoms and somatization
- Physician-experienced difficulty in the doctor–patient relationship (i.e., the "difficult patient")
- Health-related habitual behaviors—smoking, eating disorders
- Newly diagnosed, rapidly deteriorating, or frightening illnesses (e.g., HIV infection, cancer, end-stage renal disease, myocardial infarction)
- Disruptions and change in the family system—divorce, separation, death, immigration, or emigration
- Natural and social disaster or trauma—fires, floods, earthquakes, crimes
- Sexually transmitted illness
- Anniversary dates and important holidays
- Domestic violence
- Reproductive health—pregnancy, termination of pregnancy, family planning

family problems (Table 11-4). An activated patient will do the work of screening for you and immediately describe the "real problems." If the patient is reticent or the problem more obscure, the following strategies should aid the exploration.

GLOBAL FAMILY FUNCTION

Begin screening for family problems with open-ended questions about global family function (Table 11-5). The tone and content of the questions should be nonjudgmental, and even normalize the presence of problems, for example, "All families have their ups and downs, how's yours doing these days with all that is going on in your life?" An effective initial inquiry directs the patient's attention to family issues, in general leaving the patient free rein to respond.

SCREENING FOR FAMILY LIFE CYCLE PROBLEMS

If a question about global function does not provide the necessary information, ask a few screening questions about the life cycle tasks that confront the patient's family. For example, the genogram in Figure 11-2 indicates that this family will be dealing with the tasks of "the family with young children" and "the family with adolescents" (see Table 11-2). Six questions, one for each of the three tasks in these two different life cycle stages, can screen for life cycle problems (Table 11-6). However, it is likely that not all of these six questions will have to be asked to identify sources of difficulty, especially if the unique features of any particular family are used to select the initial questions.

SCREENING FOR FAMILY DIFFICULTY WITH THE PATIENT'S MEDICAL PROBLEMS AND SYMPTOMS

The presence of somatization is one of the most important indications for exploring the patient's family, because it is usually driven by the patient's and/or family's need to have the patient occupy the sick role. An effective strategy for exploring the role of symptoms and medical problems in families is to follow the sequence: *symptom—function—family response. Symptom*—"Tell me about your symptom." *Function*—"How does your symptom affect your functioning, your normal activities, and ability to do what is expected?" *Family response*—"If you can't do these things, who does? What does your family do and say?"

SCREENING WITH RED FLAG PROBLEMS

Whenever a problem associated with family dysfunction is present, the physician should screen for the family's reaction and response (see Tables 11-4 and 11-5). Many of these problems are emotionally charged and stigmatizing. Nonjudgmental, normalizing, and directive

Table 11-5. Family assessment screening questions.

Category	Example
Open-ended assessment of family problems	"How are things going with your family? How is everyone getting along?""Are you having any problems with (name the key individuals in the genogram)?"
Family problems with the patient's medical problems	"How is your family dealing with your medical problems?""How is (name the key individuals in the genogram) dealing with it. What is their reaction?"
Problems associated with family dysfunction (see Table 11-4)	"I know you have been feeling quite depressed lately, how has your family reacted to that?""What has (name the key individuals) said or done about your depression?"
Family life cycle problems	"I see you have a houseful of adolescents. I know that can be quite difficult. How have you been bearing up?"
Problems in the doctor–patient–family relationship: the compensatory alliance	"What does your family think and feel about the suggestions I have made?""What were you hoping I might say to or do about your family?"

Table 11-6. Family life cycle screening questions for families with young children and adolescents.

Stage 3—The family with young children
How are you doing with making time and space in your lives for three children?
How are you and your wife managing with child care responsibilities?
How are you getting along with the children's grandparents, *particularly your mother-in-law,** and your other in-laws?

Stage 4—The family with adolescents
How are you doing with a teenager, *your daughter,* in the house, and setting rules and expectations?
How are you and your wife doing with your work or careers?
Your youngest is going to go to school all day now. Will that change your or your wife's responsibilities or activities?
What concerns do you have about the health or functioning of your parents or in-laws, *particularly your mother-in-law?*

*Generic questions for this stage of the family life cycle are shown in regular type, questions or elements in italic are modifications *specific for the family of the father* (see Figure 11-2).

questions are therefore critical. These issues often have immediate clinical and legal implications and raise issues of confidentiality that need to be addressed.

SCREENING FOR PROBLEMS IN THE DOCTOR–PATIENT–FAMILY RELATIONSHIP

Throughout the family assessment, consider what role you may be playing in the family system and be alert to the development of dysfunctional alliances with the patient or other family members. Ask the patient or other family members what reactions the family has had to health care providers' suggestions or interventions. It is also useful to determine what the patient wants you to say to other family members. Often these hopes and expectations are implied by patients' words or behavior rather than stated, because patients may not be fully aware of what they want, are too embarrassed to ask for it, or do not feel they have permission to make the request explicit.

 CASE ILLUSTRATION 1 (CONTD.)

In response to an open-ended question about how things are going at home, Ariana immediately identifies as the major problem the stress that Estelle's illness places on her mother and the pressure her mother puts on her (Ariana) to help out. Regarding her family's reaction to her own medical problems, Ariana says her mom has difficulty understanding why she's always so sick. Ariana's sister Gladys has

come right out and said that she doesn't think Ariana's problems should be taken seriously. Ariana feels that the pressure of her mother's demands makes it difficult to think about getting involved with anyone. She blames her divorce on her ex-stepson's wildness and her ex-husband's inability to control him. Ariana thinks her mother is depressed about Estelle's illness, and suspects that she resents Estelle's continued dependence but can't admit it to herself or anyone else. Asked what she would like her physician to do in terms of her problems at home, Ariana says that she would like the physician to make her family understand that she really is sick. (Figure 11-3 shows the genogram at this stage of the family assessment.)

Treating the Patient in the Context of the Family: Communicating about & Caring for the Patient's Medical Problems

After completing the basic genogram, assessing the family life cycle stage, and screening for problems in family function, the practitioner should be able to provide basic medical care for the patient in the context of the family (Table 11-7). With the majority of families, the interventions described in this step accomplish the basic goals of family assessment and no further intervention is needed (see Table 11-3). A basic family assessment will, by itself, facilitate the following.

ENHANCING THE THERAPEUTIC ALLIANCE

Perhaps the most important consequence of conducting a family systems assessment is to enhance the therapeutic alliance among the patient, provider, and other family members. Patients' perception that their physician cares for them is probably the single most important variable in the formation of a successful doctor–patient relationship. Few things accomplish this better than talking to patients about the most important people in their lives (see Chapter 2).

COMMUNICATING WITH THE FAMILY

Family assessment enhances communication with the family about the patient's medical problems. This may involve educating them about the patient's condition, discussing self-care regimens and monitoring family involvement with the medical regimen, facilitating the family's role in decision making and advance directives, and helping the family adjust to changes in the patient's functional capacity.

ASSESSMENT AND SUPPORT

Assessing the family's emotional response to the patient's problems and providing needed support are challenging and rewarding family-oriented tasks. It is often difficult

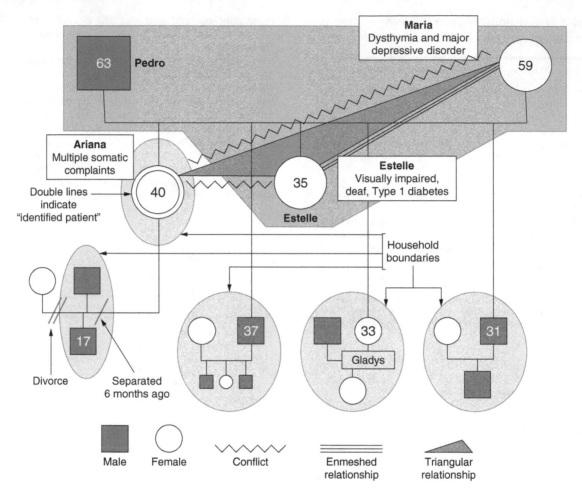

Figure 11-3. Annotated genogram for Ariana in Case Illustration 1.

for the physician to witness the emotional distress experienced by patients and their family in the face of serious medical problems. The temptation to "stick to the facts" and restrict attention to biomedical issues is both strong and understandable, especially in light of the physician's perception that he or she "can do nothing" about the emotional pain. It is important to understand that empathically listening to the family and the patient is a powerful therapeutic intervention in itself—even if it appears to "fix" nothing (see Chapter 2).

Table 11-7. Basic family interventions.

- Enhancing the therapeutic alliance by demonstrating interest and concern about the patient's family and life situation
- Communicating with the family about the patient's medical condition
- Providing information about the patient's problems: Discussing prognosis and answering family members' questions about medical problems
- Discussing self-care and enlisting family assistance with medical management
- Facilitating the family's participation in decision making about therapeutic options
- Discussing and mediating the effect of the patient's loss of function on the roles of other family members
- Providing emotional support to the patient and family
- Counseling the family about simple family system problems
- Identifying problems requiring attention from the family
- Preparing for further family assessment, intervention, and referral for further family interventions
- Working in collaboration with family therapists or other mental health specialists

It is often possible to make simple family systems interventions by suggesting that families try new behaviors.

CASE ILLUSTRATION 2

A 36-year-old man with hypertension presents to a walk-in clinic with tension headaches that have been going on for 2 weeks. The genogram interview (see Figure 11-2 and Table 11-6) reveals that he is distressed by ongoing conflict between his wife and teenage daughter about rules governing her behavior with peers outside the home. At home, the father remains silent until the fights between mother and daughter become intolerable. Their fights stop only when he complains about the headaches the fights have given him. He has never discussed his own ideas about rules for his daughter's behavior—or of family arguments—or negotiated a common position with his wife.

An appropriate intervention would be to suggest that the patient and his wife discuss the situation before the fights begin and try to develop a plan on which they both agree. If the family has the flexibility to respond to this suggestion, it may help them with the developmental life cycle challenge. If this intervention fails to help sufficiently, it may be a sign that further family assessment and interventions are required. It is important that suggestions be based on at least as thorough an evaluation as that produced by the preceding steps of this method; premature suggestions based on incomplete assessment are likely to fail.

CAREGIVER COLLABORATION

If the patient or family is receiving treatment from mental health specialists, the physician should actively collaborate, and they should consult with one another when issues come up that are relevant to the other's expertise. Patients may attempt to play one health care provider against the other; for example, they may present somatic symptoms to the mental health specialist and attempt to engage the medical provider in issues being examined in therapy. Patients or family members may complain about the therapist, especially when the family or patient is being challenged to change. Active communication between treating providers is critical if this dynamic arises (commonly referred to as "splitting").

FOCUSING ON THE DYSFUNCTION

Some problems have a clear and potentially devastating effect on the family. Focusing the family's attention on the problems associated with family dysfunction is a crucial clinical task. For example, if a patient or a member of the patient's family has a problem with alcohol abuse or dependence, it is important to assess the family's response, help the family accept the reality of the problem, and support their need to address it. Many families are waiting for just the kind of professional, extrafamiliar attention that the physician can provide. Validating their feelings, and providing information about resources such as Alcoholics Anonymous (AA), may be all that it takes to precipitate action.

However, the patient's and family's resistance to change may be so strong that basic family assessment is not enough to help them take action. In these cases, it is sometimes preferable to refer the patient to a mental health specialist without further family intervention. However, it is often necessary to proceed to the next level of family intervention to make a successful referral.

FOUR-STEP FAMILY ASSESSMENT & INTERVENTION

If serious family dysfunction is interfering with medical management, the doctor–patient relationship, or the patient's functional status and quality of life, a more intensive, four-step evaluation and intervention is required (Table 11-8). The goals of family assessment and intervention as described differ from the structural systems changes that are employed in family therapy. Even if medical providers had the time and training, they could not treat families with commonly employed techniques that require forming alliances with different family members during treatment, because this process can threaten the trust required to deal effectively with the patient's medical problems.

Step 1: Assessing the Family: "Bringing the Pain into the Room"

The previously described basic family assessment is the core and foundation of the first of the four steps of intervention with dysfunctional families (Table 11-8). The difference lies in the need to achieve three goals that go beyond a basic understanding of family functioning. The physician must (1) have a relatively complete understanding of the major conflicts or issues in the family; (2) understand how the sick role, if present (and it usually is), is functioning as a coping strategy for the patient and the family; and (3) conduct the interview so that patients can bring the full intensity of their feelings about the family problems out, that is, "bring the pain into the room."

The first step of family assessment and intervention is complete when you can say, with confidence that the patient will agree, "It seems to me that the family problems we are discussing are extremely painful, and that you have been unable to resolve them until now." Bringing the pain of the patient's life "into the room" during the interview is an important part of the process because

Table 11-8. Family intervention.

Step	Objective	Statement
Analyze, and "bring the pain into the room"	1. Understand the major conflicts in the family system. 2. Understand how the sick role functions in the family system. 3. "Bring the pain into the room," that is, help the patient (and family if present) experience the pain of their problems during the interview.	"Your [family problems] are serious and painful, and you have not been able to resolve them on your own."
Reframe	1. Direct the patient's (and family's) attention to the underlying family problems and away from the sick role establishing somatization, excessive functional impairment, or dysfunctional self-care behavior. 2. Endorse the patient's objectives while separating them from the use of the sick role to obtain them.	"*In addition to* your [symptom/problem] these family problems are equally worthy of attention." "*Even if you were in perfect health* I could understand why you would want your [family problem] resolved in a way that meets your needs."
Empathically witness	1. Provide emotional support and empowerment to the patient. 2. Enhance the therapeutic alliance.	"I am so impressed with how well you are doing despite all your problems."
Refer	1. Provide access to and educate patients about psychotherapeutic intervention. 2. Address resistance to psychotherapeutic treatments.	"You have important questions about how to improve your family situation; therapy is a way of answering those questions."

the shared knowledge will provide the rationale and impetus for the second step of the process, that is, reframing attention to the underlying family problems. The following techniques will help accomplish this first task.

Two features of the way in which family systems work, so called triangles and circles, can help guide exploration of family relationships. First, all dyadic interactions ultimately triangulate. We fully understand the way individuals interact only when we understand the series of triangular relationships they belong to. Second, families that are having difficulty, that are "stuck," engage in a repetitive or "circular" sequence of behaviors that represents the best they can do to cope with their problems. For example, in their study of adolescents with brittle diabetes or poorly controlled asthma, Minuchin and colleagues often observed the following pattern: unresolved marital conflict erupts into an argument between the adolescent's parents; the adolescent, in response to the stress of the fight, becomes acutely ill; the parents stop fighting and focus on caring for their child; the exacerbation of the child's illness resolves; the unresolved marital conflict erupts into another fight, and the process is repeated. From this point of view, it is clear that the outcome of the seemingly dyadic parental conflict cannot be understood without knowing that the child and the illness are "triangulated." It is impossible to understand the behavior of any member of this triangle without examining the interaction with both of the other two.

The triangular relationships among family members are caught up in circular patterns of interactions. The sequence of events that takes place in the adolescent's family may be described in a linear fashion, that is, parents argue, the child is upset and gets sick, the parents stop arguing to help the child, the child gets better. The interruption of the fight, however, also prevents the parents from "finishing" their fight and resolving their problems, thus, the pattern inevitably repeats. Dysfunctional families are often stuck in such a repetitive, self-sustaining pattern.

It is important to understand how the "sick role," created by the patient's symptoms, is embedded in the family system, and how the whole family participates in it. There are no pure victims or villains in such a system: The adolescent is not merely the "victim" of marital discord; the child's sick role and the acute exacerbations of illness have a powerful controlling influence on the inability of the spouses to resolve their conflicts. Looked at from a more positive vantage point, the child's illness is performing the important function of modulating a marital conflict that might otherwise threaten the integrity of the family system more completely. The symptom is the product of and serves the needs of the entire family system. Though the price is high for all involved, and this "solution" is likely to fail in the long run, it is the best that the family can do at the moment to cope with the totality of their problems.

Patient-centered emotion-supporting interviewing techniques can be instrumental in "bringing the pain into the room" during the interview. A "one-two punch" that couples a statement giving permission to express feelings, combined with an open-ended question about an emotionally charged issue, is often effective. For example, you might say to a new grandmother whose single-parent daughter is hoping for child care for her new baby, "setting limits with your children so that you can be a grandparent rather than a nanny can be difficult and even cause a lot of guilt. How's it been for you?"

Conducting a family meeting is a powerful technique for analyzing family systems. The objective of the family meeting is to have the family enact their interactions, and have other members directly report their responses to the patient's sick role symptoms and behavior. If they enact "the pain in the room," so much the better. The physician merely stops the action when it reaches its peak, concludes Step 1 with the statement, "It seems to me that the family problems we are discussing are extremely painful, and that you have been unable to resolve them until now," and moves on to Step 2, "reframing."

CASE ILLUSTRATION 1 (CONTD.)

Ariana greatly appreciated the opportunity to describe the situation at home, especially when the physician expressed sympathy for the burden that Estelle's illness placed on everyone and for the disappointment resulting from Ariana's failed marriage. The physician now had a general feel for Ariana's family. It was clear that Ariana needed to be labeled as "sick" and that every diagnostic test, referral to a specialist, and symptomatic treatment helped create a compensatory alliance establishing the sick role. Ariana, clearly feeling that the physician was on her side after the genogram interview, readily agreed to a family meeting.

During the family interview, the tremendous burden placed on the family by Estelle's visual impairment, deafness, and diabetes became painfully clear as the physician struggled to communicate with her, a process that required writing notes in letters 6 in. high, or having Ariana or her mother slowly and carefully speak so that Estelle could read their lips (Estelle was unable to read anyone else's lips, and the family had tried but failed to learn sign language). It became clear how much the family depended on Ariana and how she stepped ambivalently into the fray whenever Estelle needed attention.

When the subject turned to Ariana's failed marriage and social life, the mother (Maria) expressed some hope, immediately labeled as ridiculous by Ariana, that she (Ariana) would get back together with her ex-husband. Ariana said, "with all this,"

meaning the problems with Estelle, "how can I find time to get involved with anyone?"

Further discussion revealed that Maria was a worrier and was constantly preoccupied with whichever of her children was having difficulties, especially medical problems. Ariana's medical problems elicited sympathy from her mother, who suggested that since Ariana was no longer married, she should move back into the family house.

Ariana immediately rejected the offer and said that her medical problems were the primary reason she could not move back into the house; she didn't want her mother to see her when she was sick because her mother would worry too much. Ariana added that when she was feeling sick, she needed to stay home by herself, and at these times she didn't even answer the phone or know what was going on in her parents' house.

The physician concluded that Ariana's somatization was embedded in the repetitive pattern of events dominated by her triangular relationship with Estelle and their mother. Ariana's physical symptoms allowed her to remain connected to and receive attention and emotional support from her mother, and simultaneously allowed her to control the family's expectations that she would always be there to help with Estelle. It seemed that Ariana's reason for remaining away from her mother and Estelle was an illness, that is, something beyond her control. The desire to devote more of her life to herself, even though it was closer to the truth, would not be acceptable to either Ariana or the family.

Step 2: Reframing Attention to the Underlying Family Problems

The goal of Step 2 of family intervention, "reframing," is two-fold (Table 11-8): (1) focus the patient's and family's attention on the underlying family problems, and away from physical symptoms and sick role-justifying problems; (2) separate the patient's (or family's) objective in using the sick role from the use of the sick role as a tactic to achieve the goal. This is done by recognizing the objective that the patient is pursuing and endorsing it as something that the patient is "entitled to even if [they] are in perfect health."

REFRAMING, "IN ADDITION TO YOUR PAIN . . ."

The transition from Step 1 to Step 2 occurs when the interview has "brought the pain into the room," and patients are in touch with their distress, that is, when they agree with the first critical reframing statement, "It seems to me that the family situation you have just described is extremely painful, and that *in addition to* your [problematic symptom or behavior], this family problem is also worthy of attention."

A critical component of the first reframing statement is "*in addition to*" in contrast to either "instead of" or "because of." Even if your understanding, based upon a psychosomatic hypothesis, that family stress is "causing" the somatoform presentation, you must resist saying so. The legitimacy of the sick role and coping strategies that the patient and family currently need to function depends upon there being a "disease beyond one's control" to justify the sick role. If the family intervention begins to have effect, and healthier coping strategies are adopted, then the family will be able to relinquish sick role-based coping. Until that time they must be allowed to retain the sick role strategy. Therefore, the goal of reframing is to establish a *parallel* concern directed at the underlying family problems. Occasionally, a patient or family member will be able to make the connection themselves: "Doctor, do you think that maybe my headache is being caused by all these problems?" In such cases, the psychosomatic hypothesis can be endorsed. The mistake is to make the connection before the patient and family are ready. This will result in the all too familiar, "Doctor, you think it's all in my head. It's not in my head, my pain is real!"

REFRAMING, "EVEN IF YOU WERE THE PICTURE OF PERFECT HEALTH YOU WOULD BE ENTITLED TO . . ."

Unless your patient's objectives in occupying the sick role are antisocial, you should be able to identify an essential core of their objective that you can endorse—a new grandmother who does not want to be mistaken for a nanny, a father who wants peace in his home and rules for his teenage daughter, a young woman who does not want to become her sister's home health aide, and so on.

The second objective of reframing is to separate the objective from the tactic of occupying the sick role, and to empower the patient and family to adopt other, healthier strategies. This can be done by telling the patient, "*if you were the picture of perfect health, you would be entitled to*—be a grandmother not a nanny, have your daughter follow some agreed upon rules, set limits on your role in taking care of your sister, and so on." This part of the reframing addresses the fundamental function of the sick role, which is to establish entitlement, and uses the authority of the physician to legitimate the desired entitlement on other, healthier grounds.

CASE ILLUSTRATION 1: DISCUSSION (CONTD.)

It was relatively easy to reframe the burden of caring for Estelle as a problem worthy of attention after the painful demonstration of just how difficult it was to just have a conversation with her. It was also easy to reframe Ariana's desire to have some time for herself—a need she was unwilling to claim on her own—as something that would be important for "a woman her age" *even if she was not ill*. Ariana was willing to accept the suggestion

that her failure to develop the kind of intimate relationship she desired was also a problem worthy of consideration.

Step 3: Empathic Witnessing: "I Am So Impressed with How Well You Are Doing Despite . . ."

The most immediate way to ensure that family intervention has a positive and therapeutic effect is to "empathically witness" the patient's and family's problems and their efforts to cope (Table 11-8). If the interview has succeeded in exposing the family's distress and their best attempts to deal with their problems, the patient and family will recognize that the physician knows the family in a very intimate way. If the physician acknowledges the special nature of this awareness, and responds empathically to the patient and family, the effect can be very therapeutic. The general format for empathic witnessing is to say to the patient (or family) that having heard their story, and seen what they have to cope with, "*I am very impressed with how well you are doing despite all your problems and difficulties.*" It is helpful to remember that even if you cannot praise the patient's behavior or accomplishments, you can usually empathically witness their efforts: "I am impressed that you *want to be* a good mother to your children."

CASE ILLUSTRATION 1 (CONTD.)

The family admitted that the current situation was indeed painful and that they had not been able to solve the problem despite their best efforts. The physician was able to tell Ariana and her mother: "I am so impressed with how well you are both doing despite the tremendous problems you have had to deal with." The physician also remarked on the magnitude of the sacrifice Ariana had made, neglecting her own social life to be available to the family. The physician also commented that it was easy to understand how this area of Ariana's life might be difficult for her to deal with because of her past problems.

Step 4: Referral for Family & Psychotherapy

Referral for therapy is not always indicated. Very often a brief family intervention can empower patients and their families to address their difficulties with new energy, insight, and courage to change. However, when mental health intervention is indicated and proposed, patients and families may not readily accept it (Table 11-8).

Resistance to a mental health referral is common. Referral for therapy may make sense to the provider long before it does to the patient. Framing family problems as "in addition to" will help patients feel comfortable that therapy does not threaten their use of the sick role before they are ready to give it up. Resistance to therapy may be due to fear of dealing directly with painful and powerful emotions. Empathic witnessing and reframing can make this challenge seem more surmountable. Finally, patients may accept the reality of family problems yet not accept the fact that therapy will help: "What's talking going to accomplish?" The process of therapy may indeed seem obscure to patients and it may be useful to restate problems as questions and describe therapy as the process of looking for answers. For example, "you have a serious question to answer. You have to determine how much child care you actually want to provide, and then how to talk to your daughter about it. Therapy can help you find answers to these questions."

Sometimes, patients and their families never get to therapy. Even in that case, the reframing and empathic listening to the patient's family story have a positive effect. *After* performing a family assessment and intervention, the physician may say the following to the patient who has not followed through with referral for therapy and who returns with persistent or recurrent symptoms (as did the father in Case Illustration 2).

CASE ILLUSTRATION 2 (CONCLUSION)

"I am sorry that your headache is still bothering you. Your wife and daughter are still fighting, aren't they? It's too bad that you haven't gotten to the therapist yet. I truly wish that there was more that I could do for you. Now, why don't we check your blood pressure."

The patient—aware that the physician has witnessed the family conflict—knows that the clinician understands the importance of the conflict at home and that this understanding is empathic. Hence, the physician does not have to repeat the assessment and intervention interview, merely recall it for the patient. The physician is in a position to respect the meaning of the patient's symptoms without allowing them to divert the process of care into unnecessary testing, medication, or referrals for more evaluation.

CASE ILLUSTRATION 1 (CONCLUSION)

The physician (1) referred the family for family therapy to explore better approaches to coping with Estelle's medical problems; (2) suggested that Ariana would benefit from individual counseling to explore her difficulties in forming a satisfying intimate relationship; (3) asked Maria's physician to consider the diagnoses of dysthymia and major depression; and (4) recommended that the family try to obtain a home health aide for Estelle to give Maria a break. The family agreed to all four of these suggestions. When Ariana returned for her next visit, she still had numerous symptoms but spoke of them only briefly, allowing the physician to turn the discussion to what was going on at home. Ariana reported that the family had taken no steps toward family therapy and that she was still considering whether to go to individual therapy. She did report feeling more comfortable setting limits on her mother's expectations of assistance in dealing with Estelle, and reported success in obtaining a home health aide for Estelle. Maria had been placed on an antidepressant, made a few visits to a community mental health center, and was much less symptomatic.

Eight months later, Ariana entered individual therapy and her somatization decreased dramatically and her limit-setting improved. Eventually, she started dating and entered a steady relationship but has not married.

SUGGESTED READINGS

Carter CA, McGoldrick M, eds. *The Family Life Cycle: A Framework for Family Therapy.* New York, NY: Gardner Press, 1980.

Doherty WJ, Baird MA. *Family-Centered Medical Care: A Clinical Case Book.* New York, NY: Guilford Press, 1987.

Doherty WJ, Campbell TL. *Families and Health.* New York, NY: Sage Publications, 1988.

Haley J. *Problem Solving Therapy.* San Francisco, CA: Jossey-Bass, 1976.

McGoldrick M, Gerson R. *Genograms in Family Assessment.* New York, NY: Norton, 1985.

Minuchin S. *Families and Family Therapy.* Cambridge, MA: Harvard University Press, 1974.

Children

Howard L. Taras, MD

12

INTRODUCTION

This chapter reviews common childhood behavioral problems and suggests some management guidelines. Pediatric behavioral medicine cannot be easily disassociated from child development because many problematic childhood behaviors have developmental roots. Clinicians who work with children need to identify parents' behavioral concerns, even if these are not brought up as problems by parents. Clinicians also need to develop strategies they are comfortable with to address childhood behavioral issues with parents, so that they can lead to resolution.

UNDESIRABLE BEHAVIOR: PART OF NORMAL CHILDHOOD DEVELOPMENT

A child's ability to understand and interact with the environment is constantly evolving. To learn more about the world, a child experiments with ways of interacting with it. Most often, children test the reactions of the people to whom they are closest, their parents. Colloquial phrases such as *"the terrible twos," "she's going through a stage,"* and *"boys will be boys"* indicate that undesirable childhood behaviors are commonly accepted as "normal." But when an undesirable behavior is manifesting in your child, the normalcy can be difficult to accept. And even when the cause is well understood, many parents still need the knowledge and skills to respond to the problem behavior.

Extraordinary Stress

Behavioral problems associated with normal childhood development must be distinguished from problems with more complex causes. Aberrant childhood behaviors are often secondary to extraordinary life stresses. This applies to children who witness violence, are members of communities that have experienced a natural disaster or catastrophic event, are exposed to continuous marital discord, have a frequently absent parent (such as military deployment), have a chronic illness or

a chronically ill sibling, or who do not feel wanted. Children living under any condition that seriously threatens healthy and successful transition through a developmental stage are likely to pose serious behavioral problems.

Children, like adults, may appear to be the dysfunctional member of an otherwise healthy family unit even though the problem actually stems from family issues. This is particularly the case with childhood behaviors, because children are dependent on adults in almost every way. Take, for instance, the child who refuses to attend school. Classically, this behavior occurs when one or both parents send subliminal messages to the child to remain home. Although the primary problem is parental anxiety about separation, it is the child who exhibits the apparent symptoms.

Stresses causing unwanted childhood behavior may be relatively more subtle than those described above. For example, children of immigrants often successfully acculturate to the prevalent culture. But when these children's attitudes and behaviors are not culturally acceptable or understood by their parents, children can be perceived to be behavioral problems. Or, they may manifest true aberrant behaviors as a result of the stresses of this culture clash.

Inherent Disorders

In addition to childhood behavioral problems stemming from normal development and extraordinary life stresses, a third general category involves problems caused by disorders inherent to the child. Attention deficit disorders are the most common and well known, but conduct disorders, depression, autistic spectrum disorders, and other psychiatric diagnoses manifest during childhood. A complete history, observation, and response to treatment help the primary care clinician distinguish these from other causes of behavioral problems. The latest version of the *Diagnostic and Statistical Manual of Mental Disorders* is an excellent resource for primary care physicians trying to gauge a child's behavior in relation to a psychiatric diagnosis.

SCREENING FAMILIES FOR DIFFICULTIES WITH CHILDHOOD BEHAVIORS

Pediatric primary care providers must screen families for difficulties with undesirable childhood behaviors, sort out probable causes for the behaviors, recognize when a mental health referral is appropriate, and manage those problems that are likely to respond to simple environmental changes or to elementary behavioral management techniques.

Practitioner concern versus time constraints. Many parents do not know where to seek help for behavioral problems such as their baby's night awakenings, their toddler's tantrums, or their fourth grader's class clown behavior. They do not realize that their child's clinician can assist them. To overcome these barriers, health care providers should take every opportunity to talk about behavioral issues, although time constraints may limit the practitioner's ability to listen to extensive histories. Therefore, clinicians need to screen for behavioral information in ways that are expedient and that leave time to reflect on issues that can be discussed more fully at another time.

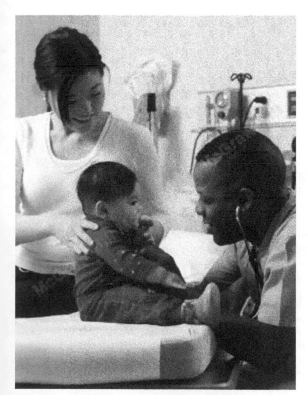

Peds doc QD-56959468.jpg: **Doctor with Mother and Child** (image from the McGraw-Hill Image Library).

Trigger questions and questionnaires. One way to elicit information from parents is to ask a preset list of key questions, specific to each age group. Use of a screening questionnaire that is mailed home in advance or that parents can answer electronically is a reliable way to elicit history. Numerous such questionnaires have been available since the 1990s. Despite their availability, they are rarely used by primary care clinicians. Some feel these questionnaires merely confirm what a clinician would suspect anyhow once the patient and family are in the office for a clinical evaluation. In addition, these screens have not yet been shown to be cost-effective. Nevertheless, brief screening tools, such as the 17-item Pediatric Symptom Checklist should be considered by clinicians prior to the child's visit or even while the family is waiting to be led to a clinical interview or examination room. These tools help clinicians gather history and distinguish between disorders and problem behaviors.

To effectively screen for childhood behavioral problems, practitioners need to develop their skills of observation and to learn to apply their natural intuitions. Parent–child interaction in the office can be an excellent indicator of problems occurring at home. When reported childhood behavior problems are combined with a clinician's suspicion that there is aberrant pattern of attachment between parent and child, this is a warning sign. Incidents in the office that induce parents to discipline their child are opportunities for clinicians to better understand the parent–child relationship and to bring behavioral management issues into discussion. Experienced clinicians have learned to become aware of subtle signs in the office that are indicative of a family's dynamics, such as how a mother holds her baby. A mother who seems uncomfortable feeding her baby, a pattern of noncompliance, or suspicion about the levels of interest mother or father show are all indicative of issues that should register concern with the clinician. Involvement of grandparents and other extended family, references parents make about their own upbringing, and other family characteristics are also worth noting. Positive impressions that clinicians form about families also provide clinically useful information.

Television, movies, video games, texting, smartphones, and computer networks have assumed central roles in our children's daily lives. It is still unclear what effect this has on children's general mood and associated behavior. There are probably both negative and positive consequences to this growing phenomenon. Excessive screen time should be a concern if it appears to be associated with the emergence of behavior problems. It is certainly worthwhile to take a history of how "wired" a child is when confronted with a history of problem behaviors.

Interviewing young children. Primary care providers can find themselves in a quandary when they try to elicit information directly from the child. Most children by age 2½ to 3 years are capable of communicating certain thoughts and feelings to an inquiring health provider. But children do not typically divulge such information to clinicians when questioned directly. Children freely offer their honest opinions on just about any topic, sensitive or banal, but they often do so when it is unsolicited. Parents themselves are often surprised when their children first reveal their feelings about a delicate personal issue to an adult with whom they are not ostensibly very close (a preschool teacher, a friend's mother in their car pool, and so on).

Primary care providers should, therefore, use tools that help children more freely and predictably disclose what's on their minds. One way is to ask children old enough to understand and comply to draw a picture, for example, to draw "anything they want," "something scary," "their family," or "the worst day at school." The position of the characters in the drawings, facial expressions, and choice of colors can yield important information about what they are thinking and may be indicative of how they are feeling and can be used as a starting point for discussion. Children often find it easier to speak about themselves when the conversation is in the third person, such as "Why would that little girl in the picture want to hit her mommy?"

To avoid alienating parents, you may go through a few such questions when both parent and child are in the room. But many children, and most of those older than age 4 years, respond differently when their parents are in the room. Explain to parents that you would like to interview the child in the same way without them. The general nature of children's responses can be discussed later with parents. Parents should be notified that this will occur, but the interviewer need not feel compelled to reveal children's specific responses to each interview item, particularly if information may be hurtful and not of therapeutic value at that time. Parents and children should know that too.

Other oblique ways of eliciting information from children are to ask open-ended questions using questions that children like to respond to: "Pretend a magical genie in a bottle wanted to grant you three wishes, what would they be?" And "If you could magically turn into any animal you wanted, what would it be?" To their response to the last question, then ask, "Well that's wonderful! And why would you be happy as that animal?"

Sentence completion games are also useful. The clinician begins the first few words of a sentence and asks the child to complete the sentence by making something up. Examples of some are given in Table 12-1. These (and clinicians can improvise on others like them) can be typed onto colorful cards so that children can choose one at a time and perceive it as a game, not a real interview. Allow the child to be imaginative with

Table 12-1. Samples of "sentence completion" items for interviewing young children.

- I really like it when . . .
- I am ashamed . . .
- I worry a lot about . . .
- My mother . . .
- I hate . . .
- It makes me sad to . . .
- It makes me happy to . . .
- People think that I . . .
- I really hope one day that I . . .

responses, and indicate that their responses can be the truth but do not have to be.

Toddlers and school-age children are often aware of the clinician's actual intent when these interviewing techniques are used. Despite this, children seem to enjoy going along with this format of questioning and appreciate having an easy way to express themselves. Children respond best when they are comfortable with the clinician. Arranging a number of office visits can help to establish that relationship.

When using drawings, questions in the third person, or questions evoking the child's imagination, it is important not to read too deeply into children's responses. Children have active imaginations: they play around with frightening ideas and with wishful thinking. Sometimes they are merely obsessed with speaking about what they have recently seen on television. To be taken seriously, responses of young children should fit into a general pattern of what the clinician suspects from parent interview and symptoms. One or two worrisome responses should not stand on their own as proof for the etiology to a problem.

Beyond the physician–child–parent triad. Many toddlers are placed in the care of a day care provider, babysitter, or relative. Virtually all children older than age 5 years of age spend a large portion of their waking hours in school. Yet despite this, clinicians traditionally rely almost exclusively on parents (and the children themselves) to gather a behavioral history. Some clinicians send questionnaires to school staff to elicit information, or they ask parents about their children's progress at school or day care. It is rare, however, for clinicians to routinely engage in direct telephone contact with child care providers and teachers. Yet these people occupy many, and occasionally most, of children's waking hours. The value of attaining parental permission to speak directly with educational professionals in a child's life cannot be overstated. Teachers and child care providers can provide valuable insight. Many have numerous years of experience with all types of children, and their observations rarely include the emotional biases that sometimes confound a parent's interpretation and recollection of details. Once a behavior plan has been recommended, a relationship with daytime caretakers may extend the plan's implementation to that setting and render it more effective.

NORMAL CHILDHOOD DEVELOPMENT

Knowledge about stages of normal childhood development can assist a clinician with understanding the etiology of a maladaptive behavior. It can allow the clinician, and in turn the parent, to attribute an undesirable behavior to a developmental stage of childhood. An understanding of child development can guide parents to respond to a child problem behavior using a strategy that is consistent with that child's stage of development. For example, it is often appropriate to just give a firm "no" to a child's behavior without any supportive reason when they are very young, but that response would be insufficient for an older child who has developed skills of reasoning.

Sigmund Freud's psychoanalytic theories emphasized unconscious and conscious mental processes that children go through. Each stage, which is several years long, is a decisive turning point where a child can become vulnerable or strong for a certain characteristic. For example, according to this theory, in the anal stage at 1½ to 3 years of age, children are personally focused on elimination and interpersonally focused on "rebellion versus compliance" with parental demands. At this stage, they may fear loss of parental love. Erik Erickson's stages are an expanded version of psychoanalytic theory, and his teachings can help clinicians and parents understand children's psychosocial development. Infants develop trust or mistrust through their experiences up to about age 18 months. In the next stage (ending around age 3 years), children develop autonomy versus doubt in themselves. And in preschool (up to age 6 years), children learn to either take initiative, or feel inhibited to do so. Through school age, children can acquire the psychological skills to feel competent in work, versus repeated frustration and feelings of inferiority. No one stage is ever really resolved completely forever, but the experience of those critical years are present in some way as the person moves throughout life.

Jean Piaget described stages of cognitive development. Though his theories have since been proven to underestimate children's abilities, they are still very useful guides. For example, until around age 7 years, children are what Piaget termed as "preoperational." They engage in make believe, and parents should not misconstrue this as lying. Complex concepts, such as cause and effect, are not yet developed. Parents must not get frustrated by trying to rationalize with them by using logic. Once well into elementary school, they are at the "concrete operational" stage, meaning they are less egocentric and understand how events outside of their own actions can lead to concrete changes. Hence, parental explanations for behavior are important for children at this age. Adolescence is marked by the increasing ability to work with abstract concepts. They test out these new skills by how they interact with their peers. They can begin to moralize about their own and others' behaviors.

MANAGEMENT AND REFERRAL

Primary care providers can and should evaluate and manage common child behavior problems in their own offices. Mental health referrals are usually unnecessary since so many undesirable child behaviors are maladaptations or manifestations of normal child development. There are occasions when the need for psychiatric assessment, psychotherapy, or play therapy is apparent from the start. But for most problems that present to primary care practitioners, children respond well to brief, solution-focused strategies. Although no single behavioral management technique works well for all children with similar problems and similar etiologies to their problems, clinicians can quickly learn to tailor their management plans to suit the individual needs of each family. These plans should be based on families' cultural characteristics, size, work schedules, and other factors. A management failure should always first be considered a problem with the behavioral management technique prescribed, not with the child or family.

It is useful for primary care clinicians to have some understanding of the underlying theoretical basis of several psychotherapeutic interventions. Expertise and even competency in any one of these therapies takes years of specialized training—which is not feasible in the primary care setting. Providing psychotherapy in the clinical setting takes numerous sessions, and for some, many years. However, just knowing the premise behind these psychotherapeutic techniques may guide a clinician on how best to frame a conversation with a child and family when they face relatively minor behavioral problems with their children.

Family therapy is based on the premise that every family is a system (see Chapter 11). When a child has a problem behavior, it can be analyzed in terms of its being one outcome of the relationships between all members of the family. By first understanding and then intervening with the nature and dynamics of the family as a system, family therapy can help parents understand the complex etiology of their child's aberrant behavior. In the primary care setting, this concept can help underpin the etiology and management of relatively minor behavior problems. For example, a clinician can rationalize inviting the entire family to the office when addressing a child who refuses to eat meals, when the problem hinges on a doting live-in grandmother who slips cookies to her granddaughter between meals. The grandmother's need to have affirmation of love by her grandchild does not necessarily need to be addressed in the clinical setting, if just raising the actions and their consequences helps to stop the behavior.

Cognitive behavioral therapy comprises a series of techniques based on the notion that it is a person's thoughts, not factors in the external environment, that primarily drive his or her feelings and behavior. When used by mental health professionals, it involves structured and directive relationship building and can take several visits before a person is able to unlearn his or her unhelpful emotional reactions to the environment. This concept can be useful for a primary care provider who is trying to coax parents to recognize that their child's obstinate "no" to every directive need not raise their parental ire. Teach parents to recognize their reaction to their child's misbehavior and how that emotional reaction to their own thinking may actually promote further such behaviors from the child.

Motivational interviewing was designed as a technique to improve treatment outcomes for people with substance abuse disorders (see Chapter 19). However, many clinicians have recognized that the philosophy and techniques of motivational interviewing can be helpful when trying to change other patient behaviors. Many people come to a health professional stating that they would like to stop smoking or lose weight, but they may be less than ready to do so. Motivational interviewing recognizes the stage of readiness the client is in. Behavioral experts in this technique learn not only to echo the client's perspective but to help the client push him or herself to the next stage. Helping someone recognize the discrepancy between their stated desire and their current predicament is an important stage in the process. This concept can be helpful to clinicians, for example, those faced with parents who state they dislike their child sleeping in the parental bed each night, but then do not seem to follow the clinician's advice. Rather than showing frustration, the clinician can show some sympathy for the parent and point out how it is not atypical to be ambivalent about changing the status quo. Encourage the parents to weigh their reluctance to change the child's nighttime behavior against the benefits they are experiencing. Allow parents to explore aloud what it will take to become more ready to accept the difficulty that comes with reversing the situation.

Emotional intelligence is defined as the ability to identify one's own feelings, to identify the feelings of others, and to solve problems that involve emotional issues. The extent to which this "intelligence" is innate versus learned is unknown. Emotional intelligence has been found to be related to, for example, having a lower risk for smoking during one's youth. Parents who provide their child with "tools" to handle emotional challenges may be able to increase the emotional ability of their child. By learning a vocabulary of words that describes emotions, such as "frustrated," "anxious," and "envious," children may become more likely to use them *in lieu* of acting out these behaviors. Clinicians can also encourage parents to foster an environment in which children will want to describe their feelings. Naturally, this is more easily accepted in theory by parents in your office than at home. Clinicians can ask about specific and recent situations at home that demonstrate the child's personality and stage of emotional maturation. By understanding these details, a clinician can offer step-by-step suggestions that are pertinent to that family's issues and that child's emotional level.

Resilience There are significant individual differences in biological sensitivity to negative and positive experiences. A child's ability to withstand or recover from a significant challenge is probably based on neurobiological and epigenetic processes. This resilience is not the only protective factor, as the resilience of that child's family or community are also factors that predict outcome. Therefore, when assessing a child, elicit a history that is larger than that of the individual child's own history.

There is growing evidence that one can promote childhood resilience through intervention during critical stages of development. Positive relationships with caring adults and effective parenting promote attachment. Learning problem-solving skills, self-regulation skills, and one's self-efficacy for success are associated with resilience. Societal factors, such as positive friends, faith (i.e., hope, spirituality, and belief that life has meaning) and effective teachers and schools appear to be correlated with resilience. A good school or child care setting, and other programs or environments where children can experience success are considered to be critical.

Advocacy Clinicians have the power to help modify environments in which all the community's children spend time, not only those children who are patients in their practices. Such environments include schools, playgrounds, parks and recreational centers, and child care centers. Clinicians can influence even the media to which these children have easy access. Advocacy can be preventive or responsive to a pattern that the clinicians have experienced in several patients of their own. Programs for which clinicians can advocate with regards to childhood behavior may be school classroom interventions, where children are taught that anger is an emotion that can be recognized before it is acted upon irrationally. Educational programs like this have helped students discuss and even act out situations that evoke their own anger and those of others. They also learn how to temper these emotions and how to de-escalate a situation.

EXAMPLES OF COMMON BEHAVIORAL ISSUES

Infancy: Night Waking

CASE ILLUSTRATION 1

Parents of a 12-week-old girl complain that their daughter rarely sleeps more than a total of 4–5 hours between 8 P.M. and 6 A.M. She may fall asleep at 8 P.M., only to awaken an hour later. She seems to fall asleep during or after short feeds and then remains awake for hours later on. Each night is a struggle of long awakened periods between short spells of sleep. Her parents note that she cries when left alone. She seems content at night when parents walk around with her.

Child development in early infancy is characterized by large fluctuations in temperament and schedules. In the first few weeks of life, infants often sleep as much during the day as at night. In the first 2 months of life, two night awakenings are common, but by 3 months of life most infants are sleeping for 5–6 hours uninterrupted. In this case, the child did not naturally "learn" the difference between night and day, and parents did not train her to do so. However, if clinicians ask parents to let their young infants cry themselves to sleep, they set parents up for feelings of inadequacy or guilt. This, in turn, strains the relationship of attachment that parents are forming with their children.

CASE ILLUSTRATION 1 (CONTD.)

On further questioning in this case, the parents reported that their baby falls asleep immediately after daytime feeds and sleeps for 3–5 consecutive hours thereafter. This baby did not adapt to an acceptable or optimal day/night schedule so their doctor recommended waking the baby up after no more than 2–3 hours of daytime sleep. Parents were to try to occupy their infant's daytime hours by walking around, talking, playing music, and offering other playful activities. It was recommended that nighttime feeds be made minimally stimulating: soften the lights, produce minimal noise, and avoid "fun" interactions at night. Although sleeping and feeding "on demand" need not always be discouraged, in this case the infant's pattern needlessly disrupted parents' well-being and this justified modification. After 5–6 days of compliance with this schedule, it became easier for parents to keep their daughter awake during the day and the parents settled for a nighttime feed at 11 P.M. before they retired and another feed at 4 A.M.

It is important to note that the likely causes for night awakenings change with developmental stages. This same sleep history told by parents of a 9-month-old child would be more likely related to the child's cognitive ability to recognize that parents still "exist" after they leave the room. At that age, if there were no other likely cause, other recommendations would be in order. A nightlight or a transitional object (favorite blanket or teddy bear) could prove to be helpful. The clinician, in this case, should devise a careful behavioral intervention schedule that includes parental reassurance for the child but may also include an allowance for the child to "cry it out" for a couple of nights.

Toddler: Aggression

CASE ILLUSTRATION 2

The parent of a 3-year-old boy reports that her son throws himself on the floor, throws objects, and screams . . . usually when he does not get his own way. This seems to happen daily. At his child care center, he has begun to bite other children when he is angry, and other parents have begun to complain about him.

Assessment of this behavior begins with elucidating, through history gathering, the extent of the child's aggression, and its likely etiology. Angry outbursts are common at 3 years of age, when children often begin to direct their anger at others. Parental response to a given level of aggression differs widely from family to family. Parental expectations of children's behavior, not solely the magnitude of the child's behavior, help define whether a behavior is a problem. Large discrepancies between childhood behaviors and parental thresholds may predict that a child will continue to be problematic in the future. A child who explores the environment very actively may be described as "curious" in one family but as "always climbing the walls" in another. A "difficult and stubborn" child in one family is "persistent—just like his successful grandpa" in another. Perhaps the more positive perspective creates a better self-image for a child and leads to fewer problems later on.

Certain questions may help clinicians assess the etiology of aggressive behavior: Is the child a cruel or unhappy child? Is the child exposed to frequent violent (physical or verbal) outbursts from others at home? Are the incidents that induce these behaviors unpredictable? Is the child cognitively not acting consistently with his or her age? Positive responses to these questions make a normal developmental etiology less likely.

When development is still the most likely cause, there are a number of possibilities to consider. First, children with well-developed cognitive abilities, but with comparatively delayed language abilities, often become frustrated with limited ways of expressing themselves. Second, children at this stage often strive for adult attention and have found aggressive behaviors to be a certain way of getting it. Third, children at this stage need to express their independence, yet some adults have not found enough acceptable ways to allow the child to do this. To ascertain the likely cause(s), clinicians should explore events surrounding these incidents of aggression. Detailed examples of what instigated the last one or two aggressive behaviors are more revealing than letting the parent say, "Oh it happens for just about anything." Always ask parents how they feel when their child acts out. Feeling like "I just don't have time for this" may be a good indication that the child is trying to get attention. If their first reaction is to feel that this is a power struggle, then the child's strivings for independence may be his or her primary incentive. Also ask what parents have done in response to misbehavior and whether this reaction worked.

 CASE ILLUSTRATION 2 (CONTD.)

In this case, the child's degree of aggression was within reason for a child at his developmental stage. His tantrums began as a result of typical frustrations experienced by children his age. Over a period of months as his parent became busier with other family needs, however, he discovered that expressing anger was an excellent way to get adult attention, and the frequency of these behaviors increased. As part of the management plan, his parent was instructed to ignore his anger and put him in his room for a few minutes when he became physically violent with others. Concomitantly, she was to increase time spent doing happier things with him, like playing games, going on walks, and having him help around the house. At day care, he was given increased individual attention during times he was behaving well. Child care providers were asked to ignore him when he was aggressive toward other children and to shower a "noticeable" amount of attention on the other child. Within a couple of weeks he stopped biting and seemed happier. Although he still had a terrible temper, these strategies gave his mother the feeling that she had some control over the situation.

Toddler: Oppositional Behavior

 CASE ILLUSTRATION 3

A 3-year-old boy refuses to go to bed on time. He prolongs bedtime rituals by making numerous requests (e.g., for water, use of bathroom, adjusting the door, etc.). He repeatedly leaves his bed. On many nights he finally falls asleep in the living room or his parents' bedroom while spending time with his parents.

 CASE ILLUSTRATION 4

A father solicits your opinion on vitamin supplements to counterbalance his 28-month-old daughter's picky eating habits. She drinks apple juice and eats hot dogs and Honey-Nut Cheerios, and little else. When these foods are not offered, she protests violently and eats nothing.

The behaviors described in these cases are typical for this age group. Toddlers commonly oppose parents for many sorts of issues, including the eating and bedtime cases illustrated here (e.g., getting dressed, putting toys away, wearing seat belt, and so on). A tendency to challenge parents' instructions subsides naturally as children grow older. But they need to be dealt with properly for those months or years they are present. When parents mistake a child's behavior as a personal offense, they react to the behavior in a way that creates additional conflict and heightens oppositional behavior. Therefore, it is important for clinicians to emphasize the developmental component. Children in both illustrative cases have learned to exploit their parents' uncertainty with what exactly is in their child's best interest. In both cases, the clinician should rule out deeper problems by interviewing the parent and, to whatever extent possible, the child. Look for unusual fears, nightmares, and other symptoms that may indicate an unusual etiology to the oppositional behavior. None was found in these two cases. Parental persistence must be designed to outlast the child's. In Case 3, it is almost always effective within 2 weeks, and often within two nights. If this child shared a room with a sibling, it would have been suggested that the sibling sleep in the parents' room until the index child's behavior became less disruptive.

CASE ILLUSTRATION 4 (CONTD.)

In the second case, the same principles were applied to other behaviors. The child was offered three wholesome meals and one snack at preset times of the day. After telling their daughter once, parents were not to engage in any discussion with their child about the volume eaten. No other foods in the house were made available to her during this behavioral management period. Between meals this girl was allowed an unlimited quantity of water, but nothing else. After a difficult period of 1½ days (thrown silverware, persistent crying, etc.), she began to nibble at new foods and to enjoy the positive attention for doing so. Although the child still enjoyed only a limited range of foods, parents were able to expand her repertoire to include broccoli, milk, and pasta.

Parents often worry about harming their child by restricting access to food after a missed meal, so they need to be reassured that this is not harmful and will ultimately improve nutrition. It is all too common for a well-meaning grandparent who resides in the home to "save" the child by sneaking her a cookie between meals (Case Illustration 4) or lying down with the child after a designated bedtime (Case Illustration 3). Such kindly motivated behaviors unwittingly prolong the child's maladaptive behavior, extending the period of inadequate nutrition and sleep. It is imperative that clinicians invite all adult household members to their offices when prescribing a management plan to ensure that all involved endorse both the intent and methods. It is useful to write behavioral management "rules" down on a prescription pad to be taped to the refrigerator door. This helps prevent conflict among adult household members that may arise later. Clinicians should also routinely recommend follow-up visits to their offices once the management plan has been implemented to monitor progress.

Toddler: Toilet Training

Children must be developmentally ready before toilet training is initiated by parents. First, physiologic sphincter control is necessary. This usually develops between ages 1 and 2 years, and parents often know when their child is beginning to sense a bowel movement because of a characteristic grimace or stance. The ability to follow sequential instructions, the motivation to imitate parents, and the patience to sit on a potty should also be present. It is reasonable to try toilet training at age 2 years if these milestones have been achieved. But disinterest or undue difficulty should alert parents to terminate their attempt and wait 2–3 months before

trying again. Some children may not be ready until age 3. Others are ready at 18 months.

Although a number of effective toilet training methods exist, only one method is described here. Place the potty in the bathroom the child typically uses and explain what it is for by drawing parallels with the toilet that parents use. The child should be encouraged with praise to sit on the potty for a couple of minutes a day, initially with diaper and pants on and after a few days, without them. The child should accompany the parent to empty soiled diapers into the potty. Parents should avoid commenting on the foul odor of the stool, as some children identify what they have produced as extensions of themselves. Gradually, the child should be asked to sit on the potty more frequently during the day, particularly if there is a time when bowel movements are likely to occur. Encourage the child to let the potty "catch" the stool. Parents should never scold a child for an inability to do this or for any "accidents." Night training, standing at urination, and using a larger toilet are secondary skills that should be introduced only after the child has mastered the basics or if the child expresses interest.

Preschooler: Sexual Behaviors

CASE ILLUSTRATION 5

A 3-year-old girl has been touching the genitals of the family's dogs and has commented on her father's genitals. One week prior to their visit to your office, the little girl was repetitively using her finger and food in a way that resembled intercourse to her astonished parents. Not knowing how to react they have been begging their daughter to stop. Surprised by their odd reaction, the child has increased such activities.

The clinician was initially and appropriately quite concerned herself by these actions. But after taking a physical examination and taking a careful history of the relationships in the families, she found no suspicions of sexual abuse, physical abuse or neglect, or recent emotional trauma within or outside the home. The clinician then instructed the parents to simply ignore the behaviors. On follow up, the clinician learned that these behaviors that started with normal childhood exploration, self-resolved within a week when they were no longer propagated with parental attention.

School Age: Primary Nocturnal Enuresis

One workable definition for enuresis is at least one bed-wetting incident weekly for a boy older than 6 years of age or a girl older than 5 years of age. It is considered secondary enuresis if a child had been dry previously for a period greater than 6 months. This is one of the most commonly asked questions of pediatric health care providers. Other urinary tract problems (infection, neurogenic bladder, and so on) can be ruled out with a basic medical examination and history. It is important to recognize that the only problems with primary nocturnal enuresis are the reactions of the child and the parent. Otherwise, it is a self-limiting condition that resolves spontaneously. If a child and his or her parents are not bothered by it, then no treatment is necessary. This is worthwhile to point out to families whenever the option for intervention is offered.

To treat this condition, it is necessary that children themselves, not only their parents, are motivated. Verify that a child is truly motivated and determine the source of motivation by interviewing the child separately. When a child is not genuinely motivated to try something new in order to be dry, clinical efforts should be directed toward other family members. Gauge parental actions and anxieties and if necessary influence them so that their actions and anxieties are not causes of unnecessary stress for their child. Children should never be punished for their enuretic disorder. Even if parents insist that their child help to change wet bed sheets, this task should be carried out with the same attitude as other household responsibilities the child has been expected to take on.

Not drinking to excess during the evening meal and afterward makes some logical sense and is easily followed. This should not be regarded as a fluid restriction for children who play sports or who live in very dry ambient air conditions. Going to the bathroom before bedtime to void is also advisable. Commercially available alarm devices assist clinicians and parents in instituting "conditioning therapy." This method is of clinically proven use. With this device, an alarm awakens the child with the first few drops of urine. Eventually, this teaches the child to awaken with the sensation of a full bladder. The child is still responsible to get to the bathroom. The alarm is usually effective when used nightly for a couple of months. Setbacks occur after removing the alarm, but these are often corrected more permanently by one further trial period with the device.

Desmopressin (DDAVP) tablets, an analog of antidiuretic hormone, is a pharmacologic therapy of choice. If children respond to this medication, they usually do so within 2 weeks. Relapses after withdrawal are not uncommon, however, and this therapy is best offered when the alarm device has failed and for temporary relief (e.g., summer camp). Imipramine has also been shown to be useful in certain circumstances. Sphincter control exercises, fluid restrictions in the evening hours, and urine retention training may be tried, but these methods have shown only limited success.

School Age: Bullying

 CASE ILLUSTRATION 6

During a routine health supervision visit of a 12-year-old girl, your customary questioning of social development reveals that this seventh grade student has been having problems with peers at school. She dislikes school and many of her classmates. Problems began about 3 months ago when another girl knocked an apple out of her hand and onto the cafeteria floor. Your patient tried to swat at the (but missed) and was reprimanded by the lunch monitor. Your patient broke into tears at that time and has since been the butt of sneaky jokes among a group of girls. False rumors about her have been spread verbally at school and through the occasional e-mail that children write to one another from home in the evenings.

Victims of bullying are likely to internalize bad situations, and it is likely that this child did not reveal much of her distress to her parents at the onset of her problems. Indications that one's child is being bullied may include an increasingly apparent dread of going to school, depressive signs, symptoms of anxiety (e.g., headaches, stomach aches), or changes in academic success. Many children who internalize threats and fears of bullying may believe they are somehow to blame for the behavior of others. Some parents and school staff members view bullying among school-age children as a normal part of growing up. Parents with this attitude need to be educated. Many parents who did not text, use Internet-based social media, or have classmates with digital cameras in school when they were growing up, can fail to recognize the plethora of new potential threats their child faces. Lack of recognition and resolution for bullying experiences and situations can result in anxiety disorders, depression, and social withdrawal.

Although some victims of bullying respond with aggression, many more are passive. Sometimes, certain personality characteristics or maladaptive behaviors have made children prone to becoming a victim of bullying. Problems such as having poor social skills, difficulty making friends, or even just being quiet, withdrawn, or shy can be sufficient. Victims are often those who easily become upset or have difficulty standing up for or defending themselves in public. Many feel more comfortable socializing with adults than with age-appropriate peers.

Primary care providers need to assess the level of entrenchment and severity for characteristics that predispose a child to being a victim of bullying behavior.

Are there signs that this occurs in more than one environment, including the home? Are improvements recalcitrant to basic interventions? Are there too few positive social interactions with one's own age group? For some, victimization is a sign that the child requires assessment and intervention of a mental health specialist.

CASE ILLUSTRATION 6 (CONTD.)

The primary care physician made a verbal agreement with the young girl and her parents that they would work together on the problem until there was no bullying at all. The girl would heretofore share her experiences with her parents, despite embarrassment, and parents would take these seriously and keep her from facing these issues alone. Parents would speak with their child's school administration and suggest a plan. Further history-taking, in this case, uncovered that this girl is an excellent artist. The parents were encouraged to consciously shower verbal praise for her artistic accomplishments as well as other successes. They were to encourage school staff to do the same. They were also to seek new opportunities for their daughter to exhibit these strengths to herself and to others.

The youngster's parents kept a record of bullying episodes and communicated these with the school principal. Eventually, enrollment in an after-school art class helped this girl develop a couple of new friendships, which lent her a sense of confidence in herself and made her less vulnerable to being bullied.

Primary care physicians must realize that the interventions tendered in this case illustration are often inadequate to turn a situation around and that schools need to play a larger role. An experience with a bullied patient presents an excellent opportunity for a primary care provider to advocate in a local school or district so that bullying is taken seriously and that promising bullying prevention programs are adopted. To be successful, a bullying prevention program requires more than one interested school counselor with a plan or policy. Interventions designed by Olweus have been relatively well researched and demonstrate encouraging results. School interventions should occur at several levels: school-wide interventions (i.e., staff training and development of school-wide rules against bullying); classroom-level interventions (i.e., regular classroom meetings and class parent meetings); and individual-level interventions (interacting on a one-to-one level with bullies and victims). School administrators and all school staff must be committed, and each site needs a coordinator responsible for assuring that the plan is carried out.

It is no less essential for primary care providers to identify patients who are bullies, as well as those who are bullied. It is also important to help parents take note of signs that their children may be bullies. Bullies and victims often share problems with friendships, but they manifest these problems in different ways. Parents and clinicians need to be alert to children who are often in trouble at school (but are great at talking themselves out of blame) and who seem to need to control their friends and peers. All too often schools' and parents' only intervention for these bullies has been to punish them. This is typically ineffective because that response alone cannot get to the core of these children's underlying problems. Strict rules, close supervision, and communication with the school are important interventions for parents to adopt. When underlying psychological problems have led to poor conduct, poor peer relationships, and emotional upheaval, and when these are not addressed during their youth, it has been found that bullies have a significantly higher chance of engaging in criminal activity later in life. Professional mental health assessment and management may be appropriate for persistent bullying behavior.

CONCLUSIONS

With the elicitation of a good history and an understanding of child development, primary care clinicians can develop reasonable hypotheses about childhood behavioral problems. Clinicians who manage childhood behavioral problems become very comfortable with a set of behavioral management protocols that can be applied to many of these common problems. Behavioral problems that require psychiatric or psychological intervention usually become apparent early in the process. Assisting families with behavioral issues that arise with their children in the primary care office improves the relationship that families develop with their primary care clinicians.

SUGGESTED READINGS

American Academy of Pediatrics; Policy Statement. The future of pediatrics: mental health competencies for pediatric primary care. *Pediatrics* 2009;124(1):410–421.

American Academy of Pediatrics; Clinical Report. The evaluation of sexual behaviors in children. *Pediatrics* 2009;124(3):992–998.

Aranda MC, Middleton LS, Flake E, Davis BE. Psychosocial screening in children with wartime-deployed parents. *Mil Med* 2011;176(4):402–407.

Brown ML, Pope AW, Brown EJ. Treatment of primary nocturnal enuresis in children: a review. *Child Care Health Dev* 2011;37(2):153–160.

Galland BC, Mitchell EA. Helping children sleep. *Arch Dis Child* 2010;95(10):850–853.

Hagan JF, Shaw JS, Duncan PM, eds. *Bright Futures: Guidelines for Health Supervision of Infants, Children, and Adolescents.* 3rd ed. Elk Grove Village, IL: American Academy of Pediatrics, 2008.

Hayutin LG, Reed-Knight B, Blount RL, Lewis J, McCormick ML. Increasing parent-pediatrician communication about children's psychosocial problems. *J Pediatr Psychol* 2009; 34(10):1155–1164.

Kellogg ND. Sexual behaviors in children: evaluation and management. *Am Fam Physician* 2010;82(10):1233–1238.

Njoroge WF, Bernhart KP. Assessment of behavioral disorders in preschool-aged children. *Curr Psychiatry Rep* 2011;13(2): 84–92.

Olweus D. School bullying: development and some important challenges. *Annu Rev Clin Psychol* 2013;9:751–780. doi: 10.1146/annurev-clinpsy-050212-185516. Epub 2013 January 3, 2013 PMID: 23297789.

Oman RF, Vesely SK, Tolma EL, Aspy CB, Marshall LD. Reliability and validity of the youth asset survey: an update. *Am J Health Promot* 2010;25(1):e13–e24.

Perepletchikova F, Kaufman J. Emotional and behavioral sequelae of childhood maltreatment. *Curr Opin Pediatr* 2010;22(5): 610–615.

Sanci L, Lewis D, Patton G. Detecting emotional disorders in young people in primary care. *Curr Opinions Psychiatr* 2010;23:318–323.

Sapienza JK, Masten AS. Understanding and promoting resilience in children and youth. *Curr Opin Psychiatr* 2011;24(4): 267–273.

Spruyt K, Gozal D. Pediatric sleep questionnaires as diagnostic or epidemiological tools: a review of currently available instruments. *Sleep Med Rev* 2011;15(1):19–32.

WEB SITES

Cambridge Center for Behavioral Studies. http://www.behavior.org/. Accessed July 2013.

"Kids Health for Parents". http://kidshealth.org/. Accessed July 2013.

American Academy of Pediatrics Web site for parents. http://www.healthychildren.org. Accessed July 2013.

Olweus School Interventions for Bullying. http://www.clemson.edu/olweus. Accessed July 2013.

Search Institute. http://www.search-institute.org. Accessed July 2013.

Adolescents

Lawrence S. Friedman, MD

INTRODUCTION

This chapter offers a practical behavioral framework to assist those who provide health care to teenagers. Stages of adolescent development along with behavioral correlates are discussed, as are suggestions for effective patient–doctor communication, interviewing, and provision of health services. From a physiologic perspective, adolescence is the interval between the onset of puberty and the cessation of body growth. In psychosocial and behavioral terms, it is the time during which adult body image and sexual identity emerge; independent moral standards, intimate interpersonal relationships, vocational goals, and health behaviors develop; and the separation from parents takes place. Although some of these tasks may begin prior to puberty and evolve into adulthood, they provide the foundation for understanding adolescent behavior.

Accessed at http://www.emilyprogram.com/blog/new-adolescent-family-intensive-program/

Health Status & Trends

Most teenagers are healthy. Compared with other age groups, mortality rates for teenagers are low. The majority of health problems in teenagers are behavior related and include unwanted pregnancy; sexually transmitted infections (STIs); weapon carrying; interpersonal violence; suicidal ideation; alcohol, cigarette, and illicit drug use; and dietary and exercise patterns. Nationally, accidents are the leading cause of death for most populations of teenagers, although homicide (often gang related) leads in some geographic locations. Socioeconomic status and population density, rather than ethnic or racial grouping, define the neighborhoods most at risk for gunshot deaths. Nonetheless, the most common reasons for acute office visits for teenagers are routine or sports physicals, upper respiratory infections, and acne. One of the major challenges to a provider caring for teenagers is eliciting a history that reveals health risk behaviors. Because most adolescent mortality and morbidity are preventable and because many behaviors such as sexual practices, diet, exercise, and substance use that result in adult disease begin in adolescence, ignoring this age group means missing a major public health opportunity.

In 1992, the American Medical Association published Guidelines for Adolescent Preventive Services (GAPS), the first set of developmentally and behaviorally appropriate comprehensive health care guidelines for adolescents, emphasizing anticipatory, preventive, and patient-centered services. Guidelines for Adolescent Preventive Services suggest that promotion of adolescent health and prevention of disease involve a partnership encompassing patients, parents, schools, communities, and health care providers. Although these guidelines have existed for several decades, and have been shown to be valuable as care standards and as quality measures, there is little evidence that they are being widely implemented.

Adolescent health outcomes—perhaps more than for any other population—are closely linked to cultural, educational, political, and economic policies at the local and national level. Handguns and bullying are both relevant examples. For example, the availability of handguns is not a problem that the health practitioner can resolve during an office visit, yet making them less available would substantially benefit the health of many teenagers. There would very likely be less depression and suicidal ideation if more schools instituted zero tolerance programs for bullying and developed programs that promoted diversity.

The Internet and all forms of related electronic communication including social networks, texting, and instant messaging have profoundly changed the way we all interrelate socially and how we receive and disseminate health-related and behavioral information. Adolescents and young adults are, and will likely continue to be, at the forefront of this communication transformation. It is essential that those providing care to adolescents understand how these communication developments might have beneficial and detrimental influences on this population. Electronic social networks are a good example. Such networks for adolescents with chronic diseases might serve as a positive influence to improve medication compliance and decrease the sense of isolation. Conversely, bullying through social networks has been the cause of depression and even suicide. It is especially important to understand these influences because there is compelling evidence that teens who feel connected to parents,

school, and community are less likely to participate in health-compromising behavior than teens who feel isolated or disconnected. It should be expected that the evolution of new forms of electronic communication will continue to play a role in how teenagers connect to all facets of their environment including those that relate to health and well-being.

STAGES OF DEVELOPMENT

Medical services for teenagers need to be appropriate for each developmental stage. Each of the three recognized developmental stages in adolescence is distinguished by physical, cognitive, and behavioral hallmarks. Not all adolescents fit perfectly into each phase, and they often progress at different rates from one phase to the next. Moreover, rates of physical, cognitive, and behavioral development may not be congruent. For example, a 14-year-old girl who is physically mature may be emotionally and cognitively unable to decide about sexual intimacy and the potential consequences.

Early Adolescence (Ages 11–14)

PHYSICAL

Rapid growth causes physical and body image changes. Many teenagers question whether their growth is "normal," and commonly there is a good deal of somatic preoccupation and anxiety. Gynecomastia, for example (a common transient problem for boys), may cause concern, and prevent participation in physical education class. Because the topic may be too embarrassing for an already self-conscious teenager, clinician-initiated reassurance is essential when the condition is identified during a physical examination. Early or later onset of puberty has widely variable effects. Early puberty may be associated with the increased likelihood of weight concern and excessive dieting and other eating disorders in girls, but it may result in greater self-esteem and athletic prowess in boys. Because self-esteem is linked closely with physical development and peer group attractiveness, teens who develop later than their peers may have self-esteem problems. Among early adolescents, questions and concerns about menstruation, masturbation, wet dreams, and the size of their breasts (too large or too small) and genitals are common. These questions need to be anticipated and specifically and carefully addressed. Endocrine disorders related to sexual maturation are likely to emerge; early diagnosis and treatment can improve health and self-esteem.

SOCIAL

In adolescence, peer group involvement increases and family involvement decreases. Friendships are idealized and are mostly same gender. Close peer relationships coupled with curiosity about body development may result in homosexual and other sexual experimentation, anxiety, and fear. Although some heterosexual relationships are initiated, contact with the opposite sex frequently occurs in groups. Often by this age adolescents have access to the Internet, participate in online social networks, and use cell phones. How they are used and potentially monitored will often become an important issue of family discussion.

COGNITIVE

The transition from concrete to abstract thinking begins. Because experience and emotion play important roles in decision making, improved cognition alone is not enough to prevent many teenagers from making impulsive decisions with little regard for consequences. Increased cognitive ability linked with the search for identity often leads teenagers to test limits both at home and at school. Daydreaming is common.

Middle Adolescence (Ages 15–17)

PHYSICAL

The issues of early adolescence may continue, although most physical development is complete by the end of this phase.

SOCIAL

Independence, identity, and autonomy struggles intensify. Peer groups may become more important than family to some teenagers and result in increasing teen–parent conflict. Experimentation with alcohol, drugs, and sex is common. A sense of invincibility coupled with impulsiveness leads to relatively high rates of automobile accidents and interpersonal violence. Suicide, impulsively linked to failed love relationships, or poor self-esteem because of difficulty finding peer group acceptance may also occur during this phase. Despite adhering to peer group norms regarding music, dress, and appearance (including body piercing, tattoos, clothes, hair color, and makeup), the expression of individuality is common. Many teenagers find identity and support in school, sports, community, or church activities. For teenagers whose support systems or community resources are inadequate, gangs may supplement personal strength and provide a sense of identity. Teenagers from alienated and disenfranchised ethnic groups are at particular risk for gang activity. In spite of slowly improving cultural acceptance, gay, lesbian, and transgendered teenagers may feel increased isolation, alienation, and bullying (see Chapter 17). This may lead to depression, sexual promiscuity, or suicide. The Internet leads to easy linkage to social networks for minority youth, such as those with chronic diseases, who in the past might have felt isolated and now can gain access to social and psychological support. Those same networks, however, also make it much easier for sexual encounters and resulting exposure to STIs or unintended pregnancy.

COGNITIVE

Improved reasoning and abstraction allow for closer interpersonal relationships and empathy in this group. Evaluation of future academic and vocational plans becomes important. Poor school performance may heighten anxiety and concern about vocational choices and lead to "escape" in drugs and alcohol. Practical guidance that identifies strengths and builds self-esteem can help avoid frustration and failure.

Late Adolescence (Ages 18–24)

PHYSICAL

Body growth is usually no longer a concern. The quest to become comfortable with one's physical appearance often continues throughout adulthood.

SOCIAL

If the adolescent's development has occurred within the context of a supportive family, community, school, and peer environment, individual identity formation and separation will be complete. In reality, however, at least some developmental issues usually remain unresolved into adulthood. Late adolescents typically spend more time developing monogamous interpersonal relationships and less time seeking peer group support. Ideally, decision making, based on an individualized value system, is modulated by limit setting and compromise.

COGNITIVE

Vocational goals should now be set in practical terms, and there should be realistic expectations about education and work.

ADOLESCENTS & THE MEDICAL INTERVIEW

A general health assessment should include a review of systems and an evaluation of health-related behavior. This should include risk factors for accidents, STIs, including human immunodeficiency virus (HIV), pregnancy, interpersonal violence (including past physical or sexual abuse), nutrition, substance use, exercise, sleep, learning, and mental health problems. Guidance about promoting healthful behaviors and preventing disease should be integrated into the discussion. Inclusion of these factors is considered community standard of care for adolescents. Documentation of health encounters ideally should be done electronically; it is therefore recommended that a standard written protocol be developed so that all elements described above can be documented and searched for quality assessment. From the patient's perspective, the clinician's inquiries and assessment of some behaviors may be viewed as embarrassing, intrusive, or trivial. It is therefore helpful to explain, prior to questioning, that (1) the same questions are asked of all patients and that (2) the encounter goal is patient self-awareness and health education. During the interview it is important to reinforce and praise healthy decisions, such as sexual abstinence.

Confidentiality

Certain ground rules are important. Ensure the adolescent that, unless homicide or suicide is threatened or ongoing abuse is reported, all conversations are confidential, and the information will not be shared with parents, teachers, or other authorities without permission. Discussions about sex and drugs should always occur in private unless otherwise requested by the patient. If the patient is accompanied by a parent, solicit parental concerns, and then ask the adult to leave the room and conduct the interview in private. It is also helpful to let the parent know (if present) about the confidential nature of the patient–clinician conversation.

Although most teenagers want to receive health information and discuss personal behavior, these discussions must generally be initiated by the physician. Many teenagers are not accustomed to interacting in such participatory, nonjudgmental conversations with adults. The willingness of a teenager to share personal or intimate information depends on the perceived receptiveness of the provider. Teenagers need to feel that they have permission to share personal, behavior-related information. For example, it is usually not difficult for patients and clinicians to discuss routine chronic medical conditions such as diabetes or asthma. Control of these conditions in some teenagers, however, may be related more to dietary indiscretions and cigarette use, than to insulin or inhaler use. Such health-compromising behaviors must be identified before they can be dealt with; comments, facial expressions, or body language indicating disapproval can undermine the patient's willingness to disclose confidential behavior (Table 13-1).

Most electronic medical record systems now include patient web-portals that allow secure communication between patient and provider. This type of system potentially makes communication easier and faster for all involved. Issues around confidentially and parental access make independent use by minors problematic, although is often supported by many parents. Future systems will likely also include embedded video (telemedicine) linkage, and the same issues related to parental control will apply. See Table 13-2 for Quality and Safety suggestions.

Legal Issues

Many practitioners worry about the legality of evaluating and treating teenagers without parental consent. Because laws vary by state, it is essential to become

Table 13-1. Interview suggestions.

1. Ensure doctor–patient confidentiality. Do not inquire about health-related behaviors in front of parents.
2. Use the HEADSS format to organize the interview.
3. Assess the patient's cognitive and developmental level through interactive dialogue.
4. Initiate discussions about behavior and offer anticipatory guidance that is culturally and developmentally appropriate.
5. Listen actively to patients' opinions and perspective.
6. Be familiar with and refer to local resources for cases of domestic violence, runaways, and substance abuse.
7. Include patients in discussing and making all diagnostic and therapeutic decisions.
8. Review the behavioral stages of development with parents. Emphasize the importance of instilling confidence and building self-esteem in their children.
9. Reinforce good behavior. Congratulate teenagers who do not use drugs and who are not sexually active.
10. Address all teenagers with respect, and be nonjudgmental about their behaviors and traits.

familiar with the applicable local statutes. Many states permit the diagnosis and treatment of teenagers with sex-, drug-, and alcohol-related problems without parental notification or consent. States do vary at the age about which teens can receive such services without parental permission. Likewise, most states permit medical care if a condition is potentially life threatening. Documentation of the rationale leading to the decision to proceed without parental permission, in a potential "life-threatening" situation, is essential.

Table 13-2. Recommendations for care quality.

1. Written documentation (electronic documentation ideal for audits) of behavior-related health risk factors
   a. Alcohol and drugs
   b. Tobacco
   c. Violence/gang involvement
   d. Seat belt use
   e. Helmet use
   f. Firearms and storage
   g. Sexual behavior
   h. Nutrition/diet /exercise
2. *Chlamydia* screening in patients who are sexually involved
3. Vaccines (assuming up-to-date with childhood vaccination)
   a. HPV males and females
   b. Meningococcal booster
   c. Tdap
   d. Influenza

Interview Organization

A comprehensive health risk assessment should cover issues dealing with home, education, activities, drug use, sexual practices, and suicidal ideation (HEADSS). Using the HEADSS format helps with organization and standardization. Assessing cognitive ability using interactive dialogue needs to be done in the first few minutes of the interview. The following interview goals and questions facilitate communication.

HOME

1. **Goal**—Determine household structure, family structure and function, conflict-resolution skills, the possibility of domestic violence, and presence of chronic illness in the family (see Chapter 11).
2. **Questions**—"Who lives where you live?" If only one parent is at home, the interviewer should inquire about the other parent's whereabouts, visitation pattern, reasons for leaving (especially domestic violence and substance abuse), and whether the teen moves back and forth between parents. Teenagers caught between divorced parents or those who feel neglected may "act out" and get into trouble to gain parental attention, sometimes in the hope that their problems will reunite separated parents. For single-parent families, the patient can be asked, "Does your mom or dad date? How do you get along with the people he or she dates?" Questions about domestic violence should include "What happens when people argue in your house?" and "Does anyone get hurt during arguments? How about you?" and "What if someone has been drinking or using drugs and they argue?" and "Have you ever seen your mother hit by anyone?" "Are there guns in your house?" If there are, ask if they are always locked and who has a key. Educate parents and patients about accidental gunshots. Ask about siblings, including their health and whereabouts. Somatization may be learned by observing a family member who receives attention for a chronic medical condition. Learning about extended family members living in the household is also important and will likely be revealed with the first question above.

EDUCATION

1. **Goal**—Identify attention deficit hyperactivity disorder (ADHD) and other learning disabilities, school performance, cognitive ability, and vocational potential.
2. **Questions**—"What grade are you in?" "What type of grades do you get?" "How do they compare with your grades last year?" Falling grades may indicate family, mental health, or substance-abuse problems. "Have you ever been told you had a learning problem?" "Can you see the blackboard?" Most teenagers respond that everything in school is okay. Specific questions about courses and content need to be asked, including the student's favorite and worst subjects and his or her career aspirations. Generally, teenagers who perform well in school are less likely to participate in multiple health risk behaviors. The teen should be asked about attendance, and truancy or other school troubles. Teenagers with drug problems may enjoy going to school because, although they may rarely attend class, school is where they visit friends and purchase or sell drugs. Students who get all "A's" should be asked about school-related stress and what would happen if they did not receive high grades. Depression and even suicide can be related to unrealistic grade expectations by teenagers and their parents.

ACTIVITIES

1. **Goal**—Evaluate the patient's social interactions, Internet use and purposes of use, interests, and self-esteem.
2. **Questions**—"What do you do for fun?" "Are you involved in school, community, or religious activities, such as youth groups, clubs, or sports?" Self-esteem is often related to successful participation in these activities. Teenagers actively involved in "productive" activities are less likely to participate in delinquent behavior. The clinician should ask about gang or fraternity/sorority membership, either of which can be a source of inappropriate peer pressure. Gangs may provide the strongest sense of family or community available to some teenagers.

Questions should be asked about dietary habits, including the frequency and amount of "junk" food, who cooks, and dieting or self-induced vomiting (see Chapter 23). It is also important to inquire about patients' physical activities, and to educate and to make recommendations about regular exercise, protective headgear, and seatbelts. Internet assessment should include types of sites visited and purpose of use.

DRUGS

1. **Goal**—Evaluate the patient's current habits, patterns of use, and the genetic or environmental risk factors (Table 13-3). Distinguish between those who drink because of social, cultural, and peer pressure, those who are genetically predisposed, and those who drink or use illicit drugs because of comorbid mental health problems.
2. **Questions**—It is less threatening to begin by asking, "Are you aware of alcohol or drug use at your school?" and "Do any of your friends drink or use drugs?" followed by "Have you ever tried alcohol or

Table 13-3. Substance abuse risk factors for adolescents.

---
1. Family history of use
2. Low self-esteem and body image
3. Depression or thought disorder
4. Antisocial personality traits
5. Peer and cultural pressures
---

drugs?" The physician should inquire specifically about cigarettes, alcohol, marijuana, recreational "pills" (e.g., ecstasy, ketamine), cocaine, lysergic acid diethylamide (LSD), crystal methamphetamine, anabolic steroids, and heroin. The quantity, frequency, circumstances, and family patterns of use are important. To learn about family drinking, ask specific questions about each parent and both maternal and paternal grandparents, including whether anyone in the family attends Alcoholics Anonymous (AA) or other self-help groups. When parents do not recognize or admit to a problem, a child may not identify them as alcoholics. The teenager should be asked to describe the parent's pattern of alcohol use. "Have you ever seen your mother or father drunk?" If the answer is yes, then ask "When and how frequently?" The CRAFFT questions (Table 13-4) have been validated as a useful brief screening test for teenagers suspected of substance abuse. Two or more YES answers on the CRAFFT indicate a significant problem.

Recognition of a parental problem is also essential. Even the best treatment program will fail if a teenager is discharged back into the home of an actively using parent. The willingness of parents to change either their own drinking or family behavior patterns is one of the best predictors of adolescent treatment success.

Table 13-4. CRAFFT* questions.

---
1. Have you ever ridden in a **C**AR driven by someone (including yourself) who was "high" or had been using alcohol or drugs?
2. Do you ever use alcohol/drugs to **R**ELAX, feel better about yourself, or fit in?
3. Do you ever use alcohol/drugs while you are by yourself, **A**LONE?
4. Do your family or **F**RIENDS ever tell you that you should cut down on drinking or drug use?
5. Do you ever **F**ORGET things you did while using alcohol or drugs?
6. Have you gotten into **T**ROUBLE while you were using alcohol or drugs?
---

*Two or more YES answers indicate a significant problem.

Among many teenagers, the use of drugs and alcohol is often not considered abnormal or dangerous. Only about 5–10% of teenage drinkers or drug users develop substance-abuse problems as adults. Because serious physical consequences, other than accidents, usually do not occur until later in life, there is little negative association with alcohol or drug use. Abused, neglected, disabled, or chronically ill teenagers may consider drugs or alcohol one of the few things that, at least temporarily, make them feel good and accepted by peers. If legal involvement, school problems, or family conflict are present, it is important to assess the role of alcohol and drugs. Even if use seems minimal, it should be pointed out that problems are best solved sober.

Referral to a substance-abuse expert is indicated when use significantly interferes with school, family, or social functioning. Anticipatory guidance should address age-appropriate concerns. Advising teenagers to stop smoking cigarettes because of the possibility of future lung cancer and heart disease is usually meaningless. Talking about wrinkled skin, bad breath, and yellow teeth is much more relevant to body image concerns and far more likely to prevent or stop cigarette use. Similarly, the association between alcohol and date rape is more important to teenage girls than are other future consequences.

Sex

1. **Goal**—Determine the level of the patient's sexual involvement and sexuality, use of birth control, protection against STIs, and any history of abuse.
2. **Questions**—An opening question such as "Have you ever been sexually involved with anyone?" is preferable to "Are you sexually active?" The word *active* is notoriously misinterpreted. Questions need to be open ended and should not assume heterosexual orientation. Assumptions about boyfriends or girlfriends inhibit discussion or questions about homosexual partners or feelings. Because teenagers frequently practice serial monogamy, the sequential number of different partners and their ages should be determined. Ask whether they have ever met anyone on the Internet for sexual reasons and the circumstances related to that encounter. A 15-year-old teenager with a peer group partner is at less risk for STIs, especially HIV, than is one with a substantially older partner. For the sexually involved, discuss birth control techniques and condoms. One of the most common reasons for not using a condom is the belief that birth control pills provide adequate protection against STIs. When appropriate, physicians should reinforce sexual abstinence with congratulations and support.

Sexual abuse is unfortunately common. A history of such incidents should be sought by asking, "Have you ever been touched sexually when you did not want to be?" Obtaining this history may be pivotal in helping a teenager who has developed abuse-related behavioral problems, such as sexual promiscuity, depression, substance abuse, delinquency, and an eating or somatization disorder.

Unwanted pregnancy among teenagers is still at epidemic proportions. Risk factors are complex but include ignorance, lack of access to family planning services, cultural acceptance, and poor self-esteem.

SUICIDE

1. **Goal**—Identify serious mental health problems and distinguish them from normal adolescent affect and moodiness. Primary risk factors are listed in Table 13-5.

   Distinguishing significant psychiatric illness from normal fluctuations in a teenager's affect is challenging. In spite of the general perception to the contrary, most teenagers are not maladjusted, and the rates of mental health problems are no higher than in adults. Few teenagers announce that they are feeling depressed or are in emotional turmoil. Depression may be reflected in sexual promiscuity, drug and alcohol abuse, or in the commission of violent and delinquent acts. Chronic somatic complaints such as headache, abdominal pain, or chest pain without an identifiable biological explanation may also indicate depression secondary to abuse.

2. **Questions**—Practitioners should identify vegetative signs of depression, such as sleep disturbance, decreased appetite, hopelessness, lethargy, continuous thoughts about suicide, hallucinations, or illogical thoughts. It should also be noted that many of these symptoms may also be caused by substance abuse. Evaluation of lethargy should be done from the patient's perspective. Energy may be low relative to the parents' desires or expectations—but sufficient for the teenager. There may be insufficient energy to clean, help with household chores, or

Table 13-5. Risk factors for major depression and suicide.

1. Prior episode of serious depression or suicide
2. Family history of suicide or mental health problems
3. History of victimization
4. Substance abuse or dependency
5. Gay or lesbian sexual identity
6. Availability of handguns (increases rate of success)
7. Recent loss of significant friends or family
8. Extreme family, school, or social stress

complete homework but plenty of energy available to play sports, go on a date, party with friends, travel miles, and wait for hours to obtain concert tickets.

CASE ILLUSTRATION 1

Lauren is a 15-year-old girl admitted to the hospital with an arm fracture requiring surgical repair. The fracture occurred during cheerleading practice while climbing a pyramid of other cheerleaders. She reported being distracted while climbing, lost concentration, and fell to the ground. During the admission history the patient was talkative and easily distracted. Although she did not report taking any medications to the admitting nurse, when asked "are you supposed to be taking" any medications, Lauren reported that she should be taking medication for ADHD (see Chapter 27). She had not taken medication for the last several days because she was staying with a friend and did not want her friend to know that she took medication.

This case illustrates several important adolescent issues. First, teenagers may concretely interpret questions. When Lauren was asked by the nurse if she was taking any medication, she answered honestly. A combination of clinical judgment at the time of interview related to Lauren's inattentiveness, knowledge that teenagers may interpret concretely, and that they may not make the connection between behavior and health consequences are all important to this case. Second, teenagers seek peer conformance. Medication compliance problems may relate to avoiding peer awareness of medications and, therefore, being labeled as different. Taking medication at school, camp, or at the house of a friend may all make a teenager feel different. Lastly, instructions about medications should be given in terms of what is important to the patient. Lauren may have known that medication was beneficial for school performance, but may not have realized that it would improve concentration with other tasks that required focus and attention.

CASE ILLUSTRATION 2

Two days after sustaining minor injuries in a traffic accident, Jeff, a 16-year-old teenager, comes to the physician's office complaining of left shoulder pain. He is accompanied by his mother, who is concerned because Jeff was also recently arrested for driving under the influence of alcohol. There is no history of medical or behavioral problems, although, on questioning, his mother describes a 12-month history of moodiness and falling school grades. Using the HEADSS format assessment, the physician assesses Jeff's health risks:

Home: Jeff lives at home with his biological mother and father. The parents are first-generation immigrants who both work full time. There are few arguments at home, and Jeff describes both parents as stoic, religious, and unemotional.

Education: Although he was an above-average student until last year, Jeff's education is now being adversely affected by his truancy and lack of interest.

Activity: Although Jeff previously played several sports at school, watching television is now his favorite activity.

Drugs: Jeff admits to using drugs frequently. He drinks alcohol at least twice a week and smokes marijuana daily. Since this use is no more frequent than that of his friends, he does not consider it excessive.

Sex: Jeff has no steady sexual partners, but has had several short-term relationships.

Suicide: Jeff denies being suicidal or depressed. When asked about significant losses, however, he becomes tearful and talks hesitantly about his older brother, a construction worker, who died accidentally 2 years ago. Since the burial, his brother was never talked about at home.

The connection between increased substance use, declining grades, and the brother's death seems obvious. Because the substance use began insidiously, and significant trouble did not occur until more than a year after his brother's death, neither Jeff nor his parents associated the events. Furthermore, this is a family that seemingly does not share emotions, and Jeff never learned how to discuss his feelings. In this case, simply learning about his drug use, home situation, school performance, and activities was not enough. The facts all confirmed his substance abuse but did not explain it. With a teenager who previously has been without significant behavioral problems, it is crucial to search for personal or family events, including losses, that underlie and precipitate behavior change.

Both Jeff and his parents must be made aware of the connection between the substance use and the brother's death. It is imperative that Jeff acknowledge his drug problem and be referred to a practitioner experienced in treating adolescents with substance-abuse problems (see Chapter 24). Although Jeff should respond to psychotherapy that addresses his grief and loss, psychotherapy may not be effective if mind-altering substances are being used concomitantly.

SPECIFIC AT-RISK POPULATIONS

Homeless & Runaway Teenagers

There is a heterogeneous group of between 500,000 and 2 million homeless teenagers in the United States. Some are homeless because their families are, some live on the streets for brief periods of time, and others find shelter with friends or relatives. Those who leave home, do not return, and no longer depend on parents for financial support or shelter constitute a significant proportion and may be more precisely called *throwaways*. Before they leave home, these teenagers have usually had repeated contacts with social service agencies and have histories of severe parental conflict and high rates of physical and sexual abuse. Family abandonment because of sexual orientation is not uncommon. The social network designed to protect them has failed, and their experience of neglect, abuse, and abandonment results in a distrust of adults and institutions.

Leaving home and living on the streets may initially be a liberating experience. Once on the street, multiple substance use is common, often becoming a short-term pleasant escape from an otherwise dismal existence. Survival often depends on trading sex for drugs, food, or shelter. Other survival techniques, such as selling drugs and theft, create risks for interpersonal violence and victimization. Poor self-esteem, depression, and suicidal ideation are common in this group. Usually—within weeks or months—the liberating experience of independence becomes one of desperation and hopelessness.

The initial medical evaluation may seem overwhelming. Many of these patients qualify for emancipated minor legal status and may be eligible for Medicaid or other entitlements. Distrust of adults, the inability to navigate a complicated health system, and reluctance to disclose personal information may, however, keep them from receiving benefits and proper health care. It is important for the clinician to prioritize such a patient's health issues and be familiar with community referral sources. Shelter, food, safety, social support, substance abuse and mental health counseling, and medical evaluation are all usually necessary. Developing a trusting working relationship is essential and may require several visits. Keeping medical appointments and complying with referrals may be complicated by a reversed sleep–wake cycle. In some cases, it may be that texting can be used beneficially for appointment and medication reminders. As with other teenagers, questions about sex and drugs are best kept in a medical context; it should be made clear that they are asked only because of their health implications. Rather than asking whether a teenager has been a "prostitute," asking, "Have you ever had sex in order to obtain drugs, food, or a place to sleep?" is nonjudgmental and will be readily understood.

Questions about sexual orientation may be confusing to a teenager with a history of sexual abuse and survival sex and may provoke anxiety and shame. These issues are best raised after a stable living situation and support system have been established.

Chronic Disease & Disability

At least 2 million teenagers in the United States have chronic disabilities or diseases. Although this is a diverse group, its members share some similar behavioral issues. Unlike other teenagers whose identity and self-esteem are molded by the acceptance of a peer group, chronically ill or disabled teenagers have limited ability to conform and often have poor self-esteem. Too frequently this leads to depression, family conflict, and social isolation.

Like those of other teenagers—issues usually revolve around physical, social, and sexual development. Frank discussions, including realistic assessments of their hopes and expectations, need to be initiated by the physician. It is crucial to identify and encourage the interests and skills that may realistically be expected to strengthen self-esteem. Predictors of successful coping include friendships with healthy as well as ill or disabled peers, parents who are not overly protective, involvement with family activities, and appropriate household responsibilities.

Chronically ill teenagers are often "noncompliant" with medical regimens. Adolescence is no less a time of experimentation, self-discovery, and testing of limits for the chronically ill teen than for other teens, and chronically ill teenagers—like others—are often noncompliant. Issues about compliance are often issues about control and of testing of limits. The struggle for independence conflicts with the limitations of the disability itself as well as the relationship with parents and health care providers. Supportive electronic social networks of teens with similar disorders might greatly decrease the sense of social isolation, and texting reminders has the potential for improving medication compliance. Table 13-6 lists some suggestions for ways of improving compliance.

Gay & Lesbian Youth

Gay and lesbian teenagers are at risk for social isolation, depression, STIs, substance abuse, and interpersonal violence. The relationships they develop with a health care provider may help them cope with the negative stereotyping they receive from other parts of society. A nonjudgmental and supportive attitude by the clinician helps lessen the weight of such cultural negativity.

Although some teenagers may volunteer information about their homosexual concerns or ideation, many do not unless they are specifically asked or given permission to do so. Some teens may have feelings of

Table 13-6. Strategies for improving compliance.

1. Have patients participate in all therapeutic and diagnostic decisions.
2. Discuss developmentally appropriate consequences of noncompliance. For instance, the renal or neurologic complications of poor diabetes control will not seem very important to a 14-year-old teenager. Emphasize the positive instead–such as how proper glucose control will allow continued participation in sports and other peer activities.
3. Parents need guidance on how to balance protectiveness with their teenager's need to make independent decisions. Role-playing in specific scenarios may be helpful.
4. When possible, communicate directly with the patient without using the parent as a conduit. Let patients know that their opinions and questions are important.
5. Refer patients and parents to local peer support groups such as diabetes, asthma, and epilepsy societies. Support groups exist for almost all chronic illnesses and can usually be found through local telephone directories or agencies such as United Way.

anxiety, shame, and guilt about same-sex experiences. Such experiences are common, especially among young adolescents who may not yet have firm sexual identity. Such experiences do not necessarily reflect future sexual orientation. The risk of HIV infection increases when gay teenage boys have older partners, who themselves may have had multiple partners. Inquiry about Internet use and actual sexual encounters is essential to get a sense of potential health risk behaviors and exposure to STIs. Table 13-7 lists some suggestions for working with gay and lesbian youth.

Table 13-7. Recommendations for addressing needs of gay or lesbian youth.

1. Assess the patient's level of comfort and self-acceptance.
2. Evaluate and discuss external stressors, such as parents, school, and the patient's social and religious environment. Refer the patient (and parents, if necessary) to mental health experts if the stressors are severe and interfere with daily activities.
3. Reassure the patient that from a medical perspective, homosexuality is a normal variant like left-handedness.
4. Refer patients to local gay youth groups for peer support; most cities and colleges provide resources for lesbian and gay youth, and telephone directories usually list local resources. Refer parents to local parent support groups, especially the local chapter of Parents and Friends of Lesbian and Gay Youth (P-FLAG).

SUGGESTED READINGS

Centers for Disease Control and Prevention. Youth Risk Behavior Surveillance—United States, 2009. *Morb Mortal Wkly Rep* 2010;59(SS-5):1–142.

Committee on Substance Abuse. Policy Statement: alcohol use by youth and adolescents: a pediatric concern. *Pediatrics* 2010;5: 1078–1087.

Elster AB, Kuznets NJ, eds. *AMA Guidelines for Adolescent Preventive Services (GAPS)*. Philadelphia, PA: Williams & Wilkins, 1994.

O'Keefe GS, Clarke-Pearson K, *Council on Communications and Media*, American Academy of Pediatrics. 2011;127:800–804.

WEB SITES

A Consensus Statement on Health Care Transitions for Young Adults With Special Health Care Needs. American Academy of Pediatrics, American Academy of Family Physicians and American College of Physicians-American Society of Internal Medicine. *Pediatrics* 2002;110;1304. http://pediatrics.aappublications.org/content/110/Supplement_3/1304.full.pdf. Accessed April 2013.

Official Position Papers on Multiple Relevant Topics. Society for Adolescent Medicine Web site. http://www.adolescenthealth.org/Position_Papers/4700.htm. Accessed April 2013.

Older Patients

Robin Telerant, MD; Elizabeth Eckstrom, MD, MPH;
Clifford M. Singer, MD; & Jay Luxenberg, MD

INTRODUCTION

We are an aging society. By the year 2020, one in five Americans will be over the age of 65 years, compared to a little over one in eight today. The oldest of the old, those aged over 85 years, comprise an increasing proportion of the elderly, and present special challenges to health care providers. The clinical care of older adults relies on knowledge of normal aging and the common diseases of old age. This chapter focuses on these aspects of mental health and illness.

NORMAL PSYCHOLOGICAL AGING

Although chronic and degenerative diseases impact quality of life, many older adults are active, engaged, and pleasure seeking. They remain curious and continue to learn throughout their lives. Temperament (i.e., energy, intensity, reactivity) remains stable, whereas personality (learned behavior patterns) undergoes refinement and change over time in most healthy adults. Predictable changes in intellect occur in most people as they age. Although judgment, knowledge, and verbal skills increase through the life span, mental functions that rely on memory and processing speed are adversely affected by aging.

Successful adaptation to old age is difficult to define and variably expressed. Signs of successful aging include acceptance of change, affectionate relationships with family and friends, and a positive view of one's life story. Another indicator is the ability to find new sources of self-esteem independent of raising children, career, physical strength, or beauty. Factors that promote successful adaptation are luck (good genes, avoiding injury) and healthy behaviors including proper diet, adequate sleep, plenty of physical activity, and good stress management. Having enough money for basic needs as well as strong kinship and extended family bonds add extra protection from disease and despair, as do spirituality, having friends and confidants, and feeling valued by society. Opportunities to be productive and assist younger generations can provide a sense of connection to one's community and a feeling of completeness.

Patients and families will often ask for advice on staying engaged and active. Many communities have senior centers, agencies, or programs that organize discussion groups, lectures, hobby groups, travel groups, book groups, adult education classes, and volunteer activities. Similar programs or groups can be created, even in the smallest communities, by forming book or knitting groups, foster grandparent services, or peer support programs. The local Area Agency on Aging may have information for specific resources and volunteer opportunities in your community.

Social conditions that contribute to demoralization in old age include highly mobile and rapidly changing communities, youth-oriented aesthetics, the deaths of friends and family members, and forced retirement. Physical conditions that limit function and increase isolation, such as urinary incontinence, chronic pain, gait and mobility problems, and hearing and vision loss also contribute to demoralization. Declining hygiene, poor nutrition, falls, alcohol abuse, social withdrawal, chaotic finances, and denial of severe health problems are clues that an older person is failing at home because of diminishing physical, emotional, or intellectual function. Recognizing these problems can be difficult. Health care practitioners may not detect problems if older patients are reclusive, try to look their best in the office, or avoid discussion of problems they face functioning at home. Often it is family members, friends, neighbors, and others who first recognize a person's functional decline. Their impressions can be very helpful to clinicians, but sometimes the family needs to be specifically asked to investigate the well-being of the patient. In extreme cases, Adult Protective Services or a local Council on Aging may be asked to investigate a patient's safety. The challenge is to obtain the needed information while abiding by Health Insurance Portability and Accountability Act (HIPAA) regulations, and obtaining the information while retaining the confidence of the patient. If time permits, a home visit may be especially revealing.

Older adults experience obstacles to obtaining medical care. Financial barriers to mental health care are compounded by the lesser coverage for mental compared to physical illness under the Medicare insurance program. This disparity is being phased out by 2014 under the Medicare Improvements for Patients and Providers Act (MIPPA). Older patients may also deliberately avoid seeking help, particularly for emotional and cognitive problems. Some seniors do not view emotional distress as something to discuss with physicians. They suffer silently or disguise their distress with physical symptoms or irritability and withdrawal from family, friends, or caregivers. Unfortunately, the prejudicial attitudes of physicians and mental health providers about mental and emotional problems in old age play into this silence and contribute to the under recognition and treatment of these disorders. Clinicians may be reluctant to prescribe treatment for problems viewed as inevitable parts of aging or they may simply consider treatment to be futile.

Providing medical care to older patients requires an understanding of normal changes in mental and emotional functioning in old age, and skill in determining when intervention is needed. Addressing the concerns of family and caregivers, accessing community services, and advising patients about end-of-life and long-term care options all require sensitivity and skill. Diagnosing mental disorders in older people is challenging as multiple clinical syndromes—including both mental and medical—often overlap. In the following sections, we will review an approach to geriatric conditions and highlight cases that illustrate how clinicians can effectively treat this population.

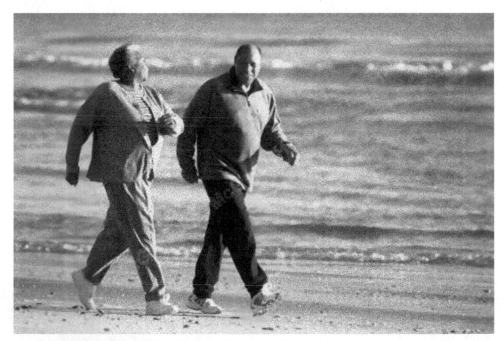

Elderly Walk.jpg (obtained from McGraw-Hill image library).

THE CLINICAL ENCOUNTER

Considerations for Communicating with Older Patients

THE CLINICAL SETTING

Seeing older adults in a primary care practice can be challenging due to the special needs of this population. Adaptations to the office setting, such as larger, wheelchair-accessible rooms, can make it easier for patients to get in and out of the examination room. Loud noises, from the waiting room or adjoining rooms, can be distracting and can limit the provider's ability to obtain a focused history. If possible, appointments should be made later in the day to allow older adults to arrange transportation. A more liberal "no-show" policy may need to be adopted as cancellations in this age group are not uncommon.

PATIENT INTERVIEW

Clinicians should inquire early in the interview whether they are being heard and understood. Projecting one's voice and speaking distinctly are helpful for many older persons, but clinicians should not assume this is necessary and shout at all patients just because they are very old. Speaking slower facilitates communication much better than speaking louder. Assistive devices, such as portable amplification (e.g., Pocket Talker*), can be invaluable in obtaining useful information. Active listening methods, such as maintaining eye contact, nodding, and paraphrasing the patient's questions and statements should be used (see Chapter 1). Attention to the light source is important; be certain not to sit or stand with your back to the window or light fixture so patients will be able to see your face. Shorter, more frequent visits for patients with many symptoms or greater need to talk will reduce the physician's frustration, improve communication, and better meet the patient's emotional needs for contact with the physician. One of the true pleasures of caring for older patients is hearing their life stories, but time constraints may mandate that this occur over several visits.

FAMILY AND CAREGIVER INTERVIEW

Most frail older patients should be accompanied by a family member or caregiver so that the clinician can obtain a complete view of the problem. If this is not possible, a phone conversation with family, once permission from the patient is obtained, can be just as illuminating. Patients with dementia may not be aware of their memory impairment and can actively deny they have any problem. They may also have limited insight into functional decline in their own activities of daily living (ADLs), depressive symptoms, or paranoid thinking. Delusional thoughts may seem perfectly logical until the family or caregiver is consulted (sometimes, of course, the patient is correct—abuse and exploitation must be ruled out). Family consultation must be pursued with sensitivity to the patient's feelings, and may need to occur outside the examination room (with permission from the patient) to avoid alienating the patient. It is during these separate interviews that clinicians can obtain more candid reports of impaired ADLs, psychiatric symptoms, and memory problems.

Assessment

HISTORY

When assessing older adults, clinicians should pay particular attention to recent changes in function and a review of the most common geriatric syndromes. These include cognitive impairment, falls, urinary incontinence, hearing loss, vision loss, malnutrition, frailty, and mood disorders. Careful medication reconciliation is one of the hallmarks of a geriatric assessment. Polypharmacy

Table 14-1. The "MOMS AND DADS" geriatric neuropsychiatry review of symptoms.*

M	Mobility	Gait and balance, recent falls, use of walking aides
O	Output	Bowel function, urine output, bladder continence
M	Memory	Emphasis on recent memory function
S	Senses	Changes in hearing and vision
A	Aches	Pain survey
N	Neuro	Neuro symptoms such as dizziness or weakness
D	Delusions	Psychotic symptoms, paranoia, hallucinations
D	Depression	Dysphoria, anxiety, fearfulness, irritability, hopelessness
A	Appetite	Food and fluid intake
D	Dermis	Changes in skin color, integrity, dental problems
S	Sleep	Problems initiating or maintaining sleep, daytime alertness, abnormal nocturnal activity

*This offers a helpful supplement to the standard organ system-based review of systems.

and medication interactions are common. Many medications can result in behavioral side effects, and many medications for mental health conditions can cause serious medical adverse events. Increasingly, vitamins, homeopathic medications, and over-the-counter therapies are being used, further complicating the picture. Alcohol use is often overlooked in this population, but abuse is not uncommon, and the results can be devastating. A careful assessment of alcohol intake is key. A useful acronym we have developed for a geriatric review of systems (MOMS AND DADS) is presented in Table 14-1.

PHYSICAL ASSESSMENT

Though a complete physical examination is always informative, there are certain elements that are especially important in older adults. General appearance and hygiene can help determine whether the patient is well cared for or able to take care of him or herself appropriately. Weight measurements are useful in assessing nutritional status. Orthostatic blood pressure measurements can help determine a patient's risk of dizziness and falls, and are particularly important to monitor if new medication is being considered. The oral examination, often overlooked in younger adult patients, can be critical in this population, as poor dentition or ill-fitting dentures can contribute to weight loss and frailty. A careful neurologic examination can pick up conditions such as Parkinson disease and Lewy Body Dementia. Gait and balance, which can be evaluated with tools like the Get Up and Go or the Tinetti Gait and Balance, should be assessed to determine fall risk. Evidence of abuse, such as suspicious bruises or injuries, or evidence of neglect should prompt an adult protective services referral through the local Area Agency on Aging or as directed by the regulations applying to your jurisdiction.

MENTAL AND COGNITIVE STATUS EXAMINATIONS

An important component of geriatric assessment is using validated tests to examine cognition and mood. Orientation, short-term memory, problem-solving ability, judgment, insight, initiative, executive function, mood, and affect are all components of a broad cognitive assessment.

The Geriatric Depression Scale (GDS) is a standardized mood rating scale that can be administered by the clinician or the patient himself or herself. The answers are "yes" or "no" rather than a five-point scale, which allows for use in an ill or cognitively impaired population. The original is a 30-question version, but a shorter 15-question version has been validated and can be a more efficient tool.

The Folstein Mini-Mental State Exam (MMSE) is the most widely used tool to assess cognition. It is a 30-point scale that can be used to screen for dementia, as well as assess severity, and monitor response to treatment. The MMSE has been translated into 10 foreign languages, making it the most useful for diverse populations; however, the MMSE is copyrighted and copies must be ordered through the company that holds the intellectual property.

There are many other useful cognitive evaluation tools that are free. The Mini-Cog, which consists of a three-word recall and clock-drawing test, is an extremely time-efficient way to do a preliminary screen for cognitive impairment. If any of the words are not recalled, or the clock draw is abnormal, further testing should be pursued. The St. Louis University Mental Status Exam (SLUMS) is a tool that may be more sensitive for detecting dementia in its earlier stages, testing orientation, memory, calculation, naming, and clock drawing. The tool is only available in English, and is free online. The Montreal Cognitive Assessment (MoCA) is another similar test, also available free online. It can be used with a diverse population as it has been validated in 21 languages and dialects.

FUNCTIONAL ASSESSMENT

One thing that sets the evaluation of older adults apart from assessment of younger patients is the importance of performing functional assessment. The ability to perform ADLs, such as bathing, dressing, grooming, eating, transferring, and toileting can be affected by medical illness and mental disorders. Instrumental activities of daily living (IADLs), such as telephone use, money and medication management, shopping, cooking, driving, and transportation are impacted by even mild dementia.

Status of ADL and IADL function needs to be assessed to determine a person's safety at home. Improvements in ADL and IADL status will demonstrate successful response to medical treatments and allow patients to remain at home and independent for as long as possible.

SOCIAL SYSTEM ASSESSMENT

When frail patients are dependent on caregivers, the caregiver's capacity and coping become the clinician's concern. Caregiving is often associated with depression and health problems. The clinician should tactfully probe for indicators of stress, feelings of burden, and breakdown in the caregiver's ability to provide care (there are a number of tools available to assess caregiver burden, such as the American Medical Association's *Caregiver Self-Assessment Questionnaire*, available on their web site). The potential for abuse should also be assessed, keeping in mind that hostile remarks and impatience are risk factors for physical aggression and neglect. Many states require physicians to report suspected abuse, and all communities are required by federal law to have Area Agencies on Aging that provide adult protective services.

ENVIRONMENTAL ASSESSMENT

Community nursing and senior care agencies can assist health care providers by making home assessments and evaluating patients' safety in their own environment. These services are often covered as a Medicare benefit, especially if the patient is homebound. Fall risk, fire safety, medication management, and hygiene concerns are among the many things that can be evaluated. Removing loose throw rugs, keeping the path to the bathroom free of clutter and lit at night, adding bars next to the toilet, and other simple interventions can markedly increase safety and prolong independent living.

QUALITY MEASURES

Assessing Care of Vulnerable Elders (ACOVE) is a program created through collaboration between Rand Health, the American Geriatrics Society, and Pfizer. ACOVE works to educate clinicians on the assessment and care of older adults. They have developed quality measures for specific geriatric conditions, including depression and dementia. The specific measures are included below in the respective sections.

DIAGNOSIS

Major Mental Disorders of Older Adults

DEPRESSION

Major depression is common in community dwelling older adults (2–4%), and even more common in residents of long-term care facilities. Depressive symptoms are even more prevalent, affecting up to 20% of older adults. Chronic medical conditions are common in this population and increase the risk of developing depression. Major depression in geriatric patients manifests in all the usual ways seen in younger adults, but nonspecific and atypical symptoms are common and may dominate the clinical presentation. Although depressed mood and hopelessness have diagnostic value, less specific symptoms may be prominent and give valuable clues to the underlying diagnosis. Anhedonia, anxiety, fearfulness, irritability, cognitive impairment, apathy, dependency, and numerous somatic complaints should prompt the consideration of depression even when the patient denies feeling depressed (see Chapter 25).

The most efficient tool for assessing mood is the two-question screener: "In the past month, have you felt depressed or down?" and "In the past month have you had little interest or pleasure in activities and/or hobbies?" If either question is answered in the affirmative, further testing is indicated. The GDS is a more complete screening tool. Scores can be followed over time to monitor progression or response to therapies.

The prognosis for depression in old age is fairly good, at least for acute symptoms, and patients need to be told this to counter the hopelessness they might feel. However, partial remissions and relapses are common, especially in patients with previous episodes of depression. Other negative predictors include persistent health problems that compromise function or comfort, poor social support, and ongoing psychosocial stressors. Antidepressant medications have been shown to improve outcomes and reduce the risk of relapse in older adults. Caution must be used when prescribing antidepressants in older adults as side effects may outweigh any gains in mood. Electroconvulsive therapy (ECT) has high efficacy rates and can be used for drug-resistant depression, as well as patients with psychotic features. There are no absolute contraindications, but many patients experience short-term memory loss after this treatment.

Cognitive impairment associated with depression may improve with remission of the mood disorder, but is predictive of an underlying dementia. Such patients need close follow up to catch the dementia early and ensure safety at home. ACOVE has developed quality measures to help clinicians treat depression effectively. These include recognizing depression, screening for suicidality, treating depression, and monitoring for response to therapy.

ANXIETY DISORDERS

Older patients have the highest per capita use of antianxiety medications. These figures are probably higher than necessary, since many of the anxious elderly are actually suffering from depression as their primary illness. Apart from depression, the differential diagnosis of anxiety in older adults includes transient apprehension and fear, adjustments to life changes, phobic avoidant behaviors,

obsessive-compulsive disorder, panic disorder, posttraumatic stress, and generalized anxiety disorder (see Chapter 26). Secondary anxiety disorders are also very common: medications, chronic obstructive pulmonary disease, and endocrinopathies are often implicated.

Although the mainstay of pharmaco therapy for anxiety in all adults are selective serotonin reuptake inhibitors (SSRIs) many patients are treated with benzodiazepines. Unfortunately, due to physiologic changes of drug excretion as well as changes to the benzodiazepine receptors, older adults are exquisitely sensitive to this class of medications and often suffer adverse side effects. Increased somnolence, unsteadiness, memory loss, and disinhibition are common, and dangerous, reactions. If there is no other option for treatment, clinicians should opt for short-acting formulations in small doses. In patients with long-term use, a taper should be attempted.

DELUSIONAL DISORDERS

Delusional thinking arises from a number of disturbances in old age. Hallucinations can be seen in end-stage dementia and delirium. Charles Bonnet syndrome is a condition that causes patients with vision loss to have complex visual hallucinations. These hallucinations are often not bothersome, and the patient frequently has insight that the visions are not real. Although there is no specific treatment for Charles Bonnet syndrome, fixing the visual deficit can stop the hallucinations. Musical hallucinosis is an auditory variant of hallucinosis associated with acquired deafness, in many ways analogous to Charles Bonnet syndrome. A primary delusional disorder of unknown etiology, previously known as paranoia, is sometimes seen in older women who live alone. Although these patients describe persecutory delusions of an intense nature, highly suggestive of schizophrenia, they do not have other manifestations of this disease, such as hallucinations, loose associations, disorganized behavior, and functional decline. Elders who do exhibit these cardinal symptoms of schizophrenia have usually had the disease for many years, although it can develop in late life. Paranoia and delusions can also be the presenting symptoms of dementia, depression, mania, and alcohol abuse.

DEMENTIA

The prevalence of dementia, or Major Neurocognitive Disorder per the DSM-V, increases with age, approaching 20% at the age of 80 years and 50% by the age of 90 years. The diagnosis of dementia is made when intellectual impairment is severe enough to affect independent functioning. Alzheimer disease (AD) is the most common cause of dementia in the elderly, and can be diagnosed with fairly good accuracy by using formal diagnostic criteria (see Chapter 30). The presence of progressive decline in recent memory, normal motor function (without weakness, ataxia, or parkinsonism), and deficits in at least one other higher cortical function (language, praxis, visual–spatial, calculations, and executive functions), is highly supportive of the diagnosis. Mild cognitive impairment (MCI) is diagnosed when cognition is impaired but function remains intact. Mild cognitive impairment, amnestic type, gradually progresses to AD in most individuals, while mild cognitive impairment of the non-amnestic type (often characterized by executive function deficits) may progress to vascular dementia or Lewy Body Dementia. Medical treatment of AD includes long-term maintenance on acetylcholinesterase inhibitors and memantine (for modest improvement in symptoms and slowing of functional decline) if the patient has shown a response, treatment of neuropsychiatric symptoms when necessary, and attention to comfort (especially pain), continence, and caregiver distress.

Many vitamins and supplements including vitamin E, vitamin B, and *Gingko biloba* have been suggested to slow the progression of the disease; but unfortunately, none has been shown to be effective in clinical trials. Vitamin E is associated with higher cardiovascular risk and for this reason, is not recommended. The best nonpharmacologic data for prevention of dementia and slowing of disease is the Mediterranean diet and a healthy exercise routine.

Prescribing atypical antipsychotic medications to treat agitation and psychosis in patients with dementia is complicated by clinical trial evidence of higher mortality risk (60–70% higher vs. placebo) and a Food and Drug Administration (FDA) warning against their use in this population. A multicenter trial funded by the National Institute on Aging indicates that the efficacy of these drugs is often limited by rapid discontinuation because of side effects. Nevertheless, the atypical antipsychotics remain in widespread clinical use, partly because of the high risk of the symptoms these drugs are used to treat, and also a relative lack of evidence for safety and efficacy of alternative medications. If used in this population, these medications should be dosed very conservatively, patients and families should be counseled on the risks, and patients should be closely monitored for side effects including sedation.

ACOVE has developed quality measures for dementia. These include screening all vulnerable elders for cognitive impairment and reviewing medication lists for possible causative therapies. They also recommend a thorough neurologic and laboratory examination in patients who screen positive for dementia. A discussion about the benefits of acetylcholinesterase inhibitors should be initiated in all patients, and a history of behavioral symptoms should be elicited. Lastly, clinicians should provide caregiver support, as burnout is common and can negatively impact both the patient and the family.

Another common dementia of older age is Dementia with Lewy Bodies (DLB). This is diagnosed when a patient manifests progressive dementia, parkinsonism (especially bradykinesia and rigidity without tremor), daily fluctuations in mental status similar to delirium, and visual hallucinations. Sleep disturbance is common, especially daytime sleepiness and excessive motor activity during rapid eye movement (REM) sleep. Dementia with Lewy Bodies accounts for 5–10% of cases of dementia, and may occur mixed with AD. Treatment of DLB involves a trial of acetylcholinesterase inhibitors and psychotropic medications for targeted neuropsychiatric symptoms. Older antipsychotic medications, such as haloperidol, must be rigorously avoided. Most clinicians will prescribe low doses of quetiapine (12.5–100 mg/day in divided doses) for delusions and hallucinations that do not respond to acetylcholinesterase inhibitors; however, this is considered off label use and the increased mortality risk noted in the black box warning does apply. For neuropsychiatric symptoms that persist after cholinesterase treatment within package insert dosing guidelines, there is some evidence that higher doses can be tolerated with improved efficacy. Parkinsonism can respond modestly to L-dopa, but L-dopa can worsen neuropsychiatric symptoms, and needs to be used with caution in patients with DLB.

Vascular dementia is another common cause of intellectual and functional decline in older adults, accounting for about 5% of dementia cases and contributing to worsening dementia in many more patients as a comorbid condition with AD. Large cortical strokes produce a stepwise decline with noticeable points of change associated with recurrent strokes. Small-vessel disease producing lacunar infarcts in subcortical structures is associated with hypertension and diabetes. Also known as Binswanger dementia, this condition produces a more gradually progressive dementia that looks similar to AD, but with more obvious gait impairment, incontinence, parkinsonism, and affect lability. Executive function and cognitive processing speed are usually affected more than memory. Circulatory problems in the absence of stroke (i.e., congestive heart failure, hyperviscosity states, and so forth) can also produce cognitive impairment. Patients with vascular dementia can potentially benefit from a trial of cholinesterase treatment.

DELIRIUM

Delirium is characterized by the acute (within hours) or subacute (within days) development of disorientation and confusion. Inability to focus and sustain attention are key to the diagnosis. Hallucinations, fearful or paranoid perceptions, fluctuating awareness, and alterations in the sleep–wake cycle are other frequent symptoms. In patients with mild delirium, the decreased level of alertness may not be obvious. Patients will often have psychomotor slowing, listlessness, and apathy. These patients may be misdiagnosed as depressed or demented, although there frequently is an underlying dementia.

Delirium is often the first symptom of medical illness in frail elderly people. The most common causes of delirium in older patients are infections (usually urinary tract and pulmonary), medications, metabolic abnormalities, alcohol or sedative intoxication and withdrawal, stroke, seizures, and heart failure. In patients with dementia, problems such as pain, fecal impaction, and urinary retention can cause rapid changes in mental status and behavior that look like superimposed delirium.

Many, if not most, older adults have at least mild delirium when hospitalized for an acute illness or surgery. An excellent screening tool for delirium is the confusion assessment method, and this should be performed on every older adult at risk of delirium. In hospital settings, delirium increases fall rates, length of stay, and risk of poor outcomes. Adequate pain control and correction of metabolic problems or infections will help shorten the time course of the delirium. Agitation, paranoia, and sleeplessness may require separate pharmacologic management (see Chapter 30). Low doses of haloperidol (0.25–1 mg every 4 hours, max 4.5 mg daily) or quetiapine (12.5–25 mg up to 2–3 times daily) is the treatment of choice in most instances. Patients should be monitored closely for cardiovascular complications. Younger patients, or those with primary mental illness, may need higher doses or alternate therapies.

SUBSTANCE ABUSE AND POLYPHARMACY

Often overlooked, substance abuse is common in older adults; alcohol abuse is the third most common mental disorder in older men. Unexplained falls, ataxia, confusion, malnutrition, burns, head trauma, and depression should prompt questions about surreptitious alcohol abuse. Prescription pain medication, sedative–hypnotic medications, over-the-counter remedies for constipation, sleeplessness, and pain; and numerous vitamins and supplements are also overused. Seeing multiple physicians and practitioners and patronizing several pharmacies are clues to the clinician that prescription abuse is likely (see Chapter 24). Polypharmacy increases the risk of adverse drug reactions, a leading cause of confusion, depression, falls, and functional decline. Frequent medication review and reduction should be part of the care of every older adult.

SOMATIZATION

Geriatric patients are not immune to somatic perceptions for which there are no known physical causes. Of course, older patients often manifest illness in vague and nonspecific ways, so an open mind is necessary when thinking through mysterious symptoms. The clinician should avoid unnecessary interventions while continuously supporting the needs of the patient to be heard and understood. Although regularly scheduled appointments with brief, focused examinations that allow the "laying on of hands" continue to be the most effective interventions, major depression and anxiety disorders commonly underlie somatization. Antidepressants and psychotherapy may improve function and a sense of well being in somatically focused patients (see Chapter 28).

CASE DISCUSSIONS

 CASE ILLUSTRATION 1

Mr. J is a 78-year-old man with hypertension and hypothyroidism, who is brought in by his daughter who has noticed a decline in his ability to care for himself. She noticed the decline after her mother, his wife of over 50 years, died 6 months ago. Since that time he has lost 20 pounds and has not been going to his weekly bridge games. He has been forgetful, initially losing his keys or missing appointments, but progressing to the point where he became lost driving in his own neighborhood. He has become increasingly disheveled.

When approached with his daughter's concerns, Mr. J reports that he thinks he is doing just fine and simply has not felt like playing bridge recently. With regard to getting lost in his neighborhood, he says he just was not paying attention. He answers questions in short phrases. His biggest concern during the visit is low back pain, which has been acting up recently. On examination, he is poorly groomed. He scores a 25/30 on the SLUMS test, missing all of the orientation questions and several of the recall questions. He scores 10/15 on the GDS.

This case highlights the difficulty in distinguishing dementia from depression. Cognitive deficits can be associated with depression. Although he may have some cognitive impairment as well, he will have to be reevaluated after his depression resolves or remits. The abrupt onset timed with the passing of his wife is more consistent with depression than dementia, which usually has a more insidious onset. Then again, his wife may have been covering for preexisting deficits that became evident after her death. Medical causes such as drug side effects and hypothyroidism should be ruled out. Some depression is normal after the death of a loved one, but his symptoms are starting to affect his ability to take care of himself. Treatment should be initiated with counseling and/or antidepressant therapy. If no response is seen, switching medications can be helpful. ECT is an option for drug-resistant depression. If his symptoms do respond to therapy, his cognition should be reevaluated as he may also have an underlying dementia.

CASE ILLUSTRATION 2

Mrs. R is an 84-year-old woman with a history of hypertension and bilateral cataracts who is brought in by a neighbor out of concern for hallucinations. Her neighbor brings her groceries once a week and notes that lately the patient has been making comments about children and animals that are not there. The patient admits that she does sometimes see one young boy and two small cats in her home. She knows they are not really there but is not bothered by them. In fact, she somewhat enjoys the company. On further questioning you find that she drinks one martini each night before bed and occasionally takes diphenhydramine to help her sleep. On presentation, she is well groomed, and aside from her vision the examination is unrevealing. She scores 24/30 on the SLUMS test but misses only the questions that require intact vision. Her attention is normal as she is able to participate in activities such as spelling words backwards and naming days of the week backwards. A laboratory workup is also unrevealing, showing no signs of infection or electrolyte abnormality.

This case highlights the differential diagnosis of a patient presenting with visual hallucinations. Dementia, delirium, psychosis, intoxication, and medication effects should all be considered in this patient. Though she had an abnormal score on the SLUMS test, her memory was intact. In delirium, inattention is a hallmark of the disease and you must see fluctuations in consciousness. Her alcohol intake and diphenhydramine use may be implicated, and these should be stopped, if possible. This patient may be suffering from Charles Bonnet syndrome if workup of the other diagnoses is negative. If medically stable, the patient should undergo surgical removal of her cataracts, as this may cure her of her hallucinations.

TREATMENT

Caring for Older Patients

MAINTAINING FUNCTIONAL INDEPENDENCE

The focus of treatment planning with the frail elderly patient is always the provision of comfort and the maintenance of independent functioning. Although there are clearly times when safety becomes paramount, as in the case of the older driver who is a hazard behind the wheel, independence is usually the shared goal of both the patient and clinician. To achieve this in the face of aging and progressive disease, treatment planning must include utilization of community care resources, skillful medical management, and rehabilitation therapies.

COMMUNITY CARE OPTIONS FOR THE FRAIL ELDERLY

Clinicians should become familiar with the services available in their community that provide case management, in-home assistance, and emotional support to older patients and caregivers. Local and county agencies providing services for seniors, private case management firms, local chapters of the Alzheimer's Association, and home health care agencies will be resources to you and your patients in arranging the services necessary to keep them at home longer than would otherwise be safe. In rural areas without these resources, family, neighbors, and lay networks of helpers can sometimes fill in the gaps and keep frail elders cared for at home. The Family Caregiver Alliance web site (www.caregiver.org) provides information on local resources supporting caregivers in every state.

Patients with round-the-clock care needs will eventually exhaust many family caregivers. Some patients with dementia-associated agitation, delusions, and misperceptions can be combative and make caregiving frustrating and occasionally dangerous. Caregivers, family, and paid professionals all face depression and health risks more than their peers. There comes a time when placement in a long-term care facility may become necessary for both the patient's as well as the family's well-being. Physicians, nurses, and other practitioners play important roles in assisting patients and families through this transition. Clinicians can help them anticipate the need to leave home for supervised living settings, familiarize them with different long-term care options in the community, and also help families with feelings of guilt experienced when they have to make the decision on the patient's behalf. This role requires clinicians to know what the patient's care needs are and what type of facility can safely meet those needs. People who need assistance only with housekeeping and cooking will do fine in retirement homes and residential care facilities. Residential care facilities may be able to administer medications and provide assistance with ADLs for additional cost. A few states allow people to provide care for up to five frail elders in a private home. These "adult foster homes" or "care homes" provide a home-like alternative to residential care facilities. Additional care needs may be met by an independent or assisted living facility. Assisted living or "independent living" facilities may provide some nursing supervision and occasionally may even have a medical director. However, the amount of nursing and medical involvement varies greatly based on state regulations and the management philosophy of the owners. These facilities are very popular with patients and families and are increasingly seen as alternatives to skilled nursing facilities because they are less expensive and much less "institution like" than nursing homes. Many assisted living facilities allow patients to "age in place" and even allow them to receive hospice-level care at the end of life without having to move to a nursing facility. However, it is important to inform patients and families that these facilities cannot generally provide the same level of nursing assessment and care that intermediate and skilled nursing facilities provide. Many patients with complex care needs will still need nursing homes, but there are now many other options for less frail patients.

MEDICAL TREATMENT PLANNING

The motto of the British Geriatrics Society, "Adding Life to Years," is useful to keep in mind when treating older patients. Comfort, meaningful engagement, and increased activity become the goals of treatment. Providing adequate pain relief, physical therapy, and treatment of depression are all integrated into comprehensive treatment plans.

Immunizations, smoking cessation, weight loss, exercise, and proper nutrition should continue to be a focus of preventive care in older adults. It is also important to explore the expectations of both the patient and the caregiver and to discuss end-of-life treatment decisions. If possible, this discussion should take place before an acute medical condition leads to interventions that may be invasive, futile, or unwanted. These "advance directives" should extend beyond cardiopulmonary resuscitation and include the patient's goals of care. If the decision is to forego these interventions, the clinician should provide assurances that the comfort of the patient will be maintained (see Chapter 40).

Given the high prevalence of mental disorders in old age, it is not surprising that the elderly are prescribed psychotropic medications at a higher rate than younger adults. Special care must be taken to start most medications at a lower dose in older patients (generally half the usual starting dose in young–old patients, i.e., 65–80 years, and a third the usual dose in old–old patients, i.e., over the age of 80 years). In the case of benzodiazepines, antipsychotics, and mood stabilizers, the effective treatment dose will also usually be one-half to one-third the dose used in younger patients. However, in the case of antidepressants, the eventual effective doses are frequently the same as those used in young adults.

FUNCTIONAL REHABILITATION

Functional rehabilitation of older patients with mental disorders following stroke, fracture, or medical illness ideally involves a multidisciplinary team approach. Mental disorders, such as depression, can by themselves induce substantial physical disability through decreased activity. The goal is to treat the mental disorder and primary disability, while preventing secondary disabilities such as immobility and incontinence, and complications such as skin breakdown and infection. The composition of the team varies widely and may include rehabilitation professionals such as physical, occupational, and speech therapists. The rehabilitation plan, like the medical plan, must have realistic goals that are individualized to the patient. This plan must be frequently reevaluated and revised as the progress of patients toward reaching their goals is reassessed. Older patients lose function rapidly when hospitalized and bedridden for even a few days, and a brief period of strengthening rehabilitation may be needed for those who lose the ability to ambulate or transfer independently while in hospital.

SUGGESTED READINGS

D'Ath P, Katona P, Mullan E, et al. Screening, detection and management of depression in elderly primary care attenders. I: The acceptability and performance of the 15 item Geriatric Depression Scale (GDS15) and the development of short versions. *Fam Pract* 1994;11:260–266.

Jacobson SA, Pies RW, Katz IR. *Clinical Manual of Geriatric Psychopharmacology*, 2nd ed. Washington, DC: American Psychiatric Publishing, Inc., 2007.

Mathias S, Nayak USL, Isaacs B. Balance in elderly patients: the "get-up and go" test. *Arch Phys Med Rehabil* 1986;67:387–389.

Niven D. *The 100 Simple Secrets of the Best Half of Life*. San Francisco, CA: Harper, 2005.

Tinetti ME, Williams TF, Mayewski R. Fall Risk Index for elderly patients based on number of chronic disabilities. *Am J Med* 1986;80:429–434.

Weiner RD, Blazer DG, Steffens DC, et al., eds. *Essentials of Geriatric Psychiatry*, 2nd ed. Arlington, VA: American Psychiatric Publishing, 2012.

WEB SITES

American Association of Geriatric Psychiatry. http://www.aagponline.org. Accessed July 2013.

American Geriatric Society. http://www.americangeriatrics.org. Accessed July 2013.

American Medical Director's Association. http://www.amda.com. Accessed July 2013.

British Society of Gerontology. http://www.britishgerontology.org. Accessed July 2013.

Canadian Geriatric Society. http://www.canadiangeriatrics.com. Accessed July 2013.

Family Caregiver Alliance. http://www.caregiver.org. Accessed July 2013.

National Institute on Aging. http://www.nia.nih.gov. Accessed January 2014.

ACOVE (Assessing Care of Vulnerable Elders). http://www.rand.org/health/projects/acove.html Accessed July 2013.

Cross-cultural Communication

Thomas Denberg, MD, PhD & Mitchell D. Feldman, MD, MPhil

INTRODUCTION

Effective clinician–patient communication involves verbal and nonverbal sharing of information across cultural and linguistic boundaries. In the medical arena, these boundaries are populated on the one side by clinicians who represent the esoteric world of biomedicine, and on the other side by patients and families who often lack familiarity with biomedical concepts and procedures and may have their own strongly held beliefs about illness—what it means, how it should be diagnosed, and how it should be treated. The goals of effective cross-cultural communication (or "cultural competency," as it is sometimes called) are threefold: (1) to understand illness from the perspective of the *patient*; (2) to assist patients in understanding diseases and treatments from the perspective of *biomedicine*; and (3) to help patients and their families navigate, express themselves, and feel comfortable within large, complex, and often impersonal health care organizations. These activities require some awareness of the wider context of patients' lives, and of how the worlds of biomedicine and the lay public interact and, at times, conflict and misunderstand each other.

Cross-cultural communication skills are best developed through practice, reflection, and reading about and interacting with diverse patient populations. Knowing a few facts about the illness beliefs of an immigrant group or ethnic minority is not enough. It is important to develop ways of perceiving and interpreting what *individual* patients say and do in the context of their previous experiences with illness, structural positions within society, and membership within particular ethnic and religious communities. True cultural awareness also involves understanding how biomedicine is itself a cultural system, and how it is likely to be perceived and (mis)understood by patients.

As the dominant form of health care in the United States, biomedicine is practiced by highly specialized professionals and relies on detailed, scientific information about the human body and the use of pharmaceutical and surgical interventions to prevent or treat anatomic and physiologic disorders and their associated symptoms. It has a definite body of knowledge, set of practices, strengths and weaknesses, nonevidence-based biases, and inherent limitations. Each of its many specialties and subspecialties has unique conventions, systems of knowledge, and ways of making sense of people and events. To patients of all backgrounds, much about biomedicine is obscure; difficulties agreeing with and accepting medical explanations and recommendations are commonplace. Therefore, the perspective that orients the discussion in this chapter is that although cross-cultural communication is especially important and challenging for immigrant and minority patients, it has relevance to *all* patients.

CULTURE & SOCIAL LOCATION

Culture

Culture refers to beliefs, values, rituals, customs, institutions, social roles, and relationships that are shared among identifiable groups of people. Typically, one's own culture is taken for granted; it feels entirely natural, consisting of those assumptions and routines that make the world what it is "supposed" to be. Unconscious learning and modeling play important roles in the acquisition of cultural assumptions and routines. Within the family, one of the most influential cultural systems, there is generally a clear-cut division of labor, regular routines such as meal and work times, explanations (or myths) about family origins, and strategies for fulfilling common goals and passing down shared values. It is also within the family that beliefs are first developed about the causes of illness, acceptable ways of expressing symptoms, and strategies for diagnosing illness and restoring health. Individuals, of course, are also shaped by, and participate in, cultures related to work, school, worship, political affiliation, social clubs, and so on, each of which may also have important—and sometimes contradictory or inconsistent—influences on beliefs about and responses to illness.

Cultures are neither pure nor static, but constantly intermix and evolve. Particularly in the United States—a highly mobile, diverse, and media-saturated society—millions of people move in and out of multiple domains, borrowing and adapting ideas and customs from other groups. Because cultural change over time and across generations is considerable, it should not be *assumed* that particular patients have certain beliefs or engage in certain behaviors solely on the basis of their last name, physical appearance, or national origin. Inferences—always open to revision—should be based on detailed knowledge of patient attributes that go beyond race and ethnicity alone.

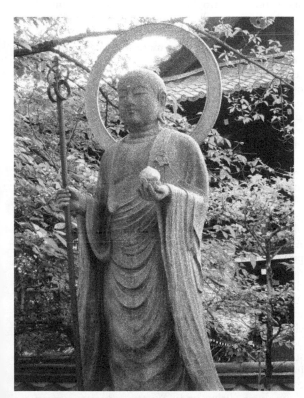

(Photo courtesy of Mitchell D. Feldman, MD, MPhil.)

THE RELATIONSHIP OF CULTURE TO RACE, ETHNICITY, AND NATIONAL ORIGIN

Some cultural competency training takes the approach that various racial, ethnic, and national groups possess distinctive cultural traits with which the clinician should become familiar to render more effective care. Commonly cited examples include beliefs in "fallen fontanelle" and "evil eye" among Latinos and "high blood/low blood" among African Americans, as well as values such as "individualism" among North Americans, and "family centeredness" among Asians. Although these generalizations (or stereotypes) may illustrate a wide spectrum of cultural influences on illness and healing, this approach is too simplistic. It implies that race, ethnicity, and national origin are the most important determinants of an individual's understanding of and response to illness, and ignores the tremendous heterogeneity among individuals *within* these groups and among individuals who may inhabit multiple groups simultaneously. Common notions of cultural competency assume that culture can be reduced to a technical skill that clinicians can develop without necessarily engaging with people in their local worlds and understanding the ambiguity and ambivalence that many people feel as a result of living within these multiple worlds.

Take the case of the United States, in which the primary racial/ethnic categories include African American, white, Asian, American Indian, Pacific Islander, and Latino. Some people may self-identify using these terms, and the labels are often important politically, but there are significant differences among people within each of these categories in terms of age, place of birth, religion, social class, sexual orientation, level of education, and so on. Conceptualizing differences in health beliefs and behaviors on the overarching levels of race and ethnicity promotes stereotyping and does little to advance more effective medical care. In general, assumptions about cultural beliefs and practices should be based on more specific identification of group membership, such as recent immigrants; particular US subpopulations such as the homeless, southern rural African Americans, or inhabitants of particular city neighborhoods.

Social Location

As we move beyond ideas of culture determined solely by race and ethnicity, knowledge of patients will be enhanced by awareness of their *social location*. Social location specifies one's position in society relative to others and is based on an amalgam of characteristics that include not only race and ethnicity, but also gender, age, immigration status, language(s) spoken, neighborhood of residence, length of time and number of generations in the United States, educational attainment, income, occupation, religion, sexual orientation, and prior experiences with racism. Gender and age are two fundamental variables that influence how patients give meaning to illness and express themselves in relation to it. Men and women, and people over the age of 50 years and under the age of 20 years, although from the same city or region, will generally belong to distinctive subcultures: they may share certain core beliefs, values, and customs, but not others. Another fundamental influence on disease risk, health behaviors, and familiarity with biomedicine is degree of acculturation. One's neighborhood of residence, with its quality of housing and schools, population density, associated level of crime, and access to public transportation, also dramatically shapes one's understanding of the world and strategies for dealing with adversity. Religion, spirituality, and membership in a community of like-minded believers also have significant bearings on attitudes toward health and illness. Historical experiences of racism can engender feelings of helplessness, anger, and distrust that may, in turn, significantly affect attitudes toward medical providers as well as interpretations of illness. Finally, the elements of social class—education, income, and occupation—have a profound influence on beliefs about illness and opportunities and strategies for restoring health.

The attributes of social location are more complete, specific, and clinically relevant than race and ethnicity alone. In this way, a clinician will not simply note that a patient is Latino, or even Mexican American, and then attempt to remember "typical" cultural traits that apply to members of this group. Instead, they will observe that the US-born patient is 20 years old, unemployed, has completed high school, speaks little Spanish, and lives with her Mexican-born, primarily Spanish-speaking, rural-origin parents in a mixed race, working-class neighborhood. Each of these characteristics, alone and in combination, provides important clues about *this* patient—clues that help in interpreting the patient's statements and symptoms and that facilitate patient education and tailored treatment.

Of course, the more experience that practitioners have with patients from a specific, narrowly defined population or community, and the greater the language concordance between practitioner and patient, the more they are likely to become aware of the health problems and themes important to that group as a whole. The ability to communicate effectively with patients from such groups can be enhanced by spending time in the local community—in senior citizen centers, at cultural and sporting events, churches, and schools—as well as by reading relevant neighborhood newsletters, ethnographies, social histories, census reports, novels, and biographies. Although such activities and materials do not constitute the normal corpus of medical duties or references, they can sensitize the clinician to the issues that are important to patients—in their own terms and from their own points of view. Detailed knowledge of a specific population as well as the ability to communicate in the patient's native language can also help the clinician understand not only the literal sense of a patient's words, but also other kinds of meanings contained in what the patient says (or chooses not to say), and in what the patient does (or chooses not to do), such as adhere to prescribed treatments.

IMMIGRANTS & ETHNIC MINORITIES

Recent immigrants bring a number of unique issues and challenges to medical cross-cultural communication. Relocating to a new country often results in dramatic alterations in social status, occupation, and daily routines; isolation from previous friendships and networks of social support; and the upending of traditional roles as older individuals rely on those who are younger to support the family, locate housing, and interpret local events. Anomie (a sense of purposelessness) and alienation (lack of feelings of belonging) can contribute to anxiety, depression, and a decreased ability to cope with the new stresses of daily life. Refugee experiences of war and natural catastrophe exacerbate these problems. The astute clinician will be aware that many individuals somatize this distress.

Recent immigrants are more likely to hold beliefs and practices that to "Western" trained physicians may seem colorful or strange. These illness beliefs and behaviors are often cited in discussions of cultural competence but are generally most applicable to elderly and/or recently arrived immigrants. Processes of globalization, including the growth of tourism, the opening of commercial markets, and the spread of popular culture from the United States and Europe, have familiarized large numbers of third-world immigrants with life in industrially advanced, capitalist societies. In addition, a substantial proportion of first- and second-generation residents quickly assimilate into US society, often because of a keen desire to "fit in" or "become American." Even among individuals who speak English poorly, are poorly assimilated, or actively resist assimilation, many will have had a significant amount of experience with biomedicine in their countries of origin. Although they may not have previously encountered the technological and organizational complexity that characterize biomedicine in the United States, they may be familiar with its reductionistic, scientific foundation, status as a profession, and its conventions for diagnosing and treating illness. It is difficult, if not impossible, to accurately gauge a patient's level of sophistication about biomedicine and "Western" disease categories through visual inspection or knowledge of the patient's race and ethnicity alone; the clinician should avoid assumptions and instead learn by observing and asking questions of the patient.

BIOMEDICINE AS A CULTURAL SYSTEM

Developing cross-cultural communication skills may involve a transition from having no insight about the role of patient culture on medical care; to accepting that a patient's culturally informed beliefs, values, and behaviors have an important influence on health, disease and treatment effectiveness; and, finally, to unconsciously integrating attention to patient culture into all areas of clinical practice. Equally important, however, is that clinicians develop an awareness of their *own* cultures and the unquestioned assumptions that are informed by their personal histories, the nonprofessional aspects of their daily lives, and the socialization imparted by their significant, lengthy engagement in biomedical training and practice.

Focusing on "culture" primarily in relation to immigrant or minority patients may convey the notion that biomedicine is itself without culture. In fact, although biomedicine is informed by scientific knowledge (a "culture" with its own values and beliefs), it is also shaped by the politics of government funding, insurance reimbursement, rivalries among specialties, as well as by competing ideologies of profit versus altruism, changing fashions and trends, best guesses, and regional biases. Biomedicine comprises many cultural worlds and languages—primary care, cardiology, surgery; the hospital, the clinic; nursing, physicians, pharmacists; and so on—that for many patients are strange, potentially threatening, and difficult to understand. Awareness of how different kinds of patients are likely to experience and interpret biomedicine is essential to enhancing cross-cultural communication. It is equally important for clinicians to be aware of their own roles in perpetuating the culture of biomedicine, and to realize the extent to which they are both the products and practitioners of this cultural system.

Table 15-1 lists several characteristics that have been associated with biomedicine and its practitioners. Tensions and misunderstandings between practitioner and patient are often strongly rooted in many of the attributes listed under (A) in Table 15-1. Often most problematic from the perspective of patients is biomedicine's tendency to sharply differentiate body from mind and to emphasize organic pathophysiology over the psychosocial ramifications and origins of illness. Nonetheless, many of biomedicine's major successes have been achieved despite—or often because of—such tendencies. These are the characteristics that set biomedicine apart from other systems of healing. They are also quite resistant to change. The clinician's goal should be to act as a cultural broker, making these features of biomedicine more accessible and understandable to the patient while at the same time exploring and attending to the psychosocial dimensions of illness from the patient's perspective.

Individual practitioners vary greatly in the degree to which they conform to the attributes of professionalism listed under (B) in Table 15-1 (see Chapter 46). Although common, none is a *predictable* feature of biomedicine in the same way as those listed under (A). A central problem, however, is that many patients have difficulty understanding or sympathizing with the attributes in either category, compounding communication difficulties and

Table 15-1. Characteristics of biomedicine and its practitioners.

(A) Biomedicine *as a system of healing rests upon and esteems the following:*
- Empiric science
- Written knowledge as opposed to oral tradition
- Rigorous and lengthy training
- Technological sophistication and innovation
- Action orientation and interventionism ("doing something rather than nothing")
- Materialism (disease in the individual, physical body rather than in the family, social group, mind, or spirit)
- Differentiating among acute illness, chronic illness, and prevention
- Reductionism (pathophysiology is molecular and anatomic; symptoms are expressions of underlying disease rather than diseases themselves)
- High levels of bureaucratic organization; complexity and subspecialization
- Team-based care
- Efficiency
- Cost containment
- "Defensiveness" or avoiding malpractice
- The prolongation of life

(B) *Many clinicians value these traits:*
- Hard work
- Self-sacrifice
- Self-reliance and autonomy
- Strong career orientation
- Status consciousness
- Respect for authority and hierarchy
- Hygiene
- Punctuality
- The physician as the expert
- Deliberateness
- Articulateness
- A clear separation between personal and work lives
- Conservatism in dress and expressions of emotion
- Quality judged by one's colleagues

(C) *Common attributions that* patients *have about biomedicine and its practitioners:*

Negative	Positive
Arrogant	Highly competent
Elite	Honest
Judgmental	Careful
Remote and inaccessible	Thorough
Narrow minded	Methodical
Difficult to comprehend	Caring
Money hungry	Accurate
Rushed	Reliable
Dogmatic	Responsible
Rigid	Impartial
Entitled	Hardworking
Uninterested in the patient as a person	Putting the patient's welfare first and foremost

leading some to hold many of the negative impressions listed under (C) in Table 15-1. This is especially true when patients desire a more personal and less professional relationship with their physicians, or when social distance compounds the patient's feelings of powerlessness. The culturally competent clinician will understand these common features and negative patient perceptions of biomedicine, recognizing when they contribute to misunderstandings and impair a patient's ability to feel at ease, communicate, and benefit from a biomedical approach.

COMMUNICATION

Communication involves the exchange, processing, and interpretation of messages—both verbal and nonverbal. In this complex process, there are myriad opportunities for miscommunication: messages can be incomplete, confusing, and contradictory; language barriers as well as emotional and physical distractions can interfere with the receipt and relaying of information; and unspoken assumptions can influence the meaning one person attributes to another's statements or actions. Much of this takes place outside of conscious awareness. With this in mind, this section reviews three fundamental aspects of communication to which the clinician should direct particular attention: (1) attempting to understand the illness from the *patient's* perspective; (2) ensuring that the patient understands, as much as possible and at an appropriate level, *biomedical* explanations of the illness and its treatment; and (3) guiding patients through the *ritualized* clinical encounter and the health care bureaucracy in ways that increase their familiarity and comfort with it.

The Patient

Barriers to health care affecting both immigrants and disadvantaged minority groups—such as lack of insurance and other financial resources, physical distance, and low literacy—often make biomedical treatment an option of last resort. Clinical consultations for such patients will frequently be more time consuming and require increased patience by the clinician. Extra effort may sometimes be needed to teach such patients to be assertive, ask questions, and raise concerns. Clinicians who treat large numbers of such patients will benefit the most from reading about and becoming personally familiar with them outside of medical settings.

EXPLANATORY MODELS

Explanatory models refer to theories of disease causation, prognosis, typical symptoms, and appropriate treatment. Eliciting patients' explanatory models of disease offers unparalleled insight into their sense of self and relationships with significant others while yielding

Table 15-2. Questions to elicit a patient's explanatory model of illness.

- What do you think caused your problem?
- What do you think you have?
- What is the name you give to this condition?
- Why do some people get this illness but not others?
- What do you think needs to be done to relieve this problem?

clues about how they are likely to interpret, resist, or accept biomedical explanations and treatments. Knowledge of the patient's perspective also facilitates the ability to ease patient fear and anxiety. Understanding the patient's *explanatory model* of illness is especially important when treating potentially debilitating chronic conditions, where nonadherence is a common concern and where the psychosocial dimensions of illness loom large.

Typically, the most important component of a patient's explanatory model is the idea of illness *causation* (see Table 15-2). To elicit this belief the clinician can ask, "What do you think caused your problem?" and then listen carefully to the answer as it is likely to reveal crucial feelings related to moral failings, discord with significant others, financial and practical challenges in daily life, and whether there is a sense of hope for the future. The clinician should not expect patients to answer questions about causation with simple and mechanistic explanations. Additional probing may also be required. For example, the clinician could follow up with questions, such as "What do you think you have? What is the name you give to this condition?" "Why do some people get this illness and not others?" "Who or what is responsible (or to blame) for this problem?" and "Do you ever think that you did (or didn't do) something to bring this on yourself, or that someone else did (or didn't do) something?" Additional questions can allow patients to elaborate on their explanatory model: "What do you think should be done to treat you?" "Do you think a complete cure is possible?" "How long will the problem last?" "What do you think needs to be done to relieve this problem?" The advantage of such questions is that they are open ended, are applicable to every patient, and can help to correct or refine initial clinical assumptions or preconceptions. They are also powerful in their ability to provide clues about what the patient may find difficult to understand or accept when it comes to explaining the illness in *biomedical* terms.

Some patients, especially recent immigrants, may be reticent about sharing their explanatory models of illness out of concern that their beliefs will be viewed as ignorant or superstitious. Alternatively, such patients may feel that they have come to hear the doctor's expert opinion, and that their own perspective is of little consequence. It is sometimes prudent to allow patients' explanatory models to emerge slowly, through gentle probing, over the course of several visits. Inference combined with direct questioning (e.g., "other patients believe X, what do you think about this?") and background knowledge of the patient's social location will often be necessary to form a coherent picture.

Shared Decision Making

Patient centeredness and involving patients in complex decisions about their health care are important goals in medical care; however, it is still the case that most medical decisions are made by physicians with little input from patients or families. In shared decision making, a patient and clinician work together to evaluate trade-offs based on the patient's values and preferences in light of the risks and benefits of various treatment options. Shared decision making is most important for preference-sensitive conditions in which there are at least two legitimate treatment options available but each has different levels of risk or types of side effects.

Imparting accurate information about the nature and course of the disease, framing numerical risks, and eliciting a patient's outcome preferences are all important for shared decision making. Successfully sharing decisions, however, also requires a consideration of cultural influences. For example, certain patients (e.g., some older patients or patients who grew up in authoritarian societies) may not wish to participate in making a final treatment decision but instead wish to be involved only in articulating preferences and in selecting the most desirable outcome. Thus, the process of promoting patient centeredness should involve directly asking patients how involved they would like to be in decision making.

In emphasizing the importance of rational decision making, traditional shared decision making approaches implicitly stress how patients "should" behave while often overlooking how they, in fact, do behave. To address these challenges, clinicians should strive to meet patients closer to where they actually begin the decision-making process. Eliciting patient explanatory models may allow patients and clinicians to consciously recognize and correct misconceptions. Sources of patient fear can be elucidated and, where possible, reassurance can be offered. Patients can also be asked to recount stories about other people who faced similar illnesses so that their attitudes and perceptions can be clarified and they can be helped to understand key differences between these stories and their own circumstances.

Sometimes there is medical uncertainty about the value of a medical test or intervention (e.g., prostate-specific antigen [PSA] screening), or there may be more than one treatment option, none of which is clearly superior in terms of prevention, cure, or control of symptoms, but each of which differs significantly in terms of cost or in the likelihood of various adverse effects on quality of life. In these instances, before taking action the clinician should attempt to gauge both the patient's desire for information as well as preferences for decision making. Studies have shown that most patients wish to be "maximally" informed about their diseases as well as medical treatments and evaluations, but there is variability in their desire to assume or share responsibility for making actual treatment decisions. Only through probing is it possible to determine how much information patients want and how much they want to share in the decision-making process. Providing too much information or attempting to make the patient accept responsibility for a medical decision can be counterproductive, but so can an approach that is overly paternalistic. One strategy is for the provider to state that there is a choice and perhaps some medical controversy or uncertainty; briefly mention the pros and cons of each option; elicit patient outcome preferences; and then wait for the patient to ask for more details, voice concerns, or express a preference.

CASE ILLUSTRATION 1

A 72-year-old World War II veteran was diagnosed with localized prostate cancer. The patient is adamant about his desire to undergo curative treatment with radical surgery after the urologist explains that the likelihood of cure is the same with radiation therapy, after he reviews the specific and significant numerical likelihood of serious side effects associated with surgery and radiation, and after he proposes that watchful waiting and active surveillance are also reasonable options. After carefully eliciting the patient's understanding of the disease and its treatment, the urologist learns, from the patient's perspective, that: "cancer is a death sentence," "the only way to cure cancer is by cutting it out," and "radiation is dangerous." By taking the time to understand the patient's explanatory model of illness, the urologist is in a position to more effectively address his misconceptions and fears, thus allowing the patient to make a more genuine, high-quality decision about his care.

Fatalism

Members of some groups, including many immigrants, may seem to be fatalistic in their attitudes toward illness. They may be passive about seeking treatment, persist in unhealthful behaviors, or accept misfortune because they believe it is preordained. It is important not to assume that this style of explaining and dealing with illness is indelibly rooted in the culture or religion of the patient's racial or ethnic group. In fact, fatalism is widespread and is common among people who have little control over the circumstances of their lives. It also emerges out of a kind of valid logic that observes that serious illness can befall even those who have no bad habits and live a "clean" or "virtuous" life. Fatalism does not usually imply a lack of interest in preventing or treating disease. Rather, it can be viewed as an idiom for describing a person's perceived powerlessness in the world, lack of hope, and even distrust. The doctor can approach this problem by acknowledging the real challenges the patient faces, and by clearly articulating the practical steps the patient can take to resolve or manage the illness.

 CASE ILLUSTRATION 2

A 56-year-old African American woman who completed a grade-school education declines colon cancer screening. On questioning, she believes that cancer is not preventable and cannot be cured. Cancer terrifies her and she therefore sees no point in learning she might have it. The clinician explains that from a medical perspective cancer takes many years to develop, and that in people aged over 50 years it can happen in a few individuals out of a hundred. She then tells the patient that the purpose of colon cancer screening—a relatively safe procedure performed thousands of times every year—is not to find a big cancer (which would be extremely unusual) but to save lives by finding a few areas (polyps) where cancer could develop and then snip them out. She provides the patient with an illustrated brochure to look over and consider.

In addition to the patient's beliefs about cancer, the clinician suspects that she distrusts the idea of doctors doing something to her that she, herself, has not requested or previously thought about. Over the course of several appointments, the clinician gently revisits the issue. A year later, the patient agrees. Trust—developed through a continuing relationship, manifest concern on the part of the clinician, and openness in explaining the purpose of medical tests—was a key factor in the patient's decision. Had the patient continued to decline screening, however, the clinician appropriately would have respected her decision, without overt negative judgment.

THE PASSIVE PATIENT

Some immigrants and older patients may be exceptionally reserved or deferential in clinical interactions, often preferring to avoid direct eye contact. The clinician should not assume that such patients are shy, uninterested, unintelligent, or uneducated simply because they avoid eye contact, agree with everything the doctor says, express a great deal of uncertainty about instructions, or are not forthcoming with information. In these circumstances, the clinician should speak clearly without reverting to an overly simplistic, commanding, frustrated, or patronizing tone of voice. Further clinic visits and gentle elicitation of questions and concerns may be necessary before the patient begins to interact more openly. The patient's behavior may reflect not only cultural norms toward those in authority, but uncertainty, fear, the expression of trust through passivity, or a desire to attain a better impression of the clinician before revealing intimate details.

 CASE ILLUSTRATION 3

An older patient, originally a schoolteacher from the Philippines, is hospitalized for community-acquired pneumonia. The hospitalization is uneventful and on the day of discharge, the medical team enters his room to review his discharge instructions. When asked for his input about preferred follow-up or his understanding of the ongoing treatment, he averts his eyes, speaks quietly, and seems unable to comprehend the discharge plan. He repeatedly asks for instructions about the various forms. The team leaves the room uncertain of his understanding. Later that morning, the pharmacist on the team returns to review his discharge medications with him. She sits down and speaks softly and respectfully. Eventually, he opens up and it becomes apparent that he understood the prior conversation completely and speaks articulately about his concerns, although he continues to avoid eye contact.

INTERPRETERS

Trained medical interpreters can greatly facilitate patient–clinician communication and improve quality of care. Unfortunately, perhaps because of economic constraints and clinicians' beliefs in their own ability to simply "get by," well-trained interpreters are underused in many medical settings, with negative consequences for patient care. For example, although clinicians with some ability in conversational Spanish may assume they understand a Puerto Rican patient's use of the term "ataque de nervios" (literally a "nervous attack"), the patient is actually referring to a culturally specific syndrome with identifiable precipitants and clear symptoms that has little to do with a "nervous breakdown." Although family members often act as de facto interpreters, this can also introduce problems. For example, a relative who "already knows" what is wrong with the patient may not wish to bother the physician with the full details of the patient's complaints, thereby omitting important symptoms. Children and adolescents are inappropriate interpreters for many reasons, including an often incomplete mastery of English, insufficient knowledge of the subtleties of translation, and issues of relationship and status.

Trained medical interpreters can provide more than literal paraphrasing: they can serve as 'cultural interpreters' by explaining patient's illness labels and idioms for the practitioner, and translating biomedical concepts and instructions into the patient's vernacular. Interpreters should be treated as full members of the health care team. Prior to the interaction, the clinician may want to meet briefly with the interpreter to review the goals for that discussion (e.g., addressing the patient's understanding of and compliance with a particular medication). In addition, the clinician should periodically stop the interview to seek clarification from the interpreter: "The patient has mentioned 'nerves' a few times. I was assuming that she felt nervous, but now I'm not so sure. Could you explain to me what she means?"

When using an interpreter, it is important to consider the physical arrangement of the participants. The clinician should always face and speak to the patient directly. The interpreter can sit next to the physician (though some patients may find this arrangement threatening), or the patient and interpreter can sit side by side. Some clinicians prefer the traditional triangular arrangement so that all parties have equal space and symbolic power, but the easy flow of conversation may be compromised as patient and provider often cannot resist the impulse to direct their attention toward the interpreter instead of toward each other.

The Clinician

Understanding illness from the patient's perspective—traditionally regarded as the essence of cultural competence—must be balanced by the equally important task of knowing how to communicate *biomedical* explanations about the disease and its treatment to the patient (i.e., serving as interpreter of biomedical culture for patients). The desire for such information is usually one of the patient's primary motivations for visiting a doctor. The clinician should offer explanations in terms the patient can understand and then gently test this understanding.

NAMING AND EXPLAINING THE DISEASE IN NEUTRAL TERMS

Naming a disease helps to transform a patient's inchoate fears into something that can be perceived and addressed directly. Speaking about disease in neutral

and mechanistic ways can also dispel feelings of shame and ideas about etiology that are rooted in personal weakness and social failure. Patients will often seize upon, and benefit from, explanations that appropriately relieve them of personal responsibility for their misfortune. Giving a specific name to a disease and explaining it in neutral terms should be regarded as one of the primary goals of communication. Reaching this point, of course, may depend upon an initial period of testing and observation.

 CASE ILLUSTRATION 4

A 65-year-old immigrant and former physician is diagnosed with cancer. The clinician is able to elicit the patient's belief that cancer often occurs in people with "repressed personalities." Believing that he brought his disease upon himself because of such a character flaw, he feels a lack of hope and is less inclined to treat the disease. He benefits from an impersonal biomedical interpretation of cancer that focuses on damaged cellular DNA leading to unchecked cellular proliferation, and treatment aimed at destroying aberrant cells.

MEDICALIZATION

Although reductionistic disease labels and explanations are often helpful, they may contribute to the medicalization of conditions whose etiologies reside in adverse environmental (e.g., polluted air and water) or social circumstances (e.g., racism, intimate partner violence, sexual abuse, and work-related stress). In other words, defining illness entirely in terms of how it adversely affects the body can direct attention away from other, more fundamental causes. It is important to remain mindful of, and at times acknowledge, the broader context that gives rise to the illness. This is often very difficult for physicians to do, in part because they are not trained to recognize these links and are limited in their ability to resolve problems such as poverty, unemployment, poor housing, or lack of education and opportunity. For example, declaring that a patient's asthma is made worse by living near a factory from which, for economic reasons, the patient cannot easily move away may imply that nothing can be done about the problem. Nonetheless, awareness of such constraints can help the clinician to better understand and sympathize with the patient and tailor therapies that are realistic and appropriate. In addition, it is extremely common for patients of all backgrounds to believe that illness is caused by breaches in the moral order, social discord, and the failure of one's self or significant others to fulfill expected roles.

Purely mechanistic biomedical explanations cannot simply replace these types of beliefs, which tend to be deeply rooted and resistant to change. Educating the patient about disease terms and pathophysiology should complement but not supersede the importance of understanding and acknowledging these other aspects of the patient's explanatory model.

"BLAMING THE VICTIM"

When it is possible to trace the etiology of disease to potentially destructive personal behaviors, such as "risky" sex, smoking, alcoholism, and drug abuse, or the worsening of disease to medical nonadherence, two pitfalls should be avoided. One is emphasizing personal culpability at the expense of helping the patient to understand the nature of the disease itself. Without adequate education, patients may have a difficult time perceiving the relationship between their behavior and the outcomes these generate, and will therefore see less reason to make changes. Although it is important to stress that certain habits are harmful and should be altered or discontinued, this should be done in a straightforward and nonjudgmental manner. The second pitfall is failing to acknowledge the personal situations and social contexts that contribute to or sustain these behaviors. Low self-esteem, depression, chronic pain, social isolation, lack of "legitimate" employment, and a strong desire to experience a sense of social belonging can contribute to many varieties of harmful and risky practices. To the extent possible, clinicians should attempt to determine the factors that perpetuate or encourage harmful behaviors and discuss these with their patients in an open and frank manner. Doing so will demonstrate empathy and concern, and help patients understand how their behavior (arising as it might for understandable reasons) should nonetheless be modified, and how this might be achieved.

COMMUNICATING BAD NEWS

Naming the disease is a cornerstone of communication in the biomedical model. However, a more flexible approach to informing patients of their diagnosis is often appropriate, particularly when the diagnosis is cancer or a terminal illness. Knowledge of a patient's social location and explanatory models of illness (including cancer), as well as in-depth questioning of the patient and family, will provide the best understanding of cultural differences and preferences. Chapter 3 offers a more complete discussion of this topic.

EVIDENCE-BASED MEDICINE AND MINIMIZING THE OVERUSE AND MISUSE OF CLINICAL SERVICES

Promoting clinician stewardship over limited health care resources and ensuring the delivery of cost-conscious, evidence-based care have become increasingly important as health care expenditures have risen to unsustainable levels in the United States. Influences that promote the overuse and misuse of clinical services include financial gain for clinicians as well as defensive medicine (ordering tests, procedures, or visits primarily in order to reduce perceived exposure to malpractice liability). Patient expectations—shaped by clinicians themselves, the popular media, direct-to-consumer advertising, and anecdotes of friends and family—are also important drivers of medical overuse. It can be a significant challenge convincing patients that more care, more expensive care, or even the latest technology do not necessarily mean better care, especially because unmet expectations for care can be associated with less patient satisfaction and reduced intentions to adhere to prescribed therapy. Nonetheless, evidence-based practice often depends on a clinician's ability to elucidate patient expectations that are unrealistic or not medically valid, the beliefs and worries that underlie these, and then on an ability to engage patients in conversations that educate and, where possible, reassure. Helping patients to feel like they have been understood is a key way of earning their trust and realigning their expectations.

 CASE ILLUSTRATION 5

A 32-year-old woman, the daughter of a prominent local philanthropist, complains of chest pain and demands that her physician obtain a stress test to make sure she is not at risk of having a heart attack. The patient, an avid runner, does not experience exertional chest pain and otherwise has no cardiac risk factors. On questioning, the physician learns that the patient recently broke up with her boyfriend and that her parents are contemplating a divorce. The physician obtains an EKG and informs the patient that it is normal. She explains to the patient that chest pain is not unusual among patients living through significant stress, that these symptoms almost always resolve with time, and that she has no risk factors for cardiac disease. She further explains that stress testing in her situation has a real likelihood of leading to false positive results, prolonged anxiety, more clinic visits, and perhaps even additional, invasive testing. Ultimately, the physician is able to help the patient understand that a stress test is unnecessary. The patient agrees to return in a week to reassess how she's feeling and consider whether referral to a therapist might be helpful.

PSYCHIATRIC DIAGNOSES

For patients of many backgrounds, profound stigma is often attached to behavioral and psychiatric diagnoses.

Labels such as "depression," referrals to psychiatrists, or prescriptions for "mind-altering" medications may be strongly resisted, interpreted as insulting by some, and may severely compromise the practitioner–patient relationship. For such patients, somatization is often the most "legitimate" way of expressing distress. If there is any doubt regarding the patient's perception of psychiatric labels and referrals, the clinician should carefully explore the meanings that patients and their families attribute to them.

 ## CASE ILLUSTRATION 6

A Mexican immigrant, working-class mother is taken aback by the pediatrician's diagnosis of "attention deficit disorder" in her child and concomitant referral to a child psychiatrist and prescription for stimulant medication. She believes these recommendations imply that her child is "crazy" and, by extension, that she, first and foremost, as well as the family as a whole, have somehow failed. Her anguish is compounded by the extreme importance she attributes to her role as a mother and homemaker. Furthermore, she holds that psychiatric medicines are "too powerful" for her child who, like all children, is "sensitive and vulnerable." She would have benefited from a discussion that elicited these beliefs in advance, followed by an approach that acknowledged her fears, reaffirmed her maternal skills and concern, and attempted gently to address her beliefs and values.

PATIENT INTERPRETATIONS OF ACUTE ILLNESS, CHRONIC ILLNESS, AND PREVENTIVE MEDICINE

Many patients do not clearly differentiate acute from chronic illness, nor do they make distinctions among curing, managing, and preventing disease. Commonly, they assume that symptoms or diseases are self-limiting or curable with a single course of therapy. This can frustrate the clinician's ability to provide education and can contribute to poor adherence. If in doubt, the clinician should determine whether patients believe a cure is possible (*not* generally the case with chronic illness) or whether patients believe the absence of current symptoms implies the absence of future disease (suggesting poor understanding of preventive medicine). Gently correcting patients' misconceptions should be viewed as an ongoing process that takes time and bears repetition.

PATIENTS WITH POOR ENGLISH LITERACY

It is estimated that up to 21% of American adults are functionally illiterate and many more are only marginally literate, limiting their ability to understand medical information and engage in meaningful discussions with their providers. Feelings of embarrassment may lead patients to conceal this problem. Strategies for managing such patients include speaking slowly, using simple terms, targeting written materials to at most a fifth-grade reading level, and using clear pictures and diagrams whenever possible. Instruments such as the Test of Functional Health Literacy in Adults (TOFHLA) can provide rapid estimates of the ability to read and comprehend common medical and lay terms. Such tools can assist clinicians in tailoring both written and spoken information, and are probably more accurate at assessing the patient's reading and numerical skills and ability to function effectively in health care settings than subjective clinician impression alone.

REVIEWING MEDICATIONS

Failure to discuss medications is one of the most frequent lacunae in practitioner–patient communication. Misunderstandings and fears about medications are extremely common and are major contributors to nonadherence. Pharmaceuticals, however, are generally the most tangible and therapeutically important products that result from the clinical encounter. Special care should therefore be given to explaining their purpose, mechanism of action, and common side effects. Eliciting patient concerns and questions to uncover erroneous beliefs is also important. This is particularly likely to benefit patients who are reticent or unable to express these concerns on their own.

Sometimes it may be helpful for clinicians to personalize information by acknowledging common challenges they face in educating and treating patients.

 ## CASE ILLUSTRATION 7

A patient has been diagnosed with hypertension. After explaining the benefits and risks of treating hypertension with medication, the physician tries to help the patient see the clinical challenge from her perspective. She explains, "As doctors, we often have difficulty helping patients understand why they should take medicines even when they have no unpleasant symptoms. Understandably, patients often hate to take medicines, especially if they feel perfectly fine. Yet medicines are important for preventing very serious problems down the road."

This kind of approach may help some patients to understand and sympathize with the challenges faced by the clinician, promoting a sense that the two are allies in achieving a common objective.

ASSESSING PATIENT UNDERSTANDING

To ensure that biomedical explanations are correctly understood, the clinician should ask patients close- and open-ended questions about their disease process and ask them to repeat instructions. For example, "Tell me what you understand about the cause of your diabetes and what you think will happen if we cannot adequately control your blood sugar. How often should you check your blood sugar? What should you do if you feel light-headed and sweaty?" Such checks will help to reinforce knowledge and understanding and identify areas that benefit from further counseling.

The Clinician as Cultural Broker and Institutional Guide

As described above, cross-cultural communication is enhanced by attention to patients' social location because it allows provisional inferences to be made about how patients, as *individuals*, are likely to interpret and respond to their illness. Initial clinical impressions are then modified by eliciting patients' explanatory models of illness. This information helps to tailor communication regarding the *biomedical* perspective. Finally, communication is further enhanced by understanding how patients perceive key features of the clinical process and by guiding them through its ritual and bureaucratic aspects.

CLINICAL RITUALS

Repetitive and predictable patterns and rules circumscribe patient–clinician interactions. In the ambulatory setting, for example, the nurse measures the patient's blood pressure and then brings the patient to see the physician, who directs the proceedings according to a predefined format of greeting the patient, asking questions in a certain order, examining the patient, and offering explanations and recommendations. The patient is given a specific place to sit and generally knows that the consultation will last a fixed amount of time. In the hospital, the medical team rounds in the morning and obtains a standard template of subjective and objective information. The basic format of these rituals is fairly simple and can be readily learned by patients and by the new initiates into the profession.

Such ritual aspects of medicine can both facilitate and impede effective communication. For example, consistency minimizes confusion about what is acceptable and unacceptable and about what will happen. Ritual offers a sense of security when patients are undressed or are sharing personal information. The ground rules and scripts of ritual are translatable from one setting to another and operate even if practitioner and patient have never met. They allow the involved actors to focus greater attention on the *content* of their exchanges and, in themselves, these rituals can be comforting and even therapeutic.

On the other hand, rituals can impair communication if patients and practitioners differ in their expectations about how they are supposed to work, or if rituals become inflexible, blind routines that leave little room for digression, variation, and opportunities for patients to express themselves freely and in fully emotional ways. This frequently happens when the clinician is pressed for time and wants the patient to provide the "facts" as tersely as possible, or when the patient yields all spontaneity of self-expression to the perceived all-knowingness and authority of the doctor. Ritual should not become so fixed that its participants become inflexible. Awareness of these pitfalls and the ability to make spontaneous adjustments to unspoken aspects of ritual can do much to enhance communication with the patient. Brief, unexpected, or even surprising disruptions to ritual—such as a joke, a doctor's personal reflection, allowing the patient to shed a tear or relate a piece of medical history during the physical examination, or briefly and politely answering a patient's personal question about the doctor or his family—can, when judiciously applied and without breaking the overall structure of the encounter, foster more effective communication and enhance the therapeutic relationship.

For almost all patients, illness is not simply an individual malady, but a social disruption that both affects and requires the involvement of significant others. The paradigmatic private, dyadic nature of biomedicine's doctor–patient relationship can also impair communication when working with patients for whom the involvement of family members is very important. When desired by the patient, and to the extent possible, allowances and arrangements should be made to incorporate the family into diagnostic and treatment plans (see Chapter 11).

INSTITUTIONAL GUIDE

Health care is often highly fragmented. The increasingly sharp separation between hospital and ambulatory medicine, a large variety of subspecialists, and the growing importance of health care "teams" means that patients often interact with a bewildering variety of individuals whom they have never previously met and whose roles are not always apparent. Carefully guiding patients—anticipating their possible confusion, explaining the function of different health care workers, and encouraging patients to ask questions at any point during their trajectory through an illness episode—can go a long way toward alleviating their fear, misunderstanding, and distrust. Providers should be especially sensitive to immigrants and other vulnerable patients who may have a particularly poor understanding of how the health care system works. Providing education about where to report for laboratory work and procedures, when results will be returned and what will be done with these, the roles of various office staff, the hours of operation, rules pertaining to the presence of children, and so on will increase efficiency, improve patient use of resources, and also increase patient trust and adherence by demystifying what seems to be a complex and threatening bureaucracy. Of note, some patients may not wish to fill out forms because of fears of deportation; it is important to be explicit about the purpose and confidentiality of medical information.

"COMPLEMENTARY" & "ALTERNATIVE" HEALERS

Despite its depth of knowledge and undeniable efficacy in many areas, biomedicine is for many patients simply *one* healing option among many others, some of which are employed simultaneously and without apparent contradiction. If the patient wishes to discuss or solicit the provider's opinion about other healing modalities, the clinician—unless there are concrete reasons to the contrary—should be willing to acknowledge the beneficial role that nonbiomedical approaches may have for the patient. If there are potential adverse interactions or side effects of "alternative" therapies, or if there is concern that potentially beneficial biomedical therapies might be thwarted by other types of healers, the clinician should express these concerns but should always respect the fact that patients are the ultimate arbiters regarding the healing modalities for which they are best suited (see Chapter 33).

RACE/ETHNICITY & GENETICS

By virtue of their race or ethnicity, patients are sometimes said to be "at risk" for certain diseases. Examples include diabetes mellitus among Native Americans, breast cancer among Ashkenazi Jews, and prostate cancer among African Americans. Particular forms of treatment are also believed to be more (or less) effective among certain racial/ethnic groups compared with others. For example, among African Americans compared with whites, it is said that the combination of isosorbide dinitrate and hydralazine is more effective for treating heart failure, angiotensin-converting enzyme (ACE) inhibitors are less effective for essential hypertension, and a therapeutic response to selective serotonin reuptake inhibitor (SSRI) antidepressants takes place at lower doses. Each of these examples is highly controversial, reflecting long-standing, often heated disputes about whether race and ethnicity are primarily social constructs or, instead, meaningful and valid surrogates for biological difference. It is beyond the scope of this chapter to summarize the elements of this debate. We believe, however, that in communicating with patients it is important for clinicians to avoid oversimplifying the relationship between race/ethnicity and genetics. Although knowledge of race or ethnicity might prompt genetic testing or detailed family history taking in particular instances, the issues are simply too complex and the evidence too uncertain in a relatively small number of conditions for clinicians to make unqualified assertions to patients that they are "at risk" for a particular illness or unlikely to respond to therapies solely on the basis of their racial/ethnic background. In very real ways, believing that one is "at risk" can unnecessarily increase stress, fear, and feelings of stigma, uncertainty, and worthlessness. When discussing with patients the possible relevance of race and ethnicity, clinicians should openly acknowledge that experts do not always agree and they should quantify and convey individual risk through a consideration of as many relevant variables as possible.

CONCLUSIONS

Cross-cultural communication can be learned and enhanced through reflection and practice with a variety of patients from different cultures. Biomedicine has its own distinct culture and practices that may be difficult for many patients to comprehend and access. Cultural stereotypes are rarely useful in clinical encounters; instead, clinicians should attempt to understand the social location of their patients as reflected in their race and ethnicity, gender, age, immigration status, literacy level, occupation, sexual orientation, and other characteristics. As their skills develop, clinicians will find enormous gratification in caring for patients who are very different from them.

SUGGESTED READINGS

Denberg, TD, Melhado, TV, Steiner, JS. Patient treatment preferences in localized prostate carcinoma: The influence of emotion, misconception, and anecdote. *Cancer* 2006;107(3):620–630.

Fadiman A. *The Spirit Catches You and You Fall Down.* New York, NY: Farrar, Strauss & Giroux, 1998.

Helman C. *Culture, Health, and Illness,* 2nd ed. Oxford: Butterworth-Heinemann, 1992.

Kaiser Permanente National Diversity Council. *A Provider's Handbook on Culturally Competent Care.* (Available for Latino, African American, Asian/Pacific-Islander, and Eastern European populations.)

Kleinman A. *Patients and Healers in the Context of Culture.* Berkeley, CA: University of California Press, 1980.

Kleinman A, Benson P. Anthropology in the clinic: The problem of cultural competency and how to fix it. *PLoS Med* 2006; 3(10):e294.

WEB SITES

NIH Cultural Competency/Health Literacy Initiative. http://www.nih.gov/clearcommunication/culturalcompetency.htm. Accessed June 2013.

Informed Medical Decisions Foundation. http://www.informed-medicaldecisions.org/. Accessed June 2013.

Women

Diane S. Morse, MD; Judith Walsh, MD, MPH; & Jody Steinauer, MD, MAS

16

INTRODUCTION

This chapter describes the broad array of behavioral issues for women using a developmental framework. We discuss expected behavioral issues occurring as part of the normal life cycle, as well as problematic ones requiring medical surveillance or intervention.

ADOLESCENCE: A TIME OF POWER IN THE MIDST OF INSECURITY

The task of adolescence is to find one's own beliefs, moving from childhood to adulthood physically and in relationships (see Chapter 13). Several events can occur during this time that will require the sensitive attention of the primary care physician, but numerous studies have demonstrated that confidentiality must be maintained for the physician to be trusted and helpful to an adolescent.

Approach to the Gynecologic Examination

Some women fear a pelvic examination, especially when they are undergoing it for the first time. Little research has been done on what strategies are best in performing a pelvic examination, but several techniques have been found to be helpful in clinical practice.

Before performing the examination, clinicians should make the patient as comfortable as possible when taking a history by asking open-ended questions, demonstrating empathetic communication skills such as eye contact and nonjudgmental reactions, and not making assumptions about sexual activity and orientation. In addition, they should ask if the patient has had a previous pelvic examination. When taking a complete sexual history, they should inquire about prior sexual abuse or challenges with past examinations.

It is useful for the clinician to describe exactly what is being done before and during the examination. Both female and male clinicians should consider offering to have a chaperone present to reassure the patient about the professional content of the examination. Other techniques include appropriate draping; using a warm, lubricated speculum; using the narrowest speculum that will allow adequate visualization of the cervix; being as gentle as possible; and encouraging the patient to use relaxation techniques including deep breathing and mental imagery, techniques which are especially useful for young women and those who have experienced sexual abuse. In addition, elevating the head will facilitate eye contact and may make it easier for some women to relax. In situations where a patient has significant anxiety, an anxiolytic medication prior to the examination may be useful.

Research has shown that the experience of the first pelvic examination influences attitudes about subsequent examinations; therefore, it is important to make the first pelvic examination as positive an experience as possible. In a study describing women's experiences of the first pelvic examination, a negative evaluation of the examination was associated with pain, embarrassment, having insufficient knowledge about the examination and what the clinician was doing, and not knowing that they could stop at any time. Taking time to provide knowledge and encourage realistic expectations of the examination may help shape attitudes about subsequent examinations.

If a gynecologic examination is being carried out on an adolescent in the context of reproductive health care or to screen for sexually transmitted infections, it is important to be aware of the legal requirements of confidentiality in the United States, which vary by state and are listed on the Guttmacher Institute website (http://www.guttmacher.org). Adolescents should be encouraged to involve their parents or guardians in medical decisions, and providers should be aware of mandatory reporting laws in the case of nonconsensual sexual activity, sex with an older adult, or other abuse.

Chronic Pelvic Pain and Vulvodynia

A condition that can affect women starting in teen or early adult years is chronic pelvic pain (CPP), which is commonly defined as noncyclical pain of at least

6 months duration that occurs in the pelvis, abdominal wall, lower back, or buttocks, and is serious enough to cause disability or require medical care. Chronic pelvic pain affects up to 15% of women and accounts for 20% of the hysterectomies performed in the United States. Up to 40% of women with CPP have other diagnoses, that may be the cause and/or effects of the CPP, such as depression, anxiety, sexual dysfunction, substance abuse, and other pain syndromes, requiring in-depth investigation into all contributing factors. A history of sexual or physical abuse, including intimate partner violence, has been identified in over 50% of CPP patients, and therefore must be included in the history (see Chapter 38). This evaluation often requires many visits, as well as providing patient education such as that provided by the International Pelvic Pain Society (http://www.pelvicpain.org/resources/handpform.aspx).

A definitive diagnosis is not made for the majority (61%) of CPP patients, but for those with diagnoses, they are more commonly of urologic or gastrointestinal than gynecologic origin. The four most common diagnoses are irritable bowel syndrome (IBS), interstitial cystitis, endometriosis, and adhesions; in these cases or other specific diagnoses, treatment is targeted at the underlying pathology. However, when no source is found, a multidisciplinary approach addressing dietary, social, environmental, and psychological factors, as well as standard medication therapy, is ideal. A recent Cochrane review supports counseling, a multidisciplinary approach to treatment, the use of injectable gonadotropin-releasing hormone (GnRH) agonist or oral medroxyprogesterone acetate, and lysis of adhesions for patients with no underlying source. Cyclic pain, although not commonly included in the definition of CPP, can be a significant problem and can be treated with similar approaches. Specifically, the levonorgestrel intrauterine device has been shown to be as effective as GnRH agonist for cyclic pain, which may also be responsive to combined hormonal contraceptives. Trigger point injections of the abdominal wall can help myofascial sources. Finally, oral analgesics may be used based on studies of benefit with other sources of pain, and some evidence supports the use of gabapentin with or without amitriptyline.

Vulvodynia is vulvar discomfort occurring in the absence of visible lesions, usually described as burning–diffuse, constant, and unprovoked, and less commonly, localized and provoked. Comorbidities associated with vulvar pain are low back pain, IBS, migraine, and fibromyalgia. Approaches to the patient with vulvar pain may include a variety of nonpharmacological modalities: education about vulvar care, addressing sexual and psychological issues, and pelvic floor physical therapy. Topical anesthetics such as xylocaine have been shown to improve pain. Tricyclic antidepressants and gabapentin have been used, although there have been few controlled trials. Topical estrogen may be helpful in women who also have vulvar atrophy. For the primary care provider, recommendations include counseling the patient about the disorder, giving emotional support, and facilitating appropriate subspecialist involvement.

SCREENING AND DETECTION OF EATING DISORDERS

Issues around Food and Eating Disorders

Eating disorders are common and challenging in young women, and the primary care physician plays an important role in their detection (see Chapter 23). The primary care physician also manages the medical complications, determines the need for hospitalization, and coordinates care. In addition, for patients with milder forms of disordered eating who may not be seeing a mental health specialist regularly, the primary care physician may have responsibility for ongoing care, including exacerbations that may mandate coordination with mental health and/or nutritional support. Although the diagnostic criteria for anorexia nervosa and bulimia nervosa are clearly defined, women may also have disordered eating that does not meet the criteria for anorexia nervosa or bulimia nervosa, but is nonetheless abnormal. In addition, two groups at particularly high risk for eating disorders include female athletes and women with diabetes.

Binge eating consists of episodes of eating a large amount of food in a discreet period of time with a sense of lack of control. The binges must have at least three of the following criteria: (1) eating much more rapidly than normal; (2) eating until uncomfortably full; (3) eating large amounts of food when not feeling physically hungry; (4) eating alone because of embarrassment; and (5) feeling disgusted, depressed, or very guilty after overeating. The episodes must occur at least twice a week for 6 months, and must not be associated with any compensatory behaviors (e.g., purging or fasting). The estimated population prevalence is 3.5% in women. Binge eating has been strongly associated with obesity; in weight control programs, an estimated 15–50% of individuals have binge eating disorder. Although many obese patients report binge eating, not all have binge eating disorder. As expected, obesity-related complications are likely to exist, and binge eating disorder may be more common in weight-cycling patients. Several studies have evaluated treatment options for binge eating disorder. The primary recommended treatment is psychotherapy, in particular cognitive behavioral therapy (CBT). Pharmacotherapy may also be beneficial but less so than psychotherapy. Medications that have been shown to be useful in reducing binge episodes include the selective serotonin reuptake inhibitors (SSRIs) and antiepileptics (topiramate).

Screening for Eating Disorders

Because many women will not seek care for an eating disorder, the clinician must remain alert for clues, such as amenorrhea, concern about weight loss by a family member, abdominal bloating, and cold intolerance. Questions that are useful in ascertaining eating habits include: "Are you trying to lose weight?" "What did you eat yesterday?" and "Do you ever binge eat (eat more than you want) or use laxatives, diuretics, purging, or diet pills?" One screening tool, the SCOFF questionnaire, may prove to be useful in screening for eating disorders. The questions included the following: (1) Do you make yourself **S**ick because you feel uncomfortably full? (2) Do you worry you have lost **C**ontrol over how much you eat? (3) Have you recently lost more than **O**ne stone (fourteen pounds) in a 3-month period? (4) Do you believe yourself to be **F**at when others say you are too thin? (5) Would you say **F**ood dominates your life? A "yes" answer to any question is worth 1 point and a score of 2 is highly predictive of anorexia nervosa or bulimia nervosa. The Eating Disorder Screen for Primary Care (ESP) has also been proposed as a screening tool. The questions include: (1) Are you satisfied with your eating patterns? (no is abnormal); (2) Do you ever eat in secret? (yes is abnormal); (3) Does your weight affect the way you feel about yourself? (yes is abnormal); (4) Have any members of your family suffered with an eating disorder? (yes is abnormal); (5) Do you currently suffer with or have you ever suffered in the past with an eating disorder? (yes is abnormal). Both of these scales need to be evaluated in broader populations.

Clinicians should remain alert for the possibility of binge eating disorder in obese patients. Questions such as, "Do you ever binge eat?" "Do you often eat alone?" and "Do you ever feel guilty or depressed after overeating?" may be useful in detecting this disorder.

Treatment of Eating Disorders: A Framework

The first step is assessment of the patient's safety, knowledge, and attitudes toward her condition by a primary care provider. She may then agree to work with one member of the treatment team, for example, a nutritionist. Similarly, counseling for developmental or family issues, or treatment for depression, may be acceptable to the patient. Family counseling may be helpful in limiting pressure from the family, as pressure may be less likely to result in changed behavior than to generate resistance from the patient. A counselor trained in treating adolescents may be able to help the patient navigate peer issues involved in the behavior. Whether or not referral to a nutritionist or psychologist is accepted, periodic medical visits to follow the presenting symptom(s)—for example, amenorrhea, low heart rate, or loss of weight—allow the primary care clinician to monitor the severity of symptoms (particularly cardiac status or other indications for hospitalization) while gently informing a patient of the medical risks of her condition. Evidence of associated medical risks, such as osteopenia, dental erosion in the case of bulimia, or concerns about fertility (particularly when the patient has low weight or is estrogen-deficient) may encourage a patient to acknowledge the diagnosis and begin full treatment. Danger signs such as bradycardia and electrolyte disturbances may mandate involuntary hospitalization.

In summary, the primary care practitioner should be equipped to detect an eating disorder, and then must work as a member of a multidisciplinary team, including a mental health professional and a nutritionist, to support weight gain as appropriate, modification of eating habits, and appropriate psychological and/or medical therapies.

YOUNG ADULTHOOD: LEAVING HOME AND PUTTING IT ALL TOGETHER

In this phase of life, individuals begin to accept financial and emotional self-responsibility, to differentiate from the family of origin, and to develop intimate relationships with peers.

Healthy Behaviors and Health Care Maintenance

Safety in relation to sexuality, substance use, contraception, motor vehicles, and preventive care are ultimately the patient's responsibility, but the physician can play an important role in establishing lifelong healthy habits and collaboration in this realm. The physician who uses gender-neutral and nonjudgmental styles of history-taking and is alert to patient cues will be more likely to be told about challenges for the patient that may have long-term modifiable consequences such as gender-identity issues, substance abuse, unsafe sex, intimate partner violence, eating disorders, and depression. Engaging with patients in partnership works best, allowing them to identify pros and cons of their choices, and supporting their ability to make changes if needed. Autonomous motivation to change and patient belief in ability to make a change are positively associated with successful changes in behavior and maintenance of those changes.

Role of Culture

Identity also includes a patient's self-definition of her cultural role within the context of her family of origin, and this can impact her health and illness behavior (see Chapter 15). If, for example, she feels great pressure to succeed as an engineer, but prefers to be an artist, this dissonance can cause stress-related symptoms that bring her to the health care system. Somatoform behavior and medically unexplained symptoms (MUS) are common across all cultures and may be reinforced in preference to the expression of emotions in some families, masking a mental health disorder.

For women, unique issues regarding culture can relate to appearance and behavior as well. Some women may feel pressure from the dominant culture regarding slender body weight, but conflict may arise if their internal or family value system and/or sex partner is concordant with a larger body habitus. Other women could be encouraged verbally and through their cultural customs to be subservient to men, though this can be manifested to varying degrees, and may or may not result in conflict. Social support may be lacking as immigrant women become more acculturated in the United States. Also, immigrants engaged in a cultural transition process may experience criticism from older relatives as they assimilate to the prevailing culture and from younger relatives or friends if they maintain connection with the culture of origin. Traditional cultures may promote respect for elders and traditional gender roles, often a family-strengthening behavior, but reinforce secrecy around family violence and abuse. It is important for physicians to remember that family violence may include intimate partner violence, violence from extended family, and honor crimes (violence toward a woman whose behavior is interpreted as shaming the family). These issues may affect women of all ages uniquely, in their traditional role in the family, and physicians should be alert for clues that problems are occurring and when warranted use direct inquiry or screening.

Pregnancy and Infertility: Psychosocial Issues

UNINTENDED PREGNANCY

Almost half of the 6.7 million pregnancies in the United States each year (3.2 million) are unintended, and more than half of these unintended pregnancies are continued. Given these statistics and the risks of neural tube defects, it is appropriate for providers to advise all women of childbearing age who are not using effective contraception to take a daily multivitamin. Unintended birth is more common in women aged 18–24 years and in lower income women, and is associated with worse maternal and neonatal outcomes than intended birth. These include late presentation to prenatal care, smoking and drinking during pregnancy, premature birth, negative pediatric mental health effects, and not breastfeeding. Nearly 40% of unintended pregnancies end in abortion; at current rates, 30% of women will have an abortion in their lifetime.

Several factors contribute to unintended pregnancy, most importantly not using effective contraception at all or consistently. Fifty-four percent of women undergoing abortion report that they had used a contraceptive, most commonly the pill or condoms, during the month they became pregnant. Forty-six percent had not used contraception, and of these women many reported concerns about contraceptives, a quarter had had unexpected sex, and 1% had had forced sex. Contraceptive nonuse was more common among black, Hispanic, poor, and uneducated women.

To help women prevent unintended pregnancy it is imperative that clinicians counsel reproductive-aged, heterosexual women who are not trying to become pregnant about contraception. They should include the highest efficacy reversible methods such as intrauterine contraception and implants in the discussion, address patient's concerns about methods, and help women choose the best method for them. Although oral contraceptives are the most commonly prescribed reversible contraceptives, they have a high failure rate of up to 8%, and require women to fill a regular prescription and take it daily. One recent study found that women, on average, do not take five pills each month, which likely contributes to its high failure rate. In contrast, the long-acting reversible methods have much lower failure rates of less than 1%.

PREGNANCY OPTIONS COUNSELING AND REFERRAL: PROFESSIONAL RESPONSIBILITY

Clinicians should provide objective, nonjudgmental pregnancy options counseling to women with newly diagnosed pregnancies. This includes asking women whether the pregnancy was intended and is desired; educating them about the options of pregnancy continuation, including adoption, and pregnancy termination; offering supportive counseling if they are undecided; and providing appropriate referrals. At times this can be challenging for individual clinicians who have strong feelings about the woman's preference. For some, they may feel morally opposed to and uncomfortable referring a woman for abortion. For others, they may feel that her desire to continue the pregnancy is not wise due to factors such as her age, resources, relationship status, or potential interference with her educational or career goals. These feelings may interfere with one's ability to provide unbiased counseling and referral for patients. This raises the issue of conscientious refusal and whether clinicians can opt out of such counseling.

The vast majority of U.S. states allow health care providers to decline direct participation in abortion services; 10 states permit clinicians to refuse to provide contraception for patients, and 6 permit pharmacists to refuse to dispense contraceptives. However, ethicists and medical organizations, such as the American Congress of Obstetricians and Gynecologists (ACOG), argue that it is the clinician's responsibility to provide a timely referral when they do not, due to conscience, provide the services the patient requests. Studies show that in practice most physicians support these guidelines. To provide women adequate counseling and referral, it may be helpful for clinicians and office staff to clarify their values about pregnancy options through facilitated discussion of different scenarios and to decide on a policy about counseling and referral.

ABORTION

Many well-designed studies have demonstrated that abortion is not associated with poor mental health outcomes. However, unintended pregnancy can be stressful for patients and requires significant psychosocial support, regardless of decision about pregnancy outcome. Women with unintended pregnancy are more likely to have a history of depression than women with intended pregnancy, and these women are at higher risk of a depressive episode at the time of or after an abortion. Thus, it is important to screen women with unintended pregnancy, regardless of their plans for the pregnancy, for depression. Also, whereas most women experience great relief after abortion, a few seek support as they grieve the loss of the pregnancy and may be referred to counseling services (http://yourbackline.org/).

When a woman seeks an abortion it is important to refer her as early as possible, because although abortion is extremely safe, its morbidity increases as women enter and proceed through the second trimester (although it is still lower than term birth). Women who have had an abortion are at increased risk of having a repeat, unintended pregnancy and therefore require extra support for choosing and using contraception effectively. Also, studies have found that two modifiable factors, intimate partner violence and substance use, increase a woman's risk of abortion and therefore warrant screening and subsequent referral.

INFERTILITY

Psychosocial stress is common in individuals struggling with infertility, increases as treatment becomes more complex, and makes discontinuation of treatment more likely. Although studies of baseline stress and conception rates with fertility treatments are mixed, a recent large meta-analysis found no relationship between baseline stress and pregnancy rates. The prevalence of psychiatric disorders also appears to be higher in infertility. Risk factors include past psychiatric illness, particularly discontinuation of medication due to anticipated pregnancy; longer duration of infertility; and history of pregnancy loss. Therefore, it is important to screen these patients for psychiatric illness, especially for anxiety and depression, as well as for the effects of infertility on various aspects of their lives and their stress levels.

Many studies have been conducted on the effect of psychosocial support—including counseling, support groups, and training in relaxation techniques and stress management—on pregnancy rates. Some studies have shown increased birth rates in patients participating in these services. A meta-analysis found an increased relative risk of pregnancy in patients participating in support groups compared with controls. Thus, it is important to screen patients seeking to become fertile for psychiatric illness and treat appropriately, and to recommend participation in a support group or similar social intervention.

Premenstrual Syndrome and Premenstrual Dysphoric Disorder

Premenstrual syndrome (PMS) is characterized by cyclic occurrences of a variety of symptoms prior to and resolving within a few days of the onset of menses. As many as 150 symptoms have been attributed to PMS, but the most common are fatigue, irritability, bloating, anxiety or tension, breast tenderness, mood lability, depression, and food cravings. Whereas up to 80% of women describe at least one PMS symptom, the more severe form, premenstrual dysphoric disorder (PMDD), occurs in only 3–8% of women and impairs daily living. Five symptoms characterize PMDD: (1) sadness, hopelessness, or being self-critical; (2) tension or anxiety; (3) labile mood interspersed with frequent tearfulness; (4) persistent irritability or anger; and (5) increased relational conflicts. Additional emotional and physical symptoms may also be present, and other psychiatric illnesses must be ruled out.

Because of varied symptoms and overlap with other conditions, a prospective daily symptom scale–demonstrating onset of symptoms around the time of ovulation and cessation of symptoms after the menses–is critical for diagnosis. Several calendars have been validated, including the Calendar of Premenstrual Experiences (COPE), in which women document symptoms daily on a 4-point Likert scale for 10 physical and 12 behavioral symptoms. A total score of less than 40 during days 3–9 of the cycle combined with a score greater than 42 during the last 7 days of the cycle is an effective screening tool for PMDD.

Treatment for PMS is approached in a stepwise fashion, first with behavioral changes and progressing to pharmacotherapy. Encouraging the patient to exercise regularly, limit salt and caffeine intake, and keep a regular sleep schedule may be beneficial. Calcium and vitamin D supplementation are associated with a lower incidence of PMS symptoms. The prospective daily symptom scale may be therapeutic as well as diagnostic by allowing the patient to be proactive in anticipating, managing, and avoiding symptoms. Since stress has been shown to increase symptoms, relaxation exercises and counseling may be effective.

Most patients with PMDD require pharmacological therapy for significant improvement. The SSRIs are considered first-line therapy and have been proven to be effective in multiple studies, for both behavioral and physical symptoms. Fluoxetine is FDA-approved for this indication at doses between 20 mg and 60 mg, with lower doses equally effective and better tolerated. Other effective SSRIs are sertraline, paroxetine, and citalopram, and all can be administered continuously throughout the month, intermittently from ovulation to the onset of menstruation, or semi-intermittently with increased doses in the late luteal phase. The benzodiazepine alprazolam can be used in the luteal phase to reduce symptoms, but with less effect than SSRIs. Patients who do not respond to SSRIs or anxiolytics can try agents to suppress ovulation; options include continuous oral contraception or contraceptive rings (the patch cannot be used continuously due to increasing weekly levels of ethinyl estradiol). One pill formulation with drospirenone improves PMS when prescribed traditionally, with a hormone-free interval, but only in comparison with placebo and only in the short term compared with other pill formulations (by 2 years symptoms are equivalent to the effects of other pills). Also, GnRH analogues, which require add-back estrogen therapy if used for more than 6 months, can treat symptoms. Other treatments showing some benefit are vitamin B6 supplementation and spironolactone.

Depression in Pregnancy

Women with a history of major depression are at highest risk of depression in pregnancy. Other risk factors include discontinuing or decreasing antidepressant medications. In the absence of suicidal or homicidal ideation, nonpharmacological treatments are advised. Psychotherapy for depression has been shown to be equally effective when compared to antidepressant medications (see Chapter 25). Often the focus of psychotherapy in this setting is on the transition to motherhood and the acquisition of the requisite skills.

The decision about prescription of psychotropic medications is complex: The risk of medication exposure to the fetus must be balanced against the risk of untreated depression for the mother, other children in the home and, ultimately, the infant. Decisions about medication include factors such as the severity of the depression, the number of prior depressive episodes, and a woman's history of response to medications. All the evidence comes from observational studies.

Overall, experts recommend sertraline as the preferred drug for treatment of depression in pregnant women.

Postpartum Depression

During the postpartum period, women can experience mood changes, including postpartum blues, postpartum depression, panic disorder, and postpartum psychosis. Transient postpartum blues are common, occur within a few days of delivery in 40–80% of women, include mood swings, irritability, sadness and crying spells, and resolve within 2 weeks. Postpartum depression has been estimated to occur in 5–9% of women. The clinical diagnostic criteria are feeling depressed or hopeless most of the day almost daily for at least two consecutive weeks, with onset usually within 1 month but up to within a year of birth. The biggest risk factor for postpartum depression is a personal history of depression. Other risk factors include lack of social support, history of miscarriage or other pregnancy loss, not breast-feeding, pregestational or gestational diabetes, and family psychiatric history. Some of the symptoms of postpartum depression such as fatigue, sleeping problems, and decreased sexual drive are common symptoms of the immediate postpartum period, making the disorder more difficult to detect. Feeling overwhelmed or guilty, being unable to care for or bond with the baby, or not sleeping even when the baby is sleeping, should all alert the clinician to the possibility of the diagnosis.

The Edinburgh Postnatal Depression Scale has been validated and used in multiple settings to screen for postpartum depression. Clinicians should ask about mood, appetite, sleep, and being overwhelmed during postpartum visits. A woman who expresses thoughts about harming herself or the baby should receive immediate evaluation by a mental health professional. When evaluating a woman for possible postpartum depression, thyroid disorders should be ruled out, as both hypothyroidism and hyperthyroidism are more common in the postpartum period.

Women with mild to moderate symptoms should be initially treated with nonpharmacological measures including sleep hygiene, education, psychotherapy, CBT, or family therapy.

There are no randomized controlled trials of pharmacotherapy for postpartum depression, so recommendations are based upon observational studies and extrapolation from the general population. Antidepressant drugs are generally initiated in the same fashion as in the usual treatment of major depression, using a medication previously effective whenever possible. The SSRIs are the drug of first choice, given their safety profile and relative low risk of side effects, with the evidence slightly favoring sertraline and paroxetine. Although there is limited evidence about antidepressant use in breast-feeding women, there are only few reports of adverse effects. The benefits of depression treatment and of breast-feeding are generally felt to outweigh the risks of the medications.

Irritable Bowel Syndrome

Young adult women may present to their physicians with IBS, as it is the most common gastrointestinal disorder seen in primary care. It is characterized by chronic abdominal pain and altered bowel habits in the absence of an organic cause. IBS is estimated to occur in 1–20% of the population with a female predominance of 1.5:1. Only about 15% seek medical care for their condition, yet the volume of patients is large and the burden to society in health care costs and missed work is significant.

The pathophysiology of IBS remains unknown. It is thought to be a disorder of gastrointestinal motility, dysregulation of the nervous system, increased visceral sensitivity, and possibly bacterial overgrowth. Psychosocial stressors have been shown to precipitate and exacerbate symptoms but are not thought to be a cause of the underlying condition. Women who have a history of physical or sexual abuse are more likely than controls to suffer from IBS and other functional bowel disease. Patients with a history of abuse have poorer health outcomes as manifested by an increase in pain, physician visits, and surgical procedures than patients without an abuse history. Although women seeking treatment for IBS are more likely to suffer from depression, anxiety, panic disorder, somatization, or other mental illness, those who do not seek treatment have the same incidence of these problems as the general population. Hence, it is unclear whether psychiatric stressors exacerbate the disease or contribute to the underlying etiology, perhaps varying in different individuals. Other conditions related to IBS include sleep disturbance, depression, and fibromyalgia. Interestingly, health-related quality of life appears to be more related to extraintestinal symptoms rather than traditionally elicited gastrointestinal symptoms in patients with IBS.

Effective treatment for IBS involves an integrated behavioral and pharmacological stepwise approach individualized to the patient's main symptom. Treatment for mild disease can involve only education, bulking laxatives, and antispasmodics. Both the SSRIs and the tricyclic antidepressants (TCAs) are effective for symptom relief in some patients but the TCAs can exacerbate constipation. Loperamide is helpful for treatment of diarrhea, but does not relieve other symptoms. Rifamaxin, a nonabsorbable antibiotic given for a short course, has been shown to relieve some symptoms of IBS. Newer treatments include alosetron, a 5-hydroxytryptamine-4 (5-HT-4) antagonist, which was removed from the market because of serious complications, but is now again available for limited use. Cognitive behavioral therapy (CBT) has been shown to be helpful in several studies. Dynamic psychotherapy and hypnotherapy have also been shown to be useful in reducing IBS symptoms, although results are somewhat mixed and effects were of short term in some studies. In the largest trial testing CBT in women, CBT was significantly more effective than education alone. Certain subgroups of IBS sufferers may be especially responsive to CBT. Simple educational interventions designed to help patients learn more about their bodies and IBS can be helpful in reducing anxiety and improving health-related quality of life. However–similar to other disorders overlapping with a history of childhood or adult abuse, sexual trauma, psychiatric comorbidities, or somatization disorder–sensitive communication strategies and avoidance of unneeded interventions are crucial.

THE MIDDLE YEARS: FAMILY AND TRANSITIONS

Women with children negotiate a myriad of changes in themselves, their children, their families of origin, and their committed relationships. In the childbearing years, depending on their own relationship situation, women need to integrate the child into a diversity of potential relationship environments: same- or opposite-sex partner, marriage, cohabitation, monogamous or non-monogamous. Relationships are mapped upon changes in the woman's emotional and physical self, career, and the rest of the family on all sides. This often requires profound multitasking. As children age, the parent(s) must accommodate varying tasks in the children's lives, helping them with their transitions, even as the parents, sometimes paradoxically, make their own transitions. Women, with and without children, are the most likely ones to care for aging parents, parents-in-law, and other older relatives. Expected physiologic changes or unexpected illness further impact women in these years. It is imperative that primary care providers anticipate these developmental processes and incorporate them into their approach to these patients.

Menopause: Managing Symptoms

Personal, cultural, and family attitudes can have a large effect on the emotional and functional impact of menopausal symptoms. A biopsychosocial approach, which includes inquiring about the impact of these developmental processes and ascertaining whether symptoms can be managed without medication, is crucial. Since publication of the results of the Women's Health Initiative, which showed increased risk of breast cancer and cardiovascular disease associated with use of estrogen/progestin, many women and their physicians are reluctant to use hormone therapy (HT) for treatment of menopausal symptoms. However, estrogen can be very helpful for the treatment of hot flashes and vaginal dryness and in the prevention of osteoporosis. Use of systemic estrogen, and progesterone if the women has a uterus, is an option that some women may choose if symptoms are severe or if other therapies are not successful. The primary care provider can help female patients sort through the multitude of options, including assessing the risks and benefits of HT, and make their own best decisions. Comorbidities such as family history of breast cancer, use of cigarettes, and personal or family history of thromboembolic disease may impact this decision.

The average age of menopause in the United States is 51 years. More than 50% of postmenopausal women experience "hot flashes," a manifestation of vasomotor instability associated with the abrupt withdrawal of estrogen. Hot flashes, also known as hot flushes, are sensations of feeling warm, frequently associated with perspiration, palpitations, and anxiety. When they occur at night, they can be manifested by night sweats, frequent awakening, and consequently, sleep disturbance and chronic insomnia. A recent meta-analysis showed that the average duration of menopausal symptoms is 4 years, so any potential treatment options must be considered within the context of this symptom duration.

Another important menopausal symptom is urogenital atrophy. The loss of estrogen causes thinning of the vaginal epithelium and may lead to vaginal irritation, dyspareunia, and increased risk of vaginal infections. When the urethra is affected, urinary frequency, incontinence, and bladder irritation or infection can also occur.

Treatment of Vasomotor Instability

Symptoms such as hot flashes and changes in sexual function can have a profound effect on a woman's mood and quality of life. Many women with mild vasomotor symptoms will try nonpharmacological interventions, such as lifestyle changes, relaxation, and exercise, but the evidence for these therapies is limited. Obesity, however, is a risk factor for hot flashes, hence weight loss may help reduce hot flash severity.

Determining the efficacy of pharmacological treatments for vasomotor instability is challenging, as about 30% of women will respond to placebo (Table 16-1). However, estrogen has been shown to be the most effective in reducing the frequency of hot flashes, associated with an 80% reduction in hot flash frequency.

Nonestrogen therapies that have been used for vasomotor symptoms include the selective serotinin reuptake inhibitors (SSRIs), the serotonin norepinephrine reuptake inhibitors (SNRIs), high-dose progestins, clonidine, gabapentin, and several complementary therapies. Several trials have evaluated antidepressants (SSRIs and SNRIs) in the treatment of postmenopausal hot flashes. Drugs that have been found to be effective include venlafaxine and desvenlafaxine (SNRIs) and paroxetine and escitalopram (SSRIs), and are generally associated with about a 60% reduction in hot flash frequency. High-dose progestins (megestrol acetate or Megace) have been associated with about a 50–60% reduction in hot flashes, although prolonged therapy can be associated with weight gain. Clonidine has been associated with about a 40% reduction in hot flashes. Gabapentin has also been associated with a reduction in hot flash frequency of about 30–45%.

Several complementary and alternative therapies have been used for treating hot flashes, although the trials are often small, short in duration, lack a placebo arm, and use variable doses. Isoflavones are contained in soy products and red clover, and have been frequently used for the treatment of menopausal symptoms; however, studies have not shown any benefit. Several herbal remedies have been promoted for hot flash reduction. Black cohosh, wild yams, progesterone cream, ginseng, dong quai, and evening primrose oil have all been used but do not have proven efficacy.

Many women go through menopause without medications, using behavioral strategies such as exercise, hydration, wearing layered loosely fitting clothes, and short daytime naps to compensate for hot flash-interrupted sleep. It is important for primary care providers to establish a collaborative relationship with patients, allowing them to discuss issues that may compound menopausal symptoms. Normalizing these sometimes stressful transitions may help a woman to accept a trial of watchful waiting or even psychotherapy to address the stress of these changes. Discussion of menopausal symptoms may not necessarily be a request for medications, but should trigger discussions about the variety of available management strategies.

Treatment of Urogenital Atrophy

The mainstays of treatment for urogenital atrophy are currently vaginal moisturizers and topical vaginal estrogen

Table 16-1. Alternatives for treatment of hot flashes compared to placebo.

Treatment	Dosage (mg/day)	Efficacy (%)
Estrogen CEE (conjugated equine estrogen)	0.625	80 vs 20–30
Paroxetine	12.5 or 25	62 vs 38
Escitalopram	10 to 20	55 vs 36
Venlafaxine	37.5	37 vs 27
Venlafaxine	75 or 150	61 vs 27
Desvenlafaxine	100	64 vs 51
Clonidine	0.1	38 vs 20
Gabapentin	900	45 vs 29

in either cream or ring form. Vaginal therapy can be safely used in most women, although there is some controversy about use in women with estrogen-dependent tumors. Regular use of vaginal moisturizers and use of lubricants during intercourse can be beneficial to relieve symptoms but do not treat the underlying genital atrophy.

Maintaining Sexual Function

It is important for physicians to inquire about sexual function; a national study of 1749 women and 1410 men aged 18–59 years found a prevalence of sexual dysfunction of 43% for women (see Chapter 32). Sexual function in women is both emotional and physical. As some women age, they experience a liberation from the responsibilities of young children, relationship struggles, and financial concerns that allows them to enjoy sex more than they ever have. This may also be due, in part, to a relative rise in testosterone, as estrogen levels decrease, that improves sexual function in some women. Others experience physiologic changes described above that diminish sexual function, such as urogenital atrophy or sleeplessness from hot flashes. Expectations may be different between male and female partners, especially if the male is able to treat erectile dysfunction medically. Besides lubrication, women can be advised to try a slower pace of sexual activity, as it is normal for reaction time to diminish with age in both genders. If estrogen is used to treat vasomotor symptoms of menopause, the relative drop in testosterone can diminish sexual drive or function in some women, and that subgroup of patients may benefit from the addition of small amounts of testosterone. A primary care physician may defer prescription of these medications to a gynecologist or endocrinologist, but should be familiar with the physiology and be able to make recommendations accordingly.

WOMEN IN LATER LIFE: SHIFTING ROLES AND OPPORTUNITIES

Women in their later years are achieving the tasks of shifting generational roles and changes in couple and family functioning. Challenges may include loss of spouse, family members, and friends, along with physiologic aging and financial concerns. Opportunities exist, however, for life review and integration, along with time for new friendships and activities. Additionally, a woman may enjoy being appreciated for her wisdom, without many of the burdensome responsibilities of younger years. A primary care provider should be prepared to assist in these challenges and supportive of the opportunities (see Chapter 14).

Osteoporosis and Falls

Both osteoporosis and falls are more common in older women than in men. More than half of all women will develop osteoporosis by the age of 80 years. Fractures are 2.2 times higher in women over the age of 65 years than they are in men. Women appear to recover more slowly from these injuries, which may contribute to increased medical costs for falls in women. Hence, prevention of falls is an important issue for older women and has several behavioral components. Interventions shown to reduce falls include muscle strengthening and balance retraining, multidisciplinary health and environmental risk factor screening and intervention programs, group exercise with tai chi, home hazard assessment, withdrawal of psychotropic medications, and vitamin D supplementation.

Fear of falling can significantly impact an older woman's life by inhibiting activities, leading to a loss of independence. In one survey, 80% of women answered that they would rather be dead than experience the loss of independence and quality of life that results from a bad hip fracture and subsequent admission to a nursing home. Clinicians caring for older women should address this fear and consider interventions not only to reduce osteoporosis risk but also to reduce risk and fear of falling. Some of the same activities that reduce incidence of falls can reduce fear of falling; these include tai chi and strength training.

Urinary Incontinence

Up to 50% of elderly women report some urinary incontinence. Daily incontinence occurs in about one-fifth of community-dwelling women aged 85 years or older. More than half of the women with urinary incontinence do not tell their health care provider about their situation and just try to live with it. The psychological morbidity from this "hidden" problem can be high. Problems may include social withdrawal, depression, and sexual dysfunction. The clinician can uncover these problems with thorough history and physical examination to assess for volume overload, constipation, musculoskeletal limitations, bladder integrity, and vaginal atrophy. Specialist referral should be considered in those with abdominal or pelvic pain, hematuria, fistula, pelvic mass or prolapse, complex neurologic conditions, and those who fail conservative management.

Several behavioral treatments are helpful in urinary incontinence. For stress, urge, and mixed incontinence, avoiding overfilling of the bladder and regular muscle contraction (Kegel) exercises are beneficial. In urge and mixed incontinence, bladder retraining in cognitively intact women along with biofeedback is effective. In cognitively impaired women, prompted voiding by a caregiver can further reduce incontinent episodes. Smoking, caffeine, alcohol cessation, and weight loss are of benefit. Anticholinergics, antispasmodics, or combinations are the most commonly used and effective pharmacological options in conjunction with behavioral treatments for urge and mixed incontinence. Topical estrogen is another potentially helpful option. If these conservative measures are not effective, specialist referral is indicated.

Cognitive Dysfunction

Cognitive dysfunction, including mild cognitive impairment and dementia, are major issues facing older women, with an estimated annual incidence for Alzheimer dementia of 0.6% for people over the age of 65 years and 8.4% of those over the age of 85 years. Women appear to be at higher risk of developing dementia and, because of women's longer life span, there are many more older women suffering from dementia than men. Prevention of dementia would be optimal in reducing the burden of this disease, and many of the prevention strategies involve behavioral approaches (see Chapter 30). Risk factors for dementia include hyperlipidemia, diabetes, hypertension, smoking, low levels of physical activity, low levels of mental activity, and poor social network. Older women should be encouraged to adopt a "brain-healthy" diet, which includes a decrease in overall fat and an increase in foods high in monounsaturated fats and antioxidants (fruits, vegetables, nuts, and cold-water fish). They should also maintain a healthy weight, get regular physical activity, participate in social activities, and exercise the mind (learn new things, read, play games, crossword puzzles, etc).

It has been hypothesized that HT after menopause would help decrease the risk of cognitive dysfunction and dementia. Several prospective population cohort studies found fewer declines in cognitive function in women taking HT. Earlier small clinical trials have shown some cognitive improvement in women taking HT, but the Women's Health Initiative actually showed an increase in cognitive decline in some groups taking HT, both estrogen-alone and estrogen–progestin groups. As this study started several years after menopause for most of the participants, no conclusions regarding early postmenopausal therapy can be made. Using current evidence, HT should not be prescribed for the sole purpose of preserving cognition.

SUMMARY

There are a number of behavioral issues in the primary care of the woman patient, and these should be integrated into preventive care and management of medical issues from a biopsychosocial perspective. Although the developmental stages women experience include challenges, there are also opportunities for fulfillment both for the patients and those who care for them.

ACKNOWLEDGMENT

We acknowledge Sangita Devaskar for her assistance with manuscript preparation.

SUGGESTED READINGS

Basson R. Women's sexual dysfunction: revised and expanded definitions. *CMAJ* 2005;172(10):1327–1333.

Boivin J, Griffiths E, Venetis CA. Emotional distress in infertile women and failure of assisted reproductive technologies: meta-analysis of prospective psychosocial studies. *BMJ* 2011;342: d223.

Cotton MA, Ball C, Robinson P. Four simple questions can help screen for eating disorders. *J Gen Intern Med* 2003;18(1): 53–56.

Hammerli K, Znoj H, Barth J. The efficacy of psychological interventions for infertile patients: a meta-analysis examining mental health and pregnancy rate. *Hum Reprod Update* 2009;15(3):279–295.

Hendrick V, Altshuler L. Management of major depression during pregnancy. *Am J Psychiatry* 2002;159(10):1667–1673.

Jones RK, Kooistra K. Abortion incidence and access to services in the United States, 2008. *Perspect Sex Reprod Health* 2011; 43(1):41–50.

Munk-Olsen T et al. Induced first-trimester abortion and risk of mental disorder. *N Engl J Med* 2011;364(4):332–339.

Murray L, Carothers AD. The validation of the Edinburgh Postnatal Depression Scale on a community sample. *Br J Psychiatry* 1990;157:288–290.

Nelson HD et al. Nonhormonal therapies for menopausal hot flashes: systematic review and meta-analysis. *JAMA* 2006; 295(17):2057–2071.

Politi MC, Schleinitz MD, Col NF. Revisiting the duration of vasomotor symptoms of menopause: a meta-analysis. *J Gen Intern Med* 2008;23(9):1507–1513.

Stones W et al. Interventions for treating chronic pelvic pain in women. Cochrane *Database Syst Rev* 2005;Issue 2. Art. No.: CD000387. DOI: 10.1002/14651858.CD000387.

Wisner KL, Parry BL, Piontek CM. Clinical practice. Postpartum depression. *N Engl J Med* 2002;347(3):194–199.

WEBSITES

Guttmacher Institute. http://www.guttmacher.org. Accessed January 2014.

The International Pelvic Pain Society. http://www.pelvicpain.org/resources/handpform.aspx. Accessed January 2014.

Backline. http://yourbackline.org/. Accessed January 2014.

Lesbian, Gay, Bisexual, & Transgender Patients

Richard E. Greene, MD, FACP; Donald W. Brady, MD FAACH; & Jason Schneider, MD, FACP

INTRODUCTION

Lesbian, gay, bisexual, and transgender (LGBT) people have become more openly accepted into the framework of society. Likewise, the medical literature has expanded its discussion of the health needs of LGBT people, though often addressing the issues from a strictly sexual behavior perspective (e.g., "men who have sex with men"). Specific knowledge and skills are essential for the health care provider to be able to ascertain the sexual orientation and gender identity of patients; communicate acceptance and understanding of LGBT health issues; screen for conditions amenable to behavioral interventions; and provide information and resources specific to the needs of LGBT patients. Providers can use these skills to provide access to competent medical care for LGBT patients.

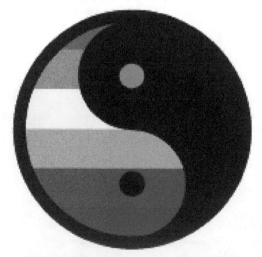

Embracing wholeness: yin-yang symbol with LGBT rainbow colors. Accessed at http://spiritualityireland.org/blog/index.php/2013/06/l-g-b-t-spirituality-taoism/

Lesbians and gay men make up anywhere from 1% to 10% of the general population—depending on the source quoted and the sampling method used in the study. In most studies, self-identified bisexuals are a small fraction of the lesbian or gay population. Whatever the exact percentage, however, in absolute terms, LGBT persons constitute a significant group of patients with unique medical, psychological, and social needs. Sexual orientation and gender identity are generally invisible. Consequently, many health care providers caring for LGBT patients do not recognize or acknowledge their unique needs.

DEFINITIONS & CONCEPTS

Sexual Orientation, Sexual Behavior, & Identity

Sexual orientation refers to sexual attraction to another person, including fantasies and the desire for sex, affection, and love. Sexual orientation is distinct from and not necessarily predictive of sexual behavior or activities. Being gay, lesbian, or bisexual assumes awareness of this sexual attraction to people of the same gender or both genders, respectively, and development of an identity based on this awareness. Emotions, psychological responses, societal expectations, individual choices, and cultural influences are all factors that form this identity. Most lesbians and gay men prefer the terms *lesbian* and *gay*, because such terms incorporate emotions, behavior, and a cultural system, as well as sexual orientation. Compared to the term *homosexual*, often interpreted as more clinical and sometimes pejorative, *gay* and *lesbian* are more accepted terms.

Sexual orientation, sexual behavior, and identity are interrelated but function independently. Most self-identified lesbians and gay men are sexually active with a partner of their own gender. However, despite this identity, some lesbians and gay men are celibate or have sexual partners of the opposite gender. In fact, most lesbians have had at least one sexual experience with a man, but would not self-identify as bisexual. On the other hand, some men and women who identify as bisexual enter into and codify long-term relationships with a partner of the opposite gender while maintaining sexual relationships with partners of the same gender. Because of the variable relationship between orientation, behavior, and identity, physicians must remain sensitive, open-minded, and nonjudgmental (see section "Provider–Patient Interactions").

Race and ethnicity have a strong influence on sexual identity and behavior. "Down low," a colloquial term coined in African American hip-hop culture, refers to nondisclosure of same-sex sexual behavior among men who identify as heterosexual. Sexual behavior in conflict with sexual identity is not unique to African American men. Men and women from racial and ethnic minority communities are less likely to identify as gay, lesbian, or bisexual because of the complex interactions of homophobia (see section "Homophobia and Transphobia"), religious institutions and influences, and cultural norms. As an example, the concept of *machismo* or masculinity is highly valued in Latino culture. A gay male Latino identity runs counter to this norm.

Gender Identity, Gender Expression, & Gender Roles

Gender identity refers to the deep-seated beliefs, emotions, and thoughts that create the self-perception of being male or female. A person is considered transgender when gender identity conflicts with biological or genetic sex. Many in the transgender community use the terms *cis-gender* (referring to a gender unchanged from birth) and *trans-gender*, (referring to a gender that changes from a gender assigned at birth), although these terms are relatively new. Gender expression is the behavioral manifestation of gender identity. Toddlers and school-age children often engage in sex-discordant gender expression normally. In transgender individuals, this conflict between sex and gender is pervasive and long lasting. The current edition of the *Diagnostic and Statistical Manual* defines transgender as "Gender Dysphoria", replacing the previous "gender identity disorder", an imperfect but important move away from characterizing transgender individuals as diseased.

The gender expression and roles that transgender people exhibit vary widely, influenced by personal preference and access to health care resources. Some transgender men and women may only desire an outward physical appearance (e.g., hair style, cosmetics, clothing) consistent with their identity. Others may seek cosmetic and/or full sex reassignment surgery. Many transgender individuals interact with the health care system actively in transition from one gender to another.

The spectrum of gender identity is distinct from sexual orientation and identity. A transgender person can have either same-gender sexual attraction, opposite-gender sexual attraction, or both. Regardless of the gender of sexual partners, transgender individuals do not necessarily identify as gay, lesbian, or bisexual.

Many LGBT patients are not comfortable identifying as one specific "letter," that is L, G, B, or T, and prefer broader terms like "Queer" or "Gender Queer." "Queer," which was formerly used as a derogatory term for LGBT people, has now been reclaimed by portions of the LGBT community as an inclusive term. Queer is often used by younger members of the LGBT community to refer to a sexual orientation outside of the usual binary. Others will still consider this an offensive term, so it is important for providers to consider an individual's feelings when using such terms and not assume one term fits each patient.

Homophobia & Transphobia

Homophobia is defined as an irrational fear of or prejudice against gay men, lesbians, and bisexuals. Transphobia is a more recent term reflecting a similar fear or prejudice against transgender individuals. In daily life, LGBT individuals experience homophobia and transphobia as interpersonal, workplace, societal, or political bias. In other words, homophobia and transphobia reflect prejudice or hatred based solely on perceptions of sexual orientation and gender identity. LGBT people often find it difficult to act in accordance with their identity for fear of bias, discrimination, or violence.

The stigma that accompanies attitudes of homophobia and transphobia contributes to chronic stress (sometimes called "minority stress") and negative health outcomes for LGBT persons. Societal discrimination both creates a disparity in social support and resources and limits access to appropriate health care resources. Internalized homophobia (i.e., self-hatred) and self-concealment can create adverse mental health outcomes. Conversely, disclosure of LGBT identity often leads to better psychological adjustment. However, if self-disclosure by an LGBT individual is not supported, it can lead to its own stressor and risk behaviors (see section "Coming Out").

Provider Bias

LGBT patients frequently report detrimental experiences with health care providers. In a survey of its members, the Gay and Lesbian Medical Association reported that more than 50% of respondents were aware of substandard care delivery because of a patient's sexual orientation. In an earlier survey of nursing students, 8–12% of those responding "despised" gays and lesbians. Several studies document negative reactions after patients self-disclose their identity to a provider and such reactions have been shown to lead to worsened health outcomes for these patients.

Each negative experience with a health care provider decreases the likelihood that LGBT patients will continue to seek health care. Providers must work to overcome judgmental attitudes and biases toward LGBT patients. The *Code of Ethics* of the American Medical Association states that professional obligation limits a physician's prerogative to choose whether to enter into a relationship with a patient, in that "physicians cannot refuse to care for patients based on race, gender, [or] sexual orientation . . . ." Health care providers must recognize that they will likely encounter patients of all orientations and identities in the daily practice of medicine (see section "Provider–Patient Interactions").

PROVIDER–PATIENT INTERACTIONS

 ### CASE ILLUSTRATION 1

Robert, a middle-aged high school teacher, comes to the doctor's office. This is his first visit, and he has not completed the intake history form. After the introductions, the physician looks at the form and prepares to take a social history.

The doctor starts the social history:

Doctor: *Are you single, partnered, married, widowed, or divorced?*

Robert: *I'm divorced, with a 20-year-old son, and I'm partnered now. His name is Tim.*

Doctor: *How long have you been together? How's the relationship?*

Robert: *Six years, and going well.*

Further questioning reveals that Tim is younger than Robert—and openly gay. Although openly gay with his friends and family, Robert is uncomfortable being that open at work; he is afraid of a scandal at school and the loss of his job. As the history taking continues, the physician asks how Robert feels about having the fact that he is gay documented in the chart. After some discussion, the two decide on a coded entry of the information. At the end of the visit, Robert thanks the doctor for being so understanding; he especially appreciates the advice to establish a durable power of attorney for health care, something that he and Tim have not discussed yet. The doctor is also happy with the visit because he has been able to screen the patient appropriately and provide him with his first physical examination in 6 years.

The provider–patient relationship is the key to providing competent and respectful care to LGBT patients.

Without a good provider–patient relationship, patients may avoid medical care. Providers who are uncomfortable working with LGBT patients, or who fail to recognize the sexual orientation of a patient, will not provide quality care. Patients who do not obtain competent primary care services, including screening and health risk and psychosocial counseling are likely to have a lower health status than their heterosexual counterparts. Providers can develop a good relationship with LGBT patients by showing an understanding of their health needs and communicating a nonjudgmental attitude.

Overcoming Barriers to Communication

Many LGBT persons are reluctant to share their sexual orientation with health care providers for fear of negative judgments and homophobic responses. Some fail to share this information even when asked directly. Unpleasant experiences with health care providers have made LGBT people more likely to avoid health care and routine screening. Even sympathetic health care providers are often uncomfortable with the interaction. They may lack experience with LGBT health issues or feel unsure as to what language to use to elicit information respectfully from these patients. When both patient and provider are uncomfortable, important information is not shared.

THE SEXUAL HISTORY

Gathering information about a patient's sexual orientation or sexual practices is often a challenge for health care providers. Asking about orientation only while taking a sexual history and not at other times can limit the opportunity to learn important details about the patient. The initial focus should be on sexual behavior, not identity, as many people with same-sex partners do not identify as gay or lesbian, and sexual orientation is a complex, multifaceted concept. Therefore, the provider should avoid questions that presume behavior or identity. Examples include: "What form of birth control do you use?" "Are you married, single, widowed, or divorced?" "When was the last time you had intercourse?" Because the options given do not necessarily pertain to them, the patient must either provide false information or awkwardly stop and explain. Needing to give such explanations can make obtaining an already challenging sexual history even more difficult for both parties. To avoid this awkwardness, or to avoid negatively impacting the provider-patient relationship, patients may play along with the assumption of heterosexuality, which may negatively impact their health care.

THE SOCIAL HISTORY

This may be a more comfortable part of the interview in which to raise issues of sexual orientation. By asking questions that do not have heterosexual assumptions, the provider can increase the opportunities for, and comfort level in, discussing these issues. Providers learn about the patient's family structure, any stressors the patient might have, and personal and community resources on which patients would be likely to draw.

SENSITIVE COMMUNICATION

Because LGBT people come in all shapes, sizes, ages, and colors, providers need to use questions that avoid bias with all men and women, not just those they suspect of being LGBT. Sensitive questions make no assumptions about sexual orientation and are easily phrased: "Are you single, partnered, married, widowed, or divorced?" "Who is in your immediate family?" "Over your lifetime, have your sexual partners been men, women, or both?"

In the initial visit with the patient, it is important to discuss explicitly the documentation of sexual orientation in the chart. Many LGBT persons keep their sexual orientation hidden for legal, employment, or child custody reasons. A direct question, such as, "How do you feel about my documenting your sexual orientation on the chart?" may be asked. When an LGBT patient does not want sexual orientation documented, providers can use a coded entry. The code serves to remind providers of the patient's sexual orientation for medical purposes but will prevent inadvertent breaches of confidentiality.

As a relationship develops between the patient and the provider, it is appropriate to inquire more deeply about a patient's gender identity or sexual practices. For example, a provider may use one of the following questions: "If you become ill, is there someone important whom I should involve in your care?" or "What percentage of the time do you practice safer sex?" Transgender individuals very early in a transition to another gender may have an appearance that is discordant from the intended gender. Others may have not yet changed the assigned sex or name on legal documents or the medical record. It is perfectly acceptable to inquire about the preferred use of personal pronouns: "What name do you prefer? Would you prefer I address you as he or she?"

Enhancing the Relationship

Providers who show a nonjudgmental attitude are much more likely to develop trusting relationships with gay and lesbian patients. Providers can improve the relationship in several simple ways: offering to include a partner in the discussions, ensuring that an LGBT patient's partner is treated as a spouse in the office and the hospital, including partners in discussions of next-of-kin policies and advance directives, and using office and hospital forms with words that do not assume a heterosexual family structure.

LESBIAN, GAY, BISEXUAL, AND TRANSGENDER PROVIDERS

Lesbian, gay, bisexual, and transgender patients often prefer working with LGBT health care providers because of the presumed absence of homophobia in the relationship. LGBT providers, however, train in the same settings as their heterosexual counterparts and, thus, may have learned communication skills without recognizing heterosexual bias. Gradually, more information is emerging about lesbian and gay health issues (though not as much about bisexual or transgender issues), and new language habits for bias-free communication are being disseminated.

Lesbian and gay providers may find themselves in a situation in which the question of whether to disclose their own sexual orientation to their patients arises. The question the providers should ask themselves is whether disclosure of sexual orientation is in the best interest of the patient. In many cases, such disclosure may be beneficial. When a patient clearly needs to understand that there will be no overt homophobia in the interaction before agreeing to remain in care, it may be reassuring to know that the provider is LGBT. As patient–provider relationships develop, patients often want more personal information about the provider. LGBT providers must weigh for themselves the therapeutic benefit to the patient, the patient's need for information, and their own level of comfort in self-disclosure. Although many LGBT physicians have reported ostracism, harassment, and professional discrimination from colleagues, teachers, administrators, and health plans, others report being open about their sexual orientation without experiencing any negative consequences.

COMING OUT

The process of discovering one's sexual orientation and/ or gender identity and revealing it to others is known as *coming out* and can occur at any age. Stage theories for coming out have been well described and have been summarized as a four-step process:

1. Awareness of homosexual and/or transgender feelings
2. Testing and exploration
3. Identity acceptance
4. Identity integration and self-disclosure

Recent research suggests that there may be different sequences of coming out for younger and older individuals, with individuals who come out in adolescence often identifying and disclosing themselves as homosexual prior to any consensual sexual experiences. The process of coming out involves a shift in core identity that can be associated with significant emotional distress, especially if family and peers respond negatively. Prevailing social attitudes also influence the experience.

Most often, individuals come out to other people in person, but some may choose to come out initially through virtual arenas, a process with its own potentially complicating factors, including issues of privacy or unintended disclosure to other individuals. Societal and internalized homophobia often causes lesbians, gay men, and bisexual individuals to perform a fatiguing "cost–benefit" analysis for each situation in which they consider coming out. This process can be even more taxing for transgender persons as each situation may involve issues of both orientation and gender identity. Data show that women who have children before coming out are slower in reaching developmental milestones in this process than either women without children or women who have children after coming out. If the costs of self-disclosure are repeatedly high, an individual may ultimately become socially isolated or revert to denying their LGBT identity. On the other hand, disclosing at work and working for more gay-supportive organizations correlates with higher job satisfaction and lower anxiety at work.

RELATIONSHIPS & STAGES OF LIFE

In 2011, the Institute of Medicine released a report that examined LGBT health and health disparities through the life stages. *Adolescence* is characterized by the transition from being a dependent child to an independent young adult. It is complicated by the physical and emotional changes that occur during puberty. *Early and middle adulthood*, here considered together, is roughly the period from the early 20s to the 60s. It begins with the ending of puberty and continues through the completion of formal education and the establishment of financial independence. For some it includes the selection of a partner and building a family, whether this means the introduction of children or a close community of friends. *Later adulthood* is then a period of continued growth but also, for many, the onset of disease. During this period, LGBT people may become dependent on health care providers and feel uncomfortable disclosing their LGBT identities. Although many of the stages that follow can occur at any stage of life, they are listed during the stage in which they most commonly occur.

Adolescents

COMING OUT

LGBT adolescents are particularly vulnerable to the emotional distress of coming out, and this distress can make adolescent development even more difficult (see Chapter 13). Adolescents who self-identify as lesbian or gay prior to consensual sexual experiences may have a more rapid progression through the coming out stages, have fewer or no heterosexual encounters, and may engage in less risky sexual experiences. Cultural factors, such as race and ethnicity, do not seem to hamper the formation of identity but may delay the integration of identity with behavior.

Parental acceptance of the adolescent during the coming out process may be the primary determinant of healthy self-esteem. Research by Ryan et al. (see Suggested Readings) demonstrated that teens that have been rejected by their families are more than eight times more likely than their cohorts to have attempted suicide. They were also more likely to suffer from depression, anxiety, and low self-esteem, to perform worse in school, and more likely to engage in risk-taking behaviors such as high-risk sexual behavior or substance abuse. Teens that come out in school may be more likely to be teased or bullied and even threatened with a weapon. In many instances, these teens feel unsupported by teachers or parents. Indeed, teens may feel fearful of or bullied by their parents or siblings and feel unsafe at home. This can lead to increased feelings of isolation, hopelessness, and suicidality.

Primary care providers need to screen for signs that adolescents are questioning their sexual orientation. These signs may include depression, diminished school performance, alcohol and substance abuse, acting out, and suicidal ideation. Providers noting these signs need to consider distress regarding sexual orientation in the differential diagnosis, along with depression and substance abuse. Providers also need to be willing to discuss sexual orientation with their adolescent patients, as their attempts to discuss same-sex attractions and homosexual orientations may be the patient's first disclosure of these feelings. If providers meet such reaching out with reticence, dismay, or contempt, then adolescents may be less likely to share their feelings with others and either revert to denial or engage in more covert, risky behaviors.

SOCIAL MEDIA

In the past, LGBT individuals have sought out others in the community by finding bars, social clubs, or community spaces frequented by other LGBT people. This is difficult in more rural areas or where the population of LGBT people is sparse or where many people are not out. The Internet, and more specifically social media, allows LGBT individuals to network with people worldwide. An adolescent is no longer isolated to his or her geographic location, but can find a social support network on the Internet on social networking sites. This access is not without risk, however. Some data show that LGBT people meeting others like themselves online also may engage in increased risk behavior (both sexual risk taking and substance abuse), particularly among men who have sex with men (MSM) who use such sites to meet sex partners. These data have so far been inconclusive and the risks must be weighed with the benefits.

Early/Middle Adults

COMMUNITY

Many LGBT individuals experience support and nurturing from their biological families after coming out to them. For others, the support network of LGBT individuals may not include their biological family, as many families do not accept the sexual orientation or gender identity of the individual. In either situation, partners, friends, and community organizations can serve as an extended family. Primary care providers should be aware of a few useful resources to which they can direct patients (some resources are listed at the end of this chapter). LGBT people in rural or suburban geographic areas may have difficulty in accessing community-based support networks available in urban environments. In a study focused on MSM, those outside concentrated urban areas were less likely to identify as gay, be in a long-term relationship, be involved in a gay community, and were more likely to be out to a smaller number of people. In rural areas, a caring, open-minded physician may be an especially important source of support for LGBT patients.

PARTNERS

Like most heterosexuals, the majority of LGBT people express a desire to find a partner and develop a relationship. And like heterosexuals, LGBT people can form and maintain long-lasting relationships. LGBT couples have commitment ceremonies and get married (in some localities), own homes together, share finances, and raise children. Physicians should be aware of local, state, and federal laws that allow LGBT individuals to codify their relationships with partners and children, ensure health care and retirement benefits, document advance directives, and secure inheritance rights.

Because of potential isolation from family, coworkers, and religious organizations, the relationship with a partner can be particularly important to an LGBT individual's well-being. As a result, discord in the relationship may be even more stressful than it might be for heterosexual couples. In times of relationship stress, an individual may have limited resources for help in coping. Primary care providers should screen for such stressors and be able to provide appropriate referrals for individual and couple therapy.

PARENTHOOD

Parenthood plays a role in the lives of many LGBT people, and the decision to become parents is usually deliberate and carefully made. LGBT individuals or couples may have children from previous heterosexual relationships or through adoption, artificial insemination, in vitro fertilization and surrogacy, heterosexual intercourse, or service as foster parents. Dual gay and lesbian couples raising children together is becoming more common.

Studies of the attitudes of gay and lesbian couples toward parenting find more similarities than differences compared with heterosexual couples. Children of gay or lesbian parents are no more likely to be gay or lesbian or to have gender identity confusion than the general population. Current evidence indicates that children of gays or lesbians develop normally and fare better in relationships where parents share responsibilities equally and have a low level of interpersonal conflict. Though they may face additional stigma in the school or community, children of gay or lesbian parents, like all children, are resilient and cope well with this challenge. Many professional medical associations, including the American Academy of Pediatrics and American Medical Association, have policies supporting same-sex, co-parent adoption.

Older Adults

COMING OUT

Because there are varying degrees of disclosure, older individuals may be "out" to themselves and a partner or close friends but no one else beyond that trusted circle. Older gay, lesbian, or bisexual individuals are vulnerable to social isolation, and primary care providers are often among the primary support resources for older individuals. Older individuals are more likely to engage in same-sex sexual experiences prior to self-identifying as gay or lesbian than adolescents and thus may be at greater risk for adverse health consequences because of risky sexual behavior. In exploring the social support network for their older patients, primary care providers need to be alert to the possibility of a lesbian or gay identity and the needs this engenders.

Loss

GRIEF

Grieving the loss of a partner may be more difficult for a lesbian or gay man if that person does not have an adequate support system. Gay men and lesbians have been particularly affected by the deaths of partners and many friends from AIDS. When a partner dies, the survivor, in effect, loses a spouse. This fact often goes unrecognized in the survivor's own social network. Frequently, the family of the deceased partner excludes the survivor or will not allow him or her to take part as a spouse in the funeral. A close-knit network of surviving friends is often neglected when a grieving family takes over funeral plans.

Occasionally, parents and family of the deceased are shocked and embarrassed to learn of the individual's sexual orientation or gender identity. In such cases, the family may feel intense guilt or the need to hide their grief, unable to share it with their support network because of embarrassment. Family members of gay or lesbian individuals can find information and support for this and other issues by contacting Parents and Friends of Lesbians and Gays, a national organization with local chapters (see the list of resources at the end of this chapter).

Primary care providers can assist surviving partners and friends in the grieving process in several ways. Providers can assist the survivor in talking about the loss and expressing his or her feelings, identify and interpret normal grieving behavior and timelines, provide ongoing support throughout the grief process, encourage the survivor to develop new relationships and support structures, and help the survivor adapt to new roles and patterns of living. In some cases, the health care provider may be the only individual in whom the survivor can confide.

ADVANCE DIRECTIVES

The durable power of attorney for health care is particularly important for lesbians and gay men. Because many are unable to marry legally, LGBT individuals need to execute these documents to appoint their partners as surrogate health decision makers. Without such a document, current law considers the next of kin as the surrogate decision maker. Completing this document is the best way to avoid tragic decision-making conflicts between a partner and the estranged family members of seriously ill patients in time of crisis. As with all patients, providers should include a discussion of advance directives in the preventive medicine check up (see Chapter 40).

CLINICAL ISSUES

The American Psychiatric Association removed homosexuality from its list of mental disorders in 1973. Psychiatric and behavioral interventions like reparative therapy, used to "cure" patients of homosexuality, have proven neither effective nor necessary. Nonetheless, primary care providers must be aware of the unique psychosocial issues that face many LGBT people.

Depression & Suicide

Multiple studies indicate a higher prevalence of depression among both gay men and lesbians. Higher rates of suicidal behavior are also evident compared with the general population, though the prevalence is equivalent between gay men and lesbians. Lesbians are four times

more likely to report suicidal ideation than heterosexual women, and gay men are six times more likely to attempt suicide than heterosexual men.

Adolescents are particularly vulnerable to depression and suicide. One report suggests that approximately one-third of gay or lesbian adolescents will attempt suicide. Much of the literature on this topic, however, comes from surveys of self-reported behavior subject to report bias. Whatever the exact prevalence of suicidality, gay, lesbian, bisexual, and transgender youth face additional risk of suicide related to coming out early, rejection by family members, rejection by religious institutions, interpersonal violence, and additional levels of marginalization (e.g., homelessness, racial and ethnic minority status).

Smoking

LGBT populations have a 1.6 times higher prevalence of smoking compared with heterosexual populations. The Women's Health Initiative survey data documented a 10–14.4% smoking prevalence among lesbian respondents, compared with 7.2% among heterosexual counterparts. The Urban Men's Health Study data indicate a 31.4% prevalence of smoking among MSM. Theories supporting the increased rates of smoking among these groups include higher levels of stress secondary to homophobia and discrimination, bars as a frequent social focus, potentially higher rates of associated drug and alcohol use, and targeted advertising by cigarette manufacturers. As with any group of patients, asking about tobacco product use is a vital part of the social history for LGBT individuals.

Substance Abuse

Inquiring about drug and alcohol use is also important for LGBT patients (see Chapter 24). A provider should specifically explore the type, frequency, and quantity of substances, and whether patients use them during or preceding sexual activity. Many substances have a disinhibiting effect on the user and may make individuals more likely to engage in unsafe sex practices. In a multivariate analysis of drug use among MSM, amyl nitrate ("poppers"), crystal methamphetamine ("crystal meth"), cocaine, and heavy alcohol use were all associated with unprotected anal intercourse, independent of partner-specific variables. Similar to many other populations, crystal meth, with its highly addictive potential, has had a profound impact on many gay men. There is a strong association between crystal meth use and prolonged, unprotected sexual activity. Although drug and alcohol use is an important issue for the entire LGBT population, there is controversy about its extent. Based on more recent literature, alcohol use among gay men is probably the same as or slightly more prevalent than among heterosexual men. Drug use is more common among gay men compared with their heterosexual counterparts. According to a comparison of a population-based sample of lesbians in the San Francisco Bay area with a control group, alcohol use appears to be no more prevalent among lesbians than among heterosexual women. There are no population-based studies of drug use among lesbians compared with heterosexual women.

Intimate Partner Violence

Contrary to some popular beliefs, battery of LGBT persons by their partners exists. The exact prevalence of battery in same-sex relationships is unknown, but recent literature suggests the rate of same-sex intimate partner violence to be at least equal to that of opposite-sex intimate partner violence. Unfortunately, gender-role stereotyping both in the likelihood of the perpetrator inducing injury (men more capable than women) and the seriousness of the violence (women are more likely to sustain serious injury) exists and likely influences the recognition of same-sex intimate partner violence, the consequences to the perpetrator, and empathy for the victim. Lesbians perceive that interpersonal power imbalances contribute to battery. They also report that many women's shelters are not responsive to their specific needs. Gay men may find it even more difficult to obtain services related to battery.

Minority stress (e.g., internalized homophobia, discrimination) negatively influences same-sex intimate partner violence perpetration and victimization among LGBT persons. There is likely a similar, if not greater, effect among transgender individuals. Health care providers should screen their LGBT patients—and all patients—for the possibility of intimate partner violence and be able to give referrals to LGBT-inclusive resources, including shelters and counselors (see Chapter 38).

Hate Crimes

Also known as bias crimes, these are words or actions directed at an individual because of membership in a minority group. The U.S. Department of Justice reports that LGBT individuals may be the most victimized group in the nation and that the incidence of hate crimes against LGBT persons is rising. Many studies report crimes ranging from verbal abuse and threats of violence to property damage, physical violence, and murder. The number of hate crimes reported by LGBT persons is increasing every year. Lesbians at universities, for example, report being victims of sexual assault twice as often as heterosexual women. Youths who report same-sex or both-sex romantic attractions are more likely to be both victims and witnesses of violence.

Perpetrators of hate crimes often include family members and community authorities. Many gay and lesbian adolescents leave home because of an abusive family member, and homeless LGBT youths are of increasing social concern. LGBT survivors of hate crimes display more symptoms of depression, anger, anxiety, and posttraumatic stress than other recent crime victims. When patients present with symptoms of depression or anxiety, providers should consider violence, including hate crimes, as a possible correlate.

EDUCATION, REFERRALS, & RESOURCES

Patient Education

This is a cornerstone of primary care. Providers who care for LGBT patients must know how to advise patients on health issues, refer them to appropriate educational and community resources, and provide appropriate reference materials to hand out at visits.

Instruction

Instruction in preventing the spread of HIV and other sexually transmitted diseases should be clear and specific to individual sexual practices. Physicians should be able to educate LGBT patients about risks and screening for cancer. They should be able to counsel patients, or refer them for counseling, about issues such as safer sex, parenting, coming out, violence, substance use, and depression.

Referrals

Referrals should include other providers and community-based resources sensitive to the needs of LGBT people. Specialists of particular importance to delivering appropriate, multidisciplinary care include gynecologists, urologists, general or colorectal surgeons, plastic surgeons, and endocrinologists. Local resources with which to be familiar include bookstores, youth groups, senior groups and retirement centers, community centers, supportive religious organizations, substance abuse treatment programs, and support groups. LGBT-oriented periodicals from a nearby urban area may have resources listed for surrounding suburban and rural regions.

Provider Education

Health care providers can obtain additional information about specific health issues and communicating with LGBT patients through textbooks, review articles, teaching videos, and workshops at both national and regional medical conferences. See below for details on individual resources.

SUGGESTED READINGS

Floyd FJ, Bakeman R. Coming-out across the life course: implications of age and historical context. *Arch Sex Behav* 2006;35(3): 287–296.

King M, Semlyen J, Tai SS, et al. A systematic review of mental disorder, suicide, and deliberate self harm in lesbian, gay and bisexual people. *BMC Psychiatry* 2008;8:70.

Mills TC, Stall R, Pollack L, et al. Health-related characteristics of men who have sex with men: a comparison of those living in "gay ghettos" with those living elsewhere. *Am J Public Health* 2001;91(6):980–983.

O'Hanlan K, Cabaj RP, Schotz B, et al. A review of the medical consequences of homophobia with suggestions for resolution. *J Gay Lesbian Med Assoc* 1997;1:25–39.

Ryan C, Huebner D, Diaz RM, et al. Family rejection as a predictor of negative health outcomes in white and Latino lesbian, gay, and bisexual young adults. *Pediatrics* 2009;123:346–352.

Stall R, Mills TC, Williamson J, et al. Association of co-occurring psychosocial health problems and increased vulnerability to HIV/AIDS among urban men who have sex with men. *Am J Public Health* 2003;93(6):939–942.

RESOURCES AND WEB SITES

1. General Resources

- Gay and Lesbian Medical Association. www.glma.org. Accessed July 2013.
  - Resources for providers and patients
  - Provider referral network
- The GLBT Health Access Project. www.glbthealth.org. Accessed July 2013.
  - Community standards of practice for provision of quality health care services for LGBT clients
  - Educational posters
- National Coalition for LGBT Health. http://lgbthealth.webolutionary.com/. Accessed July 2013.
- National Association of Gay and Lesbian Community Centers (Centerlink: The Community of LGBT Centers). www.lgbtcenters.org. Accessed July 2013.
  - Directory for centers throughout the United States
- GLBT National Help Center. www.glnh.org. Accessed July 2013.
  - National nonprofit organization offering toll-free peer counseling, information, and local resources, including local switchboard numbers and gay-related links: 888-THE-GNLH (843-4564)
- GLBT National Youth Talkline: 1-800-246-PRIDE (7743)
  - Youth peer counseling, information, and local resources, through age 25

2. Lesbian Health

- Lesbian Health & Research Center. www.lesbianhealthinfo.org. Accessed July 2013.
- Mautner Project, the National Lesbian Health Organization. www.mautnerproject.org. Accessed July 2013.
- Lesbian and Bisexual Health Fact Sheet. www.womenshealth.gov/publications/our-publications/fact-sheet/lesbian-bisexual-health.cfm. Accessed July 2013.

3. Gay Men's Health

- The CDC Gay and Bisexual Men's Health Page. www.cdc.gov/msmhealth/. Accessed July 2013.
- Gay Men's Health Crisis. www.gmhc.org. Accessed July, 2013.
- NYU Medical Center—Men's Sexual Health Project (M*SHP). www.hivinfosource.org/hivis/clinicaltrials/testingproject.html. Accessed July 2013.
  - A New York City-based group with link to low literacy STI information

4. Bisexual Health

- Bisexual Resource Center. www.biresource.net. Accessed July 2013.

5. Transgender Health

- World Professional Association of Transgender Health. www.wpath.org. Accessed July 2013.
- International Foundation for Gender Education. www.ifge.org. Accessed July 2013.
- Transgender Law Center: recommendations for transgender health care. www.transgenderlaw.org/resources/tlchealth.htm. Accessed July 2013.

6. Youth

- The Trevor Project. www.thetrevorproject.org. Accessed July 2013. 1-866-4-U-TREVOR (1-866-488-7386).
  - A national organization providing crisis intervention and suicide prevention services to lesbian, gay, bisexual, transgender, and questioning (LGBTQ) youth. Services are available by phone or online chat.
- National gay, lesbian, bisexual, transgender youth hotline: 1-800-347-TEEN
- Youth Guardian Services: on-line support. www.youth-guard.org. Accessed July 2013.
- Youth Resource: a project of Advocates for Youth. http://www.amplifyyourvoice.org/youthresource. Accessed July 2013.
- National Youth Advocacy Coalition: Youth Guide. www.nyacyouth.org. Accessed July 2013.

7. Elders

- SAGE: Services and Advocacy for Gay, Lesbian, Bisexual, and Transgender Elders. www.sageusa.org. Accessed July 2013.

8. Support and Resources for Family and Friends of LGBT People

- PFLAG (Parents, Families, and Friends of Lesbians and Gays). www.pflag.org. Accessed July 2013.
  - Promotes the health and well-being of gay, lesbian, bisexual, and transgender persons, their families and friends

9. Intimate Partner Violence

- National domestic violence hotline 1-800-799-SAFE (7233) (24 hours in English and Spanish), TTY: 1-800-787-3224
  - Local referrals, including LGBT-sensitive

- The Network La Red: Network for battered lesbians and bisexual women hotline. www.thenetworklared.org. Accessed July 2013; Hotline: 1-617-742-4911

10. General Information: National LGBT Rights and Advocacy

- Human Rights Campaign. www.hrc.org. Accessed July 2013.
  - National organization working for LGBT equal rights on federal government level
- Lambda Legal. www.lambdalegal.org. Accessed July 2013; Legal helpdesk: 1-866-542-8336
  - National LGBT legal and policy organization protecting civil rights of LGBT and people living with HIV
- National Center for Lesbian Rights. www.nclrights.org. Accessed July 2013; Hotline: 1-415-392-6257
- National Gay and Lesbian Task Force. www.thetaskforce.org. Accesssed July 2013.
  - National organization supporting LGBT advocacy efforts at state and federal levels

11. Media/brochures (for Waiting Room)

- American Cancer Society. http://www.cancer.org/search/index?QueryText=cancer+facts+for+LGBT. Accessed July 2013.
  - Cancer facts for gay and bisexual men
  - Cancer facts for lesbians and bisexual women
  - Tobacco and the LGBT community
  - Place order for free brochures by phone: 1-800-ACS-2345
- American College Health Association. http://members.acha.org/source/orders/index.cfm?section=unknown&task=1&StartRow=1&PageNum=1&SEARCH_TYPE=find&FindSpec=&continue=1&CATEGORY=BROCHURES&FindIn=. Accessed July 2013.
  - Man to man: three steps to health for gay, bisexual, or any men who have sex with men
  - Woman to woman: three steps to health for lesbian, bisexual, or any women who have sex with women

Vulnerable Patients

*George Saba, PhD; Neda Ratanawongsa, MD, MPH; Teresa Villela, MD; &
Dean Schillinger, MD*

OBJECTIVES

- Describe the elements of building a therapeutic alliance, eliciting the patient's narrative, and assessing the patient's vulnerabilities and strengths.
- Explore critical components of the therapeutic alliance: building trust, conveying empathy, and collaboration.
- Describe the relevance of the therapeutic alliance to the effective care of vulnerable patients.
- List the benefits of eliciting the patient's narrative.
- Review common psychosocial vulnerabilities and illustrate how identifying them can help create a patient-centered clinical encounter.
- Describe strategies for clinician sustainability in working with vulnerable populations.

INTRODUCTION

CASE ILLUSTRATION 1

Ms. Sviridov is a 67-year-old woman with chronic arthritis pain, hypertension, prior stroke, diastolic dysfunction, and diabetes. Despite a sizable, guideline-based medication regimen and frequent visits to both a primary care physician and a cardiologist, she has recalcitrant heart failure, requiring multiple hospital admissions. An extensive cardiac workup has been unrevealing.

Ms. Sviridov's new primary care physician asks about her life. She describes an active singing career and a rich family life in the past, and the importance of her church. She acknowledges that profound depression and concern over the welfare of her drug-abusing son, however, now interfere with caring for herself.

Ms. Sviridov's physician suggests he make a home visit. Exploring her initial refusal, he learns that her

son deals drugs from her apartment. Eventually, with the support of her physician and adult protective services, she is able to demand that her son leave. She receives support and assistance from home-health services and her church group. Her conditions stabilize and she is not rehospitalized.

Social characteristics—living in poverty, having a low level of education and limited literacy skills, being from a minority background, having no health insurance, speaking little English, among other factors—make individuals vulnerable to contracting illness and to facing overwhelming obstacles in the care of that illness. Vulnerable populations tend to experience these health risks in clusters, making both individuals and communities more susceptible to declines in health. For example, it is not uncommon for an individual living in poverty to have limited literacy skills and no health insurance; to simultaneously have diabetes, heart disease, or depression; and to smoke or to live in a community with limited access to high-quality grocers and safe outdoor space for physical activity.

Clinicians must learn to successfully engage those most at risk by virtue of this clustering. Unfortunately, vulnerable patients experience a triple jeopardy when it comes to health care: they are more likely to be ill; more likely to have difficulty accessing care, and when they do, the care they receive is more likely to be suboptimal. This reflects the mismatch between the psychosocial vulnerabilities that they bring to the clinical encounter and the knowledge, attitudes, skills, and beliefs of the clinicians caring for them, as well as the priorities and policies of the health systems in which they receive care. In this chapter, we focus on the centrality of strong provider–patient relationships to all efforts to improve the health of vulnerable patients. Three essential strategies are recommended to promote a context for effective care for vulnerable patients: building a therapeutic alliance, eliciting the patient's

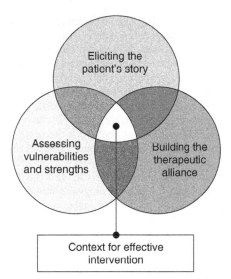

Figure 18-1. Creating a context for effective intervention in the clinical care of vulnerable patients.

story or "narrative," and assessing for the patient's psychosocial vulnerabilities and strengths. Clinicians can use a combination of these approaches to create more productive and effective interactions and relationships with vulnerable patients (Figure 18-1).

VULNERABILITY & THERAPEUTIC ALLIANCE

Psychosocial vulnerabilities can affect health and health care, either alone or in concert (see Figure 18-2). The first path is a direct one, a situation in which the vulnerability in and of itself leads to poor health. Concrete examples of this mechanism might be intravenous drug abuse and skin abscesses or intimate partner violence and head trauma. A second path is an indirect one, where the vulnerability attenuates the benefits of medical treatment on coexisting medical conditions; that is, the vulnerability presents a barrier to optimal acute, chronic, and/or preventive care, thereby accelerating disease course. Examples of this include the effects of depression on nonadherence to medications among patients with heart disease, or inability to pay for medications and poor diabetes control. The third mechanism, also an indirect one, is mediated entirely through the therapeutic alliance. In this path, the vulnerability affects components of the relationship or therapeutic alliance with the provider (such as open disclosure, mutual trust, caring, and engagement), thereby limiting the benefits of a collaborative relationship on care. Examples of this include a patient with an undisclosed illness that is inconsistent with a prescribed treatment plan; a physician whose belief systems regarding addiction impedes true engagement with a patient with a substance use disorder; or a patient with depression that impedes follow-through with a prescribed treatment plan, thereby leading to mutual frustration and blame.

What is the Therapeutic Alliance?

In the field of medicine, a therapeutic alliance exists when patient and provider develop mutual trusting, caring, and respectful bonds that allow collaboration in care and treatment. "Patient-centered" and "relationship-centered" care models build on the notion of the therapeutic alliance, and research reveals that patients reporting greater trust, increased satisfaction, and more collaborative relationships with clinicians have increased adherence to medication and treatment regimens and better health outcomes.

Key dimensions of the Therapeutic Alliance include:

- **Mutual trust**—Patients need to trust in their clinicians' integrity and competence, and clinicians need to trust that patients enter the relationship trying to do their best.
- **Empathy**—Demonstrating empathy, or recognizing and understanding the beliefs and emotions of another without injecting one's own, allows the clinician to connect emotionally with the patient without pity or over identification.
- **Respect**—Expressing respect for patients and treating them with dignity are important and require creating a context in which communication can occur as equals.
- **Collaboration**—Collaboration requires a meaningful partnership in which clinician and patient perceive that they are working together toward a common goal and committed to resolving conflicts that inevitably emerge about treatment goals.

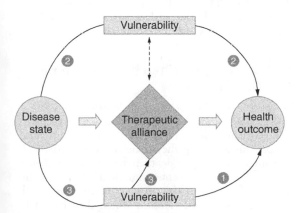

Figure 18-2. Pathways by which psychosocial vulnerabilities affect health and health care in the clinical encounter (see text for details).

The therapeutic alliance must be broadened beyond the one-to-one relationship between clinician and patient to include other important people (e.g., family; patient navigators/health coaches; consulting clinicians). Health systems can foster or erode the therapeutic alliance based on the policies they promote.

Therapeutic Alliance & Vulnerable Patients

 ### CASE ILLUSTRATION 2

Mr. Jackson is a 52-year-old man with type 2 diabetes, hypertension, and end-stage renal disease. He receives care intermittently at a public clinic. He was recently referred for dialysis but missed his appointment for evaluation. He was a construction worker and now is unemployed; he lives alone and is episodically homeless. He is African American and has two sons living in the area.

He was admitted to the Family Medicine Service of a county hospital and found to be in diabetic keto-acidosis. During the admission, the inpatient team rediscusses his need for dialysis. His initial meeting with the Renal Team ends with him becoming angry and refusing dialysis. The resident assigned to his care urges him to reconsider, and he becomes withdrawn. She attempts to arrange dialysis again, and the Renal Team, citing his history of alcohol use, his intermittent homelessness, and his lack of follow-through, declares him a "poor candidate" for dialysis.

The resident meets with Mr. Jackson to better understand his thinking. Initially he remains distant; as she expresses her concern for helping him receive the best care, he is able to express his anger at the medical system over the years. He feels he has not been given information about his illness in a manner that he understands; he is unable to implement the many self-care suggestions, given his living situation; and feels that doctors have only been interested in him if they can "learn medicine" by experimenting on him. The resident expresses her concern and regret for how he has been previously treated and offers to do her best to help him now. He is able to talk about his experience with diabetes, his fear about dying, and his desire to change. She expresses her appreciation for his willingness to be forthright and offers to become his primary care physician. She also offers to advocate for him with the Renal Team to initiate dialysis both in and out of the hospital.

A growing body of evidence suggests that it is precisely with vulnerable patients that the therapeutic alliance can have its most profound benefits. Through a therapeutic alliance, clinicians offer a professional relationship aimed at helping patients feel comfortable to be as open and honest as is necessary to receive the best care. Clinicians are permitted access to the interior of patients' lives that few other people are allowed. Using this privileged position, they can help build an alliance that empowers patients and reduces barriers to their care.

Empowerment—Vulnerable patients often experience human relationships as broken or disrupted (e.g., due to violence, immigration, mental illness, homelessness, and illness). Through the therapeutic alliance, clinicians can offer a reliable, dependable, and continuous presence that is supportive, accepting, and nonjudgmental. They can provide safety, thus allowing patients to tell the stories of their lives and illness and disclose their vulnerabilities. By examining the patients' strengths and resources, clinicians can provide a sense of dignity and hope. Through validating their experiences, clinicians can help patients feel less marginalized. In supporting patients as competent and strong, clinicians can help empower them to become actively involved in their care.

Access to care and related resources—Vulnerable patients often face limited access to health care and social services. In part, they may be unaware of what is available and may not have the facility to negotiate complex, bureaucratic systems. Clinicians are in a position to remedy both of these barriers. Through the therapeutic alliance, clinicians can help patients feel safe enough to reveal concerns or problems beyond the presenting problem, which they might not otherwise have done. For example, a patient seeking care for her diabetes may disclose that she lives with an abusive partner, drinks alcohol regularly, or is only sporadically housed. The clinician has the ability to collaborate on treatment plans and to facilitate entry into the various health and social systems that can help address vulnerabilities. The therapeutic alliance can help patients feel assured that clinicians will not abuse the disclosure of information (e.g., leading to rejection or legal action) but will help them access resources critical for their health.

What Can Happen When the Therapeutic Alliance Is Absent?

The absence of a therapeutic alliance can result in serious consequences for the health of vulnerable patients.

Trust—Clinicians often enter into relationships with patients assuming they share the same goals and will trust each other to do their best to attain them. However, many patients enter into the relationship with a degree of mistrust. This may result from personal experiences with institutions in which they have felt betrayed or unwelcome or may be rooted in broader, historical experiences of their community. Clinicians should not automatically assume that they have patients' immediate, total trust; rather, they should earn it by demonstrating trustworthiness.

Clinicians can indicate their trustworthiness by:

- *Being transparent*: Vulnerable patients often experience external intrusions into their lives and little privacy; they may not understand why clinicians ask about personal information. Explaining the context of questions that may not seem immediately pertinent to the patient's concern may dispel patients' concerns about hidden agendas (e.g., "I am asking about who you live with, not to pry, but to see who might be available to care for you following your operation."). Similarly, vulnerable patients may believe clinicians are interested in ordering particular laboratory tests, imaging studies, or procedures to learn at the expense of the patient or to increase financial resources. On the other hand, patients may fear that they are being denied particular treatments to save the health care system money. Explaining why one is recommending a particular diagnostic course or treatment regimen can build trust (e.g., "I want you to get the treadmill test, because I think it is the best way we have to know how best to help you and to decide the best treatments.").

- *Following through*: Vulnerable patients are accustomed to hearing that something will occur (e.g., appointment scheduled; prescription ordered; referral to social service made) and then learning, for whatever reason, that it did not happen. By taking the extra time to follow-through on promises, clinicians can show patients that they can be counted on to ensure the best care ("I told you I would call when I found out how to help you find housing; here's what I've learned." "My homework after your last appointment was to find out about Spanish-speaking support groups for patients with diabetes; there is one not too far from your home.").

- *Addressing concerns*: Vulnerable patients may experience clinicians as rushed, interested in their own agendas, and nonresponsive to those of the patient. By taking the time to ask and answer questions and focus on what the patient needs, clinicians can indicate that they are interested in helping the patient and can be trusted to care ("While there are many things that I want to talk to you about, what are you most concerned about?" ("I know that I am more worried about your high blood pressure than you are. I also know you are more concerned that you cannot work because your elbow is so painful. Let's work on both today.").

Caring—Poor and minority patients frequently receive care in teaching hospitals and community health centers with high provider turnover. Patients may question providers' motivation and commitment, fearing that they are educational fodder for trainees who will go on to care for the privileged. When clinicians do not offer certain treatments, patients may be suspicious about the clinicians' willingness to expend resources for them. When clinicians persuasively argue for unwanted treatments, they may fear being used as experimental "guinea pigs." Rather than risk raising concerns or disagreements with a clinician whose motives they question, patients may choose not to follow-through on recommended treatment or simply not return for care.

Respect—Perceived disrespect and discrimination due to race or socioeconomic status has been associated with lower satisfaction with the health care system and worse health outcomes among patients with chronic illness. Significant proportions of African Americans, Latinos, and Asians and those with lower educational attainment have reported that they were treated with disrespect, were treated unfairly, or received worse care because of their position in society. These perceptions influence whether patients follow recommended advice or delay needed care for chronic illness. Communicating respect is essential to convincing vulnerable patients that clinicians are willing to enter into a relationship based on equality and dignity.

Mutual agreement and collaboration—In the absence of a trusting relationship, true collaboration may be difficult to achieve. Fear of being punished or treated unfairly for speaking truthfully can lead patients to withhold their beliefs and values about a suggested treatment or to refuse to follow through on a recommendation. Clinicians, in turn, feel frustrated and mistrustful when they wonder if they are being misled or if patients really care about their health.

Shared decision making is often promoted as a model for mutual agreement and collaboration. However, research with diverse populations suggests that clinicians and patients, seemingly engaged in the cardinal behaviors of shared decision making, may still not perceive that a collaborative partnership exists between them. Indeed, being treated with respect and dignity may be more important than engaging in shared decision making, and may itself lead to positive outcomes (i.e., higher satisfaction, adherence, and receipt of optimal preventive care).

BUILDING A THERAPEUTIC ALLIANCE WITH VULNERABLE PATIENTS

There are no simple, protocol-like statements or behaviors that we can employ to make another human being feel cared about or respected. However, if clinicians consciously strive to transmit a sense of trust, caring, and respect, along with a desire to enter into true partnership, they increase the likelihood of forming productive relationships with patients. Some guidelines to consider in this process include the following:

- **Demonstrate commitment to the relationship**. Clearly state your desire to be available to your patients within the scope of your practice (e.g., "I will be your regular doctor. Here is my telephone number with a voice mail; I check it daily and will get back to you as soon as possible."); be clear about what you will do for the patient between visits (e.g., "I will check into support groups and tell you at our next appointment."); and follow-through as promised.

- **Allow for the humanity of the patient and the clinician to emerge**. The humanity of the health care worker and the patient should be expressed and elicited. This may include the sharing of beliefs, values, and feelings as they relate to the clinical issues facing them (e.g., express concern about suffering, *"I am sorry you have to deal with this pain;"* offer self-disclosure to identify a shared history or common interests with the patient, *"As a parent, I can't imagine how incredibly strong you had to be to escape with your children."*).

- **Elicit patients' stories or health "narratives."** This interviewing approach can provide critical insights into a patient's illness model, allow for expression of the patient's humanity, and uncover important psychosocial vulnerabilities (see section "Eliciting the Patient's Story or 'Narrative'").

- **Search actively for patients' strengths and resources**. We commonly focus on what is wrong or dysfunctional in the patient's life. Just as vital as the search for deficits is the identification and validation of the strengths and resilience each patient has (e.g., *"You have been through a lot of suffering in your life; how have you been able to survive?" "Who gives you the strength to deal with difficult things?"*). Reflecting on how the patient has used these resources in previously difficult times can provide a positive starting point for healing (e.g., *"You have talked about turning to God when dealing with other major crises in your life; have you thought of doing that now?"*). The power for healing does not rest solely with the clinician, but must involve an empowered patient and family (e.g., *"Your sister gave you strength to leave an abusive relationship; can she help now in dealing with your diabetes?"*).

- **Express caring overtly**. When patients describe difficult or painful experiences, clinicians can acknowledge the patient's perspective (e.g., *"I can't imagine how difficult your life has been;" "What you have lived through sounds so frightening;" "I know you're afraid of going through these tests and treatments; is there anything I can do to make it less scary?"*). A number of nonverbal behaviors and verbal statements can also express that we care: (1) body language (e.g., *sitting in proximity; a focused, unhurried posture*); (2) active listening and reframing (e.g., *"It sounds to me that you felt betrayed by the people you trusted most; am I right about that?"*); (3) support (e.g., *"I know you are trying very hard to live on your own now; I think you are doing great, and I want to do whatever I can to support you."*); and (4) validation (e.g., *"You are right to feel that you do not deserve to be abused."*). Caring can also be communicated in a number of indirect ways, such as making an unexpected phone call to follow-up with a patient in crisis (e.g., *"I know you had your colonoscopy yesterday, and I wanted to see how you are doing."*). Not all patients (nor all clinicians) are comfortable with touch. Some patients may even believe clinicians are afraid to touch them. Respectful physical contact during painful or uplifting moments can help cement a mutual human connection.

- **Create a context for conflict to emerge and get addressed**. We need to convince patients that when they have beliefs, opinions, or ideas different from ours, we will welcome discussing them. We must allay any fears patients have that voicing disagreement will incur displeasure or even punishment from the provider. A corollary to this is that patients need to understand that they can change their minds about treatment plans and decisions at any time. Patients need repeated reassurance and reminders that disagreement will not cost them the provider's regard and care (e.g., *"I will not be angry or upset if you disagree; it would be very helpful to know how you really feel, because together we can figure out the best thing to do."*). Building a therapeutic alliance does not require clinicians to deny their viewpoint but to adopt nonthreatening ways of communicating differences with their patients.

- **Clarify boundaries**. Vulnerable patients may often experience considerable intrusion into their personal lives by government institutions or social service agencies. They may be required to disclose more information than others, and then find it shared across agencies without their knowledge or permission. We should clarify why we are inquiring about certain information (e.g., *"I want to ask more specifically about your family because they seem important in your care, and I want to understand how they help you."*) and what is confidential or required to be shared (e.g., *"I will keep whatever you tell me confidential unless I think you may harm yourself or someone else; then I must tell others to protect you from any harm."*).

We should also clarify our own boundaries; it is not uncommon for a relationship between a clinician and a patient to evolve into one of unhealthy dependence or unrealistic expectations. For example, as we learn more about the hardships our patients face and their difficulty navigating the system, we may feel tempted to reach out to them differently than we would for nonvulnerable patients. We may be inclined to give them a pager number or even our home phone because we want to improve access; we might lend them money or give them a ride. While these behaviors might not, in and of themselves, prove problematic, they do represent a crossing of boundaries that are commonly set with patients and signal us to reflect upon and to consider potential consequences. We can avoid creating problematic relationships by remaining mindful of the role we play in the therapeutic relationship and by regularly reflecting on our interactions. Communicating with colleagues about our patient challenges (including boundaries) can provide a critical and supportive perspective as we strive to make appropriate decisions in building the therapeutic relationship.

- **Address the therapeutic alliance directly**. When caring for a patient who is doing poorly clinically but receiving optimal "medical" management, we should consider if the therapeutic alliance needs attention. We can directly state our desire to have a strong relationship and a real sense of partnership. We can ask if the patient would want any changes in the relationship, reassuring them that speaking honestly is not only acceptable, but essential to working together.

ELICITING THE PATIENT'S STORY OR "NARRATIVE"

What is the Patient's Perspective?

Many factors—individual, familial, societal, spiritual, and cultural—shape a person's concepts and experiences of health and illness. These inform an individual's sense of responsibility as a patient, expectations of health care providers and family members, and the meaning of healing and recovery. Personal concepts of health determine what preventive and self-care behaviors are considered appropriate, which symptoms seem worrisome, and when to seek help from health care professionals. These explanatory models encompass the meaning of the illness, the presumed cause, its proposed trajectory, the degree of hope of cure, and how treatment should be conducted (see Chapter 15).

The same factors that influence how people think about health and illness also impact other aspects of their lives, and eliciting information about these influences can uncover perspectives important to health care. For example, how individuals make decisions about health care may resemble how they make decisions about parenting or work; the process for how a family decided to immigrate to the United States may be very similar to how they will approach a difficult treatment decision; one's explanation of life difficulties and the narrative of how one has prevailed over them

may illustrate how one will face challenging health problems as well. Illness may be framed hopefully or pessimistically; patients may identify themselves as efficacious or as victims; they may prefer being independent or isolated or they may find strength in support from others.

Potato Eaters, by Vincent van Gogh, 1885. https://images.nga.gov/en/search/do_quick_search.html?q=potato+eaters Accessed July 4, 2013. National Gallery of Art, Open Access Images.

Importance of Eliciting the Patient's Perspective

Patient's perspectives—a complex mixture of very personal beliefs, values, and assumptions reflecting multiple influences—can determine how they develop a relationship with their clinician, and whether they feel understood and respected or misunderstood and discounted. Clinicians, in turn, have their own individual perspectives on health and illness, and ascribe specific meaning to their role as healers. Assuming a shared understanding and not exploring the differences may in fact lead to greater distance and misunderstanding. Eliciting patients' perspectives allows for accurate empathy and can uncover interests or experiences common to both patient and clinician, thereby reducing the social distance that often impedes the development of a therapeutic alliance.

Eliciting the patient's story can also improve patient trust, satisfaction, and adherence. It enriches and brings meaning to interactions and allows providers to be more effective and engaged.

Furthermore, sometimes the way people frame their illnesses can cause suffering. Within the context of a strong therapeutic alliance it is possible, as part of the healing process, to recast some narratives. A patient who feels incompetent, for example, might grow, through learning to control his illness, to feel capable and empowered in realms beyond the medical.

ASSESSING & ACKNOWLEDGING PSYCHOSOCIAL VULNERABILITIES

Much of clinical training and guideline development focuses on pathophysiology, disease, diagnosis, and treatment. Seasoned clinicians, however, are acutely aware of the gap between the outcomes that are expected (e.g., from reading textbooks or following guidelines) and the outcomes that are actually achieved in practice. While there are many reasons for the observed variation in quality and health outcomes, one of the most important and frequently least appreciated factors is the patient's social context. A wide range of psychosocial vulnerabilities can impinge on a patient's ability to carry out the treatment plan and interfere with the therapeutic alliance (see Table 18-1).

When faced with a patient who is doing poorly from a clinical standpoint, many clinicians do not reflect on the psychosocial factors that may be influencing the patient's course. They may simply throw up their arms and attribute a patient's clinical decline to his or her social milieu in a global or at times derogatory fashion, referring to such a patient as "nonadherent," a "difficult patient," or a "social nightmare," without digging deeper. Such clinicians often believe that addressing psychosocial problems is "not my job," stating, "I can't fix his social problems." Still others may not have the communication skills to uncover underlying psychosocial problems, or to address them and integrate this

Table 18-1. Generating a differential diagnosis of psychosocial vulnerabilities.

Violence
Uninsured
Literacy and/or Language barriers
Neglect
Economic hardship
Race/Ethnic discordance, discrimination
Addiction
Brain disorders (e.g., depression, dementia, personality disorder)
Immigrant
Legal status
Isolation/Informal caregiving burden
Transportation problems
Illness model
Eyes and Ears (vision and hearing problems)
Shelter

Table 18-2. Common pitfalls in assessing for vulnerability.

- Failing to recognize the contribution of psychosocial vulnerabilities to the patient's illness.
- Failing to acknowledge vulnerability and to explore how vulnerability may be affecting care.
- Failing to address specific vulnerabilities.
- Failing to integrate knowledge of vulnerability into treatment plans.
- Failing to recognize the shame and stigma associated with vulnerabilities.
- Neglecting to identify and acknowledge strengths, resilience, and range of resources.

knowledge into treatment plans to forge a more genuine, engaged therapeutic alliance.

Screening for psychosocial vulnerabilities is central to caring for patients in any setting and at many points during the process of care, particularly when treatments appear to be failing. Some vulnerabilities will be apparent from the first encounter, whereas others may be hidden. For some problems, it is not until a collaborative relationship has been established that a patient might feel comfortable enough to disclose sensitive information. Similarly, patients may perceive a problem to be irrelevant to their health and neglect to discuss it. When assessing for areas of vulnerability, the clinician should be nonjudgmental, allowing the patient to respond at his or her own pace. Using open-ended questions and responding to patient cues may enable a patient to reveal the important nonclinical factors that may be impeding progress (see Table 18-2).

It is important to raise four important *caveats* about assessing for psychosocial vulnerability. The first is that in the pursuit of identifying vulnerability, the clinician should be reminded of the importance of simultaneously identifying and acknowledging an individual's *strengths, resilience,* and range of *resources,* such as one's belief in a higher power or support from a religious community; or the love and support provided by a spouse, friend, or pet. Reviewing and reflecting patients' past experiences of overcoming difficulty and helping them identify patterns of success is critical to building self-efficacy and developing a therapeutic alliance in the face of vulnerability.

Second, vulnerability is *context dependent.* For example, in countries with universal health care coverage, lack of insurance simply does not contribute to vulnerability. Conversely, absence of interpretation services may exacerbate the effects of limited English proficiency when compared to settings with medical interpretation; presence of a methadone treatment program or a mobile treatment van in one's clinic may mitigate the untoward health effects of heroin addiction and housing instability, respectively. As such, the effects of vulnerability on health care can be influenced by altering the context in which caregiving takes place, which most frequently means adapting the clinical encounter. This suggests that when caring for vulnerable populations, clinicians and systems should also perform *self-assessments*, and carefully explore the ways in which the caregiving context can be adapted to best attenuate (or even eliminate) the health effects of vulnerability.

Third, in the process of assessment, the clinician should be sensitive to the concerns of patients with respect to shame and stigma. It is clear that a number of factors listed in Table 18-1 may elicit feelings of shame, such as having limited literacy, being marginally housed, having mental illness, or being addicted.

Fourth, after identifying vulnerability, the clinician should not forget the important step of exploring with the patient, in a supportive and nonjudgmental manner, how the vulnerability may be affecting health and care and how to mitigate these effects. Only by doing so can the clinicians develop a more effective treatment plan while simultaneously enhancing the therapeutic alliance.

SUSTAINABILITY IN BUILDING THE THERAPEUTIC ALLIANCE WITH VULNERABLE PATIENTS

There are several additional strategies that may be especially useful in developing and sustaining a therapeutic alliance with socially vulnerable patients. These include *showing* patients in concrete ways that you care (i.e., "going the extra mile"); *advocating* for patients with the myriad bureaucracies with which they struggle; *connecting* them to appropriate community resources (e.g., immigration lawyer, domestic violence counselor, exercise groups); *networking* with others, including family, friends, public health, and community resources, so as to encourage them to support the patient's efforts to achieve health; and engaging in *self-disclosure* to narrow social distance and encourage the sharing of personal stories.

Building a therapeutic alliance with vulnerable patients comes with both special rewards and challenges. Working with the underserved allows a clinician to apply his or her skills to assist those who are most in need, fulfilling one of the basic humanitarian ideals in medicine. Developing a therapeutic bond with patients that do not represent the "typical patient," or that many consider too difficult to manage, can be rewarding in and of itself, often involving a process of shared discovery and reflection.

It is not uncommon, however, for even seasoned clinicians to be overwhelmed by the many challenges inherent to caring for vulnerable patients. Developing patterns of codependency, such as repeatedly "rescuing"

patients from the decisions that are in their control, may be a prelude to clinician "burnout." In addition, the work environment plays an important role. Although clinicians in underserved clinical settings report serving higher proportions of medically and psychosocially complex patients, they are more likely to report a chaotic work environment and less likely to feel in control. In these contexts, clinicians who perceive high proportions of challenging patient encounter have higher odds of burnout and reduced job satisfaction.

Clinicians should be aware of signs of "burnout," such as exhibiting their anger and frustration at patients or staff, or developing an overly passive style of patient engagement.

To minimize burnout and maximize sustainability, clinicians caring for vulnerable populations may draw on personal, interpersonal, and environmental supports. In a qualitative study exploring why clinicians work in underserved clinics, clinicians cited the importance of personal motivators (such as opportunity for personal growth and concordance of service with self-identity and mission-based values); career motivators (such as work–life balance and loan repayment assistance); and environmental factors, primarily supportive interprofessional colleagues and teams.

Clinicians who have been able to sustain therapeutic relationships with vulnerable patients and maintain fulfilling careers in the care of vulnerable populations tend to (1) elicit patients' agendas so as to establish an understanding of patient expectations, (2) set realistic goals for what they can accomplish and share these goals with their patients, (3) limit what they aim to accomplish in any given encounter and see their work with patients as evolving over a long period of time, (4) continually clarify boundaries, (5) maintain a sense of curiosity and discovery about the patients' clinical and personal profile, (6) acknowledge that many of the problems experienced by vulnerable patients are structural/societal in nature, and not always a result of patient choice, (7) engage in public health-related or social advocacy efforts to affect structural determinants of health, (8) seek the advice and support of colleagues who share common ideals and practices, and (9) engage with interprofessional colleagues to draw on their expertise as part of an integrated team. Health care systems wishing to recruit and retain clinicians caring for vulnerable populations should provide opportunities for clinicians to develop these intrapersonal and interpersonal skills and enhance the clinical resources that allow clinicians to feel successful in this work.

CONCLUSIONS

A strong therapeutic alliance creates a trusting context for patient care, contributes to a higher quality of care, and can improve patient safety. Building a therapeutic alliance, eliciting the patient's narrative and assessing for vulnerabilities and strengths are critical to creating this context. Fostering the therapeutic alliance requires developing trust, conveying empathy, and collaborating about treatment goals. Depending on the skills, attitudes, and orientation of clinicians and the systems in which they work, the clinical encounter can increase social distance and exacerbate the effects of vulnerability on health, or it can lead to productive engagement with patients to mitigate or even eliminate the effects of vulnerability on health. Though it may be especially challenging to develop and sustain a therapeutic alliance with those who are socially vulnerable, the benefits to patient and clinician can be profound.

KEY CONCEPTS

- Vulnerable patients often experience fragmentation and disconnection in their lives and in their health care.
- The therapeutic alliance is an important means to reduce the effects of vulnerability on health outcomes.
- Eliciting the patient's story or perspective is an effective means to uncover health beliefs, develop shared meaning, enable empathy, and enhance the therapeutic alliance. It also serves to uncover patient vulnerabilities and reveal patients' resilience.
- By identifying vulnerabilities and acknowledging these to the patient and to other clinicians involved in the patient's care, clinicians will be better equipped to develop effective treatment plans.
- Though it may be especially challenging to develop and sustain a therapeutic alliance with those who are socially vulnerable, the benefits to patient and clinician can be profound.

CORE COMPETENCY

Eliciting the Patient's Perspective

- Let patients know that hearing their perspective is important to you.
- Explain that you think discussing family, coping styles, and their personal story is important to patients' health.
- Take the time necessary, and use the time well.
- Set a climate of interest, concern, and calm.
- Use an inquiry style that fosters more, not less, information.
- Maintain a high degree of curiosity; be aware of patients' verbal or emotional cues.

- Follow up on cues—such as *"It seemed that talking about that brought up some feelings for you. Why is that?"*
- Use open-ended questions and reflective statements.
- Discover the patient's explanatory model.
- Ask the Kleinman questions:

  What do you call the problem? What do you think has caused the problem? Why do you think it started when it did? What do you think the sickness does? How does it work? How severe is the sickness? Will it have a short or long course? What kind of treatment do you think you should receive? What are the most important results you hope to receive from this treatment? What are the chief problems the sickness has caused you? What do you fear most about the sickness? (Kleinman, 1988)

- Consider the interpersonal context of patients' general health care framework.
- Focus on the meaning of what patients are saying.
- Avoid using technical, medical jargon.
- Do not try to gather the entire perspective in one appointment, but try to gain some insight every time.

DISCUSSION QUESTIONS

1. Discuss clinical experiences you have had with vulnerable patients in which the presence or absence of strategies such as building a therapeutic alliance, eliciting patients' narratives, and assessing for vulnerabilities and strengths influenced the process and perhaps the outcome of their health care.

2. Consider what structural and health policy changes would need to be made to better incorporate the strategies of building a therapeutic alliance, eliciting patients' narratives, and assessing for vulnerabilities and strengths into the day-to-day clinical care of vulnerable patients.

3. What are some of the most surprising or fascinating nonmedical pieces of information you learned about the last patient you cared for and how did it influence either the treatment plan or your relationship with the patient and his or her family?

4. Discuss how personal beliefs, values, and assumptions about vulnerable patients affects your ability to create a context for effective care using strategies such as building a therapeutic alliance, eliciting patients' narratives, and assessing for vulnerabilities and strengths.

5. What special rewards and challenges have you encountered in caring for vulnerable populations and what strategies would help you sustain therapeutic alliances with your patients and families?

SUGGESTED READINGS

Beach MC, Sugarman J, Johnson RL, et al. Do patients treated with dignity report higher satisfaction, adherence, and receipt of preventive care? *Ann Fam Med* 2005;3:331–338.

Bennett JK, Fuertes JN, Keitel M, Phillips R. The role of patient attachment and working alliance on patient adherence, satisfaction, and health-related quality of life in lupus treatment. *Patient Educ Counsel* 2010;85:53–59.

Blanchard J, Lurie N. R-E-S-P-E-C-T: patient reports of disrespect in the health care setting and its impact on care. *J Fam Pract* 2004;53:721–730.

Copper LA, Roter DL, Carson KA et al. A randomized trial to improve patient-centered care and hypertension control in underserved primary care patients. *J Gen Intern Med* 2011;26: 1297–1304.

Fuertes JN, Boylan LS, Fontanella JA. Behavioral indices in medical care outcome: the working alliance, adherence, and related factors. *J Gen Int Med* 2008;24:80–85.

Goudge J, Gilson L, Russell S, et al. Affordability, availability and acceptability barriers to health care for the chronically ill: longitudinal case studies from South Africa. *BMC Health Services Res* 2009;9:75.

Hayashi AS, Selia E, McDonnell K. Stress and provider retention in underserved communities. *J Health Care Poor Underserved* 2009; 20(3):597–604 .

Kleinman A. The Illness Narratives: Suffering, Healing and the Human Condition. New York, NY: Basic Books, 1988.

Lyles CR, Karter AJ, Young BA, et al. Provider factors and patient-reported healthcare discrimination in the Diabetes Study of California (DISTANCE). *Patient Educ Couns* 2011, doi:10.1016/j/pec2011.04.031.

Moskowitz D, Lyles CR, Karter AJ, et al. Patient reported interpersonal processes of care and perceived social position: The Diabetes Study of Northern California (DISTANCE). *Patient Educ Couns* 2011, doi:10.1016/j.pec.2011.07.019.

Odom Walker K, Ryan G, Ramey R, et al. Recruiting and retaining primary care physicians in urban underserved communities: the importance of having a mission to serve. *Am J Public Health* 2010;100(11):2168–2175.

Piette JD, Bibbins-Domingo K, Schillinger D. Health care discrimination, processes of care, and diabetes patients' health status. *Patient Educ Couns* 2006;60:41–48.

Saba GW, Wong S, Schillinger D, et al. Shared decision-making and perceived collaboration in primary care. *Ann Fam Med* 2006;4:54–62.

Schillinger D. Improving chronic disease care for populations with limited health literacy. In:Nielsen-Bohlman LEA, ed. *Health Literacy: A Prescription to End Confusion*. Washington, DC: Institute of Medicine, National Academy Press, 2004, pp. 267–284.

Varkey AB, Manwell LB, Williams ES, et al. Separate and unequal: clinics where minority and nonminority patients receive primary care. *Arch Intern Med* 2009;169(3):243–250.

WEB SITES

American Academy on Communication in Healthcare. http://www.aachonline.org. Accessed July 2013.

SECTION IV
Health Related Behavior

Behavior Change

Daniel O'Connell, PhD

Photo by Hank Christensen (www.hankchristensen.com).

INTRODUCTION

Many of the common contemporary health problems such as diabetes, heart disease, and cancer, are related to patients' lifestyles and specific behaviors. To treat patient's health issues, clinicians must encourage reduction or elimination of destructive behaviors (e.g., smoking and alcohol dependence), promotion of healthier behaviors (e.g., weight control, regular exercise, stress management, safer sex), and adherence to medical regimens intended to treat acute or chronic illness (e.g., taking medications, dietary restrictions, checking blood glucose). Clinicians are hardly alone in their influence on patients' behavior.

Patients' social networks, their personal histories, genetics and life circumstances, as well as the media and broader societal forces also shape behavior. Not everyone's vision of the good life involves careful attention to healthy behavior. Many patients prefer a medication or procedure over behavior change to ameliorate a problem. All this can leave clinicians unclear about how much they are supposed to be pressing for behavior change and what are the limits of their influence in the brief context of the patient encounter.

Fortunately, work done in the field of behavioral medicine in the past 30 years has great practical application for clinicians and patients alike. In this chapter, we will incorporate the contributions from the most researched approaches to behavior change: the *Stages of Change Model, Motivational Interviewing, Self-Efficacy, Social Influence, Willpower, Goal Setting, Mindfulness, Self-Monitoring,* and *Contingency Management.* The objective is to use this research as the basis for a practical approach to influencing patients that respects both the complexity of human behavior and the resources and limitations of the medical encounter.

BEHAVIOR CHANGE MODELS

The *Stages of Change Model* introduced the idea that people move through a succession of five relatively distinguishable stages in making changes in behavior (in addition to *Relapse* if they revert to old behaviors after an initial period of success). Quickly determining the patient's stage of change with regard to specific behaviors allows the clinician to focus where further discussion or assistance would be most valuable. Many of the other behavior change models and strategies work well when integrated into this framework. The stages are outlined in Table 19-1.

The following descriptions and examples more fully illustrate each of the stages of behavior change:

Precontemplation: The patient gives little thought to the problem and how best to solve it (e.g., adolescent drinks heavily, but is apparently oblivious to consequences).

Contemplation: The patient thinks about the problem and the potential methods, costs, and benefits involved in trying to address it, but makes only inconsistent stabs at changed behavior (e.g., dietary changes that last only a few days before relapse).

Preparation: The patient now commits to a specific course of action and timetable (e.g., patient decides to join Weight Watchers this month with a girl-friend from work).

Action: A plan is being carried out on a regular basis with relatively clear goals and strategies being pursued (e.g., walking at least 30 minutes in the morning or evening 5 days a week).

Table 19-1. Stages of change and patient characteristics.

Stage	Patient Characteristics
Precontemplation	The problem exists, but the patient minimizes or denies it.
Contemplation	The patient is thinking about the problem and the costs and benefits of continuing with the problem or trying to change.
Preparation	The patient commits to a time and plan for resolving the problem.
Action	The patient makes daily efforts to overcome the problem.
Maintenance	The patient has overcome the problem and remains vigilant to prevent backsliding.
Relapse	The patient has gone back to the problem behavior on a regular basis after a period of successful resolution.

Maintenance: Successful changers begin to incorporate *Action* stage behaviors into a "new normal" way of living. Ongoing effort continues, but now feels less like a temporary alteration of familiar and normal behaviors and more incorporated into a sustainable lifestyle and identity (e.g., alcoholic with 5 years of sobriety).

Relapse: There is a consistent return to problem behaviors and attitudes after an initial period of successful change.

Clinicians typically associate behavior change with the action stage, yet fewer than 20% of patients report readiness to take action on a health behavior change in the next 30 days (e.g., quit smoking or start a weight loss program). Clinicians can increase patients' readiness to take action, as well as improving the action they eventually take, by encouraging them to contemplate, choose, and then commit themselves to a specific plan, carry through and modify the plan when needed, and incorporate new behavior into healthier lifestyles or recover from relapse and get going again. Moving from contemplation to maintenance in smoking cessation, for example, has been shown to take years on average. The goal of each clinician–patient conversation is to catalyze movement through the stages, and most of the patient's work is done outside the visit, as they think about, plan, commit, and then carry out the new behaviors with the guidance and encouragement from their clinicians. The indented examples that follow illustrate ways in which the clinician can converse with the patient in various stages, beginning with precontemplation.

Clinician: Sounds like we are agreed that your cholesterol level is a worry, but taking into account the possible side effects, you would prefer not to start a medication now to try to bring it down. (patient nods) Well, here is a handout that describes the problems caused by elevated cholesterol and options for treating it. I encourage you to look through the section on diet and exercise and decide how much and what kinds of changes you are ready to commit to. Does that seem like the right step for you now?

People typically start out in the *Precontemplation* stage. They already have the problem (e.g., drinking excessively, smoking, gaining weight, elevated blood sugar), but appear unaware or unconcerned about it. Awareness often builds in response to some "bad news" (e.g., physical symptoms, clothes that do not fit, restrictions on smoking, media focus on a health issue, a routine blood pressure check, or laboratory test). Any and all of these may prompt patients to start thinking more about the problem and weighing the pros and cons of trying to address it, moving them into the *Contemplation* stage. The clinician prompts this movement into contemplation by asking open-ended questions that require exploration and self-reflection by the patient or family in the office and later at home.

Clinician: What concerns do you have about your alcohol use? (Pause for response) Is there anything about it that worries you? (Pause for response) What is your wife most worried about? (Pause for response and empathize if contentious issue at home). What has happened to make this such a concern to her? (Pause for response) How important is her concern to you? (Pause for response). You may want to ask your family if there is anything about your drinking that worries them, as a way of helping you decide how important this really is. Is that something you would be willing to consider?

Depending on the specific problem, there may be validated screening questions that fit in nicely here, for example, CAGE or MAST (Michigan Alcohol Screening Test) screening for alcohol, brief screening inventories for depression such as the Patient Health Questionnaire (PHQ-9) or anxiety, or the SOAPP (Screener and Opioid Assessment for Patients with Pain). Providing normative data is a potent stimulant for further contemplation and helps patients in weighing the pros and cons of change.

Clinician: I have a brief questionnaire that can be helpful in determining to what extent depression is contributing to the constant tiredness you reported. Why don't you take a moment to complete it and we will score it together and see what it suggests to us.
Clinician: Tommy is at the 95th percentile for weight for a 9-year-old at his height, Mrs. Mason.

What do you and your husband think about that? (Pause for response) Have you noticed Tommy expressing any concern about this weight? (Pause for response). Tommy, I am wondering how you feel about your weight?

Contemplators often make inconsistent efforts to change, lacking the planning and determination needed to sustain them. Unfortunately, they often come to the wrong conclusion about why change has not followed (e.g., "I guess I don't have the willpower"). Over time they may either get stuck in ambivalence and procrastination, or move forward to become increasingly *committed* to a specific plan, goal, and timetable. To help, the clinician can encourage contemplators to come to a conclusion from their self-reflection.

Clinician: We have talked about the pros and cons of starting insulin for a few visits now. Given the laboratory results today and your readings at home, I wonder if you have come to your own conclusion about what must be done next to get you out of the danger zone?

Although making a commitment is essential, the plan must be put into action to produce the desired dividends. In the *Action* stage, people are "doing it" on a regular basis (e.g., walking a mile five times a week, closely following a diet plan, adhering to a medication regimen). To succeed they must keep their specific plan and intentions front and center and muster sufficient resolve and willpower to overcome moment-to-moment temptations to slip back into old behaviors. Recent research about *willpower* has brought some objectivity into what has in the past been either overvalued or dismissed as an artifact. Willpower can be thought of as the energy, focus, or commitment that fuels the capacity to make the previously determined choice in challenging situations. Willpower grows by mindfulness, clarity of intentions, anticipation, and preparation for challenges, as well as by modifying one's environment when not in the throes of immediate temptation (cool situations) to avoid overtaxing one's capacity for self-control in more tempting (hot) situations.

Clinician: So, as you plan for how to use your willpower to best effect, think about how your commitment not to buy high-calorie foods in the less tempting setting of the supermarket makes it easier to resist the urge to consume high-calorie snacks in the more tempting situation in front of the television that evening.
Clinician: What do you think you may need to change in your social life, if you are going to stay out of situations where the temptation to drink or use drugs could be really strong?

Clinician: You will need to be especially mindful of your intentions as you sit down to a meal. What ideas do you have for how to bring your intention to say "no" to seconds clearly into your mind at that crucial moment?

Contrast this kind of contemplation, anticipation, and commitment planning to the "New Years Eve Resolution" marked by good intentions, but lacking the underpinning for adherence in the face of even mild temptation. Such failure is often misattributed to "a lack of willpower," when actually it was a failure of clear intention and plan clarification and preparation that left the person unprepared at the first hint of temptation.

The initial conversion of *Preparation* into *Action* is usually a time of high effort and little payoff. Think about the first week of exercising after a long layoff. Patients do best when they have anticipated this and have a ready response that can head off second thoughts (e.g., "Pain is the weakness leaving my body. My decision to exercise is already made, and I am not going to remake it every morning!"). On the other hand, it is common to discover that some intensification of effort or the addition of other behaviors to the mix must be made to the action plan if desired results are to be attained (e.g., walking a mile a day will lead to some improvement in fitness, but without reducing caloric intake it is unlikely to lead to significant weight loss). *Self-monitoring* research points to the importance of patients tracking the data carefully (about their actions and their results) and using that information in moments of choice and when reevaluating their action plan if desired results are slower in coming than expected.

Clinician: Sounds like you were hoping to have continued to lose weight at the same rate as when you started out, but you know about the body's natural mechanisms to resist further weight loss. What changes in your action plan do you think you might need to make to continue burning off more calories than you are taking in, now that you seem to be experiencing some of those set point issues?

Contingency management research has always highlighted the importance of having rewards lined up for the accomplishment of intermediate and larger milestones to motivate the initial and continued efforts at change. People may come up with these rewards naturally (e.g., "When I have lost 15 pounds I will buy myself some new outfits."). It can also be helpful for the clinician to anticipate and encourage the patient to build rewards into their action efforts.

Clinician: Be sure to reward yourself periodically for the efforts you are making. For instance, in addition to all the health benefits it will bring you, what do you thing would be a fitting reward for getting your hemoglobin A1c below 7?

In the *Maintenance* stage patients try to incorporate their *Action* stage behaviors into a sustainable new lifestyle. Depending on the problem they are addressing, maintainers may be able to reduce some of the frequency and intensity of action stage effort (e.g., attending fewer Alcoholics Anonymous [AA] meetings, or allowing previously forbidden foods back into their diet in a controlled manner) and still hold onto improvements they have made. This is a challenging transition. Patients may have secretly been hoping that the intensive efforts of the Action stage would be time-limited, but many behavior and lifestyle changes must be maintained indefinitely if improvements are to be sustained. In the Maintenance stage, those behaviors tend to come more naturally if people increasingly identify with the new lifestyle and can remind themselves to enjoy the improvements their efforts have produced. It is also necessary for their immediate social network to adapt or be reconfigured to support the new behaviors and routines (e.g., Long-term sobriety depends on building associations with people and activities that do not encourage drug and alcohol use. Family members must learn to not inadvertently encourage overeating, and the changer must learn how to gracefully say "no" to well-meaning offers of unnecessary food.). Self-monitoring is very important as the path to relapse often begins with a series of slips that are not recognized and not recovered from swiftly (e.g., a cigarette or two after putting the kids to bed, giving oneself permission to exercise less as winter weather sets in and the outdoors is less inviting).

Clinician: Congratulations on all you have accomplished. Are these changes starting to feel like a better lifestyle for you?
Clinician: What have you noticed is the amount of exercise and calorie control you need to continue before your weight starts to increase again?
Clinician: How is your social life different, now that you are committed to staying sober?

Unfortunately, any single attempt at behavior change offers a high risk of *Relapse* (e.g., weight regained, exercise abandoned, substance use renewed, etc). Relapsers may feel discouraged and stuck, or alternatively may remain committed to change and primed for another try. The clinician can help by reframing relapse as a time for regrouping, taking the lessons learned and planning the next action.

Clinician: So you were able to quit smoking when you were pregnant with Tommy but little by little slipped back into smoking in the year afterwards?

Is it still clear in your mind that smoking will cause health problems for you and the baby? (Pause for response). How were you able to resist the urge to smoke for those 9 months? (Pause for answer) I wonder if some of those same strategies might work for you again if you decide that quitting is still best for you and your family. What do you think?

In the examples above, each stage of readiness to change has been addressed in a different way by the astute clinician. Appropriate clinician strategies for each of the stages are summarized in Table 19-2.

Research in *motivational interviewing*, *intrinsic motivation*, and *psychological reactance* has revealed that people are inclined to resist coercion and have trouble maintaining behavior changes that do not meet internalized values and goals. Unfortunately, typical attempts at influence (by doctors, parents, teachers, etc) are often limited to "pushing" types of interactions involving lecturing, explaining, exhorting, criticizing, inspiring, or threatening dire consequences if change does not occur. Much of this can feel like unwanted external pressure and coercion to the patient. Researchers have found little support for the sustained effectiveness of a heavy-handed, coercive or even inspirational approach. On the contrary, reactance theory shows how people, who might otherwise have admitted their concern over a problem, may instead feel compelled to defend their

Table 19-2. Stages of change and clinician strategies.

Stage of Change	Patient Characteristics	Clinician Strategies
Precontemplation	Denies problem and its importance. Is reluctant to discuss problem. Problem is identified by others. Shows reactance when pressured. High risk of argument.	Ask permission to discuss problem. Inquire about patient's thoughts. Gently point out discrepancies. Express concern. Ask patient to think, talk, or read about situation between visits.
Contemplation	Shows openness to talk, read, and think about problem. Weighs pros and cons. Dabbles in action. Can be obsessive about problem and can prolong stage.	Elicit patient's perspective first. Help identify pros and cons of change. Ask what would promote commitment. Suggest trials.
Preparation/ Determination	Understands that change is needed. Begins to form commitment to specific goals, methods, and timetables. Can picture overcoming obstacles. May procrastinate about setting start date for change.	Summarize patient's reasons for change. Negotiate a start date to begin some or all change activities. Encourage patient to announce publicly. Arrange a follow-up contact at or shortly after start date.
Action	Follows a plan of regular activity to change problem. Can describe plan in detail (unlike dabbling in action of contemplator). Shows commitment in facing obstacles. Resists slips. Is particularly vulnerable to abandoning effort impulsively.	Show interest in specifics of plan. Discuss difference between slip and relapse. Help anticipate how to handle a slip. Support and reemphasize pros of changing. Help to modify action plan if aspects are not working well. Arrange follow-up contact for support.
Maintenance	Has accomplished change or improvement through focused action. Has varying levels of awareness regarding importance of long-term vigilance. May already be losing ground through slips or wavering commitment. Has feelings about how much the change has actually improved life. May be developing lifestyle that precludes relapse into former problem.	Show support and admiration. Inquire about feelings and expectations and how well they were met. Ask about slips, any signs of wavering commitment. Help create plan for intensifying activity should slips occur. Support lifestyle and personal redefinition that reduce risk of relapse. Reflect on the long-term—and possibly permanent—nature of this stage as opposed to the more immediate gratification of initial success.

behavior when criticized, pressured, or coerced. The rhetorical question is an example of such a thinly described "push" (e.g., "Don't you think . . . ?"). Motivational interviewing has shown instead how "pulling or attracting" by eliciting the patient's ideas, values, feelings about the problem, and potential solutions produces greater change with less strain in the clinician–patient relationship than the "pushing" strategies clinicians typically used. The clinician's role is to help the patient gather the relevant data from which to weigh the pros and cons of change, determine the importance and urgency of change, and then commit themselves to a reasonably effective course of action when they are ready.

This motivational approach is accomplished through an interview style that encourages expressions of empathy for the challenges at each stage, curiosity about feelings and ideas, and respect for the patient's ownership of the problem and autonomy in deciding when and what to do next. Listening for and highlighting "change talk" (in which patients themselves are providing the arguments for change and exploring how it might be accomplished) can be very effective. Expressing concern instead of control, and curiosity rather than command, are the hallmarks of this approach. Although the clinician is often the one providing the worrisome information that precipitates the behavior change conversation, pulling rather than pushing is usually the best way to promote patient self-reflection and to build internal (and therefore sustainable) motivation to consider change. Using the rhythm of *provide–elicit–provide* keeps the patient active in the conversation, rather than a passive recipient of a "push" lecture. This strategy works when the clinician offers succinct pieces of information or feedback and then immediately elicits the patient's response before deciding what next to provide.

> **Clinician:** What went through your mind as I described your most recent lab values and blood pressure readings and the risks associated with them?
> **Clinician:** What do you already know about the relationship between the extra weight you are carrying and the problems you are having with sugar control and high blood pressure? (The question suggests the connection while encouraging the patient to come up with the self-motivational evidence.)
> **Clinician:** It sounds like you would love to lose weight, but at the same time you are pessimistic that you could keep the weight off based on your past experience (feedback and elicit response). Tell me more about that.

The clinician is not abdicating responsibility to provide information, guidance, and set limits when a patient's request or ongoing behavior is unsafe. On the contrary, behavior change is sometimes catalyzed when clinicians, and other important people in the patient's life, have made clear the limits of what they can support or tolerate.

> **Clinician:** Having discussed this with you, I am starting to see that we have two problems to contend with here. One is that you continue to feel a great deal of discomfort and the second is that the narcotics are not the safest and most effective way to help you with that discomfort. I could not allow myself to continue to prescribe a medication that is likely causing more harm than good. Are you open to an alternative approach? (Clinician does not try to immediately push or sell alternatives, but instead allows the patient to participate in the discussion as a way to reduce the risk of reactance. While the patient is not being given the choice to continue to get narcotics from this clinician, the clinician is acknowledging the patient's autonomy to work together on an alternative approach or seek a second opinion if desired.)

Self-efficacy theory predicts that for the individuals to become more motivated for a change they must become sufficiently *convinced* both that the change is in their best interest and also that the specific change being considered would be *effective* in meeting their objective (e.g., "Is losing weight really necessary for me? *And* If I were able to follow a Mediterranean or low-fat diet, etc, would I really lose significant amounts of weight?"). Self-efficacy research also reminds us that people must feel sufficiently *confident* that they can reliably perform the changed behavior before they will commit themselves to action. The effective clinician is not just working to help the patient feel convinced that change is needed or desirable, but also helping the patient create manageable and achievable steps that can be embraced with confidence. Ultimately, the change must strike the patient as sufficiently *important* that it feels worth all the effort, which for many behavior changes is considerable! These are continuous variables (more/less/sufficiently) rather than all or none. Increased conviction that the change is important and necessary, combined with building confidence that the specific steps are doable, ultimately results in the tipping point being reached where the patient is willing to commit to a course of action.

Depending on the patient's stage of change, the clinician could promote further contemplation of the problem and potential solutions, encourage commitment to a specific course of action already contemplated, help tailor the patient's current actions to accelerate desired outcomes, or assist incorporation of successful actions into the patient's ongoing lifestyle. Assessing and building conviction is usually the place to start, since a patient who is not sufficiently convinced that the problem is important is unlikely to think much about how to solve it or what the challenges might be.

Clinician: I am concerned that your hemoglobin A1c has gone up further. How worried are you about that? (Provide–elicit). What do you think might have caused that? (Pause for an answer). What do you think may be needed to turn that around? (Many patients already have a good idea what might be needed). How confident are you that you could start to make those changes today? (Pause for an answer).

Clinician: If you are reasonably convinced that change is needed, then let's think about a plan that you feel reasonably confident you could start out with. What ideas do you have about that? (Asking the patient to start the exploration of specific behavior changes helps prevent the "yes, but" dynamic that can get triggered when the clinician is the one offering the ideas first.

Clinicians can help increase the confidence of individuals who feel that even a desired change is impossible for them. For the *Contemplation* or *Preparation* stage patient, clinicians can encourage thinking about or researching or imagining the specifics of a plan they are reasonably confident the patient could carry out. Making this a thought experiment often can catalyze the process.

Clinician: If you were to decide to get more exercise, what are some ways you could imagine doing this that you feel most confident you could stick with? For instance, you might consider joining a health club, getting an exercise machine, finding a friend to jog or walk with? What can you picture about any of those alternatives?.

For the *Preparation* stage patient, the clinician is encouraging a choice or commitment in the face of inevitable uncertainties about how things will actually go. *Contemplation* can become prolonged when the patient is searching for certainty about the "best way" rather than accepting that consistent adherence to any reasonable plan is better than the endless search for the perfect plan.

Clinician: Sounds like you are not confident that you would be able to make time for exercise after you get home to your family in the evening. (Provide feedback and elicit). I am wondering when else you could fit in exercise? (Pause for patient's ideas) For instance, some of my patients tell me that it is more possible to exercise some mornings before work, or on some lunch breaks, or to stop on the way home a few evenings each week, because they know they will not be able to get out again once they get home in the evening. What do

you think of something like that for you? (A "Yes, but . . . " response would signal that the patient needs to do more contemplation work before commitment is possible.) You may want to ask your family when it would be easiest on them for you to make time for more regular exercise and perhaps lay out for them why this is so important to you. Is that something you can imagine doing this week?

Clinician: Picture yourself cutting back the number of cigarettes you smoke from 20 to 15 a day for the next 2 weeks and then going down to 10 a day until we talk again in a month. Does that seem doable to you when you try to picture it?

Asking patients to rate their conviction, confidence or the importance of a change on a 1–10 scale can add clarity. It is helpful for deciding whether offering data that might help convince the patient of the *importance* of change would be most helpful, or instead helping them to build a plan they feel more *confident* they can carry out is the better use of time.

Clinician: On a scale of 1–10, with 1 being unimportant and 10 indicating that almost nothing is more important, where would you now place the importance of using protection when having intercourse? (Pause for response) Can you tell me a little more about why you rate it a 4 rather than a 2, for instance? (Asking the patient to indicate why the selected number is higher than a lower number can elicit the level of importance, however small, the patient attributes to the change. A follow-up question shifts the focus to further considerations that could strengthen the patient's sense of importance.) What would it take to move your rating from a 4 to a 7?

For the *Commitment* stage patient, the clinician probes for the readiness to move into action in the foreseeable future. Research in *goal-setting* highlights the value of setting specific targets and timetables as one moves into action and keeping regular track of both the actions themselves and their desired outcomes. Publicly announcing a commitment to specific behaviors and outcomes has also been shown to impact outcomes more powerfully than private commitments, and so can also be encouraged.

Clinician: If you let your family know your intention to cut down on the amount you are eating, they may be in a better position to serve smaller portions, not encourage you to finish up leftovers and perhaps they can support you in other ways without just nagging you.

Clinician: You will know that you are really committed to change when you don't think of reminders as nagging, but instead see them as just-in-time prompts that can help you be more mindful of what you already intended to do in a situation. Like when your wife reminded you that you had decided to limit yourself to two drinks when you go out socially.

For *Action* stage patients, the clinician inquires about challenges to their consistency and helps them either adjust to a more manageable action plan (i.e., one in which they have more confidence they can persist) or intensifying or including more elements in their current action plan if desired results are not coming quickly enough.

> **Clinician:** It sounds like you continue to believe that walking 2 miles every evening is the best plan for you, but then you find yourself re-making the decision to get going every evening. I imagine that the voice that says "But maybe not tonight?" is not unexpected and you could plan for that voice as well. You might simply remind yourself, "I already made that decision and always feel better for having done it!" and then just put on your walking shoes and go. Eventually getting regular exercise could feel like the normal way to live and you will wonder how you ever lived without it. Does that make sense? (Clinician listens for a "yes, but" which would call for switching from advice giving to pulling for the patient's ideas.)

Here is an example involving smoking that incorporates some of the elements described above:

> **Clinician:** Where are you now in your thinking about quitting smoking? (Determining current stage.)
> **Clinician:** How convinced are you that stopping smoking will be necessary to help you breathe with less effort now and also slow down the progression of symptoms in the future? (Check conviction about value or importance of change.)
> **Clinician:** Now that we have talked about the over-the-counter and prescription aids that can help to reduce those initial cravings for nicotine, how confident are you that you could get through those first few months without cigarettes? (Check confidence about a specific method of change.)

Recent research is highlighting the extent to which an individual's behavior is influenced by and even comes to match those in their *social networks*. For example, heavy drinkers often associate with other heavy drinkers for whom this level of drinking is normal. We see similar effects in smoking, other drug use, weight issues, effort at schoolwork, sexual behavior, etc. It is useful for patients to reflect on and plan for (contemplation work)

the challenges that will come if they begin to express desires and behaviors in contrast to peers. On the positive side, a change in the behavior of a person in the patient's social network can be expected to promote contemplation of change by the patient. The clinician can inquire about the behavior of people in the patient's social network as a way to encourage emulation of healthy behavior, or as a heads up that the patient must prepare for some disapproval if starting a behavior change challenges the status quo of those they associate with most closely.

> **Clinician:** Do you know anyone who has successfully _____? Tell me more about that.
> **Clinician:** As you think more about changing this behavior, who do you anticipate will be most supportive and where do you think you might expect some resistance? (Pause for response) How could you handle that?
> **Clinician:** Many people do best when they have a companion to exercise and diet with. Is there someone you think is ready to take action with you, perhaps at home or at work, or a friend who is also concerned about this?

Sometimes clinicians feel they are shirking their duty if they do not take a strong prescriptive stance about their patients' unhealthy lifestyle and behavioral issues. The key is to integrate the responsibility to advise and encourage, with an empathic, concerned, and curious demeanor, drawing patients into a more active exploration and ownership of the problem. Here are some examples of how a clear recommendation for behavior change can be made empathically rather than judgmentally within a collaborative, rather than clinician-centered framework.

> **Clinician:** Probably the best things you could to reduce the chances of another heart attack would be to quit smoking and get your cholesterol under control. Tell me what goes through your mind as I say that to you?

Expressing increasing levels of concern is another way that clinicians can meet their obligation to alert patients to potential health consequences while not provoking either the embarrassment or reactance, which could fuel resistance.

> **Clinician:** I am increasingly concerned that your poorly controlled blood sugars are already doing damage and dragging you still closer to all the serious problems you told me earlier that you wanted to avoid. What do you think can be done to turn this around?
> **Clinician:** I agree that no one is more concerned about your child's well-being than you. I just worry

that you could blame yourself if Caitlin gets a serious case of one of these illnesses that widely validated research tells us vaccination could have safely prevented. How concerned are you about that aspect of the risk of vaccinating or not vaccinating?

Clinician: I imagine that learning you are pregnant is a big deal all by itself. On top of that, here I am telling you that things like alcohol and cigarettes could really hurt your developing baby. Tell me what is going through your mind as you hear all that?

People almost always feel two ways about behavior change. *Ambivalence* is normal. Patients see discomfort and disruption of their familiar routines in the short term, balanced against the hope of desirable outcomes in the longer term. The effective clinician asks about and empathizes with this ambivalence by inviting the patient to talk about the resulting stalemate and its effects. This is better done with open-ended rather than rhetorical questions (e.g., "Don't you think that …?"). Here is an example of exploring ambivalence:

Clinician: It sounds like you are weighing the burden of time and effort involved in exercising regularly against the upset you feel with yourself for not doing more to reduce your risk of another heart attack? How do you imagine you will ultimately decide what to do?"

Clinicians can translate their sense of urgency into an expression of concern that the patient's goals may not be met unless the ambivalent impasse is resolved and a tipping point is reached in favor of change. Using the language of "I am concerned" emphasizes the desire to be helpful over the tone of judgment that people so easily hear and resent.

Clinician: I am just concerned that you will feel more and more like an invalid unless you can get yourself out of the house for some activity every day. But what do you think?

Clinician: I am just concerned that without restarting the home stretching and conditioning program, you will continue to feel limited by this back pain and perhaps end up choosing the surgery that you told me initially you wanted to avoid. (Pause for response.)

Clinicians often wonder how best to shift the discussion toward behavior change for a patient who is not bringing up behavioral and lifestyle contributors to health issues (common in *Precontemplation*). A natural lead-in is to make statements linking the patient's concerns to their behavior as the clinician's reasons for pursuing the behavioral issue. For example, if a female patient asks for birth control, the clinician can use her concern about pregnancy as a basis for asking how else

she had been protecting herself when having sex. This may lead naturally to a discussion about using condoms with new partners, an issue that was not on her agenda for this visit. If a patient comes for his annual physical it makes sense to ask, "Is there anything you have been doing which you think has inadvertently gotten in the way of your being more healthy?"

A discussion of smoking cessation with a patient hospitalized for chronic obstructive pulmonary disease (COPD) is an example of how bridging between symptoms and behavior can come about naturally:

Clinician: Let me ask you about a few behaviors that usually worsen COPD and create the kind of crisis that led to your admission. For instance, how do you think your smoking might be affecting this?

Clinician: I imagine it was pretty scary to feel that you couldn't get a breath. How important is it to you to avoid another breathing crisis like that one? (Pause for response). Is that important enough to make the effort to quit smoking now? (Searching for the intrinsic motivation rather than over-relying on "doctor's orders" or other "pushing" behaviors that we have described earlier.)

As mentioned earlier, the *self-efficacy* construct offers a very helpful diagnostic and planning metric for the clinician in deciding what to pursue next in the limited time of the encounter. The clinician can ask the patient to rate himself from 1 to 10 on how convinced he is that his smoking is a problem at this time (or stated differently, how convinced he is that quitting smoking would be helpful right now). If the patient is barely convinced that the change is valuable at this time (e.g., "I don't see how that would really help."), then exploring his understanding of the impact of smoking on his COPD will be the place to start. If the patient is already convinced that the change would be very valuable (e.g. "I know that smoking is killing me, but I have never been able to quit for more than a few days."), then the clinician's time is best spent talking about ways to enhance confidence that the patient can accomplish it.

Clinician: What aspect of quitting smoking has been the most difficult for you? (Pause for answer) Let's see what we might have to offer to help with that.

These same open-ended and scaling questions about conviction, confidence, and importance can be used with almost any health behavior. Here are more examples of questions to assess conviction, confidence, and importance:

Clinician: How convinced are you that the medication is essential for keeping your moods from swinging so dramatically from depression to mania?

Clinician: How confident are you that you could calmly set clearer limits about your children's behavior? (Pause) What affects your confidence that you can talk with them calmly when they are misbehaving? (Pause for answer). Knowing that managing your own anger is the biggest challenge for you, let's think for a moment about what can help with that. Make sense?

Clinician: Well it sounds like you are already pretty convinced that smoking is bad for you and the grandkids, and it is very important for you to get to care for your grandchildren, but your daughter won't allow that if you are smoking at home. Still, the idea of gaining even more weight is really putting you off. So to help you feel more confident that you could quit smoking, we would need to find some way to reduce that initial craving for cigarettes without your gaining a large amount of weight. Tell me what you already know about things that can help with craving, and I will fill in the blanks.

Clinician: How convinced are you that doing those stretching and strengthening exercises will reduce your back pain? (Pause for response). So, even though you do think they could help over the long term you are pretty worried that they will make the pain even worse with your back already being so irritated. That is understandable. Would it help you feel more confident if I demonstrate how you could start out doing the stretches in a way that would not make your pain worse?

Clinician: Being in the hospital allows patients time to plan for the lifestyle changes that will be essential for their recovery. What ideas do you have already about changes that will be important for you to make after discharge?" (Pull before push, ask before tell.)

CONCLUSIONS

Although clinicians are convinced that behavior change would be helpful in many patient conditions, they often lack confidence in their ability to influence patients' behavior in brief medical interviews. The goal of this chapter has been to map out pragmatic approaches that can be utilized in even the briefest encounters to have a positive influence on the patient's behavior. Assessing a patient's *Stage of Change* promotes a more focused examination or hospital room conversation by pointing up where the patient's next efforts would most productively be directed to promote movement toward behavior change. *Motivational interviewing* teaches the demeanor of empathic and respectful curiosity that acknowledges patients' autonomy while exploring the ambivalence that marks all difficult choices. The clinician learns to pull from the patient self-motivational thoughts and feelings rather than push at the patient with lectures, threats, and inspiration. *Reactance theory* reminds the clinician of the natural urge to resist coercion, and research on intrinsic motivation makes clear that for change to be initiated and sustained individuals must relate the effort and outcome to their own goals and values, ultimately deciding if the effort is sufficiently important. Research on *goal setting* emphasizes that the most effective actions are ones in which the patient has clearly identified goals and monitors both behavior and outcomes on a regular basis. *Willpower* is a necessary but limited commodity in the patient's life. It is built on the underpinning of careful contemplation of the problem and ways to overcome it, a clear commitment to a specific course of action, mindfulness and anticipation of temptations to slip and relapse, and modification of the environment to make the right choices easier and the wrong choices harder. *Social Learning Theory* teaches that behavior changes when both conviction and confidence cross a threshold that tips toward action. At each stage of change the clinician must understand what is affecting patients' conviction that the problem requires attention as well as their confidence that success is possible. The principle and reality of *patient autonomy* reminds us to respectfully inquire about, thoughtfully attempt to influence, and ultimately accept the patient's decisions about how important a change is for them. We must accept that a patient's behavior is affected by many forces and influences, one of which is us. The more clinicians can link up with and build upon the broader array of motivators and resources for healthier behavior and lifestyle, the more they will enjoy this fundamental aspect of effective patient care.

SUGGESTED READINGS

Baumeister R, Tierney J. *Willpower.* New York: Penguin Press, 2011.

Miller WR, Rollnick S, eds. *Motivational Interviewing: Preparing People for Change.* The Guilford Press, New York, 2002.

Prochaska JO, Norcross JC, DiClemente CC. *Changing for Good.* The Guilford Press, New York, 1994.

Rollnick S. Readiness, importance and confidence: critical conditions of change in treatment. In:Miller WR, Heather N, eds. *Treating Addictive Behavior,* 2nd ed. Springer US, New York, 1998.

Rollnick S, Mason P, Butler C. *Health Behavior Change: A Guide for Clinicians.* Churchill Livingstone, New York, 1999.

WEB SITES

Transtheoretical Model Cancer Prevention Resource Center, University of Rhode Island. http://www.uri.edu/research/cprc/transtheoretical.htm. Accessed February 2013.

The Motivational Interviewing Page. http://www.motivational-interview.org/. Accessed February 2013.

Patient Adherence

Veronica J. Sanchez, PhD & M. Robin DiMatteo, PhD

INTRODUCTION

In the context of medical treatment, the term adherence refers to a patient's success in following the recommendations of a health care provider for disease prevention and treatment. Nonadherence (also called noncompliance) refers to a patient's failure to follow these recommendations, such as by not filling a medication prescription or by stopping the medication before being instructed to do so, improperly using a medical device, carrying out prescribed behaviors (e.g., specific exercises) incorrectly, or entirely ignoring medical advice (such as to avoid certain foods, or to engage in disease screening). Nonadherence can be purposeful or not. The term "unintentional nonadherence" is used to describe cases in which patients believe (mistakenly) that they are adhering to what has been prescribed, whereas "intentional nonadherence" is used for cases in which patients choose to disregard treatment recommendations completely or to modify their prescribed regimens.

Across a variety of disease conditions, 25% of patients (on average) do not adhere to prevention and disease management activities (including taking medications, going to medical appointments, obtaining screening, exercising, and/or dieting); for some medical conditions, adherence can be as poor as 50% or less. Adherence is a behavior that is strongly connected to health outcomes. On average, the odds of a good health outcome for patients who are adherent are 2.88 times higher than for nonadherent patients. Nonadherence can take a significant toll not only on patient health outcomes but also on providers and the health care system. At the interpersonal level, the inability to achieve health care goals due to nonadherence can be frustrating for both patients and their providers, and from a societal standpoint, nonadherence produces a significant economic burden (between $290 and $300 billion annually in the United States alone). In addition, the number of medical visits wasted annually in the United States as a result of nonadherence is estimated to be at least 240 million.

According to the World Health Organization, adherence is affected by many factors such as: (1) the health care system including the provider–patient relationship, (2) the patient's disease type and severity, (3) the type of treatment regimen and its complexity, (4) patient characteristics, and (5) socioeconomic factors. This chapter will focus on the interplay of these factors in understanding the role of the provider–patient relationship and communication quality in effective methods for promoting adherence and chronic disease management among all, including the most vulnerable, patients. These include patients of ethnic minority status, low socioeconomic standing, low education level, and/or low health literacy. Emphasis will be placed on targeting individual patients' needs to promote adherence through the use of a recently devised heuristic model offered by DiMatteo and colleagues, called the Information–Motivation–Strategy Model©.

OVERVIEW OF THE INFORMATION–MOTIVATION–STRATEGY MODEL©

Although the elements of the Information–Motivation–Strategy Model© (IMS Model) were first introduced in the early 1980s, there was insufficient empirical research on which to build support; now, many large-scale empirical trials and meta-analytic reviews provide evidence for the framework of the model. The primary purpose of the IMS Model is to provide health care providers with a valid and practical rubric for remembering and using three broad elements of care that are essential for improving patient adherence. The three components of the IMS Model are Information, Motivation, and Strategy. They reflect the fact that patients can follow only treatments they have been informed about and which they understand; patients will adhere only to treatments they are motivated to adhere to; and patients only do what they are able to within their resource limitations and available strategies.

Information

The information component emphasizes the importance of the knowledge held by patients about their condition and its treatment, and suggests that this knowledge depends most upon effective provider–patient communication. Patients are unlikely to follow a treatment unless its importance is clear to them and they fully comprehend the care instructions. Unintentional nonadherence commonly stems from failure at this stage in the process of care. Research from hundreds of studies indicates that for many patients, their level of health literacy is low and their ability to understand the health information they receive is inadequate. Therefore, health care providers have a responsibility to communicate effectively with their patients and to inform them thoroughly, as well as to check on how well patients understand the information that they are given. A meta-analysis found that in more than a hundred empirical studies, good physician communication skills were associated with increased patient adherence. To encourage patient adherence, health care providers should focus considerable attention on communicating information effectively and on determining patients' degree of understanding of the treatment regimen. When interacting with vulnerable patients, adequate communication is especially challenging because low health literacy, language barriers, and low levels of education can hinder patients' full and accurate understanding of what they must do to care for themselves. Health professionals need to identify any specific barriers to communication and attempt to build patient trust in the therapeutic relationship, promote shared decision making, listen to patients, and allow patients to offer essential information on how they plan to follow through with their medical recommendations (see Chapter 18)(Figure 20-1).

Motivation

The motivation component of the model highlights the notion that patients will only follow treatments that they believe in and are motivated to pursue. Therefore, a major goal of health care providers should be to work with each patient to develop a treatment plan to which the patient can be fully committed. Health care providers should keep in mind that patients' beliefs about the value of a treatment (such as about the risks, benefits, and efficacy of treatment) and their sense of confidence that barriers to adherence can be overcome are crucial to influencing their motivation to adhere. In addition, patients' beliefs in the consequences of nonadherence are important; if nonadherence is perceived as likely to produce problematic health outcomes, patient adherence will be higher than if consequences are not believed or fully understood. Cultural factors, including social group norms, may also impact adherence; providers need to be aware of and sensitive to their patients' cultural beliefs and practices so that treatment recommendations do not conflict with cultural norms.

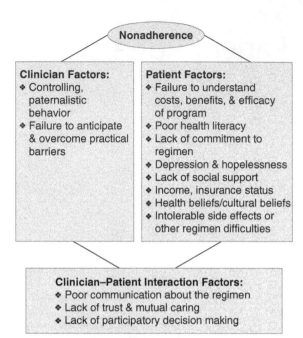

Figure 20-1. Clinician-patient barriers to adherence.

Furthermore, it is important to note that motivation to adhere may be especially compromised in disadvantaged patients who experience cultural barriers between them and their physicians. If patients and their physicians are not of a similar cultural background, for example, physicians should learn about their patient's culture to find the best way to help motivate them to adhere; providers should be careful to avoid introducing cultural impediments to adherence (see Chapter 15). Lastly, patients often desire to participate in the process of caring for their health; thus, it is beneficial to promote shared decision making between physicians and patients within the context of a strong therapeutic relationship. Doing so would allow providers to openly discuss patients' beliefs, concerns, confusions, and apprehensions about treatment regimens.

Strategy

Finally, the strategy component of the model underscores the fact that patients must be capable of adhering and have the resources necessary to follow the prescribed treatment. Patients need the tools and strategies necessary for effectively following their treatment, as well as the capacity to overcome any barriers to adherence that may arise. Thus, another important task for health care providers is to help patients identify and surpass obstacles to adherence. The concrete barriers patients face might include the financial cost of a medication, difficulties in remembering the medication schedule or in dealing with the treatment complexity, coping with unpleasant side effects, and the challenge of accommodating changes in lifestyle such as diet and exercise. Social support from family and friends is instrumental in helping patients adhere to treatments. In this context, social support is useful in terms of the assistance that individuals who are close to a patient can provide. A patient's relative, for example, can help overcome barriers to adherence by providing transportation, helping with medication affordability, offering child care to attend medical appointments, and reminding the patient to take medications. Past research has found that family cohesiveness can positively influence patient adherence, and that family conflict can threaten it severely. Providers should know their patients well enough to evaluate whether and how the people who are close to a patient can assist in promoting adherence; providers should also help their patients identify other formal systems of aid, including workplace-based interventions and community-based resources. Obtaining aid is particularly valuable for patients of low socioeconomic status. Disadvantaged patients may need help from their health care providers in building a social support network (if, e.g., they are recent immigrants) and with acquiring financial resources for covering the cost of medical care expenses (such as the costs of medications and medical devices if no insurance coverage is available).

Understanding how the three components of the IMS Model can be applied to promote patient adherence may be facilitated by the use of a case illustration.

 ## CASE ILLUSTRATION

Lucy is a 62-year-old married Hispanic female with hypertension, adult-onset diabetes mellitus, and obesity. She lives with her husband who is ill and has two loving and supportive adult children who live nearby. She has not been feeling well for the last couple of weeks and decided to see her physician, Dr. Ruiz, at the nearby publicly funded clinic. Lucy has seen Dr. Ruiz twice before and she likes her and feels that they are developing a good relationship. Dr. Ruiz sees Lucy as a friendly and generally optimistic person.

During their second medical visit, Dr. Ruiz determined that Lucy has not been adhering to the treatment regimen prescribed by her previous physician. Dr. Ruiz prescribed two medications to control her diabetes and hypertension, offered Lucy a detailed explanation of how to take the medications, and described any serious side effects that Lucy should report. Next, Dr. Ruiz discussed the behavioral changes that Lucy would need to engage in—to check her blood sugar levels daily (before and after

each meal), improve her diet (e.g., consume less sugar and salt and more vegetables), and incorporate light exercise into her daily routine (e.g., 30-minute walks). As Dr. Ruiz explained these changes to Lucy, she realized that Lucy had trouble understanding how to take her medications and how to interpret her blood sugar levels. Lucy did not believe that she needed to take medications when she felt well. Furthermore, Lucy was concerned about how she would be able to cook healthier meals and go out for walks; her time and attention were consumed by concerns for her husband's health.

APPLICATION OF THE INFORMATION–MOTIVATION–STRATEGY MODEL©

Stage One: Achieving Patient Understanding of Treatment

One of the primary reasons for nonadherence is that patients do not understand what they are supposed to do when a physician provides them with a treatment regimen. Lucy speaks Spanish fluently but is limited in her understanding of English and in her ability to speak it. Medical terminology and treatment descriptions are difficult to understand, even in her native language (i.e., she has low health literacy). Dr. Ruiz tries to speak to Lucy in terms that she can grasp, and employs a communication feedback loop (or teach-back method). She carefully explains to Lucy what having diabetes and hypertension means for her health and the importance of taking her medications, eating healthy foods, and exercising regularly. Subsequently, Dr. Ruiz can ask Lucy to state in her own words what she has understood. Then, Dr. Ruiz can try to make clear anything that Lucy has not comprehended. This process may continue until Lucy has achieved an adequate level of understanding. These techniques can be used with a medical translator as well. Good communication can help compensate for factors that inhibit proper patient understanding of medical information and can increase the likelihood that a patient adheres to treatment. Furthermore, patients who, like Lucy, tend to be disadvantaged feel empowered by understanding the medical dialogue and would be more capable of making decisions jointly with their physician and implementing their treatment regimen.

Stage Two: Motivating Patients to Adhere

A second reason why patients may not adhere to their treatment is that they may lack the motivation to do so. If Lucy did not understand the information provided by Dr. Ruiz (if stage one of the IMS Model is not effectively employed), she would likely not believe that untreated diabetes and hypertension are serious threats to her health. She may also not believe that she must take her medications and change her diet and physical activity level to remain healthy. Dr. Ruiz would need to motivate Lucy to adhere by helping her accept the seriousness of her conditions and recognize the efficacy of treatment. She can do so by prompting Lucy to discuss her beliefs and any negative attitudes that she may have about her treatment. Once Lucy believes that the benefits of adhering outweigh her concerns, Dr. Ruiz can work with Lucy to state a firm commitment to focus her efforts on adhering to the treatment, and Dr. Ruiz can provide encouragement to build Lucy's sense of her own capability and efficacy in caring for herself.

Stage Three: Creating a Feasible Strategy for Attaining Patient Adherence

A third key obstacle for achieving patient adherence is that patients sometimes lack a workable strategy for following their prescribed treatments. Lucy is preoccupied with worrying about her husband's illness and needs. She does not know how she will incorporate into a manageable daily routine the many tasks—including taking her medications on schedule, checking her blood sugar level before and after each meal, buying fresh vegetables, and cooking healthy meals instead of those that are typical for her Hispanic culture. She worries that she cannot go out for walks, tend to her housekeeping, and care for her husband. In addition, she has a very limited financial budget and is not sure that she can afford three expensive elements of her treatment: the device for checking her blood sugar level, her medications, and healthy food options. Lucy is also uncertain about her ability to remember to test her blood sugar throughout the day and to take the correct medication at the accurate time.

Dr. Ruiz can try to help Lucy address all of her concerns by first assessing all of the resources that are available to Lucy. Upon asking Lucy about close relatives, Dr. Ruiz would learn that Lucy has two adult children who live fairly nearby. She could then ask about Lucy's willingness to ask her children for assistance with bringing her groceries or helping her care for her husband, and Dr. Ruiz would realize that Lucy can potentially obtain considerable social support from her children. With regard to taking her medications, Dr. Ruiz, or her nurse, could write out a simple schedule in Spanish for when to take which medications, and Lucy could place it on her refrigerator. Dr. Ruiz could also suggest that Lucy keep the device for measuring her blood sugar levels in the kitchen where she typically eats her meals. Moreover, she could inform Lucy of financial assistance programs or discount programs where she can sign up to obtain medications and medical equipment at either no cost or at reduced prices. Dr. Ruiz or members of her team could also provide Lucy with ideas for how to adjust her current cooking style to one that slowly introduces healthier options to her traditional cuisine. Lastly, Dr. Ruiz or the team could assist Lucy with finding the best times throughout the week when she can go out for a walk and achieve the goal of increased physical activity. A general summary of the suggested care for vulnerable patients using the IMS Model is provided in Table 20-1.

Table 20-1. Adherence challenges for vulnerable patients and potential solutions using the IMS Model©.

Model Component	Challenges	Suggested Care
Information: Patients need to *know what to do* to adhere.	Low health literacy, low education level, and language barriers can severely challenge adherence. Patients may have limited understanding of the treatment regimen but remain reluctant to ask questions.	Physicians should thoroughly explain the treatment in terms the patient can understand, utilizing medical team members to work with the patient. Providers should use a communication feedback loop, having patients express their understanding while physicians clarify any confusion. Medical translators should always be present when needed.
Motivation: Patients need to *want to adhere.*	Ethnic minority patients may experience culture-based obstacles to adherence. They may have difficulty believing in the importance of adhering and reconciling their cultural beliefs with the treatment plan.	Physicians should allow patients to express their concerns and negative attitudes about the treatment. Physicians should listen, be culturally sensitive, and help patients to understand the reality of their conditions, the efficacy of the treatment, and their capability to adhere.
Strategy: Patients need help to *be able to adhere.*	Patients of low socioeconomic status may lack necessary resources and have difficulty affording their medications and medical devices. They may have many competing demands on their time, and many practical limitations that stand in the way of adhering.	Physicians should offer patients information about sources of financial assistance for their medication, and help them determine how to draw on the social support resources available to them. Physicians should address all patient barriers for implementing their treatment regimen.

CONCLUSIONS

The IMS Model asserts that patient knowledge, belief in and commitment to a treatment, and capability to adhere are essential for maximizing adherence. Nonadherence is a multifaceted problem and addressing it requires the involvement of health care providers, patients, and the other individuals who are a part of a patient's social support network. The implementation of the three components of the IMS Model can have a positive influence on the process of care for all patients, particularly those who are most vulnerable, and can improve the physician–patient relationship, communication quality, and favorable health outcomes.

SUGGESTED READINGS

Cutler DM, Everett W. Thinking outside the pillbox- medication adherence as a priority for health care reform. *NEJM* 2010; 362(17):1553–1555. PMID: 20375400.

DiMatteo MR, Haskard-Zolnierek K, Martin LR. Improving patient adherence. A three-factor model to guide practice. *Health Psychol Rev* 2012;6(1):74-91. DOI:10.1080/17437199. 2010.537592

DiMatteo MR, Haskard-Zolnierek K, Williams SL. Health beliefs, disease severity, and patient adherence. A meta-analysis. *Med Care* 2007;45(6):521–528. PMID: 17515779.

Haskard-Zolnierek KB, DiMatteo MR. Physician communication and patient adherence to treatment. *Med Care* 2009;47(8): 826–834. PMID: 19584762.

ACKNOWLEDGMENTS

Supported by a Robert Wood Johnson Foundation Investigator Award in Health Policy Research (PI: M. Robin DiMatteo) and by the Committee on Research of the U.C. Riverside Academic Senate.

Tobacco Use

Nancy A. Rigotti, MD

INTRODUCTION

Cigarette smoking is the leading preventable cause of death in the United States, responsible for an estimated 443,000 deaths per year, or one in every five deaths. Physicians often care for the health consequences of their patients' tobacco use, and it is equally important for them to prevent smoking-related disease. There is no safe level of tobacco use. Smoking as few as one to four cigarettes per day increases the risk of myocardial infarction and cardiovascular mortality. Smoking cigarettes with reduced tar and nicotine content does not protect against the health hazards of smoking. Smoking cessation treatment is one of the most cost-effective actions available to clinicians.

The prevalence of cigarette smoking in the United States rose rapidly in the first half of the twentieth century and peaked in 1965, when 40% of adult Americans smoked cigarettes. Since then, smoking prevalence has been cut in half, reaching 19% of adults in 2011. This dramatic decline reflects growing public awareness of the health risks of tobacco and decades of public health efforts to discourage tobacco use. More recently, smoking prevalence has stabilized but the pattern of tobacco use has changed. Twenty percent of current smokers do not smoke every day, and the average smoker smokes only 15 cigarettes daily. Combining cigarette smoking with other tobacco products, especially smokeless tobacco, is increasingly reflecting the impact of expanding restrictions on places where smoking is allowed. The rising cost of cigarettes has led increasing number of smokers to use small cigars that have lower tobacco excise taxes and to buy tobacco in bulk and roll their own cigarettes.

Tobacco smoking starts during childhood and adolescence. Nearly 90% of smokers begin to smoke before the age of 18 years and 99% start by the age of 26 years. The rates of tobacco use in men and women, once very different, are now similar, with 16.5% of adult women and 21.6% of adult men smoking cigarettes in 2011. In the United States, smoking is more closely linked to education than it is to age, race, occupation, or any other sociodemographic factors. Educational attainment is a marker for socioeconomic status, and these data indicate that smoking is a problem that is concentrated in lower socioeconomic groups. Smoking is also more prevalent among individuals with comorbid psychiatric disorders and substance abuse disorders.

HEALTH CONSEQUENCES OF TOBACCO USE

Cigarette smoking increases overall mortality and morbidity rates and is a cause of cardiovascular disease (including myocardial infarction and sudden death), cerebrovascular disease; peripheral vascular disease; chronic obstructive pulmonary disease; and cancers at many sites, including the lung, larynx, oral cavity, esophagus, bladder, kidney, pancreas, and uterine cervix. Approximately 30% of tobacco-related deaths are due to cardiovascular disease. Lung cancer, once a rare disease, increased dramatically during the twentieth century, becoming the leading cause of deaths due to cancer among men in 1955 and among women in 1986. Lung cancer incidence is now declining among both men and women, reflecting the decline in smoking prevalence by US adults that occurred decades earlier.

Smoking is associated with many pregnancy complications, especially low birth weight (<2500 g). This is primarily attributable to intrauterine growth retardation (IUGR), although smoking in pregnancy also increases the risk of preterm delivery. Other adverse pregnancy outcomes linked to smoking are miscarriage (spontaneous abortion) and stillbirth. Smoking during pregnancy affects children even after birth. Sudden infant death syndrome is two to four times more common in infants born to mothers who smoked during pregnancy. Cognitive deficits and developmental problems in childhood are also linked to maternal smoking during pregnancy.

Cigarette smoking also increases a woman's risk of postmenopausal osteoporosis and fracture. Smokers have higher rates of upper and lower respiratory infections, diabetes, peptic ulcer disease, cataracts, macular degeneration, and sensorineural hearing loss than nonsmokers. Smokers have more prominent skin wrinkling than nonsmokers, independent of sun exposure. Smoking causes the majority of residential fire deaths.

The health hazards of smoking are not limited to those who smoke. Nonsmokers are harmed by exposure to the smoke produced by nearby smokers, a phenomenon called secondhand smoke (SHS). According to the 2006 US Surgeon General's Report, there is no safe level of exposure to SHS. The children of parents who smoke have more serious respiratory infections during infancy and childhood, more respiratory symptoms, and a higher rate of chronic otitis media and asthma than the children of nonsmokers. Among adults, chronic SHS exposure increases a nonsmoker's risk of lung cancer and coronary heart disease. An estimated 3400 lung cancer deaths and 69,000 heart disease deaths in US nonsmokers are attributable to SHS exposure. Even after tobacco smoke has dissipated it leaves a residual of chemicals on clothing and surfaces in the area where tobacco was smoked. This phenomenon, called thirdhand smoke, allows for even more prolonged exposure to tobacco toxins.

Van Gogh Skull with a Burning Cigarette. http://commons.wikimedia.org/wiki/File%3AVan_Gogh_Skull_with_a_burning_cigarette.jpg Attribution: Vincent van Gogh [Public domain], via Wikimedia Commons HTML. Attribution not legally required.

HEALTH BENEFITS OF SMOKING CESSATION

Smoking cessation has health benefits for men and women of all ages, even for those who stop smoking after the age of 65 years or who quit after the development of a smoking-related disease. Smoking cessation decreases the risk of lung and other cancers, heart attack, stroke, chronic lung disease, and peptic ulcer disease. After 10–15 years of abstinence, overall mortality rates for smokers approach rates of those who never smoked. The risk reduction for cardiovascular disease occurs more rapidly than the risk reduction for lung cancer or overall mortality. Half of the excess risk of cardiovascular mortality is eliminated in the first year of quitting, whereas for lung cancer, 30–50% of the excess risk is still evident 10 years after quitting and some excess risk remains after 15 years.

The benefits of stopping smoking translate into a longer life expectancy for former smokers compared with continuing smokers. Smokers who benefit the most are those who quit when they are younger, have fewer pack-years of tobacco exposure, and are free of smoking-related disease. The health benefits of smoking cessation far exceed any risks from the small weight gain that occurs with cessation.

SMOKING BEHAVIOR

Cigarettes and other tobacco products are addictive because they contain nicotine, a drug that creates tolerance and physical dependence in habitual users with symptoms of nicotine withdrawal when smoking stops. Nicotine withdrawal symptoms include: (1) cravings for a cigarette; (2) irritability; (3) restlessness; (4) anger and impatience; (5) difficulty concentrating; (6) anxiety; (7) depressed mood; (8) excessive hunger; and (9) sleep disturbance. These symptoms begin within a few hours of the last cigarette, are strongest during the first 2–3 days after quitting, and gradually diminish over a month or more. Other than craving for a cigarette, the symptoms are nonspecific, and many smokers fail to recognize them as nicotine withdrawal. The severity of nicotine withdrawal is variable across smokers and is related to the level of prior nicotine intake. Smokers who smoke more than 20 cigarettes daily or smoke their first cigarette within 30 minutes of awakening are likely to suffer from nicotine withdrawal symptoms when they try to quit.

The discomfort of nicotine withdrawal is one reason smokers fail in their efforts to stop. However, the attractiveness of smoking is attributable to more than nicotine dependence. Smoking is also a habit, a behavior that has become an integral part of a daily routine. Smokers come to associate cigarettes with enjoyable activities, such as finishing a meal or having a cup of coffee. These actions trigger the desire for a cigarette in smokers who are trying to quit. Smokers also use cigarettes to cope with stress and negative emotions, such as anger, anxiety, loneliness, or frustration. Quitting smoking represents the loss of a valuable coping tool for many smokers.

SMOKING CESSATION

Over half of the living Americans who have ever smoked have now quit smoking. According to surveys, 70% of the remaining smokers would like to stop smoking and half of them tried to do so in the past year. However, most quit attempts fail, in part because only one in three smokers trying to quit use any assistance when quitting, despite the existence of effective treatments that improve the success rate of a quit attempt.

Approximately 25% of smokers who use state-of-the-art treatment are not smoking 1 year after their quit attempt, though many more smokers quit for a short time and then relapse. Most relapse occurs in the first week of a quit attempt. In contrast, only 6% of smokers who try to quit without assistance succeed for 1 year. Behavioral scientists regard smoking cessation to be a learning process rather than an action requiring a discrete episode of will power. Smokers learn from mistakes made during a prior attempt at quitting, thereby increasing the likelihood that the next attempt will succeed. Psychologists have identified a series of cognitive stages through which smokers pass as they move toward nonsmoking: (1) initial disinterest in quitting; (2) thinking about health risks and contemplating quitting; (3) preparing to quit in the near future; (4) currently taking action to stop smoking; and (5) maintained nonsmoking (see Chapter 19).

Surveys of former smokers reveal how and why they stop smoking. Fear of illness is the reason most often cited. However, awareness of health risks alone is not sufficient to motivate smoking cessation. Over 90% of current smokers know that smoking is harmful to their health, yet they continue to smoke. Many smokers rationalize that they are immune to the health risks of smoking until these risks become personally salient. Current symptoms (e.g., cough, breathlessness, and chest pain), even if they represent minor illness rather than the onset of a smoking-related disease, stimulate change in smoking behavior more powerfully than does fear of future disease. Illness in a family member may also motivate smoking cessation. The price of cigarettes and the social unacceptability of smoking are other frequently cited reasons.

SMOKING CESSATION METHODS

Evidence-based clinical guidelines for smoking cessation were released by the US Public Health Service in 2000 and updated in 2008 (http://www.ahrq.gov/professionals/clinicians-providers/guidelines-recommendations/tobacco/clinicians/update/treating_tobacco_use08.pdf). These guidelines identify two methods, psychosocial counseling and pharmacotherapy, as having strong evidence of efficacy. Each is effective individually, but combining the two produces higher cessation rates. There is no strong evidence to support the efficacy of hypnosis or acupuncture for smoking cessation.

Psychosocial Support

Effective psychosocial support provides smokers with both practical behavior change strategies and also support and encouragement as part of treatment. Cognitive behavioral treatment methods address the barriers to quitting smoking that are rooted in habit. These methods are effective in aiding smoking cessation. In a typical program, smokers monitor their cigarette intake to identify the things that trigger the smoking, change their habits to break the link between the trigger and smoking, and learn to anticipate and handle the urges to smoke when they occur. The counselor also provides social support to bolster the smoker's confidence in the ability to stop smoking.

Psychosocial support was originally developed for delivery in individual or group settings. To broaden the reach of behavioral treatment, in-person methods were adapted for delivery by telephone and found to be effective. Cognitive behavioral treatment techniques can also be packaged into booklets or videotapes for use at home. These techniques have also been adapted for delivery using newer communication tools, including websites, text messaging, mobile phone applications, and social media. Most of these programs are new and their effectiveness is not yet demonstrated.

Pharmacological Treatment

Seven products have been approved by the US Food and Drug Administration (FDA) as smoking cessation aids and rated as first-line drugs by the US Public Health Service tobacco treatment guidelines (Table 21-1). These include five nicotine replacement products, bupropion (an atypical antidepressant), and varenicline, a nicotine receptor partial agonist. Nortriptyline and clonidine have also shown efficacy for smoking cessation in clinical trials but have not been submitted for approval by the FDA for this indication and are considered second-line drugs by the US Public Health Service guideline panel.

Nicotine Replacement Therapy

The rationale of nicotine replacement therapy (NRT) is to supply nicotine in a form other than a cigarette to block the symptoms of nicotine withdrawal. Nicotine replacement permits the smoker to break the smoking habit first and begin to taper off nicotine. Five forms of

Table 21-1. Pharmacotherapy for smoking cessation.*

Name	Dosage per Day	Recommended Duration of Use
Nicotine Replacement Products		
Transdermal nicotine patch	1 patch/24 h 21 mg (smoke ≥10 cig/d) 14 mg (smoke <10 cig/d)	8–12 weeks
Nicotine gum	9-12 pieces/d 2 mg (smoke < 25 cig/d) 4 mg (smoke ≥ 25 cig/d)	
Nicotine lozenge	9 pieces/d (max 20) 2 mg (smoke 1st cig >30 min after waking) 4 mg (smoke 1st cig < 30 min after waking)	3 months
Nicotine nasal spray	1–2 doses/h (min 8/day, max 40/day)	3–6 months
Nicotine inhaler	6-16 cartridges/day	3–6 months
Bupropion SR	150–300 mg/day‡	3–6 months
Varenicline	1mg BID#	3–6 months

*Products approved by the U.S. FDA as smoking cessation aids. †Chew as needed or one piece every 1–2 h while awake
‡Start 1-2 weeks before quit day. Use 150 mg/day for 3–5 days then 150 mg twice a day.
Start 1-3 weeks before quit date. Up titration of dose: 0.5 mg/day for 3 days, 0.5 mg twice daily for 4 days, then 1 mg twice daily

nicotine replacement are approved for use in the United States. Nicotine in the form of a gum, a transdermal skin patch, and an oral lozenge are sold without prescription. A nicotine nasal spray and an oral inhaler are prescription-only products. Of all these products, the nicotine patch produces the most constant blood level of nicotine, a substantially different pattern from the fluctuating nicotine levels produced by cigarette smoking. The gum, lozenge, inhaler, and nasal spray produce nicotine levels that vary more than the patch but less than smoking a cigarette. They provide more control over nicotine level. The nicotine supplied by the gum, patch, or nasal spray is sufficient to reduce nicotine withdrawal symptoms, but does not reproduce the rapid rise in nicotine blood levels that results from smoking a cigarette.

Randomized, placebo-controlled trials demonstrate that nicotine gum, patch, lozenge, inhaler, and nasal spray all reduce symptoms of nicotine withdrawal at approximately double the rates of smoking cessation compared with placebo. Combining the patch with another NRT product is safe and more effective than using a single NRT product. The effectiveness of all products depends on the instruction and counseling that accompany it. This is particularly true for the gum, nasal spray, and inhaler, which require careful instruction for proper use. Adherence is less of a problem with the nicotine patch. Any NRT product is more effective if used with some behavioral smoking cessation support. Clinicians should refer smokers to these resources when they recommend or prescribe NRT products.

Nicotine replacement is safe to use in smokers with stable coronary artery disease. There are no data on its safety for use in smokers with unstable cardiovascular disease (myocardial infarction in the past 2 weeks, unstable angina, or life-threatening ventricular arrhythmias), although it is clearly safer than continuing to smoke. Nicotine does increase heart rate and blood pressure, causes vasoconstriction, and is thrombogenic. However, a smoker who substitutes NRT for cigarettes avoids exposure to carbon monoxide and to oxidant gases generated by burning tobacco.

TRANSDERMAL NICOTINE PATCH

The nonprescription nicotine patch contains a reservoir of nicotine that is released at a fixed dose and is absorbed through the skin. On the morning of the quit day, the smoker applies the first patch and removes it 24 hours later. A new patch is applied to rotating skin sites each morning afterward for 2–3 months, although there is evidence that prolonging use beyond 3 months produces better long-term results. Smokers who smoke 10 or more cigarettes (half of a pack) daily start with the 21-mg patch; lighter smokers start with the 14-mg patch. After 4–6 weeks, the smokers progressively switch to a lower dose patch. The most common side effect is local skin irritation, which rarely requires discontinuation of treatment and can often be managed with topical steroids. Vivid dreams or insomnia can be managed by removing the patch at bedtime. Long-term dependence on the nicotine patch rarely occurs.

NICOTINE GUM

Nicotine gum is available without prescription in 2-mg and 4-mg strengths and in several flavors. Smokers who smoke more than 25 cigarettes daily use the 4-mg gum; all others use the 2-mg gum. Proper chewing technique is essential for the nicotine released by chewing to be absorbed through the oral mucosa as intended, rather than being swallowed. The gum should not be chewed like regular gum. Initially, it should be chewed only long enough to release the nicotine, producing a peppery taste, and then placed between the gums and buccal mucosa to allow for nicotine absorption. When the taste disappears, the gum is chewed again until the taste reappears, then "parked" again. After 30 minutes, it is discarded. The smoker should not eat or drink while the gum is in the mouth, and should avoid beverages, especially acidic beverages (e.g., coffee) for 30 minutes of gum use. Common side effects include those related to nicotine (nausea, dyspepsia, hiccups, dizziness) and to chewing (sore jaw, mouth ulcers). The product is approved for use as needed to handle urges to smoke, but its onset of action is slower than smoking. Most patients chew fewer than the recommended 9–12 pieces daily. Consequently, many experts use fixed-dose schedules (e.g., chewing one piece for the first 30 minutes of every hour) to achieve blood nicotine levels adequate to prevent withdrawal. It is used for 3 months. Long-term dependence on the gum is uncommon.

NICOTINE LOZENGE

A nicotine lozenge whose pattern of nicotine delivery resembles the gum is sold without prescription in 2-mg and 4-mg doses. Smokers whose first cigarette of the day is smoked within 30 minutes of awakening should use the 4-mg dose; others use the 2-mg dose. In randomized controlled trials, it doubles cessation rates compared with a placebo lozenge. It is placed in the mouth between cheek and gum. Nicotine in the lozenge is gradually absorbed through the oral mucosa over 30–40 minutes. The user should not eat or drink when the tablet is in the mouth. The lozenge differs from the gum in that no chewing is required, making it easier to use properly. People with dentures or poor dentition who generally cannot use the gum can use the lozenge. A smoker uses a lozenge as needed to control cravings, usually every hour or two, and uses it for 3–6 months. A mini-lozenge formulation that is smaller and dissolves more rapidly than the original nicotine lozenge is now available.

NICOTINE INHALER

The nicotine inhaler, sold only by prescription in the United States, is a handheld device containing nicotine in a plug that is vaporized when the smoker inhales. The nicotine is absorbed by the oral mucosa rather than in the lungs. Therefore, the inhaler delivers nicotine in a pattern similar to the gum or lozenge with peak nicotine levels reached 20 minutes after the start of use. The inhaler mimics the hand-to-mouth behavior of cigarette smoking, a feature that appeals to some smokers. The inhaler doubles the cessation rate compared to placebo in randomized trials. Side effects are minimal; throat irritation and cough are the most common.

NICOTINE NASAL SPRAY

Nicotine nasal spray is sold only by prescription. Nicotine is more rapidly absorbed from the nasal mucosa than it is through the oral mucosa, but less rapidly absorbed than through the lungs when a cigarette is smoked. The nicotine nasal spray doubles cessation rates compared with a placebo spray in randomized controlled trials, but has a high incidence of side effects (nose and throat irritation, watery eyes, sneezing, and cough). Careful instruction is required for its proper use. The dose is one spray in each nostril as needed; this delivers a dose of 1 mg of nicotine. It is used for 3–6 months.

Bupropion

Bupropion is an antidepressant with dopaminergic and noradrenergic activity. In its sustained-release form (Zyban, Wellbutrin SR), bupropion doubles smoking cessation rates compared with a placebo and is FDA approved for smoking cessation. The most serious side effect is a reduction in the threshold for seizure. The risk of seizure is 1 in 1000 patients or less, but the drug is contraindicated in patients with a seizure disorder or predisposition. Common side effects are insomnia, agitation, headache, and dry mouth. Doses of 150–300 mg/day for 7–12 weeks are effective for smoking cessation. The drug is started 1 week before the smoker's quit date to allow for blood levels to stabilize before quitting occurs. Bupropion reduces but does not eliminate weight gain after smoking cessation (see section below "Weight and Smoking Cessation"), but the effect disappears when the medication is stopped. Nonetheless, this effect may appeal to smokers who are concerned about postcessation weight gain.

Varenicline

Varenicline is a selective partial agonist at the $\alpha 4 \beta 2$ nicotinic receptor, the subtype of nicotine receptor in the brain that appears to mediate nicotine dependence. It is thought to have a dual mechanism of action. As a partial agonist, it partly relieves nicotine withdrawal symptoms. In addition, if a smoker using varenicline smokes a cigarette, the drug blocks the nicotine in cigarette smoke from binding to the nicotine receptor, thereby making smoking less rewarding. In randomized controlled trials comparing the drug with placebo and with bupropion, varenicline produced a higher long-term cessation rate than both and nearly tripled the cessation rate compared with placebo. Nausea is the most common side effect, occurring in nearly 30% of subjects in clinical trials. In practice, it can often be managed successfully by taking with food and a full glass of water. Varenicline is used for 12 weeks at a dose of 1-mg bid, starting with a 1-week gradual up-titration in dose to minimize nausea. The quit date should be set at least 1 week after starting the drug to allow blood levels to stabilize before quitting occurs, but delaying the quit date until 4 weeks after starting the drug might produce even better results.

Concerns about varenicline's safety appeared after the drug was marketed in 2008. In 2009, the FDA reviewed case reports for all smoking cessation drugs and reported that varenicline and bupropion, but not NRT, were "associated with reports of changes in behavior such as hostility, agitation, depressed mood, and suicidal thoughts or actions." Bupropion and varenicline were both required to add boxed warnings about this to their labels. So far, an association between varenicline and behavior changes has not been observed in randomized clinical trials or observational studies of smokers starting varenicline. In 2011, the FDA reaffirmed their position that the benefits outweigh the risks in most cases. An association of varenicline with an increased incidence of cardiovascular outcomes such as heart attack was observed in one meta-analysis, but not in the second one. In both studies, the absolute risk of an adverse cardiovascular event was very low, with or without varenicline. Clinicians who prescribe varenicline should monitor patients' behavior and mood, especially those with current or past psychiatric diagnoses. Combination NRT is an alternative for individuals in whom varenicline is considered potentially risky.

Nortriptyline and Clonidine

Nortriptyline, a tricyclic antidepressant, has demonstrated efficacy for smoking cessation in randomized controlled trials. A meta-analysis found that its efficacy resembled that of the atypical antidepressant bupropion. Nortriptyline is not FDA approved as a smoking cessation aid. Hypotension and dry mouth are the most common side effects. There is no evidence to support the use of any other antidepressants or any antianxiety agents for smoking cessation.

Clonidine, a centrally acting α-adrenergic agonist, is used to treat craving for psychoactive drugs other than nicotine. In randomized, placebo-controlled trials, both oral and transdermal clonidine reduced withdrawal symptoms and increased rates of cessation. Clonidine is not FDA approved for smoking cessation, and side effects (sedation, dizziness, and dry mouth) generally limit its use in practice.

BARRIERS TO SMOKING CESSATION

Weight & Smoking Cessation

Smokers weigh 5–10 lb less than nonsmokers of comparable age and height. When smokers quit, 80% of them gain weight. The average weight gain of 10–15 lb (4.6–6.8 kg) poses a minimal health risk, especially when compared with the benefits of smoking cessation. Women and heavier smokers (>25 cigarettes per day) gain more than men and lighter smokers. The mechanism is incompletely understood, but a nicotine-related decrease in metabolic rate and possibly increases in food intake appear to be largely responsible. The best approach to the problem may be to help smokers accept a small weight gain and reassure them that the expected amount is less than they may fear. A vigorous exercise program reduces postcessation weight gain and promotes cessation. Smokers who use nicotine gum or bupropion gain less weight than those who quit with a placebo and this may help weight-concerned smokers to make a quit attempt.

Social Support

Smokers with nonsmoking spouses are more likely to quit than smokers whose partners smoke. Smokers whose efforts to stop are supported by partners, family, and friends are more likely to succeed than smokers without this support. Those who live with smokers can ask them to restrict smoking to outdoor areas to provide a smoke-free home. Formal cessation programs provide an additional source of social support that can be valuable when a smoker's own environment is not supportive of quitting.

Depression and Other Psychiatric Disorders

Stopping smoking represents a loss for many smokers. Cigarettes have been reliable "companions" as well as coping tools. Transient sadness is common and requires no special treatment. Acknowledgment that this is normal can be helpful. There is, however, a strong association between smoking and mood disorders. Smokers have more depressive symptoms than nonsmokers and are more likely to have a history of major depression. Depressed smokers are less likely to stop smoking than nondepressed smokers, but smoking cessation treatments appear to work in smokers with mood disorders. Early evidence suggests that adding a mood management component to standard treatment might increase treatment success. Clinicians should be alert to the possibility of depression in smokers. If present, it should be treated concurrently with tobacco use. Smokers with a history of depression should be watched for the reemergence of symptoms during smoking cessation.

Substance Use

There is a high rate of smoking among individuals who abuse alcohol, cocaine, heroin, and prescription opioids. As with depression, substance abuse should be considered as a potential comorbid disorder in smokers who repeatedly try and fail to quit. Even among smokers who do not abuse alcohol, drinking is frequently an ingredient in relapse situations. Smokers attempting to quit are commonly advised to avoid alcohol temporarily after quitting.

THE PHYSICIAN'S ROLE

Because smoking begins early in life, preventing young people from starting is a task for physicians who care for children and adolescents. The challenge for physicians taking care of adults is smoking cessation. Physicians have the opportunity to intervene with smokers, because each year they see an estimated 70% of the smokers in the United States. They also see smokers at times when their symptoms have caused them to be concerned about their health and, therefore, more likely to be willing to change their smoking behavior. For example, one-third of smokers stop smoking after a myocardial infarction; this can be increased with brief counseling by a physician or nurse. For women, pregnancy encourages smoking cessation. Approximately 30% of female smokers stop smoking while pregnant, although many resume smoking after delivery. Other smoking-related conditions may also provide "teachable moments" when smokers are more receptive to advice to stop smoking.

Providing brief advice to stop smoking to all patients seen in the office increases patients' rates of smoking cessation. Although advice alone is effective, randomized controlled trials in general medicine and family practices have demonstrated that supplementing advice with brief counseling in the office is more effective. Counseling smokers in an office practice is as or more cost-effective than other accepted medical practices. Brief interventions prompt smokers to attempt to quit, and physicians should then make sure that smokers attempting to quit are linked to effective treatment.

SMOKING CESSATION COUNSELING STRATEGY FOR OFFICE PRACTICE

Evidence-based clinical guidelines for smoking cessation treatment by primary care providers recommend that the primary care of adults should include a routine assessment of smoking status in all patients, strong advice to all smokers to quit, assessment of a smoker's readiness to quit, assistance for those smokers who are ready to stop, and follow-up for all smokers. The guidelines have been organized into a five-step protocol for use in office practice (Table 21-2).

Table 21-2. Smoking cessation counseling protocol for physicians.

1. **ASK**—about smoking at every visit: "Do you smoke?"
2. **ADVISE**—every smoker to stop.
   a. Make advice clear: "Stopping smoking now is the most important action you can take to stay healthy."
   b. Tailor advice to the patient's clinical situation (symptoms or family history).
3. **ASSESS**—readiness to quit: "Are you interested in quitting?"
4. **ASSIST**—the smoker in stopping smoking.
   a. For smokers ready to quit
      (1) Ask smoker to set a quit date within 4 weeks.
      (2) Offer pharmacotherapy.
      (3) Refer for psychosocial support to free telephone quitline (800-QUIT-NOW) or in-person counseling program. Especially recommended for smokers with other substance use, depression, poor social support for nonsmoking, or low self-confidence in the ability to quit.
   b. For smokers not ready to quit
      (1) Discuss advantages and barriers to cessation, from smoker's viewpoint.
      (2) Advise smoker to avoid exposing family members to passive smoke.
      (3) Indicate willingness to help when the smoker is ready.
      (4) Ask again about smoking at the next visit.
5. **ARRANGE**—follow-up visits.
   a. Make follow-up appointment 1–2 weeks after quit date.
   b. At follow-up, ask about smoking status.
   c. For smokers who have quit:
      (1) Congratulate!
      (2) Ask smoker to identify future high-risk situations.
      (3) Rehearse coping strategies for future high-risk situations.
   d. For smokers who have not quit:
      (1) Ask: "What were you doing when you had that first cigarette?"
      (2) Ask: "What did you learn from the experience?"
      (3) Ask smoker to set a new quit date.

Source: Adapted from the U.S. Public Health Service Guideline Treating Tobacco Use and Dependence (http://www.ahrq.gov/professionals/clinicians-providers/guidelines-recommendations/tobacco/clinicians/update/treating_tobacco_use08.pdf)

1. **ASK:** Someone on the clinical team should routinely ask all patients at every visit whether they smoke cigarettes and document smoking status in the health record.

2. **ADVISE:** Regardless of a smoker's degree of interest in quitting, it is the physician's responsibility to deliver clear advice to each smoker about the importance of stopping. The message should be strong and unequivocal; for example, "Quitting smoking now is the most important health advice I can give you." If appropriate, advice should be tailored to the clinical situation, either current symptoms or family history. For example, smokers can be informed that they will have fewer colds or less asthma if they stop smoking. Advice is more effective when phrased in a positive way; for instance, emphasizing the benefits to be gained from quitting rather than the harms of continuing.

3. **ASSESS:** Assess a smoker's interest in stopping. Categorizing smokers in this way is a clinically useful approach that helps the physician to determine which counseling strategy is appropriate and to set achievable goals. Although the clinician's overall goal is to assist the smoker to stop permanently, a realistic goal for a single office visit is to move the smoker to the next stage of readiness to stop.

4. **ASSIST:** Help the smoker quit. The physician's approach should vary according to the smoker's readiness.

   - *If the smoker is interested in quitting*, the physician should ask whether they are ready to set a "quit date," a date within the next 4 weeks when they will stop smoking. If so, the date should be recorded in the chart and on material given to them to take home. The physician should discuss with the patient what approach is most likely to be successful considering the smoker's level of nicotine dependence and past experience in trying to quit. Both behavioral treatment and pharmacotherapy should be offered. Behavioral treatment can be provided by referring the smoker for group, individual, or telephone counseling for smoking cessation. Free telephone counseling for smoking cessation is accessible nationwide by calling a central number (800-QUIT-NOW). The physician should be prepared to discuss the management of barriers to cessation if the smokers ask. More intensive treatment is indicated for smokers who have been unsuccessful in previous attempts. The options include referral to a formal smoking cessation program and pharmacotherapy. Smoking cessation programs provide intensive training in behavioral smoking cessation skills combined with social support from the counselor and other group members. Combinations of pharmacotherapy and

behavioral counseling are more effective than either one alone.

   - *For smokers not interested in quitting or not ready to set a quit date*, the physician should elicit the patient's views about the benefits and harms of smoking to the individual smoker. With this perspective, the physician can provide missing information about health risks and correct misconceptions about the process of smoking cessation. The discussion should focus on short-term benefits rather than distant risks, and the physician should be prepared to discuss common barriers to smoking cessation. The clinician should advise the smoker not to expose family members to passive smoke and suggest that help is available when they are ready to quit.

5. **ARRANGE:** Randomized trials have demonstrated that arranging follow-up visits to discuss smoking increases the success of physician counseling. Smokers should be asked to return shortly after the quit date to monitor progress; this is especially important for smokers using pharmacotherapy, so that side effects and nicotine withdrawal symptoms can be monitored.

   - *If smokers are not smoking at the follow-up visit*, they should be congratulated but warned that continued vigilance is necessary to maintain abstinence. The level of nicotine withdrawal symptoms should be assessed, and if indicated, treated by starting or increasing pharmacological treatment. To help prevent relapse, patients should be asked to identify future situations in which they anticipate difficulty remaining abstinent. The physician can help to plan and rehearse coping strategies for these times. Further follow-up visits or telephone calls should be offered.

   - *If the smoker has not been able to remain abstinent*, the physician's role is to redefine a failure into a partial success. The patient can be told that even 1 day without cigarettes is the first step toward quitting and be reminded that it takes time to learn to quit, just as it took time to learn to smoke. To help the patient learn from the experience, the physician should ask about the circumstances that preceded the first cigarette smoked after the quit date, what was learned from the experience that could be used for the next attempt to quit, and whether a new quit date should be set.

Health Care Systems

The responsibility for providing smoking cessation treatment in outpatient practice should not lie only with the physician. A system-level approach in which different members of the care team each have a specific role is effective and reduces the burden on the individual practitioner. In this model, the five tasks listed above are done collaboratively by different individuals with adequate training, institutional support, and reimbursement by health insurers. For example, a patient's smoking status can be assessed by a staff member in the clinic or hospital before the physician sees the patient and a reminder left in the medical record to prompt the physician to discuss smoking. The physician's prime role is to give advice to quit, assess readiness to quit, and direct the smoker to effective resources, such as medication, or community resources, such as telephone quitlines and formal cessation programs. Other personnel may assist the physician's efforts in referral and provide counseling and medication instruction.

SUGGESTED READINGS

Fiore MC, Baker TB. Treating smokers in the health care setting. *NEJM* 2011;365:1222–1231.

Fiore MC, Jaen CR, Baker TB, et al. *Treating Tobacco Use and Dependence: 2008 Update.* Clinical Practice Guideline. Rockville, MD: U.S. Department of Health and Human Services. Public Health Service, 2008.

Food and Drug Administration. *Public Health Advisory: FDA Requires New Boxed Warnings for the Smoking Cessation Drugs Chantix and Zyban.* http://www.fda.gov/Drugs/DrugSafety/PostmarketDrugSafetyInformationforPatientsandProviders/DrugSafetyInformationforHeathcareProfessionals/ucm169986.htm. Accessed January, 2014.

Hajek P, McRobbie HJ, Myers KE, Stapleton J, Dhanji AR. Use of varenicline for 4 weeks before quitting smoking: decrease in ad lib smoking and increase in smoking cessation rates. *Arch Intern Med* 2011;171(8):770–777.

Kruse GR, Kelley JH, Linder JA, Park ER, Rigotti NA. Implementation of an electronic health record care management system to improve tobacco treatment. *J Gen Intern Med* 2012;27(12):1690–1696. doi: 10.1007/s11606-012-2174-6. Epub August 4, 2012.

Prochaska JJ, Hilton JF. Risk of cardiovascular serious adverse events associated with varenicline use for tobacco cessation: Systematic review and meta-analysis. *BMJ* 2012;344(e2856):1–11. doi:10.1136/bmj.e2856.

Rigotti NA. Strategies to help a smoker struggling to quit. *JAMA* 201217;308(15):1573–1580 . doi: 10.1001/jama.2012.13043.

Rigotti NA, Clair C, Munafò MR, Stead LF. Interventions for smoking cessation in hospitalized patients. *Cochrane Database Syst Rev* 2012;(5):CD001837. doi: 10.1002/14651858.CD001837.pub3. Review.

Schroeder SA. A 51-year-old woman with bipolar disorder who wants to quit smoking. *JAMA* 2009;301:522–531.

Smith SS, McCarthy DE, Japuntich SJ, et al. Comparative effectiveness of 5 smoking cessation pharmacotherapies in primary care clinics. *Arch Intern Med* 2009;169:2148–2155.

U.S. Department of Health and Human Services. *The Health Consequences of Involuntary Exposure to Tobacco Smoke: A Report of the Surgeon General.* 2006.http://www.surgeongeneral.gov/library/reports/secondhandsmoke/index.html. Accessed July2013.

WEB SITES

Centers for Disease Control Web site. http://www.cdc.gov/tobacco (comprehensive web site of information about tobacco use, prevention, and cessation). Accessed January 2014.

U.S. National Cancer Institute Web site. http://www.smokefree.gov (tips for preparation, quitting, and staying quit). Accessed January 2014.

U.S. Public Health Service Tobacco Cessation Guideline Web site. http://www.ahrq.gov/professionals/clinicians-providers/guidelines-recommendations/tobacco/clinicians/update/treating_tobacco_use08.pdf (U.S. clinical guidelines). Accessed January 2014.

The National Alliance for Tobacco Cessation and the Mayo Clinic. http://www.becomeanex.org/ (A free web-based quit smoking program that includes detailed tips and advice from former smokers.) Accessed January 2014.

Obesity

Robert B. Baron, MD, MS

INTRODUCTION

Obesity is one of the most common problems in clinical practice. Defined as a body mass index (BMI) of greater than 30 kg/m^2, over 33% of adult Americans are obese. An additional 35% are overweight, with BMIs between 25 and 30 kg/m^2. Almost one-third of children are overweight or obese. Because obesity is at the center of chronic disease risk and psychosocial disability for millions of Americans, its prevention and treatment offer unique patient care and public health opportunities. If all Americans were to achieve a normal body weight, it has been estimated that the prevalence of diabetes would decrease by half, whereas hypertension, coronary artery disease, and various cancers would decrease by 10–20%.

Obesity is often one of the most difficult and frustrating problems in primary care for both patients and physicians. Considerable effort is expended by primary care providers and patients, often with little benefit. Weight-loss diets, for example, even in the best treatment centers, result in an average 5–10% reduction in body weight. This lack of clinical success has created a never-ending demand for new weight-loss treatments. Approximately, half of women and one-quarter of men are "dieting" at any one time, spending billions of dollars each year on diet books, diet meals, weight-loss classes, diet drugs, exercise programs, "fat farms," and other weight-loss aids. The challenge for health care providers is to identify those patients with obesity who are most likely to benefit medically from treatment and most likely to maintain weight loss, and to provide them with sound advice, skills for long-term lifestyle change, and support. For patients not motivated to attempt a weight-loss program, health providers must continue to be respectful and empathic and focus on other health concerns. Whenever possible, providers should emphasize prevention of obesity and further weight gain and the importance of physical fitness independent of body size.

DEFINITIONS

Obesity is defined as an excess of body fat. Body fat can be measured by several methods including total body water, total body potassium, bioelectrical impedance, and dual-energy X-ray absorptiometry. In clinical practice, however, obesity is best defined by the BMI—body weight divided by height squared (kilograms per square meter). The BMI correlates closely with measures of body fat and with obesity-related disease outcomes. According to the National Institutes of Health (NIH), an individual with a BMI lesser than 18.5 kg/m^2 is classified as underweight, 18.5–24.9 kg/m^2 as normal, 25.0–29.9 kg/m^2 as overweight, and greater than or equal to 30.0 kg/m^2 as obese. Obesity is further classified as class I (BMI 30–34.9 kg/m^2), class II (BMI 35–39.9 kg/m^2), and class III or extreme obesity (BMI $\geq$40 kg/m^2). The term "morbid obesity" is best avoided for those with class III obesity since obesity-related morbidity can occur at any obesity level.

PREVALENCE OF OBESITY

Globally the prevalence of obesity doubled between 1980 and 2008. According to the World Health Organization, in 2008 10% of men and 14% of women in the world were overweight, compared with 5% for men and 8% for women in 1980. The prevalence of overweight and obesity were highest in the Americas and lowest in South East Asia. (though there is emerging evidence that the BMI cut-off point in Asian populations for overweight should be 22 kg/m^2).

While overall the prevalence of obesity in the United States has increased dramatically over the last four decades in both adults and children differences between demographic groups are common. In women aged 40–59 years, for example, obesity is substantially more common in black and Hispanic women (52% and 47%, respectively) than in white women (36%). Similarly in teens, blacks and Hispanics (28% and 17.5%, respectively) have higher rates of obesity than whites (14.5%). Other subpopulations have dramatically increased rates of overweight and obesity. Eighty three percent of patients with mental illness, for example, are obese or overweight. Geographic differences in prevalence are also prominent in the United States. Obesity is more common in the southeastern United States than in other regions.

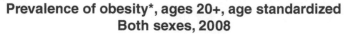

Prevalence of obesity*, ages 20+, age standardized
Both sexes, 2008

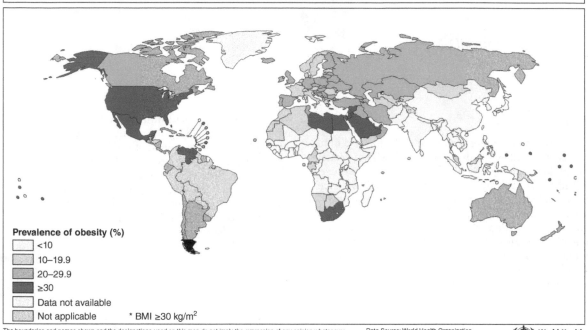

Prevalence of obesity (%)
- <10
- 10–19.9
- 20–29.9
- ≥30
- Data not available
- Not applicable   * BMI ≥30 kg/m²

The boundaries and names shown and the designations used on this map do not imply the expression of any opinion whatsoever on the part of the World Health Organization concerning the legal status of any country, territory, city or area or of its authorities, or concerning the delimitation of its frontiers or boundaries. Dotted lines on maps represent approximate border lines for which there may not yet be full agreement.

Data Source: World Health Organization
Map Production: Public Health Information
and Geographic Information Systems (GIS)
World Health Organization

World Health Organization

Global prevalence of obesity among adults aged 20 years and over. **World Health Organization** (http://www.who.int/about/licensing/en/).

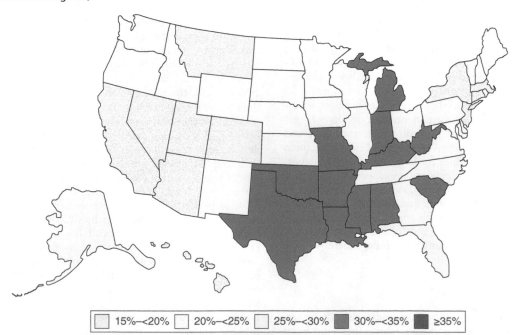

15%–<20%   20%–<25%   25%–<30%   30%–<35%   ≥35%

Prevalence of self-reported obesity among US adults (Behavioral Risk Factor Surveillance system, 2011). http://www.cdc.gov/obesity/data/adult.html

HEALTH CONSEQUENCES OF OBESITY

The relationship between body weight and mortality is curvilinear, similar to other cardiovascular risk factors. Most studies have demonstrated a J-shaped relationship, suggesting that the thinnest portion of the population also has an excess mortality. This is primarily due to the higher rate of cigarette smoking in the thinnest group except in the elderly, in whom malnutrition and being underweight is predictive of excess mortality independent of cigarette use. Recent analysis of the National Health and Nutrition Examination Study (NHANES) has suggested that overweight individuals may not have as much excess mortality as previously described and that the impact of obesity on mortality overall may be decreasing over time. Racial and ethnic factors may also impact the relationship of weight and mortality. In African Americans, the weight associated with the point of lowest mortality is greater than in whites, whereas in Asian Americans it is lower.

The increase in total mortality related to obesity results predominantly from coronary heart disease (CHD). Although it is not fully established that obesity is an "independent" risk factor for CHD, obesity is clearly an important risk factor for the development of many other CHD risk factors. Obese individuals aged 20–44 years, for example, have a three- to four-fold greater risk for type II diabetes, a five- to six-fold greater risk for hypertension, and twice the risk for hypercholesterolemia. The obese also have an increased risk for some cancers, including those of the colon, ovary, and breast.

As a result of these conditions, mortality from all causes for persons with class I obesity (BMI 30–34.9 kg/m^2) is 20% greater than for those with a normal BMI. Individuals with class II obesity, BMI 35–39.9 kg/m^2, have an 80% increase in mortality from all causes. Mortality for extreme obesity, although less well studied, is estimated to be at least double that of normal weight individuals.

Obesity is also associated with a variety of other medical disorders, including degenerative joint disease of weightbearing joints, diseases of the digestive tract (gallbladder disease, gastroesophageal reflux disease), thromboembolic disorders, cerebrovascular disease, heart failure (both systolic and diastolic), respiratory impairment including sleep apnea, and skin disorders. Obese patients also have a greater incidence of surgical and obstetric complications, are more prone to accidents, and are at increased risk of social discrimination. Several studies have also shown a rate of depression higher in the obese than in normal weight subjects and a higher rate of binge eating disorder.

In addition to the total amount of excess body fat, the location of the excess body fat (regional fat distribution) is a major determinant of the degree of excess morbidity and mortality due to obesity. Increased upper body fat (abdomen and flank) is independently associated with increased cardiovascular and total mortality. Body fat distribution can be assessed by a number of techniques. Measurements of skin folds (subscapular and triceps) reflect subcutaneous fat. Measurement of circumferences (waist and hip) reflect both abdominal and visceral fat. Computed tomography (CT) and magnetic resonance imaging (MRI) scans measure subcutaneous and visceral fat. Clinically, measurement of the waist and hip circumference is most useful, especially in individuals with BMI 25–35 kg/m^2. A circumference in men greater than 102 cm (>40 in.) and in women greater than 88 cm (>35 in.) can be used to identify individuals at increased risk of developing obesity-related health problems.

ETIOLOGY OF OBESITY

Numerous lines of evidence, including both epidemiologic studies of adoptees and twins and animal studies, suggest strong genetic influences on the development of obesity. In a study of 800 Danish adoptees, for example, there was no relationship between the body weight of adoptees and their adopting parents but a close correlation with the body weights of their biological parents. In a study of approximately 4000 twins, a much closer correlation between body weights was found in monozygotic than in dizygotic twins. In this study, genetic factors accounted for approximately two-thirds of the variation in weights. Studies of twins reared apart and the response of twins to overfeeding showed similar results. Studies of regional fat distribution in twins have also shown a significant (but not complete) genetic influence.

Genetic studies have confirmed a clear relationship between genetics and obesity in both animals and humans. In humans, at least 24 genetic disorders, such as the Prader–Willi syndrome, are associated with obesity. Studies suggest that genetic influences may impact both energy intake (control of appetite and eating behavior) and energy expenditure.

Differences in the resting metabolic expenditure (RME), for example, could easily result in considerable differences in body weight as RME accounts for approximately 60–75% of total energy expenditure. The RME can vary by as much as 20% between individuals of the same age, sex, and body build; such differences could account for approximately 400 kcal of energy expenditure per day. Recent evidence suggests that the metabolic rate is similar in family members, and, as expected, individuals with lower metabolic rates are more likely to gain weight. Differences in the thermic effect of food, the amount of energy expended following a meal, may also contribute to obesity. Although some investigators have shown a decreased thermic effect of food in the obese, others have not.

Environmental factors are also clearly important in the development of obesity. The "built environment" refers to the impacts of urban sprawl, traffic congestion, and the associated sedentary lifestyle of the population as people spend more time in cars and in gridlock driving to work or shopping. The US Centers for Disease Control (CDC) estimates that urban sprawl due to lack of adequate land use planning is associated with increases in obesity, cardiovascular disease, and type 2 diabetes (see Chapter 9). Decreased physical activity and food choices that result in increased energy intake also clearly contribute to the development of obesity. Medical illness can also result in obesity, but such instances account for less than 1% of the cases. Hypothyroidism and Cushing syndrome are the most common. Diseases of the hypothalamus can also result in obesity, but these are rare. Major depression, which more typically results in weight loss, can also present with weight gain. Consideration of these causes is particularly important when evaluating unexplained, recent weight gain. Numerous medications can also result in weight gain including antipsychotics such as clozapine, olanzapine, and risperidone, antidepressants such as amitriptyline and cyproheptadine, anticonvulsants such as valproate, carbamazepine, and gabapentin, and diabetic medications such as insulin and thiazolidinediones. Of note, each of these categories of medications includes drugs that do not cause weight gain. Weight gain is also common following smoking cessation. On average, patients gain 4–5 kg within 6 months of quitting smoking but some patients may gain much more.

PATIENT SELECTION FOR WEIGHT LOSS

The BMI should be measured and recorded at each clinical encounter. As with other clinical abnormalities, patients should be nonjudgmentally informed of their BMI and how it conforms to definitions of overweight and obesity. Patients who are told that they are overweight or obese by their clinician are more likely to classify weight as a health concern and have greater desire and more attempts to lose weight.

Weight loss is indicated to assist in the management of obesity-related conditions, particularly hypertension, diabetes mellitus (type II) and prediabetes, hyperlipidemia, and metabolic syndrome in any patient who is obese (BMI >30 kg/m^2). Many patients with BMI 25–30 kg/m^2 who have one of these conditions or significant psychosocial disability also often benefit from weight reduction.

Weight loss to prevent complications of obesity in patients without current medical, metabolic, or behavioral consequences of obesity is more controversial. In young and middle-aged individuals, particularly those with a family history of obesity-related disorders, treatment should be based on the degree of obesity and body fat distribution. Such individuals with upper body obesity (increased waist circumference) should be considered for treatment; those individuals with lower body obesity and no significant consequences of obesity can be reassured and monitored. Many such patients, however, desire weight loss for psychological, social, and cosmetic reasons. A careful discussion of the risks and benefits of weight loss in such instances helps patients make informed decisions about various weight-loss strategies.

A medical or psychosocial indication for weight loss is necessary but not sufficient to begin treatment. Treatment must be designed in the context of the patient's readiness to change. The Transtheoretical Model of Change, also commonly known as the Stages of Change Model, is a useful framework for helping patients to modify their behavior. Developed and applied initially in smoking cessation, the model has also been used to modify eating and exercise behavior. It defines behavior change as a process of identifiable stages including precontemplation, contemplation, preparation, action, maintenance, and relapse. By understanding the patient's stage of readiness to change, the clinician can work specifically with each patient to move him or her to the next stage (see Chapter 19).

Clinical assessment should also focus on how the current attempt compares with previous attempts; a realistic assessment of the patient's goals for the amount and rate of weight loss; the extent to which outside stressors, mood disorders, or substance abuse might impair the attempt; and the degree to which others can provide support. Patient readiness to change can be further assessed by requiring the patient to complete specific pretreatment assignments. For example, patients can be asked to complete a 3-day diet record and to submit an exercise plan that includes both the type of aerobic exercise the patient plans to begin and how the patient plans to fit it into his or her schedule. When obesity coexists with other significant psychiatric disorders, particularly depression, binge eating disorder, and substance abuse, treatment should initially be directed at the concurrent disorder.

DIET THERAPY

The goal of diet therapy for weight loss is to achieve a daily energy deficit whereby energy intake is less than energy expenditure. Daily energy expenditure can be estimated based on age, gender, and activity level. Two thousand calories (kcals) per day is often used as a reference level, but different individuals' requirements may vary by hundreds of calories per day. The goal of most weight-loss diets is to achieve an energy deficit of approximately 500 kcal/day. Since a pound of fat equals approximately 3500 kcal, this will result in approximately 1 lb of weight loss per week.

Meta-analysis of randomized studies of dietary therapy to achieve weight loss have demonstrated an average weight loss of 5–10% of the starting weight in patients followed for 3 months to 1 year. Follow-up for up to 5 years suggests average long-term weight loss of 2–4% of initial weight. Of note, all studies have a substantial variation of response. Some patients, approximately 20%, are able to lose substantially more weight and keep it off for longer periods of time. Studies of commercial weight-loss programs also demonstrate modest amounts of weight loss but with wide variations. Weight Watchers, for example, reports 3.2% weight reduction at 2 years.

The optimal composition for weight-loss diets has been the subject of numerous clinical trials and, of course, thousands of popular weight-loss books. Most nutrition guidelines such as the Dietary Guidelines for Americans, recommend a low-fat, high-fiber, "balanced" diet. This approach emphasizes consumption of a wide variety of foods to achieve a balanced mix of macronutrients, that is, 20–35% of total calories from fats, 45–65% of total calories from carbohydrates, and 10–35% of total calories from protein. These ranges are substantially wider than earlier federal guidelines and allow for flexibility in diet design. The DASH (Dietary Approaches to Stop Hypertension) Eating Plan, originally developed for treatment of hypertension, is an example of a balanced diet that meets these macronutrient ranges and is supported by federal guidelines. A Mediterranean-style diet can also be used to achieve an energy deficit for weight loss and remain within these ranges.

Numerous clinical trials have compared this balanced approach with low carbohydrate diets such as the Atkins Diet and South Beach Diet. These studies have consistently shown equivalent amount of weight loss independent of the macronutrient composition of the diet. Rather than nutrient composition, weight loss was predicted by adherence to the diet. Satiety, hunger, lipid levels, insulin levels, and other metabolic factors were also found to be equivalent despite large differences in macronutrient composition. Similar findings have been published with comparisons of the very low-fat Ornish diet, the Zone diet, and other diets with various combinations of macronutrients. Thus, patients can be reassured that almost any whole food diet can result in safe weight loss as long as the patient consistently follows the diet.

An important alternative in the dietary treatment of obesity is the use of safe and effective very low-calorie diets (VLCDs). Previously known as protein-sparing modified fasts and protein-formula liquid diets, these diets restrict calorie intake to less than or equal to 800 kcal/day. Patients ingest only prepackaged, often liquid, food that provides adequate protein, vitamins, and minerals. Additional intake is limited to 2–3 quarts of calorie-free beverages per day. The major advantage of these diets is the "complete removal of patients from the food environment" to facilitate short-term adherence. In addition, the significant energy deficit results in rapid weight loss, usually 2 lb/week, encouraging the patient to continue. Ongoing concerns about these diets include their cost, side effects, and long-term results. Clinical trials suggest that the use of 800-kcal VLCDs can lower cost and prevent most of the significant side effects associated with the lower-calorie (400–600) VLCDs, including gallstones and fluid and electrolyte disorders, with equal long-term efficacy.

As with standard diet therapy of obesity, VLCDs require adherence during the diet, and long-term nutritional and behavioral changes to maintain weight loss. Well-planned programs that combine VLCDs with nutrition education, behavior therapy, exercise, and social support report improved long-term results. For example, an average weight loss of 55 lb with 75% and 52% of the loss maintained at 1- and 2 1/2-year follow-up, respectively, and maintenance of an average of 24 lb after 2- to 3-year follow-up have been reported. Meta-analysis of published VLCD trials suggest that while initial weight loss is greater with VLCDs than standard diets, both approaches have equal long-term results. As with other approaches, however, there is a wide variation of response with VLCDs, and some patients can achieve long-term weight loss. Because of the quicker and greater amounts of weight loss, VLCDs may be particularly useful in situations in which rapid weight loss is clinically indicated such as preoperative treatment (joint replacement, transplant surgery, bariatric surgery) or for initial management of severe medical conditions (severe sleep apnea, poorly controlled diabetes, heart failure, or coronary artery disease).

Recent studies have helped elucidate predictors of long-term weight maintenance after diet therapy for weight loss. Most important has been information from the National Weight Control Registry. This cohort of individuals who have lost an average of 33 kg and maintained the loss for 5 years report consumption of low-calorie, low-fat diets averaging approximately 1400 cal/day; high levels of physical activity averaging 60 minutes/day; regular self-monitoring of body weight; eating breakfast daily; and maintaining consistent dietary patterns on weekdays and weekends.

HEALTH CONSEQUENCES OF DIETING & WEIGHT LOSS

Surprisingly, few studies have examined the effects of weight loss on morbidity and mortality. Studies examining the effect of weight loss on cardiovascular risk factors generally show beneficial changes with weight loss as predicted. Descriptive studies on mortality, however, show inconsistent results. Such descriptive studies are unable to clarify if changes in mortality are caused by the weight change, if disease or other factors that contribute to disease, such as cigarette smoking, cause weight loss, or if both are related to a third factor. No randomized trials of long-term effects of voluntary weight loss on mortality have been published.

Because so many Americans are dieting at any one time, and having so little long-term success, considerable interest has focused on the potential adverse effects of weight cycling ("yo-yo" dieting). Numerous adverse effects of weight cycling have been hypothesized, primarily from animal studies. These include making further weight loss more difficult, increasing total body fat and central obesity, increasing subsequent calorie intake, increasing food efficiency, decreasing energy expenditure, increasing levels of adipose tissue lipolytic enzymes and liver lipogenic enzymes, increasing insulin resistance, increasing blood pressure, and increasing blood cholesterol and triglyceride levels. Most experts currently feel that these phenomena occur inconsistently, if at all. Descriptive studies that have addressed this question by looking at the impact of weight fluctuations on CHD incidence, CHD mortality, and total mortality have shown mixed results.

There is also debate over whether weight-loss diets cause eating disorders or binge eating. Although a history of dieting often precedes the development of eating disorders, there is no evidence proving a causal link. In addition, approximately 50% of individuals with binge eating disorder report that binging preceded dieting. There is also some evidence to suggest that successful weight loss may reduce binge eating in the obese (see Chapter 23).

Thus, there is only indirect evidence suggesting that dieting has negative health effects. This remains an important question, however, and reinforces the idea that casual attempts at quick weight loss should be avoided. At present, however, committed attempts at long-term weight loss should not be discouraged because of adverse health effects or the potential of regaining weight.

Dieting also has a significant effect on energy balance both during and after weight loss. As every successful dieter has observed, the rate of weight loss slows during the course of dieting. Because this can be quite discouraging to the unwary patient (or uninformed health care provider), it is important to inform the patient prior to initiating a weight-loss diet that this is likely to occur. Weight loss is most rapid during the initial days of hypocaloric feeding due to changes in sodium and water balance caused by early loss of glycogen and protein (both contain water) and, depending on the degree of calorie deficit and type of diet, loss of sodium associated with ketonuria. Following this initial phase, weight loss depends on the extent of energy deficit. With time, however, the rate of weight loss slows again as the body's metabolic rate decreases and the energy deficit becomes smaller. This change in metabolic rate can be two to three times greater than that predicted from changes in body weight. The lower the energy content of the diet, the lower the metabolic rate. Although it was initially suggested that exercise occurring during a period of hypocaloric feeding could prevent this decrease in metabolic rate, recent studies have suggested that it has no direct effect during hypocaloric feeding (but exercise may increase the postdiet metabolic rate by preserving lean body mass).

Following the period of hypocaloric feeding (resumption of normal energy intakes), the resting metabolic rate increases, but to a level below that observed before beginning the diet. This reduction is in part a reflection of the loss of lean body mass and in part due to additional, poorly understood effects on energy metabolism. Overall energy expenditure is further reduced due to a decrease in the thermic effect of food (the individual eats less) and in differences in physical activity (it takes less energy to perform the same amount of activity for a smaller person). Thus, to maintain weight loss, individuals need to consume less energy than before dieting and increase energy expenditure by increasing the amount of physical activity.

EXERCISE

Exercise offers a number of significant advantages to patients attempting to achieve long-term weight loss. First and foremost, exercise increases energy expenditure, helping to create the energy deficit necessary for weight loss. Unfortunately, the amount of energy expended during most aerobic exercises (e.g., walking, jogging, and swimming) for the typical periods performed (30 minutes four to five times per week) is modest, approximately 1000–1500 kcal/week. Thus, exercise can be predicted to have little effect on short-term weight loss. Clinical trials reflect this modest effect: some studies demonstrate weight loss with exercise alone or extra weight loss when exercise plus diet is compared with diet alone, but other studies do not show such an effect. In a meta-analysis of 43 studies, exercise combined with diet lead to 1.1 kg greater weight loss than diet alone. Studies comparing high-intensity exercise to low-intensity exercise demonstrated a 1.5 kg greater weight loss.

The importance of exercise for successful maintenance of weight loss is more clearly established. As discussed above, an hour per day of exercise was one of the predictors of long-term weight maintenance in the National Weight Control Registry. In addition to the cumulative effect of increased energy expenditure, exercise affects the composition of the body substance lost during weight loss. When exercise is directly compared with diet, or when exercise plus diet is compared with diet alone, exercise results in greater preservation of lean body mass. That is, for each pound of weight lost, less fat and more muscle are lost during weight-loss programs without exercise. This is particularly important as the body's RME (a major portion of the total daily energy expenditure) is closely correlated with lean body mass.

The observation that much of the long-term effect of exercise is through preservation of lean body mass has resulted in an increased interest in the potential role of resistance training (e.g., weight lifting, and circuit training). Preliminary results suggest that resistance training during dieting does result in maintenance of lean body mass compared with the result from dieting alone. Thus, highly motivated patients can be instructed to add resistance training to their aerobic exercise program.

Regular aerobic exercise results in a number of other benefits to the obese patient, including improved cardiovascular training effect (increased exercise tolerance), decreased appetite (per calorie expended), a general sense of well-being, decreased blood pressure (in hypertensives), improved glucose metabolism and insulin action (in diabetics), improved blood lipids (in lipid disorders), and, in the long term, decreased mortality from cardiovascular disease and all other causes.

Young patients with mild-to-moderate obesity can be started directly on a regular aerobic exercise program. Patients are commonly instructed to select two exercises and to perform either one of them six times per week for 30–60 minutes/day. Patients are taught to take their pulse and to generate a sustained tachycardia at 70–80% of their maximum predicted heart rate. Sedentary patients, older patients, and patients with severe obesity are instructed to begin walking programs without initial concern about meeting target heart rates. In these patients, the focus is on frequency and duration, rather than intensity. As weight loss proceeds and patients become used to exercising regularly, they can be advanced to formal aerobic programs.

BEHAVIOR THERAPY & SOCIAL SUPPORT

Sustained weight loss requires long-term changes in eating and exercise behavior. Patients must learn specific skills to facilitate decreased calorie intake and increased energy expenditure. Behavior therapy, combined with diet and exercise, forms the core of the most standard "lifestyle modification" approaches to weight management. Behavior therapy can be implemented in groups or in individual therapy. Trained psychologists and dieticians commonly lead such efforts, but office-based clinicians can often learn to use many of the same techniques.

Intensity of interaction appears to be one of the predictors of success. In the highly successful Diabetes Prevention Project, for example, lifestyle modification was taught in 16 individual sessions over 24 weeks.

Meta-analysis of 36 studies of behavior therapy for weight loss showed that behavior therapy alone resulted in significantly greater weight loss, a decrease of 2.5 kg, than placebo. When behavior therapy was combined with diet and exercise and compared to diet and exercise alone, the combined treatment also resulted in greater weight loss in five of six studies. Two studies compared cognitive behavioral therapy (CBT) plus diet and exercise with diet and exercise alone. In these studies, the combined treatment lost 4.9 kg more.

Standard behavior therapy relies on specific techniques to teach the skills needed to change problematic behaviors.

1. Goal-setting: Patients are taught to set specific quantifiable, realistic goals at the outset of behavior therapy and during each week of therapy. Succeeding at meeting realistic goals creates a sense of self-efficacy and can reinforce further change.

2. Self-monitoring: Patients are taught to monitor both food and beverage intake and physical activity. Specific attention must be directed at teaching patients how to estimate portion sizes since patients may underestimate intake by 50%. The context, degree of hunger, and emotional state of each time of eating is also recorded. This may allow eating-related factors to be targets for modification. Patients are also instructed to record all programmed physical activity. Additional monitoring of physical activity can be done with pedometers.

3. Stimulus control: Patients are instructed to identify stimuli that increase the likelihood of both desired and undesired behaviors. Particular emphasis is placed on attempting to modify nonfood cues that are associated with eating. Similarly, simple techniques such as keeping certain problem food out of the house may be useful.

4. Cognitive skills: Patients are taught skills for problem solving and cognitive restructuring. Patients are asked to identify problems, consider potential solutions, list the advantages and disadvantages of each, select a feasible solution, and evaluate the results. Cognitive restructuring involves identification of dysfunctional thoughts that interfere with goals and replacing such thoughts with more rational ones. Formal CBT can also be used as part of weight management. Cognitive behavioral therapy places more emphasis on cognitive change, rather than behavioral change, as the primary focus of treatment.

Social support is an additional essential component for any successful weight-loss program. Most successful programs use peer group support. Diet partnerships and financial incentives are effective for some patients. Involvement of family members is also important. A comprehensive review of published results of weight-loss programs strongly suggests that close provider–patient contact is a better predictor of success than the particular weight-loss intervention.

MEDICATIONS FOR TREATMENT OF OBESITY

Medications for the treatment of obesity are widely available over the counter, via the Internet, and by physician prescription. A CDC survey suggested that 7% of Americans used nonprescription weight-loss drugs. Among young obese women and among those on prescription weight-loss medications the use of nonprescription weight-loss medications was 28.4% and 33.8%, respectively.

A variety of weight-loss medications are available by prescription in the United States. These include various amphetamines (Drug Enforcement Administration schedule II), benzphetamine and phendimetrazine (schedule III), and phentermine, diethylpropion, mazindol, and orlistat. Most obesity experts agree that there is no current role for the schedule II or III drugs. Orlistat, at half the prescription dose, is available for over-the-counter use in the United States. Two additional medications, lorcaserin and the combination of phentermine and topiramate were approved by the Food and Drug Administration (FDA) in 2012. Sibutramine was withdrawn from the market in the United States in 2010 due to a large randomized controlled study that showed a 16% increase in cardiovascular events in patients in the medication group.

Lorcaserin is a selective serotonin receptor agonist. In one randomized, year-long study of over 3000 adults, the medication resulted in an additional loss of initial weight of approximately 3.5% compared with placebo. Common adverse events include headache, dizziness, and nausea. Other concerns include attention and memory disturbances, depression, priapism, and serotonin syndrome. No increase in valvulopathy (as seen previously with other serotonin receptor agonists) has been reported. The medication is contraindicated in pregnancy.

A combination medication consisting of phentermine and topiramate, is also approved by the FDA for weight loss. A study of over 4000 subjects showed a 8.9% greater loss of initial weight than in patients on placebo. However, concerns persist about the increased heart rate seen in the group on medication and an increased incidence of cleft lip. Other side effects include mood disorders, increased suicidal thoughts, insomnia, impaired concentration, other cognitive dysfunction, paresthesia, dizziness, dysgeusia, constipation, and dry mouth. This medication is also contraindicated in pregnancy and is only available in certified pharmacies to facilitate careful postmarket monitoring.

Considerable controversy exists about the efficacy of and indications for these medications. Numerous clinical trials, some up to 2 years in duration, demonstrate statistically significant weight loss in subjects who take an obesity medication compared with placebo. Total loss of initial weight is modest, averaging about 5% greater than placebo. There is no convincing evidence that any one of these medications results in more weight loss than others. Although some studies also show improvement in obesity-related metabolic abnormalities (e.g., blood sugar, blood pressure, and lipids), these reductions are also small and are substantially less than those achieved with hypoglycemic, antihypertensive, or lipid-lowering medications. In addition, no studies have yet demonstrated that weight loss achieved with medications results in reductions in obesity-related mortality or cardiovascular disease outcomes.

The NIH guidelines state that the FDA-approved weight-loss drugs may be useful as an adjunct to diet and physical activity for patients with BMI greater than or equal to 27 kg/m^2 and obesity-related risk factors or diseases, and for any patient with BMI greater than or equal to 30 kg/m^2. Based on the modest efficacy noted above, however, these guidelines have not been widely implemented by clinicians. Prescriptions for weight-loss drugs should be limited to patients adhering to weight-loss diets and physical activity. In addition, weight loss in the first month of use correlates highly with weight loss at 12 months. Thus, for patients in whom no weight loss is achieved within the first month of use, weight-loss medications should be discontinued.

SURGERY FOR WEIGHT LOSS

Surgery for weight loss is typically considered the last resort for patients with severe obesity. The NIH guidelines state that weight-loss surgery may be an option for carefully selected patients with BMI greater than or equal to 40 or greater than or equal to 35 kg/m^2 with comorbid conditions. Such patients must be at high risk for obesity-related morbidity and mortality, must have failed medical therapy, must have stable psychiatric status, and must be fully committed to lifetime lifestyle changes.

In recent years, the use of surgery to treat obesity has grown substantially. With implementation of new techniques and the use of less invasive approaches, obesity surgery is now one of the fastest growing operations in the United States. A majority of procedures are now done laparoscopically and some are being done as an outpatient procedure.

Available surgical procedures include: malabsorptive procedures such as duodenal switch and biliopancreatic diversion; restrictive procedures such as vertical banded gastroplasty, adjustable gastric band, and sleeve gastrectomy; and combined procedures such as roux-en-Y gastric bypass. Most centers have avoided malabsorptive procedures, despite excellent weight loss, due to concerns of potential metabolic and nutritional sequelae analogous to those observed with jejuno-ileal bypass procedures in the past. Restrictive procedures, particularly the laparoscopic adjustable gastric band are gaining in popularity. Advantages include reduced perioperative morbidity and mortality compared to other procedures. Weight loss is less than other procedures, however, and intermediate and long-term complications are greater. Complications include prolapse of the stomach through the band, infected reservoir sites, heartburn and regurgitation, and severe esophagitis. Approximately one-third of banding procedures require conversion to a roux-en-Y bypass.

The roux-en-Y bypass is the most common bariatric procedure in the United States. Weight loss, approximately one-third of initial weight, is greater than with purely restrictive procedures. Serious perioperative complications are greater, however, and include bleeding and gastrojejunostomy leaks. Perioperative mortality occurs in 0.3% of cases, even in the best centers, and has been shown to be substantially higher in open procedures (compared to laparoscopic procedures), in patients with a history of thromboembolic disease, sleep apnea, and impaired functional status, and in older and sicker patients. Approximately 4% of patients will have early complications including deep venous thrombosis, surgical reintervention, or spend greater than 30 days in the hospital. Intentional weight loss of 5–10% of initial weight before weight loss surgery is associated with reduced perioperative complications.

Longer term complications include nutritional deficiencies of fat-soluble vitamins, especially vitamin D, iron, B_{12}, folate, and calcium. Weight regain over time is also commonly observed. In one study, weight loss at 10 years decreased from 38% at year 1 to 25% at year 10.

Beneficial effects of weight loss surgery include marked improvement in diabetes, hyperlipidemia, hypertension, sleep apnea, and other obesity-related symptoms. Overall mortality over 11 years is improved by 24%, but the number needed to treat to prevent one death per year is approximately 850 patients.

MANAGEMENT OF OBESITY IN THE HOSPITAL

Due to the high prevalence of obesity and obesity-related morbidity, and the increasing use of operative procedures to treat obesity, such patients are increasingly cared for in inpatient and critical care settings. In most respects, care is similar to that of nonobese patients; however, severely obese patients require special attention in several aspects of care. Technical procedures may be more difficult in the obese patient including intubation, tracheostomy, and vascular access. Blood pressure monitoring requires use of cuffs with bladders large enough to cover 80% of the arm circumference. Undersized cuffs can overestimate blood pressure significantly. Dosing of some medications must be adjusted in obese patients due to the larger volume of distribution for lipophilic drugs. Some drugs should be dosed according to the ideal body weight, others according to the actual weight, and some according to an intermediate weight. Similar issues are encountered with nutrition support in the obese patient. Use of the actual body weight in common energy estimation equations such as the Harris–Benedict equation is likely to overestimate energy requirements. If indirect calorimetry is not available to measure energy expenditure, the use of the ideal body weight, or an intermediate dosing weight, is less likely to result in complications of overfeeding.

SUMMARY

Obesity and obesity-related illnesses are a major public health crisis. Currently available treatments with diets, exercise, and behavior therapy provide limited efficacy for most patients. Some patients, however, can achieve long-term weight loss. Currently approved medications demonstrate limited efficacy. Surgical treatment of obesity is the most effective treatment but is associated with substantial risk and long-term complications. Given the lack of effective therapy, preventive measures are essential. Broad and ambitious public health approaches are required to impact the obesity epidemic. For most individual patients, dietary changes that emphasize calorie reduction by consuming smaller portions, more plant foods, fewer high-calorie beverages, and less fast food are necessary even to maintain current weight. Similarly, striking increases in daily physical activity are needed to maintain body weight and achieve fitness.

SUGGESTED READINGS

Baron RB. Telling patients they are overweight or obese: an insult or an effective intervention? *Arch Intern Med* 2011;171(4): 321–322. PMID: 21357808.

Flegal KM, et al. Prevalence of obesity and trends in the distribution of body mass index among US adults, 1999-2010. *JAMA* 2012;307(5):491–497. PMID: 22253363.

Gortmaker SL, et al. Changing the future of obesity: science, policy, and action. *Lancet* 2011;378(9793):838–847. PMID: 21872752.

Hite AH, et al. Low-carbohydrate diet review: shifting the paradigm. *Nutr Clin Pract* 2011;26(3):300–308. Review. PMID: 21586415.

Kirk SF, et al. Effective weight management practice: a review of the lifestyle intervention evidence. *Int J Obes* 2012;36(2): 178–185. PMID: 21487396.

Ogden CL, et al. Prevalence of obesity and trends in body mass index among US children and adolescents, 1999-2010. *JAMA* 2012;307(5):483–490. PMID: 22253364.

Post RE, et al. The influence of physician acknowledgment of patients' weight status on patient perceptions of overweight and obesity in the United States. *Arch Intern Med* 2011;171(4): 316–321. PMID: 21357807.

Puhl MR, et al. The stigma of obesity: A review and update. *Obesity* 2009;17(5):941–964. PMID: 19165161.

Rao G. Office-based strategies for the management of obesity. *Am Fam Physician* 2010;81(12):1449–1456 . PMID: 20540483.

Sacks FM, et al. Comparison of weight-loss diets with different compositions of fat, protein, and carbohydrates. *N Engl J Med* 2009;360(9):859–873. PMID: 19246357.

Tice JA, et al. Gastric banding or bypass? A systematic review comparing the two most popular bariatric procedures. *Am J Med* 2008;121(10):885–893. PMID: 18823860.

Tsai AG, et al. Treatment of obesity in primary care practice in the United States: a systematic review. *J Gen Intern Med* 2009; 24(9):1073–1079. PMID: 19562419.

Wang YC, et al. Health and economic burden of the projected obesity trends in the USA and the UK. *Lancet* 2011; 378(9793): 815–825. PMID:21872750.

WEB SITE

Centers for Disease Control and Prevention (CDC) page on obesity. http://www.cdc.gov/obesity/index.html. Accessed April 2013.

Eating Disorders

Steven J. Romano, MD

INTRODUCTION

The eating disorders, including anorexia nervosa and bulimia nervosa, continue to receive appreciable clinical and research attention, paralleling an increase in their prevalence over the past few decades. Disturbances in eating behavior are, of course, not new. Historical documentation of anorexia nervosa dates back to the early Christian saints. Binging and purging, although distinct from our current concept of bulimia nervosa, took place in the lives of ancient Romans.

The eating disorders are best viewed as clinical syndromes rather than specific diseases, as they do not result from a single cause or follow a single course. As psychiatric syndromes, they are defined largely by a constellation of behaviors and attitudes that persist over time and have characteristic complications contributing to physical and psychosocial dysfunction. Because of the complexity and breadth of contributing factors, as well as the extent of comorbid psychopathology, knowledge of the behavioral characteristics of the eating disorders can lead to improved recognition and implementation of effective treatment strategies. In light of the complicated interplay of psychiatric, psychosocial, and medical consequences, treatment beyond initial medical stabilization generally requires referral to specialists. Importantly, though, the primary care physician is in a position to identify at-risk behaviors that may contribute to the development of eating disorders, particularly in adolescent and young adult females.

MULTIDIMENSIONAL MODEL

A comprehensive multidimensional model best illustrates the role various factors play in the genesis of clinically significant eating disturbances. In this schema, also referred to as a stress–diathesis model, psychological, biological, and sociocultural stressors contribute to the development of the syndrome (see Chapter 34).

Psychological factors include personality features, such as the anorectic's obsessive-compulsive qualities, constrained affect, and sense of ineffectiveness, and the bulimic's impulsivity. They also include the influence of developmental stressors and family dynamics. Body dissatisfaction, combined with other psychological, behavioral (in particular, dieting), or biological vulnerabilities, appears to be an important contributor and may identify those at greater risk.

Biological factors are most often due to the adverse effects of starvation, malnutrition, and purging behaviors, including vomiting and the misuse of laxatives and diuretics. Restrictive dieting and subsequent malnourishment may contribute to the development or exacerbation of comorbid psychiatric conditions, such as anxiety and depression. In addition, a preexisting biological vulnerability is supported by neurophysiologic investigations showing dysfunction of serotonin, dopamine, and norepinephrine neuromodulator systems; a small number of patients with anorexia develop amenorrhea preceding significant weight loss suggestive of hypothalamic dysregulation. The additional contribution of components of the peripheral satiety network is being elucidated. Genetic findings are suggestive and support evidence of substantial heritability, but require further investigation given the complexity of these conditions.

Sociocultural factors figure prominently in the etiology of the eating disorders. The idealization of thinness contributes to dieting behavior, often beginning in early adolescence. Of note, dieting is almost always present as a precipitant to the development of an eating disorder. Adoption of Western ideals of beauty and accompanying dieting behavior is contributing to an increased prevalence of eating disorders in ethnically diverse populations both in the United States and globally. Other precipitants include periods of illness leading to weight loss; in vulnerable individuals, this may be followed by willful dieting.

THEORETICAL CONSIDERATIONS

Conceptual models aid in understanding the etiology and possible sustaining factors involved in the genesis and persistence of eating disorder behavior. Important models include those derived from learning theory and neurophysiologic abnormality or dysfunction.

Cognitive behavioral theory, which is derived from learning theory, states that cognition influences behavior in a predictable manner. Cues, both internal and external, can provoke behavioral outcomes through activation of cognitive sets. A change in negative cognition, therefore, influences a change from dysfunctional to healthy behavior. Thoughts that overvalue weight, food, and diet, especially the idealization of thinness, lead to the perpetuation of compromising responses, such as heroic dietary measures and abuses of substances believed effective for weight reduction. The coupling of such cognitions and behaviors affects self-esteem and may severely impair an individual's psychological state. Cognitive behavioral therapy has been effective in achieving symptom reduction and improvement in both medical and psychological status.

The search for specific biological markers that may help identify patients with eating disorders has focused increasingly on neurotransmitters and other neuromodulators. Research findings suggest that dysfunction in various neurotransmitter systems, including serotonin, dopamine, and norepinephrine, as well as opioids and cholecystokinin (CCK), might play a role in the development and maintenance of the eating disorders. Rationale for the examination of these hormones and other substances derives from our understanding of the pathways modulating appetitive behavior, including hypothalamic regulation and the known connection between the gastrointestinal tract and the central nervous system. The complexity of these disorders, including the stress of eating disorder behavior on physiology, however, makes it unlikely that a neurophysiologic hypothesis alone can explain the etiology and maintenance of these complex syndromes.

CASE ILLUSTRATION 1

Amy, a 15-year-old high school sophomore, presented to her pediatrician at her mother's insistence with vague complaints of abdominal pain and bloating, particularly after meals. Though she answered all questions posed, she was rather reserved and hesitant to embellish her responses. A review of systems revealed infrequent constipation and a history of two nonconsecutive missed periods over the last 6 months, a departure from her generally regular periods since onset of menses at the age of 13 years. Vital signs were notable for a pulse of 54 and a sitting BP of 85/60 mm Hg. She was 5 ft. 4 in. tall and weighed 102 lb, 9 lb less than what was recorded at the time of her annual examination, approximately 8 months ago. Physical examination

was without significant findings. In particular, there were no findings suggesting focal abdominal pathology.

In private, Amy's mother told the pediatrician that Amy was less socially engaged over the last several months, preferring solitary activities such as studying or going out with friends or family. She also noted that Amy appeared to be using a treadmill in the basement for extended periods of time, and was concerned that she may have lost "a few pounds" recently. This would not ordinarily concern her, but Amy was also skipping meals with the family and had become "so picky" with regards to food choices. She was concerned that Amy was establishing unhealthy eating and exercise habits.

When presented with her mother's concerns and the clinical information by her pediatrician, Amy insisted that there was nothing to worry about, and denied voluntary attempts to lose weight. She did admit, though, that she was concerned about the amount of food her mother was serving at dinner, and that she had begun to avoid "fattening" foods and desserts, insisting that it was for health reasons. She reluctantly added that she was concerned that her hips were "too large" for her frame, and was hoping that continued exercise might minimize this perceived defect. She was unconcerned about her irregular periods, even though the pediatrician explained that it was unhealthy and likely due to her recent changes in weight, exercise, and eating habits. Following discussion with Amy and her mother, the pediatrician gently insisted that Amy and her family speak to a psychiatrist with experience in diagnosing and treating eating disorders, as he was concerned that Amy was developing anorexia.

ANOREXIA NERVOSA

Description

Anorexia nervosa is a relatively rare disorder affecting less than 1% of young women and a much smaller percentage of young men. Its most striking behavioral manifestation is the willful restriction of caloric intake secondary to an irrational fear of becoming fat, frequently in concert with a grossly distorted view of one's self as overweight, even in the presence of severe emaciation. Patients often exhibit a phobic response to food, particularly to fatty and other calorically dense items. They develop an obsessive preoccupation with food, eating, dieting, weight, and body shape, and frequently exhibit ritualistic behaviors involving choosing, preparing, and ingesting meals (e.g., cutting food into very small pieces or chewing each bite a specific number of times).

Early in the course of the illness, patients begin to restrict many food items, as is typical of most dieters. As the disorder progresses, though, the anorectic's menu becomes grossly constricted and he/she demonstrates greater rigidity. Minor variations in meal content can produce tremendous anxiety. Unlike the average dieter, the anorectic continues his/her pursuit of thinness to the extreme and becomes dependent on the daily registration of weight loss. This fuels even more restrictive dieting. Extreme dieting is often complicated by other weight-reducing behaviors. Exercise is frequently compulsive, and hyperactivity in underweight patients is a curious but often-encountered concomitant. Weakness, muscle aches, sleep disturbances, and gastrointestinal complaints, including constipation and postprandial bloating, are common physical findings. Amenorrhea, reflecting endocrine dysfunction secondary to malnourishment, is generally present.

Some anorectics engage in bulimic behaviors, including binging and purging. This binge–purge subtype of anorexia nervosa contrasts with the purely restricting subtype described earlier. Often, purging behavior, such as self-induced vomiting or the misuse of laxatives and diuretics, is seen in the absence of binging. The coupling of purging with self-starvation compounds the medical consequences of the disorder. Furthermore, anorectics, particularly adolescents, generally minimize their symptoms and the negative consequences of their disorder and are thus rarely motivated for treatment. The characteristics of the illness, both medical and psychological, are intensified with weight loss, further frustrating attempts at engaging the patient in a meaningful therapeutic process. Family and friends become increasingly anxious, angry, and at times alienated, as their loved one regresses. Superficial compliance, as is sometimes seen, belies a profound resistance. Anorectic patients can be challenging to treat as they cling tenaciously to their beliefs and behaviors.

Psychosocial dysfunction is common in patients with anorexia. Although educational performance may not be affected in adolescent patients, social relations become increasingly constricted, and sexual interest is generally diminished or absent.

Differential Diagnosis

The pathognomonic features of anorexia nervosa, namely the intense fear of becoming fat coupled with the relentless pursuit of thinness, are generally absent in other medical and psychiatric conditions. The term *anorexia*, which itself refers to absence of appetite, is a misnomer in the case of the syndrome of anorexia nervosa. True anorexia, such as that encountered in many medical conditions or diseases, would be accompanied by other signs or symptoms of those illnesses (as in gastrointestinal disease or many cancers).

Lack of appetite or decreased intake, with or without subsequent weight loss, is encountered in a number of psychiatric disorders. These include depression, hysterical conversion, other psychosomatic disorders, schizophrenia, and certain delusional disorders, but each of these is associated with a cluster of other substantiating symptomatology. Some patients with obsessive-compulsive disorder (OCD) may exhibit what appears to be bizarre behavior around food, eating, or meal preparation, but, on further exploration, their behavior is in response to obsessional ideation, for example, the fear of contamination. Such patients, in contrast to those with anorexia nervosa, generally admit their discomfort with the need to perform such compelling and often excessive or senseless acts.

In summary, although comorbid psychopathology may be encountered in patients with anorexia nervosa, including symptoms of depression or OCD, the hallmark of anorexia nervosa (the morbid fear of becoming fat and the relentless pursuit of thinness) is absent in other psychiatric syndromes. In none of these syndromes does the goal of weight loss drive the behavior.

Medical Complications & Treatment

Treatment of anorexia nervosa is initially directed at correcting the acute medical complications and is followed by supportive nutritional rehabilitation. Most medical consequences resolve with nutritional rehabilitation and the discontinuation of purging behaviors. Exceptions include persistent osteopenic changes in those who have experienced extended periods of malnourishment and suppression of growth in severe cases of adolescent anorexia.

In many cases of anorexia associated with significant weight loss (15–20% or more of ideal body weight) a structured inpatient facility is necessary to maintain an adequate level of medical surveillance and sustain a steady rate of weight gain. On admission to an inpatient treatment facility, laboratory screening should include tests for electrolytes, liver function, amylase (elevated in patients who purge), thyroid function, a complete blood count with differential, and a urinalysis. Common laboratory findings include leukopenia with a relative lymphocytosis, metabolic alkalosis with associated hypokalemia, hypochloremia, elevated serum bicarbonate levels, and, occasionally, metabolic acidosis in patients who abuse large amounts of stimulant-type laxatives. An electrocardiogram should also be obtained, since emaciation and associated electrolyte disturbances can contribute to significant cardiac abnormalities, especially in those who purge. Hypokalemia can lead to arrhythmia and the risk of cardiac arrest.

Acute medical conditions generally requiring immediate attention include electrolyte disturbances and dehydration, both of which are readily reversible. In most cases, initiating oral intake of fluids and food reverses minor disturbances in electrolytes and establishes adequate hydration. More severe cases, for example, patients with significant hypokalemia, may require intravenous hydration and parenteral replacement of depleted electrolytes, with daily electrolyte checks until the patient's condition stabilizes. Care should be taken to avoid overhydration and the consequences of excess fluid retention in vulnerable individuals. Importantly, treatment must ensure prevention of purging behaviors in patients with this history, as persistence of purging will alter electrolyte and fluid balance.

In patients who are significantly underweight, use of a liquid supplement, initially as replacement for solid food, helps ensure necessary caloric intake. When given in divided feedings throughout the day, it may decrease the patient's sense of postprandial discomfort and early satiety, both frequent consequences of extended caloric restriction and semistarvation. Further, this approach to refeeding decreases the inevitable manipulations around food choices. Replacement of solid food with a liquid supplement may also lessen the patient's phobic avoidance of food and the subsequent anxiety around meal choices.

Psychotherapeutic Interventions

Given the lack of motivation and strong resistance to treatment exhibited by the majority of patients with anorexia, it is helpful to initiate behavioral strategies as soon as any acute medical condition is stabilized. Initial behavioral interventions, tied to daily weight gain in increments of no less than 0.25 lb or 0.1 kg, include obtaining visits from family or friends, lessening physical restrictions, and increasing involvement in activities on and off the unit. It is important that all contingencies be tied to daily weight gain, which is measured each morning at the same time and in like manner, as this is a quantifiable observation not open to argument or discussion. A milieu supportive of such interventions helps to motivate the patient and exerts pressure toward positive change.

As the patient reaches a target weight range and establishes some degree of commitment to treatment, solid food can replace the liquid supplement. The ability of the patient to maintain weight through normalization of intake marks a transition to less structured treatment, such as a partial hospitalization program or outpatient follow-up.

Other treatments applicable to both inpatient and outpatient settings include individual psychotherapy and family intervention. The initial focus in family therapy should be on psychoeducation and obtaining the support of family members. The dynamics that may be contributing to the patient's eating disorder should be identified and, when possible, resolved. Such treatment often requires extensive contact beyond any acute interventions.

Individual psychotherapy is of limited value in the early stages of treatment, as the anorectic individual is generally unmotivated and, due to cognitive disturbances secondary to self-starvation, not capable of meaningful therapeutic work. Supportive therapy during this acute stage is often helpful in allaying anxiety and encouraging adherence to treatment. The more focused cognitive behavioral and interpersonal therapies are generally more effective when the patient has begun to gain weight and is beyond acute medical risk. Cognitive behavioral therapy focuses on the particular disturbing or distorted thoughts that contribute to the patient's maladaptive behavior and helps the patient establish more effective behavioral alternatives. It may also be effective in dealing with the central psychological features of anorexia nervosa, such as disturbance in body image. Interpersonal therapy may also be helpful. It focuses on interpersonal conflicts rather than specific eating disturbances. Following stabilization and resolution of the acute crisis, including achievement of weight restoration, patients often require longer-term psychotherapeutic interventions.

Pharmacotherapy

Pharmacological therapy can play an adjunctive role in the management of both primary eating symptoms and their comorbid psychiatric features, including anxiety and depression. Such treatments should focus on particular target symptoms or behaviors. No single medication is consistently effective in managing the primary psychiatric disturbances of anorexia nervosa. Antidepressants, especially the selective serotonin reuptake inhibitors (SSRIs), can alleviate depressive symptoms and, due to their ability to regulate obsessive-compulsive symptomatology, may help reduce the preoccupations and ritualistic behaviors encountered in most anorectics. Low doses of atypical antipsychotics may sometimes be employed in severely obsessional or agitated patients, but side effects, including movement disorders and metabolic aberrations, limit their utility. Anxiolytics, especially benzodiazepines, should generally not be given to anorectics, as they are prone to development of addiction.

BULIMIA NERVOSA

 CASE ILLUSTRATION 2

Cynthia, a 28-year-old single attorney with no significant medical or surgical history, presented to her primary care physician with complaints consistent

with gastroesophageal reflux. Symptoms included substernal burning sensations and regurgitation occurring several times a week, particularly following a large meal. She also reported occasional sharp chest pains lasting only a few seconds, not associated with shortness of breath or other signs or symptoms suggestive of cardiac origin. Other complaints noted on review of symptoms were general myalgia and fatigue, both experienced "a few days a week." She was on oral contraceptives, and stated that she took the suggested dose of an over-the-counter (OTC) laxative for constipation one or two times a week. Vital signs were normal, and she was afebrile. The only positive finding on physical examination was bilateral, nonpainful enlargement of the parotid glands. An electrocardiogram showed normal rate and rhythm, with nonspecific T-wave changes. Routine blood work was drawn, and a prescription for a proton pump inhibitor was given for symptoms of gastroesophageal reflux.

A review of Cynthia's laboratory values the next day revealed an elevated amylase and a serum potassium of 2.7. The laboratory abnormalities, together with the enlarged parotids and her presenting complaints, suggested self-induced vomiting. During a telephone call to Cynthia that day, her physician expressed concern and probed for confirmation. Cynthia hesitantly admitted to having a 5-year history of binging and purging, the latter by both self-induced vomiting and the use of a diuretic, furosemide, which she had been receiving from her OBGYN for menstrual complaints. She reluctantly agreed to return to the office for repeat electrolytes, as well as for a referral to an eating disorders clinic nearby.

Description

Bulimia nervosa affects approximately 2–3% of young women and 0.2% of young men, although bulimic behaviors may be encountered in many more patients. Bulimia nervosa is generally precipitated by periods of restrictive dieting. Bulimic individuals engage in regular episodes of binge eating, followed by compensatory behaviors to counteract the weight gain from ingested calories. Binge eating is characterized by the rapid consumption of large amounts of food over a short time, usually 1–2 hours. It is associated with a sense of being out of control and is often followed by feelings of guilt or shame and other dysphoric affective states, such as depression or anxiety. Some patients report alleviation of dysphoria or even emotional numbing during or immediately following the episode, although this is short lived. During a binge, a few thousand to as many as 15,000 kcal or more may be consumed. Sometimes

trigger foods, often a fattening sweet such as chocolate, precipitate a binge, although the overall content of food consumed, by macroanalysis of nutritional content, varies. The bulimic individual generally binges in private; grossly overeating is humiliating. Embarrassment can lead to varying degrees of social avoidance or isolation.

Contributing further to avoidance behavior is the need to compensate for eating, frequently by purging. Most bulimic individuals induce vomiting during or after a binge, and some also use laxatives or diuretics. A minority of patients employs laxatives or diuretics alone. Nonpurging compensatory behaviors include compulsive exercising and restrictive dieting or fasting between binges.

Another characteristic of bulimia nervosa is patient dissatisfaction with body shape or weight. This may evolve into a significant degree of obsessional preoccupation, with self-evaluation overly influenced by these physical concerns. It can have a profound effect on self-esteem and is evidenced in part by comorbid depressive symptomatology in the majority of patients. Impulsive behavior is encountered in many individuals with bulimia nervosa and at times leads to substance abuse, sexual promiscuity, and theft.

Differential Diagnosis

Few medical or psychiatric disorders can be confused with bulimia nervosa. More frequently, signs of self-induced vomiting or use of diuretics or laxatives in a young woman who does not admit to binging or purging behaviors lead the primary care clinician to search for another primary medical diagnosis. Signs and symptoms associated with gastritis, esophagitis, dehydration, or electrolyte disturbances result in primary care or emergency room visits, postponing psychiatric consultation. If the patient is underweight, amenorrheic, and is binging and purging, he/she has anorexia nervosa of the binge–purge subtype rather than bulimia nervosa.

Medical Complications & Treatment

The majority of medical complications due to bulimia nervosa are consequences of purging behaviors. Self-induced vomiting can lead to gastritis, esophagitis, periodontal disease, and dental caries. Gastric dilatation and gastric or esophageal rupture are rare medical emergencies. Metabolic alkalosis with the development of clinically significant hypokalemia in patients who vomit is not unusual, and serum electrolytes show typical indices. When present, electrocardiographic changes are significant. Arrhythmias can lead to cardiac arrest if hypokalemia and related disturbances are not corrected. Use of diuretics cause similar disturbances. Metabolic acidosis can develop in patients who use a significant number of stimulant-type laxatives. Dehydration, sometimes requiring intravenous hydration, can accompany each of the aforementioned purging behaviors. More often associated with bulimic behaviors are general physical complaints such as fatigue and muscle aches. Long-term use of the emetic ipecac can lead to myopathies, including cardiomyopathy, the latter a rare cause of death in patients with bulimia.

Most patients with bulimia nervosa can be treated as outpatients or in more structured partial hospitalization programs. An individual with an acute medical condition, however, such as dehydration or symptomatic hypokalemia accompanied by electrocardiographic changes, requires hospitalization for medical stabilization. Patients who have failed outpatient treatment and continue to binge and purge frequently, and those with significant depression and associated suicidal ideation, may require inpatient treatment.

Psychotherapeutic Interventions

Helping patients recognize the negative consequences of their behavior and dispelling myths about the efficacy of many of their dietary maneuvers, especially the usefulness of laxatives, diuretics, and self-induced vomiting, may be enough to motivate them to decrease the frequency of bulimic behaviors. Similarly, self-monitoring intake with the use of food diaries and normalization of meal patterns can lead to short-term gains in control of bulimic symptoms. Time-limited psychotherapy, focused specifically on the disturbed eating patterns, can be conducted in an individual or group format and is often useful. More traditional exploratory psychotherapies, which are generally not time limited, do not predictably affect outcome but may play a role in the treatment of underlying or persistent difficulties following improvement or resolution of bulimia.

Cognitive behavioral therapy is an established treatment for bulimia nervosa and can lead to both acute reductions in symptoms of binging and purging and longer-term maintenance of gains. It targets the behavioral manifestations and challenges the cognitive distortions typically encountered in these patients. In cognitive behavioral therapy, identifying disordered behaviors is the first step toward productive intervention, because behavioral consequences follow specific cues. To intervene, one must recognize the various cues and respond to them deliberately rather than automatically. Cues affecting eating disorder patients are either internal or external. Internal cues include physiologic ones; most significantly hunger, as well as emotions and thoughts. External cues encompass a broad array of experiences from sensual, such as sight or smell, to situational. Cues lead to consequences that are either positive or negative; both can be reinforcing.

Following the identification of cues, associated responses can be addressed more specifically and in greater detail. Responses consist of thoughts, feelings, and behaviors. Helping the patient understand that thoughts and feelings affect behavioral responses to a cue is of great significance because both thoughts and feelings can be altered through cognitive behavioral techniques. For each cue identified, patients are taught to delineate the various response components and to evaluate the appropriateness of each. Although schematically simple, many eating-associated responses are automatic, and learning to identify the cues and various responses requires much practice.

During cognitive behavioral therapy patients are taught to recognize that behaviors follow cues and responses to cues can be broken down into thoughts, feelings, and behaviors. What patients think and feel about a cue dictate whether their response is adaptive or maladaptive. How they feel is influenced by how they think; therefore, the restructuring of thoughts is of primary importance. Eating disorder patients manifest certain patterns of distorted thinking; these patterns negatively influence feelings and fuel the maladaptive behaviors. These various styles of thinking are identified, and strategies to challenge and ultimately to alter the distortions are developed.

A simple example helps illustrate the applicability of cognitive behavioral therapy. A common cue that frequently leads to a bulimic response is the normal sense of fullness. Rather than recognizing satiety as a normal physiologic response, the eating disorder patient often misinterprets this cue, stating instead, "I feel fat." This distorted thought, unchallenged, is associated with negative feelings and often leads to dysfunctional behaviors. Rather than the appropriate response to fullness, understanding that it is temporary and will pass, patients believe they must compensate for being "fat" and rid themselves of the meal through purging or compensate for the caloric intake through exercise. Such a response causes the cycle to reassert itself.

Pharmacotherapy

Pharmacological management may play a significant role in treatment and, unlike in anorexia, can more predictably affect outcome. Many antidepressants, including SSRIs, monoamine oxidase inhibitors (MAOIs), and tricyclic antidepressants (TCAs) are effective in treating bulimia. (Dietary proscriptions limit the usefulness of MAOIs, and lethality in overdose limits treatment with TCAs.) They reduce symptoms of depression and anxiety as well as the frequency of binging and purging. Bupropion is the only antidepressant that is contraindicated, as the metabolic imbalances precipitated by purging can make the patient more prone to seizures.

SUMMARY

Eating disorders represent a broad spectrum of psycho-pathologic features. They are best understood in terms of multiple etiologic factors influencing the development of clinical syndromes. Understanding the complexity of these disorders, the behaviors associated with them, and their comorbid psychiatric features aids in their recognition and treatment. Focusing initially on control of these primary eating disorder behaviors helps reduce the likelihood of psychological morbidity. It also limits the medical complications that frequently develop in these conditions. Interventions to control behavior range from response prevention (for patients placed on special inpatient wards) to cognitive behavioral therapies for more motivated patients. Behavioral control may be augmented through pharmacological management as well as other psychotherapies (psychoeducational and interpersonal) that help reduce the role that sustaining factors play in the maintenance of these disorders.

SUGGESTED READINGS

Attia E. Eating disorders. *Ann Intern Med* 2012;156(7):ITC4-1.

Goldstein DJ, ed. *The Management of Eating Disorders and Obesity*, 2nd ed. Totowa, NJ: Humana Press Inc., 2005.

Halmi KA, ed. *Psychobiology and Treatment of Anorexia Nervosa and Bulimia Nervosa*. Washington, DC: American Psychiatric Association Press, 1992.

Halmi KA. Eating disorders. In:Hales KE, Yudofsky SC, Talbott J, eds. *American Psychiatric Press Textbook of Psychiatry*, 5th ed. Washington, DC: American Psychiatric Association Press, 2008, Chapter 23.

Kaye W, Strober M, Jimmerson D. The neurobiology of eating disorders. In: Charney DF, Nestler EJ, eds. *The Neurobiology of Mental Illness*. New York: Oxford University Press, 2004, pp. 1112–1128.

WEB SITE

Academy for Eating Disorders Web site. http://www.aedweb.org/. Accessed January 2014.

Alcohol & Substance Use

Elinore F. McCance-Katz, MD, PhD and Derek Satre, PhD

Picasso's "Absinthe drinker". Pablo Picasso: "L'Absinthe," 1901. Accessed at: http:/rss.listal.com/list/absinthe-green-fairy-art.

INTRODUCTION

Physicians are well aware of the harm that the use of drugs and alcohol brings to their patients and families. The prevalence of substance use disorders exceeds 20% in ambulatory practices and is even higher in hospitalized patients. Those affected include everyone from adolescents, teachers, and shipyard workers to doctors themselves. Physicians report that conversations with patients about drinking can be stressful and conflict laden, and that many patients are unmotivated to change their behavior. Physicians' negative feelings sometimes derive from their own family experiences or from encounters with intoxicated patients who can be hostile, uncooperative, and occasionally violent. These dynamics, combined with the sense that substance abuse may not really be a "medical" issue, tend to keep physicians from addressing alcohol and substance use disorders in their patients.

Evidence from many sources provides reason for optimism, however, and shows that clinicians who take a few moments to thoughtfully structure their interventions with patients can reduce harm, lower medical care costs, lessen morbidity for patients and families, strengthen patients' family and social relationships, and enhance patient self-esteem and emotional stability. Indeed the recovery rate from substance abuse, 30–40% of treated patients, exceeds that from most other chronic illnesses. Recovering patients often credit their clinicians with being a primary factor in their recovery and with literally saving their lives. For physicians, participating in the identification and treatment of substance abuse can be as gratifying as helping patients recover from leukemia or pneumonia.

Primary care medicine is increasing its role in addressing alcohol and drug problems, since the majority of individuals with alcohol or drug abuse usually avoid seeking care from specialized chemical dependence programs. Two important recent developments are significant in this regard. The first is a push for early identification and treatment of alcohol and drug abuse before those problems become severe. The Screening, Brief Intervention and Referral to Treatment (SBIRT) model is a public health approach promoted by the National Institutes of Health to encourage universal primary care screening and intervention when needed. This screening now qualifies for Medicare reimbursement. The second important movement is the increasing recognition that alcohol and drug use problems are often chronic relapsing conditions and need to be managed medically, with ongoing monitoring in primary care settings and referral when needed to specialized chemical dependency services. Physicians have a key role to play in this process. In this chapter, we will discuss identification and management of substance use problems, and how physicians' interactions with patients can enhance their coping with these problems.

Chemical dependence (nontobacco-related addictive disease) is a chronic, progressive illness affecting 24.8% of Americans at some time in their lives (lifetime prevalence) and approximately 6.5% of Americans at any given point in time. Heavy drug or alcohol abuse precipitates a vicious cycle of increased use associated with behavioral and social problems. Heavy drinkers are at elevated risk for hypertension, gastrointestinal bleeding, sleep disorders, major depression, hemorrhagic stroke, cirrhosis of the liver, and several cancers. The insidious development of tolerance to intoxication, cognitive deficits from high doses, and dysphoria leads to social impairment. Relationship problems are exaggerated when friends and family resent the (apparently) voluntary nature of overindulgence. Addicts can become adept at ignoring reality and suppressing negative feelings. Lengthy periods spent in brain-altered states result in the dramatic neurophysiologic changes of addiction and withdrawal. Further, emotional isolation may develop when those suffering from addiction make excuses for their behavior, direct blame onto others, and show hostility when sensible limits are discussed. Physicians have an important role to play in mitigating these adverse consequences.

 CASE ILLUSTRATION

Jim is a 50-year-old factory worker with high blood pressure. He has a follow-up visit with the doctor who has been his primary care physician for the past decade. He mentions that he recently received his second "driving under the influence" (DUI) citation and considers it unfair. His probation officer ordered Jim to undergo alcohol counseling at the local alcohol treatment center. Jim has no interest in counseling but he thinks he must attend to keep his driver's license, needed to get to his job.

Jim cannot remember his father, but knows he had serious drinking problems and left the family when Jim was 4 years old.

Jim began drinking as a teenager and got up to a 12-pack of beer per day. He cut back once he got out of his twenties, since "that was going nowhere" but still drinks four to six beers daily—at his club or playing pool or cards with his buddies, and up to two six-packs per day on the weekend. (Based on his self-report and national survey data, only 3% of American men drink more than Jim.)

You have asked Jim the CAGE questions (Table 24-4) in the past, and at that time he said that when he was

a lot younger he needed to cut down, and he drank eye-openers in the morning, again in the distant past. He said he was not annoyed because of criticism of his drinking, and that he never felt guilty or remorseful after drinking. Now, as you ask questions, he seems irritated.

You decide to begin your assessment of Jim's current situation by asking him the CAGE questions again. You ask about cutting down:

Jim: *Look, doc, my father may have been alcoholic, and many of my buddies drink a lot more than me, but I'm not an alcoholic, and I can take it or leave it.*

Rather than confronting him with the considerable evidence already available that indicates his situation qualifies as at least alcohol abuse and possibly dependence, you decide to use an empathic style and reflect his apparent feeling state as well as the content of his declaration.

Doctor: *Jim, I see this is a sensitive topic, as it is for most people, and I get it that you are convinced that drinking is not a problem for you.*

Jim: *I quit several times when my wife complained, no problem. But 2 years ago she took the kids and left, saying that they couldn't live with me unless I quit drinking. I don't understand women!*

You have important new data about drinking and about Jim's life, and Jim feels understood rather than interrogated.

On repeated checks over the past couple of years, Jim has had an elevated MCV, but the rest of his complete blood count, metabolic panel, and liver function panel are repeatedly normal. He tells you his blood alcohol concentration was 0.22 (220 mg/dL, 0.08%, is now the "legal limit" in all US states) when he was cited.

Your physical examination shows Jim's blood pressure is controlled, and you find no evidence for new medical problems or active withdrawal from alcohol. You agree to continue his lisinopril:

Doctor: *We have talked about alcohol quite a bit today, Jim. On a scale of 0–10, how interested are you in quitting drinking at this time, where 0 means not at all and 10 means quitting is a top priority?*

Jim: *I'm quitting until I get my license back, no problem.*

Doctor: *You feel you are in full control of your alcohol intake.*

Jim: *I'm fine, doc, and thanks for checking.*

Doctor: *I am pleased that you are ready to quit now, and I know you have been successful in the past. Also, I'm concerned, because I think you may have an alcohol use disorder that will require your attention even after you get the license back . . . What are your thoughts about that?*

DIAGNOSTIC CATEGORIES

Drug and alcohol problems exist on a continuum (Table 24-1). At times, diagnosis may be elusive because of scant or imprecise information. Nevertheless, experts agree on an evidence-based classification system that is useful in guiding physician actions. Patients on the severely afflicted end of the continuum, with the prototype syndrome formerly known as *alcohol* or *drug dependence*, but now diagnostically classified as severe alcohol or drug use disorder in the Diagnostic and Statistical Manual of Mental Disorders, Fifth Edition (DSM 5) (often called *alcoholism* or *drug addiction*, respectively), suffer medical and social consequences from uncontrolled use. A striking 5–10% of adults develop this syndrome. **Physical dependence** and **withdrawal syndromes** imply *drug dependence* virtually 100% of the time.

People toward the center of the continuum, with problems of modest severity, have mild-moderate *drug or alcohol use disorder (alcohol or drug abuse)*, a maladaptive pattern which leads to impairment or distress. Note that what distinguishes the patient with a mild-moderate substance use disorder (drug abuse) from the patient with severe drug abuse disorder (drug dependence) is not the **nature** of the problems, but the **frequency, persistence, and pervasiveness** of the problems. Thus, both *drug abuse* and *drug dependence* may include health problems (e.g., stroke from cocaine use, hypertension from alcohol use, oversedation from benzodiazepines), legal problems (e.g., arrests for DUI or violence), family dysfunction, and performance problems at school or work.

At the milder end of the continuum, conceptualization of alcohol and drug use problems has been broadened to include patterns of substance use that do not meet strict diagnostic criteria but which put patients at risk for adverse health consequences. These patients have been described as "at-risk," or "hazardous" users.

Table 24-1. Descriptors for the continuum of drug and alcohol use.*

"Hazardous use" has approximately the same meaning as "at-risk" use.[†]
"Abuse" of alcohol or drugs is a maladaptive use pattern leading to impairment or distress diagnostically classified as mild-moderate substance use disorder*.
"Dependence" on alcohol or other drugs is a maladaptive use pattern leading to impairment or distress, more pervasive and persistent than for abuse, and often (but not necessarily) including physical dependence and withdrawal symptoms diagnostically classified as severe substance use disorder.

*See DSM 5 (2013)
*See Fiellin et al. (2000).
[†]See Table 24-3 for alcohol amounts; any use of illicit drugs is "at risk"; see text for prescription drug use.

These people use too much, but have not developed important negative consequences. Physicians should intervene with them on the basis of the quantity of intake. In contrast, intervention with patients with "abuse" or "dependence" is made because of negative consequences and high quantity of use. Most, but not all people who experience serious life consequences use very excessive amounts, but the decision about how vigorous to be with interventions is made on the severity of problems, not on the amount consumed. Data about both amounts and consequences should be sought, but the full meaning of the data about amounts cannot be established until the physician obtains a clear picture of adverse consequences or lack thereof.

Regarding alcohol, expert consensus is that *moderate drinking* is defined by quantity of intake (not more than 14 drinks per week for men and 7 for women), a social setting for drinking, and amount consumed at one time (not more than 4 drinks per occasion for men and 3 for women). Drinking above these limits is called "at risk" or "hazardous," and is likely to cause harm, according to long-term studies. "At-risk" drinking is very common. According to the National Institute on Alcohol Abuse and Alcoholism (NIAAA), approximately 3 out of 10 adults in the United States drink at levels that put them at risk for physical and mental health problems.

"At-risk" prescription drug use includes patients on mood-altering drugs or medications with abuse liability or prescription pain medications for more than 3 months. The majority of patients using long-term sedative drugs to manage insomnia, anxiety, depression, and other disorders, as well as those using narcotics to treat chronic pain, develop neither problems nor dependence. Similar to drinkers and users of illicit drugs, however, 10–20% do experience problems such as falls, oversedation, drug interactions, drug overdoses, or symptoms of dependence, such as taking more medication than prescribed. Therefore, physicians need to be alert to potential problems arising from long-term medication use. In addition, of course, physicians need to be alert to the possibility that patients may be using medications for other than as indicated, for example, use of pain medications to enhance mood, or obtaining medications from more than one physician.

WORKING EFFECTIVELY WITH PATIENTS

Although the brain effects of addictive drugs vary in neurochemical mechanisms, timing, intensity, and potential toxicity, the severe substance use disorder is similar across the various drug classes and specific drugs. Addictions to alcohol, heroin, cocaine, methamphetamine, benzodiazepines, and other abused substances are variants of the underlying disease of substance dependence. Any differences in strategies for managing abuse of these various substances stem from the legal and social consequences of obtaining and using the particular drug, and its potential medical complications. Consequently, screening, assessment, and management of drug addictions other than alcohol are similar to strategies for alcohol-use disorders. A caveat to these general principles relates to prescription drug abuse, which may involve physicians' interpersonal and intrapersonal vulnerabilities, beliefs, and prescribing preferences and habits.

Promoting Behavior Change

Several methods for promoting behavior change in patients with substance use problems have emerged from research. A key first step is screening all patients for hazardous alcohol or drug use patterns or substance use disorders. For those with indications of hazardous substance use or abuse, several approaches may be utilized depending on the severity of the problem. These include *brief intervention, motivational interviewing, shared decision making, relationship-centered care*, and *autonomy support* (see Chapter 19 for a full discussion on behavior change). The fundamental **principles** derived from this research are as follows:

- Generally speaking, the physician takes responsibility for calibrating and adjusting interventions so that patients can hear information and feedback that create or amplify differences between the way life is now and the goals and values patients espouse. Using an empathic and caring style, the physician shows that discrepancies between the actual and the potential might be minimized if patients change their alcohol and drug use patterns.
- Patients will not change until they are ready, and ambivalence about change and/or resistance to change is normal.
- Physicians can best promote change by maintaining an empathic and relationship-centered style. Taking a strongly persuasive stand usually fails to promote change.
- Only the patient can take responsibility for change and effect change. Physicians can promote change by providing information (both feedback about the patient's health and information about resources), by showing attentiveness and listening carefully to the patient's ideas about both the pros and the cons of possible changes, and by helping boost the patient's self-confidence about change.

The fundamental **content messages** physicians should include in interviews are as follows:

- I am concerned that your drug use may be hurting you and others you care about.

- Most people use a lot less than you, or abstain.
- For better health, you should curb (or cease) your drug use.
- The key choices are up to you.
- I will give you my best advice, which is based on expert consensus and my experience with other patients with similar problems.
- I want to collaborate with you, even if progress is slow or intermittent.

The fundamental **process strategies** physicians should follow are as follows:

- Maintain dialogue when giving information and recommendations; use a *tell, ask, tell* strategy.
- Make clear recommendations, but do not try to persuade patients.
- State explicitly that you will advise, but that the patient decides.
- Establish the patient's commitment to any plans on which you agree.
- Never argue with patients and do not try to overcome resistance, reluctance, rebellion, or rationalization. Use reflection to respond to these manifestations of ambivalence.
- Support the patient's self-confidence.

Two key steps can assist physicians in doing a better job with substance-abusing patients. The first is to intervene as soon as any clue suggests that an alcohol or drug use problem might be present; do not wait until the evidence is glaring or a patient's health has begun to suffer. Physicians can better limit serious consequences of substance use by broadening their focus from the detection of dependence or addiction to include the detection of hazardous or risky patterns of use.

The second key step is to conduct those interventions using techniques specifically structured to promote behavior change, as described below. We will discuss first the process of deciding which patients require interventions, and then discuss principles, content, and strategies of effective physician–patient interactions.

IDENTIFYING SUBSTANCE USE PROBLEMS

Studies show that "brief interventions" can be structured for "at-risk" users as well as those who have developed mild, moderate, or severe substance use disorders. Adjusting interventions to problem severity is helpful, and consequently we suggest simple strategies that separate healthy users from potentially problematic ones and help clinicians assess severity. Subsequent sections advise physicians what to do in each case. In the steps below, we incorporate the National Institute on

Table 24-2. NIAAA screening question on hazardous drinking frequency.

How many times in the past year have you had five or more drinks in 1 day (men); four or more drinks in 1 day (women)?

Alcoholism's *Clinician's Guide: Helping Patients Who Drink Too Much,* which is a very useful reference and includes procedures also relevant to screening and treatment of drug use. These steps can be recalled using the "4 A's"—Ask, Assess, Advise, and Assist.

Step One: Ask about Alcohol and Drug Use

Step one is to ask **about alcohol and drug use**. Prescreen every new patient with two questions: "Do you sometimes drink beer, wine, or other alcoholic beverages?" and "When was your last use of marijuana or other drugs?" If the answer is "No," "Never," or "Years ago," leave this topic. If patients belong to an abstinent subgroup with past problems, they often disclose this spontaneously.

For patients who report any alcohol use, ask the National Institute on Alcohol and Alcoholism recommended **single question about hazardous drinking** (Table 24-2). If positive (five or more drinks in a day for men; four or more in a day for women), quantify the drinking behavior. Determine a weekly average by asking: "On average, how many days a week do you have a drink?" and "On a typical day, how many drinks do you have?" Drinking above "safe limits" (Table 24-3) means the person is at least an "at-risk" user.

The National Institute on Drug Abuse has developed a similar stepped screening approach. The first step is to ask patients which drugs they have used in their lifetime (including major categories of illegal drugs as well as prescription psychotropics other than as prescribed); and of these, which if any have been used in the past 3 months.

Step Two: Assess for Substance Use Disorders and Substance-Related Problems

For patients who drink alcohol over recommended limits or who report drug use in the past 3 months, the next step is to determine if patients meet criteria for a substance use disorder. See Table 24-1 for a summary of diagnostic criteria.

If any dependence screen is positive, or if intake exceeds safe limits, or if another clue from examination or the family suggests a drinking or drug problem, the clinician needs more detail to clarify the extent of the problems. A search for characteristic negative consequences is warranted and not time consuming if thoughtfully structured. The physician decides when to conduct this inquiry based on priorities for the present encounter; however, because alcohol and drug use produces many symptoms and affects many other illness conditions, at least a brief inventory when the issue initially surfaces is imperative. Asking patients about the symptoms in Table 24-4 as they relate to alcohol use provides ample data for the primary assessment, and the NIAAA Clinician's Guide organizes this inquiry very well. Protocols for drug use assessment are less well developed than those for alcohol. Patients can be assessed further by inquiring how much money they spend a week on drugs, the frequency of use, consequences of use, and how many days or weeks they have abstained in the past 12 months.

Interviews with others, including family, nurses, or social workers, enlarge the inquiry if the patient furnishes insufficient data. Records from other physicians or hospitals may contain unanticipated information that helps determine a diagnosis. Obtaining a thorough evaluation allows the physician to discuss impressions in a compassionate manner. In fact, experimental data show that thoughtful diagnostic conversation itself produces beneficial therapeutic effects. Additional assessment approaches, including laboratory testing, are described below.

Table 24-3. "Hazardous" or "at-risk" alcohol intake limits.

Men: More than 14 drinks* per week, or more than 4 drinks per occasion.
Women: More than 7 drinks* per week, or more than 3 drinks per occasion.

*In the United States a drink is 12 oz beer, 5 oz wine, or 1.5 oz (bar shot) of hard liquor.

Table 24-4. Examples of possible alcohol- and drug-related problems.

- Somatic: Gastritis, trauma, hypertension, liver function disorder, or new-onset seizure.
- Psychosocial: Symptoms of anxiety, depression, insomnia, overdose, or a request for psychotropic medications.
- Alcohol-specific: Any spontaneous mention of drinking behavior, such as "partying" or hangover, family history, Alcoholics Anonymous attendance, arrests for driving while intoxicated, withdrawal symptoms, tolerance, blackouts.

Table 24-5. CAGE screening test for alcohol dependence risk.

Have you ever felt that you should **Cut down** on your drinking?
Have people **Annoyed** you by criticizing your drinking?
Have you ever felt bad or **Guilty** about your drinking?
Have you ever had a drink first thing in the morning to steady your nerves or get rid of a hangover? (**Eye-opener**)

Table 24-6. Reflection.

Description: Tell the patient the message you heard (or perceived nonverbally). Always statements, not questions, agreement or disagreement, judgment, and so on. Always brief: Reflector may have to choose among several messages to be brief.
Examples: "I see, you think that none of your problems is related to drug use." "Alcohol really helps you to sleep." "That I think these abnormal liver tests stem from alcohol is confusing to you, because you drink so little." "You seem irritated with my continuing to discuss drug use."

The CAGE test (Table 24-5) is a thoroughly studied screen. Studies show that substituting "alcohol or drug use" for "drinking" in the screen is effective. Any positive response should prompt a more thorough assessment. Two positive responses to the CAGE indicate a high likelihood of dependence.

A helpful tool that can be used to gather greater information about alcohol use patterns is the Alcohol Use Disorders Identification Test (AUDIT) (Appendix 24-A). The AUDIT is a 10-item instrument developed by the World Health Organization to screen for alcohol-related problems and to quantify severity. The NIAAA Clinician's Guide also includes the AUDIT Questionnaire, with suggestions for its use and scoring in clinical practice.

Step Three: Advise and Assist

For patients whose pattern of use indicates that they are either at risk of alcohol or drug problems or who already meet criteria for abuse or dependence, the next steps include strategies to help patients reduce or eliminate drug use. As described below, interventions vary based on the extent of substance use and whether or not dependence symptoms are present. In delivering brief interventions the components we describe in this chapter can be remembered using the acronym FRAMES:

Feedback is given to the individual about personal risk or impairment.
Responsibility for change is placed on the patient.
Advice to change is given by the provider.
Menu of alternative self-help or treatment options is offered to the patient.
Empathic style is used in counseling.
Self-efficacy or optimistic empowerment is engendered in the patient.

Responding Effectively to Challenge, Resistance, & Ambivalence

We introduce the skill of "reflection"—paraphrasing the patient's message or meaning—(Table 24-6) at this

moment because quite frequently, as physicians ask screening and clarifying questions, patients show resistance and challenge. Physicians can improve the quality of the data as well as minimize tension by responding to irritation or resistance with reflections. This approach has been described extensively as "Reflective listening," a key component of Motivational Interviewing.

Physicians who can gently reflect back the resistance, ambivalence, or challenge they receive from patients generate an atmosphere of alliance and partnership. Reflection shows a desire to fully understand the patient, demonstrating acceptance of the person and a willingness to listen. Reflection is neither aggressive nor defensive, and helps to minimize arguing, hostility, and negativity. Simple reflection gives the patient full choice over what to say next (whereas questions seek answers, and giving advice stakes out a position, as does agreement or disagreement, and statements of values). In fact, studies demonstrate that reflecting negative, resistant, or reluctant statements helps engage patients in dialogue (see Chapter 1).

Especially when the patient seems negative or hostile, reflection is not an intuitive response. Studies show that doctors usually respond by asking questions, giving advice, persuading or arguing the point, or shifting the interview focus. With practice and attentiveness, physicians can reflect back patients' expressions of ambivalence, resistance, or challenge.

Jim: I drink a lot because of the neuropathy and pain in my feet, so that I can sleep.
Doctor: So, alcohol helps you a lot.
Jim: Well, it's probably not so good for my liver.
Doctor: You feel some conflict about getting sleep at the expense of hurting your liver.
Jim: The drink seems to produce nothing but problems.

As this example illustrates, an empathic reflection that recognizes patients' reasons for using substances can allow them to move forward and admit potential downsides to their pattern of use. Physicians can equally reflect patients' statements about feeling, thinking, attribution, choice, action, or behavior. Reflection helps the physician by encouraging patients to share more of their perspectives, feelings, and thoughts; it thus engenders more trust and a feeling of safety in both persons. As patients who initially show disinterest, hostility, a sullen demeanor, or confusion reveal more of themselves, physicians become less judgmental and critical, more inclined to join patients and to support them. Patients who feel joined become better able to listen to their doctors, and have more strength to take responsibility for attempting change that might at first seem unimaginable. Reflection is useful in all interview stages, whether the physician seeks more information about drug use and its consequences, additional psychosocial information, or wishes to develop sensible management strategies for a patient.

PHYSICAL EXAMINATION & LABORATORY STUDIES

Physical and laboratory examinations are useful adjuncts to structured interviewing. *Odor of alcohol* is alarming, and distinctly abnormal in medical encounters. If alcohol is easily smelled in the room, the blood alcohol level (BAL) is likely greater than 0.125 mg/dL, and a less dramatic odor indicates a BAL between 0.075 and 0.125 mg/dL. The nose is a good breath analyzer. Alcohol on the breath is a convincing sign, and always signals a serious alcohol disorder.

Intoxication (slurred speech, incoordination, and/or emotional lability) in any encounter is worrisome, and means a high likelihood of drug or alcohol disorder, even in the emergency department. To underscore this important point, assume that the 10% of the population who are alcohol- or drug dependent are intoxicated once a week (it is often more than once), and assume that the 60% who are not abusers or dependent are intoxicated once yearly (it is often less than once). Thus, in a year, from a population of 100, 30 abstainers yield no episodes of intoxication, 60 users (not in trouble) yield 60, and 10 dependent people yield 520! Further, moderate users seldom become as intoxicated and are more likely to use in controlled environments (e.g., where someone else can drive). Intoxicated people in the emergency situation are not healthy users or drinkers who "have had one too many."

Further, with respect to alcohol, if the odor of alcohol is apparent, and if the patient manifests no evidence of intoxication, *tolerance* to alcohol effect is present. Tolerance indicates brain adaptation to intoxicating alcohol levels, which is caused by heavy drinking, is inevitably toxic, and usually means that the patient is physically dependent on alcohol. Withdrawal symptoms (see Management of Withdrawal) indicate additional brain dysfunction, and are easier to discern than

tolerance. The same reasoning holds for drugs other than alcohol, but our ability to quantify their use or blood levels, as well as our ability to detect intoxication (except for sedatives or opiates), is limited, so tolerance must be inferred less directly from the patient's history.

Other physical and laboratory findings (see general medicine textbooks for the multitudinous possibilities) are poor screening tests, as they have either low sensitivity or specificity, or both. Once again, more data are available about alcohol than for other drugs. Alcohol has a broad range of toxic effects and an abnormality may prove useful in context. First, an unexplained finding may begin a fruitful investigative process. For example, despite a negative response to the alcohol screening question, the concerned physician of a young woman with palmar erythema continued the assessment, allowing the patient to reveal her alcohol problem. Second, in the presence of a clue, physical or laboratory findings substantially raise the posttest probability, and physicians should order appropriate tests, such as mean corpuscular volume (MCV) and liver enzymes (include alanine aminotransferase [ALT], aspartate aminotransferase [AST], and γ-glutamyl transpeptidase [GGT], the most sensitive to alcohol intake). For example, a 55-year-old man with chronic pulmonary disease was admitted for atrial fibrillation. His wife complained about his drinking, and an elevated MCV, AST, and ECG confirmed not only alcoholism but also "holiday heart" (alcohol-induced arrhythmia after binge drinking). Carbohydrate deficient transferring (CDT) is a more specific marker of heavy alcohol use and can be used to monitor abstinence for the patient needing ongoing treatment for a severe alcohol disorder (alcohol dependence).

Illicit drugs are readily detectable in urine; however, the ability to identify them varies with the technique used. Drugs that may not be included in routine panels include hydrocodone, oxycodone, methadone, buprenorphine, anabolic steroids, and short-acting designer drugs. Marijuana can be detected for up to 30 days in the urine of daily smokers (for 1–3 days in intermittent smokers), but all other illicit drugs are cleared within 72 hours; for example, a positive test for cocaine indicates use within the past 2–3 days. Simply being near a marijuana smoker never produces a positive urine test (it can be detected by mass spectroscopy, but levels are well below the cut-off levels of routine urine testing). Urine drug screening for recent alcohol use (last 48–72 hours) can be determined using the ethyl glucuronide/ethyl sulfate test. This test must be specifically ordered as it is not part of a routine panel of drugs tested. Further, ethyl glucuronide and ethyl sulfate are metabolites of alcohol that result from hepatic metabolism. This test will not be positive in urine that has been contaminated by ethanol-producing bacteria and so is considered to be specific for alcohol use.

MANAGEMENT OF WITHDRAWAL

Treatment of alcohol or drug withdrawal is of special concern to the medical practitioner. Other urgent complications such as arrhythmia, alcohol or viral hepatitis, bleeding, gastritis, pancreatitis, skin abscess, sepsis, and overdose are covered in appropriate medical textbooks. Alcohol and opiate withdrawal are the most common withdrawal disorders, and physicians can manage many patients in outpatient settings if the withdrawal syndrome is mild in severity. Important parameters that patients should meet for adequate treatment in the outpatient setting include a commitment to abstaining from all mood-altering drugs during withdrawal (except as prescribed for withdrawal) and an expressed willingness to engage in continuing treatment. Homeless people or others not living with someone who can help monitor medication and symptoms in case of adverse events, those with significant polysubstance use, and those with important or unstable medical or psychiatric illness should not be treated as outpatients.

With regard to alcohol, when physical dependence develops, initial withdrawal symptoms of anxiety, sleep disorder, and tremor are mild, sometimes not attributed to alcohol, and easily relieved by drinking. As time passes, alcohol less reliably controls symptoms, and intoxication is fleeting, occurring only at high BAL (>250 mg/dL). Withdrawal is not an all-or-nothing state, and addicted patients experience symptoms whenever their BAL falls. The altered neurophysiology in the brain "perceives" a drop in BAL as disruptive to the new steady-state condition of addiction, and expresses the disruption through withdrawal symptoms. Soon, the person drinks steadily to alleviate withdrawal, but relief is brief. The range of BAL at which the individual feels "not sick" diminishes, and severe withdrawal, even delirium tremens, may develop despite a BAL of 300 mg/dL or more.

Outpatient treatment can be attempted in mild withdrawal. Physicians should hospitalize patients with clouded sensorium, fever, hyperventilation, a concomitant medical problem (e.g., hepatic failure, pancreatitis), or a history of alcohol withdrawal-related seizures, or if the patient has three risk factors for severe withdrawal (Table 24-7). Degree of tremor, anxiety, tachycardia,

Table 24-7. Risk factors for severe alcohol withdrawal.

- Drinking around the clock.
- Daily consumption of a fifth of liquor, a case of beer, or more than a half-gallon of wine.
- Heavy drinking for more than 5 years (on most days).
- Poor nutrition.
- Heavy sedative, cocaine, or opiate use.
- History of severe withdrawal within the past 2 years.

Table 24-8. Medication for outpatient alcohol withdrawal

Day 1: Give 25–50 mg chlordiazepoxide initially, then 25–50 mg every 4–6 hours, if needed. Alternatively, in those with hepatic impairment, give lorazepam 1-2 mg initially; then 1 mg every 4 to 6 hours as needed.

Day 2: Give 25 mg chlordiazepoxide every 4–6 hours. Alternatively, give lorazepam 1 mg every 4 to 6 hours.

Day 3 Give 25 mg chlordiazepoxide every 6–8 hours. Alternatively, give lorazepam 1 mg every 6-8 hours.

Day 4: Give 25 mg chlordiazepoxide or lorazepam 1 mg every 12 hours

Day 5: Give 25 mg chlordiazepoxide or lorazepam 1 mg; then discontinue.

Patients should be evaluated daily when undergoing outpatient alcohol medical withdrawal as severe withdrawal not controlled by the recommended doses can be associated with complications including seizures or the development of delirium tremens. Those with ongoing withdrawal symptoms despite medication should be admitted to the hospital to safely complete withdrawal.

Admit for inpatient withdrawal treatment if the patient drinks or uses other drugs during taper.

and stomach symptoms are poor predictors of need for inpatient care. When outpatient management is feasible, pharmacological support helps with symptom relief (Table 24-8) and must be integrated with patient education and referral options designed to help patients change entrenched behaviors. Medical withdrawal from alcohol should not be attempted on outpatients unless a responsible significant other has been identified who will stay with the patient and ensure that the medications for the patient are administered according to the physician's instructions. If there is not such a support system, a patient should be admitted to the hospital or residential substance abuse treatment facility where 24 hour skilled staff are available.

With regard to opiate withdrawal, physicians can be helpful. Patients who use high doses of opiates, including those who have become addicted to prescription opioid analgesics and those who inject heroin, experience intolerable craving during withdrawal. Relatively few patients succeed in medical withdrawal from opioids without intensive follow-up treatment including use of an opioid antagonist medication, naltrexone (given orally or by injection), and ongoing psychosocial treatment to address the dysfunctional behaviors of the drug-abusing lifestyle. Except for physicians who have obtained a waiver from the Drug Enforcement Administration that permits them to provide office-based treatment of opioid dependence and who can then dispense or prescribe buprenorphine/naloxone as a

Table 24-9. Protocols for Medical Withdrawal from Opioids.

				Day					
Clonidine with naltrexone induction	1	2	3	4	5	6	7	8	9
Clonidine	0.1-0.2 mg every 4 h; Not to exceed 1.0 mg in 24 h	0.1-0.2 mg every 4 h; not to exceed 1.2 mg in 24 h	0.1-0.2 mg every 4 h; not to exceed 1.2 mg in 24 h	0.1-0.2 mg every 4 h; not to exceed 1.2 mg in 24 h	**Taper**	**Clonidine reduce dose by 50% daily**	**Dose**	Begin naltrexone if opioid free for at least 7 days	
Naltrexone								25 mg/d	50 mg/d
Buprenorphine/naloxone withdrawal procedure									
Buprenorphine/naloxone *Note*: Patient must be in mild opioid withdrawal prior to first dose which should be given at the physician's office and the patient monitored for at least 2 hours.	Bup/nlx 2/0.5-4/1 mg sublingual 2 h later; if well tolerated give a second dose of Bup/ nlx 4/1 mg	12/3 mg	16/4 mg	Start	Taper	Complete	in	13 days	

Adjunctive medications for opioid withdrawal
Prochlorperazine 5-10 mg up to twice daily for nausea and vomiting
Dicyclomine 10-20 mg every 6 hours as needed for intestinal cramping
Loperamide 2 mg as needed for loose stools not to exceed 8 doses in 24 hours or Kaopectate 60 cc after each loose stool
Ibuprofen 600-800 mg up to three times a day for severe muscle or joint pain
Clonidine should not be given if the patient becomes dizzy after taking it

withdrawal or maintenance treatment specifically for opioid dependence, doctors should never give any opiate drugs for treatment of withdrawal. Provision of opiates by well-meaning clinicians is never successful, and federal law prohibits the prescription of opiates for treatment of opioid dependence. People who are ready to stop abusing oral opioids (especially prescription pain medications) can also be treated with clonidine, benzodiazepines, and antiemetics for a few days to a week or two as outpatients if buprenorphine/naloxone treatment is not an option (see Table 24-9 for a suggested regimen). Patients should check with the physician face to face every 2–3 days until symptoms are minimal, and during the withdrawal process make initial contact with a professional treatment program. The patient will relapse unless support in coping with psychosocial aspects of dependence is available. We underscore this crucial point: treatment of withdrawal is not treatment of drug dependence.

Patients who are both alcohol and benzodiazepine dependent or who are opioid and benzodiazepine dependent or those who are prescribed benzodiazepines from their physician are not candidates for outpatient medical withdrawal. Their medication needs are likely to be significantly higher than for a patient dependent on alcohol or opioids alone. The use of high doses of benzodiazepines during medical withdrawal procedures can be medically dangerous and such patients should be referred for inpatient treatment.

INTERVENTION STRATEGIES

Early intervention is more important than certainty about diagnosis. Physicians should always share their concern when they perceive a potential problem with drugs or alcohol. Effectiveness is more dependent on intervening early with the style and skills we discuss, rather than waiting to get the diagnosis exactly correct. Habits and addictive cycles are complex and entrenched, so starting earlier with effective brief interventions is better than waiting. The strategies described below are drawn from the National Institute on Drug Use (NIDA) and NIAAA Clinician's Guides for brief interventions for alcohol drug problems in primary care settings as well as the Motivational Interviewing treatment model of Miller and Rollnick.

Assess Patients' Current Readiness to Reduce Substance Use

As we move from data gathering to sharing information and planning, we like to begin with an assessment of interest in changing alcohol or drug use. An inquiry regarding current readiness level can also open a useful dialogue that can serve to increase motivation. For example:

Doctor: How interested are you in making a change in your marijuana use at this time, on a scale of 0–10?
Jim: Well, I would say about a 2.
Doctor: Why would you say a 2 and not 0?
Jim: I am a little concerned about how much money I have been spending on it every week.
Doctor: Tell me a little more about how marijuana may be impacting your finances and what your concerns are.

As this example illustrates, it is helpful to listen carefully for what patients report as their specific reasons for change. Miller and Rollnick refer to this as "change talk." Whereas a physician is typically most concerned about the impact of alcohol or drug use on health, often patients are more concerned about other issues that nevertheless are important sources of motivation to reduce use, as in the example here in which the patient is more concerned about the financial cost of drug use. Listening for change talk is an important strategy for physicians to use, allowing patients to make the case for change in their own words. As shown above, the physician responds with reflection or a request for elaboration.

Support Autonomy

Patients must make commitments and decisions in an atmosphere that genuinely tolerates and respects the full expression of ambivalence, resistance, and uncertainty, with respect to both facts and feelings. Physicians create such an atmosphere when they show they are listening to patients' perspectives without judgment by simply reflecting what they hear, and by reminding patients that they are in charge of all the important decisions, and free to take whatever action (or inaction) they choose. That is, physicians recognize patients' autonomy, while simultaneously offering their own expertise, clear recommendations, and support. A more explicit autonomy supportive statement (to Jim, above) could have been:

Jim: I'm quitting until I get my license back, no problem.
Doctor: It is your choice whether you wish to make any change in your drinking. I will always give you my best advice, and you make the final decisions.

CREATE DIALOGUE

True dialogue is difficult in conversations that involve substantial differentials in perspectives, expertise, and/or power. Patients tend either to defend a point of view or to be passive and silent. Clinicians can encourage dialogue by consciously employing a format of "tell, ask, tell, ask," which supports taking turns and results in a dialogue. Briefly provide (i.e., "tell") advice or information, and then "ask" patients what they think about it, or how it feels to hear it, or what they intend to do about it. Keeping the "telling" brief helps clarity, and "asking" allows the patient to choose a "change-enhancing" or "change-obstructing" response. The manner in which patients respond to the "ask" also suggests which next steps will likely be helpful. Generally, "change-enhancing" responses include statements of agreement, commitment, or optimism, and these suggest that exploring the facts might be helpful. Generally, "change-obstructing" responses, such as statements of disagreement, reservation, pessimism, defensiveness, noncommittal statements, and all questions that do not ask for clarification of meaning, suggest that the clinician should reflect back the response as the next step in the conversation. Reflection invites patients to look inside themselves, and encourages motivation and attention to discrepancy between patients' current situation and stated goals. Both "asking" and making reflections foster exploration and choice.

DIALOGUE ABOUT INFORMATION

Tell information about what is known about drug problems in an impersonal "objective" or "scientific" way. Here are some examples:

- "Research shows that treatment helps," or
- "Steady drug use changes brain function," or
- "Having a high tolerance for alcohol means that a person is deprived of the early warning system that tells him to stop drinking before the alcohol level gets so high as to be dangerous," or
- "95% of men drink less than 35 drinks per week," or
- "Many people are terrified to imagine stopping drug use," or
- "Being sick in the morning until after a drink means a person's brain has become hooked on alcohol," or
- "Men with any close relative with drinking problems have an almost 50% chance of developing serious problems themselves," or
- "Guidelines from extensive research show that drinking more than 14 drinks a week is risky."

Next, *ask* what patients think of this information, and how it might apply to their situation.

Tell information about the patient's situation as a fact, a number, or score, rather than a conclusion:

- "Three of your liver tests are abnormal," rather than "alcohol has damaged your liver," or
- "Your alcohol level when you arrived in the emergency room was 0.160," rather than "You were drinking heavily before you came into the emergency room," or
- "You have a serious infection in your arm," rather than "You got this infection because you were injecting," or
- "You mentioned three important things—that your relationship with your wife is going poorly, that you

are having a lot of stomach trouble, and that you lost your license to drive," rather than "Alcohol is wrecking your marriage, your career, and your body," or

- "You are very shaky and sick to your stomach until you can get another pill," rather than "You are addicted to tranquilizers," or
- "You have quit drinking several times," rather than "Your relapses show you are addicted."

Next, *ask* what the patient thinks of this information. Think about whether the patient's response to the "*ask*" is "change-obstructing" or "change-enhancing."

DIALOGUE ABOUT RECOMMENDATIONS; *TELL* ADVICE CLEARLY, BUT NOT HARSHLY

Then, after discussing relevant information, *tell* advice tentatively, as part of a search for a suitable and attainable action option before the next visit. "Wagging one's finger," actually or figuratively, tends to push patients into a corner, it highlights any feelings of shame or stigma, and it inhibits discussion. Physicians who display a posture of "I know what is right for you," without regard to cautions that apply to science (today's truth is tomorrow's fiction, and every case is unique), make patients defensive, and encourage arguments.

Useful advice has two other characteristics. First, give an objective rationale derived from a broader database than this case; and second, make your advice consistent with your assessment of your patient's willingness to consider it. The following specific examples illustrate these ideas.

- "The option that I recommend, based on data in the medical literature, and my experience with experts who have advised me about similar patients, is that you stop drinking all alcohol. Of course, no one can be certain that this is the right thing for you to do, or that it will work for you," or
- "Most people find that talking with people in Alcoholics Anonymous (AA) is helpful. AA might or might not be right for you. I recommend you go there."

Ask what the patient thinks of the advice. Commanding or ordering instead of checking the result of giving advice ensures poor adherence, as patients will not do things that they do not choose to do. If clinicians push ahead and try persuading patients in spite of reluctance, they foster continued ambivalence, raise resistance to change, and begin an enervating downward spiral in which both participants become further demoralized and discouraged.

Doctor: Jim, one option that I recommend, based on my experience with experts who have advised me about similar patients, is that you take this opportunity to stop drinking all alcohol, and actively participate in the counseling. Of course, no one can be certain that this is the right thing for you to do, or that it will work for you.

Jim: Thanks for your concern, Doc, but I know I'm OK; I'll quit for now, zoom through the stupid counseling thing, and get my license right back.

Doctor: We have different perspectives, Jim. Your focus is on the license, while mine is on the big picture of alcohol effects over the years.

Jim: Doc, you know me pretty well, so maybe there is some truth in what you say.

Doctor: Since alcohol can have important effects on blood pressure, let's check your pressure while you are off alcohol and then continue our conversation about your license and drinking as well.

Here is another example of how this discussion might proceed.

Jim: Thanks for your concern, Doc, but I know I'm OK; I'll quit for now, zoom through the stupid counseling thing, and get my license right back.

Doctor: Jim, I appreciate that you are thinking about this matter, but are not interested in making a longer commitment right now. Before your next appointment with me, which I will schedule for about 6 weeks, I wonder if you would be willing to take careful note of both the good things about drinking and the not-so-good things about drinking? Think a bit about the good things and the not-so-good things about NOT drinking, too. Then, I'd value the chance to seek a deeper understanding of the total picture, and help you make the best decision you can for yourself, as time goes by.

(Jim's response might surprise you)

Jim: You know, a fellow at work has been pushing me to go to AA, and I almost went with him after I got my DUI (driving under the influence; suggesting that Jim is or was more worried than he declares now).

(You might act on this hypothesis)

Doctor: It seems that we agree that it might be good to do something differently right now. Many people learn a lot about themselves when they go to a few AA meetings with an open mind. Would you be willing to go to one meeting a week until I see you again in a month or so?

CONFIRM RESULTS OF DIALOGUE

Finally, physicians need to be explicit that agreement has been reached on a specific plan. Check with patients that they are indeed committed to the plan and confident that they can carry it out. Set a specific timetable to follow up.

Doctor: "So, you are going to abstain until you get your license, and we'll meet to check your pressure and talk in about a month, right?"

Doctor: "You plan to go to six Alcoholics Anonymous meetings in the coming month, and we will talk about what you learn at your next appointment."

Doctor: "You decided to seek buprenorphine treatment from the city clinic. I'll send them a note about your diabetes and anemia, and I look forward to seeing you again after you get started there."

HELPING TO MAINTAIN CHANGE OVER TIME

At the follow-up visit, it is important to ask about any behavior change that the patient may have agreed to in the interim, even if the patient indicates that they are not yet ready to cut back on alcohol or drug use at the present time. For example, if the patient agreed to track how much they are drinking or to consider pros and cons of cutting back (as in the example above), continue the dialogue to help continue building patient motivation for change.

Many patients come to physicians having already made changes in drinking and drug use. These patients will benefit from thoughtful physician follow-up regarding those changes. Begin by acknowledging that change is difficult, and support any positive change, or efforts to change. Listen to patients' perspectives on their situation, and encourage reflection about both goals and strategies. Reaffirm your willingness to assist and talk, address any coexisting psychiatric disorders, and renegotiate the goals and plans when appropriate.

PHARMACOLOGICAL CONSIDERATIONS

Pharmacotherapies for Alcohol Use Disorders

Currently there are three medications approved by the US Food and Drug Administration for the treatment of alcohol dependence (severe alcohol use disorder). These include disulfiram (DIS), naltrexone (both oral and injectable formulations) and acamprosate. All can be useful treatments in selected patients in the context of an office-based practice.

Disulfiram is an aldehyde dehydrogenase inhibitor that inhibits the metabolism of acetaldehyde, a metabolite of alcohol, leading to a noxious reaction that includes flushing, palpitations, and headaches when alcohol is ingested following DIS administration. Disulfiram has been reportedly associated with nonadherence rates of 80% in a veteran sample with alcoholism and without intervention to assist with compliance. However, in this study fewer drinking days were reported in those who did adhere to DIS treatment, and there was a significant relationship between adherence and complete abstinence. Disulfiram is a medication that requires complete abstinence from alcohol. It is best reserved for those who have either failed other alcohol pharmacotherapies or for highly motivated individuals for whom complete abstinence is a requirement. Disulfiram is also contraindicated in pregnancy, in those with significant liver disease, esophageal varices, a history of gastrointestinal bleeding, or in those with psychosis, impulse control problems, or suicidality. A once daily dose of DIS 250 mg will inhibit aldehyde dehydrogenases within 12 hours to a degree at which a DIS/alcohol reaction will be observed should alcohol be ingested. The aldehyde dehydrogenase enzymes are fully inhibited in 3 days. Further, patients must generate new enzymes that metabolize alcohol before they can drink again without experiencing the DIS/alcohol reaction, and this will require at least 6 days following the last dose of DIS.

Naltrexone is a mu-opioid antagonist medication that is approved as a treatment for both opioid dependence and alcohol dependence. Naltrexone is thought to decrease craving for alcohol because it blocks some of the pleasant and reinforcing effects of alcohol by preventing the stimulation of opioid receptors and the reduction of dopamine release in the ventral tegmental area (VTA). Naltrexone is given at a dose of 50 mg orally daily, and there is also an injectable form of the medication given once monthly at a dose of 380 mg. The most common side effects with naltrexone treatment are stomach upset and headache. The medication can be started at a lower dose (12.5-25 mg/day) if this is a concern. Naltrexone has been associated with hepatotoxicity in some, usually at doses much higher than those approved by the FDA, but this has led to recommendations of baseline liver function tests and follow-up tests approximately every 3 months. Because naltrexone is an opioid antagonist, it should not be used in those who will need opioid medications for pain relief or who are already receiving treatment with opioid pain relievers.

Acamprosate is an anticraving medication which stabilizes excitatory glutamatergic neurotransmission that is altered during withdrawal from alcohol and is also FDA approved for the treatment of alcohol dependence. Like DIS and naltrexone, it has no abuse liability, and no sedative/hypnotic or muscle relaxant properties. One difficulty for some patients is the need to take this medication three times daily making adherence a difficulty in some cases. Acamprosate is renally cleared and can be an option for patients with alcohol use disorders complicated by serious liver disease or for patients who are likely to need ongoing opioid pain medications. Because DIS, naltrexone, and acamprosate are not controlled substances and have no mood-altering effects, these medications are easily prescribed by primary care clinicians who can provide medical care for alcohol use disorders in addition to other medical illnesses.

Pharmacotherapies for Opioid Dependence

There are two pharmacotherapies available for the treatment of opioid dependence which can be prescribed by primary care providers. The first is naltrexone, the opioid antagonist drug that blocks mu-opioid receptors and thereby blocks the effects of an opioid drug with agonist effects that might be ingested by a patient with opioid dependence. The dose of naltrexone to be used in the treatment of opioid dependence is the same as for alcohol dependence treatment—50 mg daily. Similarly, injectable naltrexone has been approved as a once monthly injection for treatment of opioid dependence at a dose of 380 mg. As in the treatment of alcohol dependence, the same provisos regarding side effects and potential adverse events are present for the opioid-dependent population who should be made aware of the risks/benefits of naltrexone treatment. It is important to know that naltrexone can precipitate opiate withdrawal in a patient who is physically dependent on opioids and who ingests this medication. Therefore, it is important to document last dose of opioid, no current use (which can be verified by urine toxicology screening), and resolution of opiate withdrawal symptoms and their temporal relationship to the first dose of naltrexone to be given. In general, once a patient has been completely tapered from the opioid they have been using and no longer have significant withdrawal symptoms, naltrexone can be started. Naltrexone can be started at a dose as low as 12.5–25 mg daily for those who experience gastrointestinal upset with this medication, and this can be continued for several days before increasing to the standard dose of 50 mg daily.

The second medication that can be used in primary care for the treatment of opioid dependence is buprenorphine or buprenorphine/naloxone. Buprenorphine is an opioid partial agonist medication that can be prescribed to treat opioid addiction, including addiction to prescription opioid pain medications or to heroin. Because buprenorphine is an opioid partial agonist, it has lesser effects on respiration at high doses, making it safer in an overdose situation. The exception to this is when buprenorphine is combined with other central nervous system sedative drugs, such as benzodiazepines, where serious adverse events and even death can occur. In addition, because buprenorphine is a partial agonist, it is thought to have less reinforcing effects than those of full mu-opioid agonists. Because of this, the FDA listed buprenorphine and buprenorphine products on Schedule III, making it possible for physicians to prescribe this medication from office-based practices to treat opioid dependence. However, only qualified physicians who have received a waiver from the Drug Enforcement Administration allowing them to prescribe such medications approved by the FDA to treat opioid dependence may prescribe buprenorphine. This usually requires a training of 8 hours in assessment and treatment of substance use disorders with a focus on opioid dependence, co-occurring mental illness, use of buprenorphine in clinical practice, and treatment of special populations with opioid dependence with buprenorphine. These trainings are available through the Center for Substance Abuse Treatment/SAMHSA (see www.pcssb.org, www.pcssmat.org or www.samhsa.gov) for physicians. The formulation of buprenorphine to be used in treatment of opioid dependence is buprenorphine/naloxone. Buprenorphine and buprenorphine/naloxone are taken sublingually. The addition of naloxone to the buprenorphine tablet is meant to discourage diversion of the drug to injected use. Naloxone, an opioid antagonist, is not active when ingested sublingually, but if buprenorphine/naloxone were to be injected by an opioid-dependent person who had recent opioid use, the naloxone would precipitate opiate withdrawal. Buprenorphine/naloxone is effective at clinical doses in the range of 12/3–16/4 mg sublingually daily and the upper dose approved by the FDA is buprenorphine/naloxone 24/6 mg. Buprenorphine/naloxone induction is required to start treatment in an opioid-dependent person. The patient must come to the office in mild–moderate opiate withdrawal before the medication can be initiated. The reason for this is that buprenorphine has a very high affinity for mu-opioid receptors and will displace other opioids that are occupying the mu-receptors. However, as a partial mu-opioid receptor agonist, buprenorphine will not provide the agonist effects that the patient is accustomed to and so can precipitate opiate withdrawal in a patient who has recently ingested opioids. Determining when to start buprenorphine is not difficult when a rating scale of opiate withdrawal severity is used (see www.pcssb.org—Clinical Guidances or www.samhsa.gov) and the patient receives rapid relief from opiate withdrawal once the first dose of buprenorphine is administered. All opioid-dependent patients will need ongoing psychosocial therapy and support from family/concerned others. Referral to Narcotics Anonymous groups can also be useful for support. It is important to be aware that prescribing buprenorphine/naloxone alone is not sufficient to treat opioid dependence. Further, although buprenorphine/naloxone can be used for medical withdrawal (see Table 24-9), maintenance treatment for at least 6 months to 1 year or as long as the patient is benefitting from the treatment is recommended to prevent relapse. It is also worth noting that methadone cannot be used to treat opioid dependence/addiction from office-based settings; rather this medication can only be given from federally regulated narcotic treatment programs for the treatment of opioid

dependence. In determining which medication might be the best choice for patients with opioid dependence, it is best to discuss their expectations of treatment: Are they willing to be medically withdrawn from opioids? Are they concerned about taking a medication that produces physical dependence? Is their goal to be free of medications that are mood-altering? If the answers to these questions are "no," then buprenorphine/naloxone might be the better medication choice. If the answers to the questions are "yes," then naltrexone might be the better choice.

Many addiction specialists agree that these drugs can be helpful for patients who commit to abstinence, and cannot remain sober. Because patients may imagine that these medications will provide a miraculous cure, the physician should promote this additional step toward abstinence, and also steer the patient toward an improved recovery regimen. The primary care physician should refuse to prescribe unless the patient undertakes additional action steps, for example, toward more involvement with addiction professionals or self-help groups. It is always a good idea to provide a listing of local resources, including specialized substance abuse treatment programs and self-help group meetings in the local geographic vicinity, for patients and family to take with them.

Referral to Specialized Treatment

Substance abuse treatment programs provide patients with specialized care, and physicians should refer any patients who do not make progress on changing substance use patterns in the primary care setting. Whether patients are making progress is more important to the need for referral than the apparent level of problem or the specific diagnosis of at-risk use, abusive use, or dependent use. Substance-dependent patients may benefit from access to medical withdrawal services and multidisciplinary counseling opportunities. Treatment programs can also help patients initiate contact with community-based self-help organizations, halfway houses, and intensive counseling, sometimes in an inpatient setting. Programs with co-occurring disorders treatment capabilities (i.e., the ability to provide treatment for both substance use disorders and other mental disorders) are able to serve patients with additional psychiatric problems known to occur frequently in those with substance use problems, more comprehensively than any physician's office. Physicians in these specialized treatment programs will be more familiar with, and so better prepared to treat, more complex patients with co-occurring substance use disorders complicated by mental illness. Findings from the 2009 National Survey on Drug Use and Health underscore the need for such programs as referral centers for the primary care physician who has identified a patient with multiple disorders. This survey reported rates of mental illness in those with substance use disorders to be 43% (versus a rate of mental illness in those without substance use disorders of 18%), and the rate of substance use disorders in those with mental illness was 16.5–26% depending on the severity of the mental illness (those without mental illness have an overall rate of substance use disorders of 6.5%).

Patients will often resist following through on a referral for specialized treatment. A helpful strategy is to confirm the patient's intention and commitment to follow through, as discussed in the sections above on making choices, supporting autonomy, and giving advice. An additional strategy is to emphasize your need for a second opinion from a specialist, just as might be the case with referral to a cardiologist. Set up the appointment before the patient leaves the office. Tell the patient you will send a referral letter summarizing your views and asking for advice from the specialist. Let the patient know that you will speak with the specialist after the assessment, and that you would like to participate in the treatment plan. It may also be helpful to indicate that outpatient treatment programs often have flexible options in the services they offer—for example, intensive or less intensive services, day or evening programs—and to encourage patients to get an appointment with a program even if they are not sure that they are ready for abstinence.

Many communities have programs for patients with special needs, such as adolescents, women, abusers of particular drugs (methadone treatment for opioid dependence/severe opioid use disorder with evidence of physical dependence on opioids is the best-known example), and patients with severe psychiatric problems. Self-help alternatives to AA and other mutual help groups exist in many communities; Rational Recovery is one example, and Women for Sobriety is another. These resources are available to help primary care providers obtain all of the treatment needed by a patient with substance use problems, in addition to any other medical illnesses that might be present. The primary care clinician can then be the provider to coordinate all of the interventions and treatment resources needed by these patients.

SUGGESTED READINGS

Barth KS, Malcolm RJ. Disulfiram: an old therapeutic with new applications. *CNS Neurolog Disord-Drug Targets* 2010;9(1):5–12. PMID:20201810.

Fiellin DA, Ried MC, O'Connor PG. Screening for alcohol problems in primary care. *Arch Intern Med* 2000;160:1977–1989.

Han B, Gfroerer JC, Colliver JD. Associations between duration of illicit drug use and health conditions: results from the 2005-2007 national surveys on drug use and health. *Ann Epidemiol* 2010;20(4):289–297. PMID:20171900.

Knopf A. SAMHSA pushes all providers for MI and SUD assessments. *Alcoholism and Drug Abuse weekly.* 2011.http://www.alcoholismdrugabuseweekly.com/sample-articles/samhsa-pushes-all-providers–mi-sud-Assesments.aspx. Accessed April 2013.

McCance-Katz EF. Office based treatment of opioid dependence with buprenorphine. *Harvard Rev Psychiatry* 2004;12:321–338. PMID:15764468.

Miller W, Rollnick S. *Motivational Interviewing: Helping People Change.* (3rd ed.) New York: Guilford, 2002.

NIAAA. *Helping Patients who Drink Too Much: A Clinician's Guide.* Washington, DC: Government Printing Office, 2005. (NIH; (301):443–3860; www.niaaa.nih.gov).PMID:19621845.

Substance Abuse and Mental Health Services Administration. *Results from the 2009 National Survey on Drug Use and Health: Volume I. Summary of National Findings* (Office of Applied Studies, NSDUH Series H-38A, HHS. 2010.

Willenbring ML, Massey SH, Gardner MB. Helping patients who drink too much: an evidence-based guide for primary care physicians. *Am Fam Physician* 2009;80(1):44–50. PMID:19621845.

American Psychiatric Association. (2013). *Diagnostic and statistical manual of mental disorders* (5th ed.). Arlington,VA: American Psychiatric Publishing.

WEB SITES

Clark WC, Parish S. *Alcohol: Interviewing and Advising. Module in Doc.com: An Interactive Learning Resource for Healthcare Communication.* American Academy on Communication in Healthcare. http://doccom.aachonline.org/dnn/Home.aspx. Accessed April 2013.

National Institute on Alcohol Abuse and Alcoholism (NIAAA). www.niaaa.nih.gov. Accessed April 2013.

Substance Abuse and Mental Health Services Administration: http://www.samhsa.gov/. Accessed April 2013.

Physicians' Clinical Support System-Buprenorphine. www.pcssb.org. Accessed April 2013.

Prescribers' Clinical Support System for Opioid Therapies. www.pcss-o.org. Accessed April 2013.

NIAAA Clinician's Guide: Helping Patients Who Drink Too Much. http://pubs.niaaa.nih.gov/publications/Practitioner/CliniciansGuide2005/guide.pdf. Accessed April 2013.

National Institute on Drug Use (NIDA). Screening for Drug Use in General Medical Settings. http://www.nida.nih.gov/nidamed/quickref/screening_qr.pdf. Accessed April 2013. Providers' Clinical Support System for Medication Assisted Treatment. HYPERLINK "http://www.pcssmat.org" www.pcssmat.org. Accessed January 2014.

Appendix 24-A The Alcohol Use Disorders Identification Test (AUDIT)

AUDIT

PATIENT: Because alcohol use can affect your health and can interfere with certain medications and treatments, it is important that we ask some questions about your use of alcohol. Your answers will remain confidential, so please be honest.

For each question in the chart below, place an X in one box that best describes your answer.

NOTE: In the United States, a single drink serving contains about 14 g of ethanol or "pure" alcohol. Although the drinks below are different sizes, each one contains the same amount of pure alcohol and counts as a single drink:

 12 oz. of beer (about 5% alcohol) = 8-9 oz. of malt liquor (about 7% alcohol) = 5 oz. of wine (about 12% alcohol) = 1.5 oz. of hard liquor (about 40% alcohol)

Questions	0	1	2	3	4	
1. How often do you have a drink containing alcohol?	Never	Monthly or less	2 to 4 times a month	2 to 3 times a week	4 or more times a week	
2. How many drinks containing alcohol do you have on a typical day when you are drinking?	1 or 2	3 or 4	5 or 6	7 to 9	10 or more	
3. How often do you have 5 or more drinks on one occasion?	Never	Less than monthly	Monthly	Weekly	Daily or almost daily	
4. How often during the last year have you found that you were not able to stop drinking once you had started?	Never	Less than monthly	Monthly	Weekly	Daily or almost daily	
5. How often during the last year have you failed to do what was normally expected of you because of drinking?	Never	Less than monthly	Monthly	Weekly	Daily or almost daily	
6. How often during the last year have you needed a first drink in the morning to get yourself going after a heavy drinking session?	Never	Less than monthly	Monthly	Weekly	Daily or almost daily	
7. How often during the last year have you had a feeling of guilt or remorse after drinking?	Never	Less than monthly	Monthly	Weekly	Daily or almost daily	
8. How often during the last year have you been unable to remember what happened the night before because of your drinking?	Never	Less than monthly	Monthly	Weekly	Daily or almost daily	
9. Have you or someone else been injured because of your drinking?	No		Yes, but not in the last year		Yes, during the last year	
10. Has a relative, friend, doctor, or other health care worker been concerned about your drinking or suggested you cut down?	No		Yes, but not in the last year		Yes, during the last year	
					Total	

Note: This questionnaire (the AUDIT) is reprinted with permission from the World Health Organization. To reflect drink serving sizes in the United States (14 g of pure alcohol), the number of drinks in question 3 was changed from 6 to 5. A free AUDIT manual with guidelines for use in primary care settings is available online at **www.who.org**

SCORING THE AUDIT

Record the score for each response in the blank box at the end of each line, then total these numbers. The maximum possible total is 40. Total scores of 8 or more for men up to the age of 60 years or 4 or more for women, adolescents, and men over the age of 60 years are considered positive screens. For patients with totals near the cut-points, clinicians may wish to examine individual responses to questions and clarify them during the clinical examination.

Note: The AUDIT's sensitivity and specificity for detecting heavy drinking and alcohol use disorders varies across different populations. Lowering the cut-points increases sensitivity (the proportion of "true positive" cases), whereas increasing the number of false positives. Thus, it may be easier to use a cut-point of 4 for all patients, recognizing that more false positives may be identified among men.

SECTION V
Mental & Behavioral Disorders

Depression

*Stuart J. Eisendrath, MD; Steven A. Cole, MD; John F. Christensen, PhD;
Damara Gutnick, MD; Mary Raju Cole, RN, MS, APRN
& Mitchell D. Feldman, MD, MPhil*

INTRODUCTION

Depression is common, disabling, and often unrecognized in general medical practice. Even when recognized, physicians frequently do not provide systematic, longitudinal evidence-based management. And from the perspective of the patient, stigma and other psychosocial barriers such as negative expectations often diminish adherence to treatment recommendations. Despite robust documentation that depression is quite treatable and the widespread availability of evidence-based guidelines, overall outcomes remain poor.

This chapter focuses on the core knowledge and skills needed by general medical practitioners to effectively assess and manage major depressive disorder (MDD). We briefly address other related mood disorders: dysthymic disorder, adjustment disorder with depressed mood, depression secondary to general medical conditions, bipolar disorder/bipolar depression, and melancholia. We emphasize the routine use of a brief patient self-assessment tool, the nine-item Patient Health Questionnaire (PHQ-9), for diagnostic and ongoing management purposes. Widespread adoption of this one practice innovation may provide the pivotal leverage needed to improve outcomes for depression.

MOOD DISORDERS: MAJOR DEPRESSION & RELATED CONDITIONS

Major depressive disorder (MDD) is associated with considerable disability, morbidity, and mortality. Epidemiologic studies demonstrate that depression causes more disability and social and role impairment than most other chronic illnesses, such as diabetes, arthritis, hypertension, and coronary artery disease. The World Health Organization has identified major depression as the fourth leading cause of disability worldwide and projects that it will become the second leading cause of worldwide disability by 2020. Major depression is also a well-documented and common comorbidity in many other chronic conditions: for example, heart disease, stroke, diabetes mellitus, cancer, Parkinson disease, arthritis, pulmonary disease, and others. Furthermore, when present as a comorbidity, depression accounts for significant increases in disability, morbidity, and mortality.

The etiologic and sustaining relationships between depression and these other conditions appear to be bidirectional. For example, preexisting depression has been established as a predictor of future atherosclerotic coronary artery disease, cerebrovascular disease, diabetes, and osteoporosis, and conversely, significant physical illness predicts higher prevalence of major depression compared with individuals without physical illness. Depressed patients with heart disease (coronary artery disease, congestive heart failure) have worse medical outcomes including increased risk of reinfarction (after myocardial infarction [MI]) and up to a three-fold increase in all-cause mortality (especially after MI), even after controlling for all other identifiable and measurable cardiac risks (such as overeating, sedentary lifestyle, smoking, and other predictors of poor outcome). Patients with diabetes and depression have worse glycemic control, more microvascular and macrovascular complications and greater all-cause mortality.

Major depression is associated with adverse health habits, such as smoking, poor diet, overeating, and sedentary lifestyle, these in turn contribute to the onset of general medical illness and/or poor outcomes in illness. Conversely, functional impairment stemming from these chronic illnesses predispose to development of new depression. From an etiologic perspective, variables such as genetic vulnerability, childhood adversity (neglect and abuse), and stressful life events all contribute to the development of depression itself as well as to lifestyle risks such as obesity, sedentary behavior, and smoking that themselves predispose to chronic general medical illnesses.

Chronic care of general medical illness requires self-management behaviors to optimize treatment, for example, special diets, exercise regimens, medication changes, daily glucose monitoring, blood pressure checks, and limiting potentially harmful behaviors, such as smoking and risky drinking. Studies show that depression adversely impacts self-management, at least partly due to the fact that depressed patients are more likely to be nonadherent than nondepressed patients. Depressed diabetic patients have decreased adherence to diet and suffer more lapses in refills of oral hypoglycemic medications. Depressed patients with heart disease or stroke show decreased adherence to treatment recommendations such as taking daily aspirin and participating in exercise rehabilitation programs. This nonadherence in post-MI patients predicts increased rehospitalizations and mortality. Major depressive disorder, with or without general medical comorbidity generally is a chronic, recurring illness, with varying cycles of exacerbation and remission. Furthermore, these exacerbations or new episodes of depression tend to occur more frequently and with greater severity as the patient ages.

Dysthymic disorder is a less severe but more chronic form of depressive illness that is also associated with significant disability, and is even more likely to go undiagnosed than major depression. This disorder is diagnosed when depressed mood and at least two other symptoms of depression have been present "more than half the days" during the previous 2 years. Dysthymic disorder has been shown to respond to treatment with antidepressant medication. Patients with dysthymic disorder have an increased risk of experiencing a major depressive episode.

Adjustment disorder with depressed mood involves a reaction to an identifiable stressor, such as divorce or job loss. It presents with a sad or depressed mood, a level of impairment greater than expected for most individuals facing that specific stressor and is diagnosed within the first 6 months after the stressor has occurred. A "normal" reaction to a distressing life event should not be diagnosed as an adjustment disorder. When a stressor precipitates a depressive condition that meets the severity and symptom criteria for major depression, the diagnosis of major depression is made, regardless of the condition's etiologic relationship to an identifiable stressor.

Mood disorders due to a general medical condition (or substance) refers to psychiatric syndromes judged to result from the direct physiologic consequence of a general medical condition (e.g., hypothyroidism), substance use (e.g., amphetamine withdrawal), or medication (e.g., interferon). Treatment focuses on resolution of the underlying general medical problem or withdrawal of the offending medication, although specific psychiatric treatment may also be useful.

Bipolar disorder is a common and severe mental illness, occurring in about 3–4% of the general population, causing significant disability, and carrying 80–85% genetic heritability. Bipolar I disorder refers to patients with a history of at least one episode meeting full criteria for major depression and at least one other distinct episode meeting criteria for mania. Other bipolar spectrum disorders such as bipolar II disorder (a condition marked by episodes of major depression and at least one documented episode of hypomania, not mania) and cyclothymic disorder (no episodes meeting full criteria for either major depression or mania/hypomania) are probably much more common, thought to occur in approximately 4–6% of the population.

Bipolar depression refers to an episode of illness meeting criteria for major depression in a patient with a history of either mania or hypomania. It can be very difficult for physicians to differentiate an episode of major depression from an episode of bipolar depression because the two conditions are phenotypically identical, that is they present the same signs and symptoms. It is extremely important, however, to distinguish between major depression and bipolar depression because the two conditions, though they present with the same symptoms, should be treated very differently. Studies in primary care indicate approximately 25% of patients presenting with symptoms that suggest the diagnosis of major depression actually suffer from bipolar depression.

Evidence for the best treatment of bipolar depression, however, is still somewhat limited and controversial. Only two medications, quetiapine and a combination product (olanzapine and fluoxetine) have received Food and Drug Administration (FDA) approval for the treatment of bipolar depression. Lamotrigine has FDA approval for maintenance treatment of bipolar depression, but is not yet approved for acute bipolar depression. Many experts recommend treating bipolar depression with a combination of a mood stabilizer (e.g., lithium, valproate, or carbamazepine) plus an antidepressant. Experts agree, however, that bipolar depression should *not* be treated with an antidepressant alone. Such "unopposed" treatment (i.e., antidepressant without mood stabilizer) increases the likelihood of precipitating an affective switch from depression to mania. Failure to elicit a history of mania or hypomania by the physician can lead, therefore, to potentially serious consequences by (mis)treating the condition with an antidepressant alone, thereby increasing the chances of a "switch" into mania or hypomania, with attendant risks of erratic or irrational behavior, poor judgment in social, occupational, economic, or interpersonal situations, psychosis, and even suicide. The section below on differential diagnosis provides physicians with some guidelines to help them make the diagnosis of bipolar depression in patients presenting with the symptom profile of major depression.

Melancholia is a severe form of major depression, often but not necessarily, associated with psychosis ("psychotic depression"). The symptom profile of melancholia includes lack of mood reactivity to usually pleasurable stimuli, loss of pleasure in all (or almost all) activities, distinct quality of depressed mood, diurnal variation in mood (worse in the morning), early morning awakening, marked psychomotor retardation or agitation, significant weight loss, and excessive or inappropriate guilt. This subtype of major depression is most closely associated with the so-called "biological markers" of depression, that is, nonsuppression of endogenous cortisol after administration of exogenous dexamethasone (DST), blunted thyroid-stimulating hormone (TSH) response to exogenous IV administration of thyrotropin-releasing hormone (TRH), and characteristically abnormal sleep physiology (including prolonged sleep latency, early-onset rapid eye movement [REM], increased total REM, and increased REM density). It appears that presence of melancholic features may predict preferentially better response to tricyclic medications (vs. the selective serotonin reuptake inhibitors [SSRIs]). The presence of melancholic features predicts a positive response to electroconvulsive therapy (ECT).

EPIDEMIOLOGY

Epidemiologic studies demonstrate a lifetime prevalence of major depression in 7–12% of men and 20–25% of women. The point prevalence of major depression in a community sample is 2.3–3.2% for men and 4.5–9.3% for women. Reasons for these gender differences have not been fully elucidated, but both biological and sociocultural factors are involved. Numerous studies report a 10–15% prevalence of major depression in ambulatory medical settings with a substantially higher rate (20–40%) in patients with coexisting medical problems, particularly in those with diseases associated with strong biological or psychological predispositions to depression (e.g., stroke, Parkinson disease, traumatic brain injury, diabetes, coronary atherosclerotic disease, pancreatic cancer, and other terminal illnesses).

Prevalence of depression varies among age groups. Recent data point to a cohort effect through which current "baby boomers" experience the highest rates of

depression of any previous generation. Although the most current epidemiologic findings show a surprisingly low 1-year prevalence rate of major depression in the elderly (1–2%), the rate of major or minor depression in elderly patients who seek treatment in primary care practices is 5%, with rates ranging from 15% to 25% in nursing home residents. Major depression is often misdiagnosed in elderly primary care patients as signs of aging, and cognitive impairment may also complicate accurate diagnosis. Some medications commonly prescribed in the elderly population may actually precipitate the onset of depression or cause symptoms like fatigue and poor concentration, which may mimic depressive symptoms.

Because the usual age of onset of depression is under the age of 40 years, an apparent first episode of depression in an older patient should prompt a thorough evaluation to exclude other underlying disease and/or medication effects.

ETIOLOGY

Major depressive disorder represents a heterogeneous group of disorders. It is likely that future research will eventually provide diagnostic specificity to these disorders, leading to more targeted and effective treatments. For present purposes, however, the clinical manifestation of a major depressive episode should be considered a final common psychobiological pathway among multiple candidate etiologic determinants. Dramatic advances, however, in genetic, anatomic, physiologic, and immunologic studies already point the way toward a more precise biological understanding of this common and disabling condition.

THE EMERGING BIOLOGY OF DEPRESSION: ADVANCES IN GENETICS, ANATOMY, PHYSIOLOGY, & IMMUNOLOGY

Recurrent major depression has been shown to have a heritability of 35–40%, and genetic linkage studies have begun to identify specific regions of the genome thought to be candidates for carrying depression susceptibility. One particularly interesting candidate gene is the serotonin transporter gene (5-HTT), which makes functional sense since many antidepressants seem to work through binding to the 5-HTT protein. Recent gene by environment studies have explored the relationship between heterozygous and homozygous states and response to negative life events. While the results are not clear, this type of exploration illustrates the potential impact of genetic and environmental interactions.

Twin studies on depression in women indicate that genetic factors play the strongest etiologic role in depression, followed by recent (as opposed to early environmental) negative life events. Animal studies, on the other hand, demonstrate that early environmental stress predisposes to biological abnormalities associated with depression that may not emerge until adult life.

Postmortem pathologic studies, along with functional and structural imaging studies, converge in locating anatomic loci of depressive illness in the hippocampus, the dorsolateral prefrontal cortex, the anterior cingulate cortex, and the amygdala. Animal and human studies confirm volumetric decreases in the hippocampus in depressive illness in individuals with a history of adverse childhood events. Antidepressant medications appear to induce neurogenesis (increases in volume) in the hippocampus, possibly through increases in brain-derived neurotrophic factor (BDNF).

From the physiologic point of view, a considerable body of emerging evidence now conceptually and experimentally points to dysregulation of distributed brain networks and second messenger abnormalities as the underlying neurobiological abnormalities in recurrent mood disorders. This contrasts with earlier theories postulating that straightforward monoamine neurotransmitter deficits (e.g., decreases in norepinephrine, serotonin, and/or dopamine) serve as the biological substrate of depression. Lastly, immunologic studies have consistently found abnormalities of cytokines associated with depressive illness. Advances in all these biological correlates of depression hold great promise for the development of more specific and more effective treatments of depressive disorders in the not too distant future.

SOCIAL & PSYCHOLOGICAL FACTORS

High Stress & Low Support

From a societal perspective, significant life stress, and/or lack of social support predisposes to development of MDD. Life stress that involves loss, for example, death of a parent or spouse, the end of a relationship, and events involving loss of self-esteem, such as termination from a job, create particular vulnerability for depression. Low social support, both independently and in the face of significant stress also predisposes to depressive disorder. Low *perceived* social support, that is, the

extent to which an individual *believes* himself or herself to lack a supportive social network, creates a higher risk than any absolute or objective measure. (It is worth noting that these same risk factors of high stress and low support tend to increase risk for all illnesses, whether psychiatric or general medical illnesses.)

The stress caused by natural disasters also increases the vulnerability of survivors to depression. While the psychiatric impact of such disasters includes increased prevalence rates of posttraumatic stress disorder (PTSD), substance abuse, and other conditions, the increased rate of depression itself is significant and measurable. For example, children and adults in the tsunami-affected areas of southwestern Thailand showed significantly increased and persistent rates of depression—ranging from 6% to 30% depending upon level of exposure and level of life disruption. Similarly, war has always been a stressor with major mental health consequences. For example, the US ground troops in Iraq have shown an increase in prevalence of depression from 11.4% prior to deployment to 15.2% after deployment.

With increased life expectancy and the aging of the population in the United States, spousal caregiving of persons with disability, including dementia, is increasing. Caregivers (most often the female partner) of spouses with chronic neurodegenerative illnesses (e.g., Alzheimer disease) experience extreme physical and emotional burden. The role of caregiver presents a situation of both high stress and increasingly low support (as the caregiver progressively loses any emotionally meaningful relationship with the patient). Up to 40% of caregivers of patients with progressive dementia suffer from significant depressive symptoms or major depression.

Postpartum "blues" typically occurs in 50–80% of women within 1–5 days of childbirth and lasts up to 1 week. This "normal" reaction should be distinguished from postpartum depression, which occurs in 10–15% of women in the first 3–6 months after childbirth. Postpartum psychosis, which occurs in 0.5–2.0/1000 deliveries and typically begins 2–3 days after delivery, and is most common in individuals with a personal or family history of bipolar disorder. Postpartum psychosis is a highly acute psychiatric illness that usually requires mood stabilizers such as neuroleptic medications or lithium, and psychiatric referral (see Chapter 16).

DIAGNOSIS

The criteria for major depression require that five of nine symptoms be present for a 2-week period (Table 25-1). One of these nine symptoms must be either a persistent depressed mood (present most of the day, nearly every day) **or** pervasive anhedonia (loss of interest or pleasure in living).

Table 25-1. Diagnosis of major depression.

1. Depressed mood
2. Anhedonia (lack of interest or pleasure in almost all activities)
3. Sleep disorder (insomnia or hypersomnia)
4. Appetite loss, weight loss; appetite gain, weight gain
5. Fatigue or loss of energy
6. Psychomotor retardation or agitation
7. Trouble concentrating or trouble making decisions
8. Low self-esteem or guilt
9. Recurrent thoughts of death or suicidal ideation

Five symptoms from the above are required to make the diagnosis of depression and must include depressed mood and/or anhedonia. The symptoms must have been present most of the day, nearly every day, for 2 weeks.

Clinicians should realize that a depressed mood is not synonymous with major depression and is neither necessary nor sufficient for a diagnosis of major depression. Sadness (or tearfulness) does not constitute major depression (four other symptoms described in the following paragraph are necessary), and, conversely, major depression can be diagnosed without the presence of depressed mood (if pervasive anhedonia is present), a presentation that is more common in the elderly.

Organizing these nine symptoms into clusters of four hallmarks can facilitate clinical evaluation: (1) depressed mood; (2) anhedonia; (3) physical symptoms (sleep disorder, appetite problem, fatigue, and psychomotor changes); and (4) psychological symptoms (difficulty concentrating or indecisiveness, guilt or low self-esteem, and thoughts of death). Physical symptoms predict a favorable response to biological intervention. For example, when middle insomnia is present (awaking at 3 or 4 A.M. with an inability to return to sleep) and when a diurnal variation in mood is present (feeling more depressed in the morning), patients are more likely to respond to biological interventions.

The Fallacy of "Good Reasons"

Depression is often mistakenly believed to be an "expected" result of stressful life events. Studies of individuals under stress (e.g., terminal cancer or natural disaster) do show rates of major depression above the general population rate, but these rates do not exceed 50%. Although sad or depressed affect is an expected accompaniment of a stressful event, the full syndrome of major depression certainly does not appear in everyone. Thus, life stressors may seem to provide "good reasons" for sadness, but a stressful event, in itself, should not be considered a rationale to withhold depression treatment. If a major depressive syndrome emerges following a stressful life situation, the medical provider should treat it appropriately. This is similar to treating other medical conditions that have a "good reason," such as hypovolemic shock from a gunshot wound—the etiology is evident but the condition clearly requires treatment.

The term *reactive depression* has historically suggested a mild syndrome without a biological substrate, resulting from a psychosocial precipitant, and treatable with psychotherapy alone. None of these assumptions is true. Stressful events can precipitate very severe depressions; a biologically predisposed individual may suffer major depression in response to a minor life event; a major depression following a life stressor may develop a biological substrate; and a major depression from a life stress may respond to biological therapy as well as or better than it responds to psychotherapy. *Thus, the presence or absence of identifiable precipitants is irrelevant to the diagnosis of major depression*, which can be treated pharmacologically whether or not the condition resulted in part from psychological stressors. Depression is a frequent, but *not* an inevitable consequence of a stressful life event. When major depression is present, it should be treated aggressively.

The Confound of Overlapping Etiology

A comorbid general medical condition (such as cancer or Parkinson disease) may seemingly "cause" many of the physical symptoms of major depression, such as fatigue, anorexia, or psychomotor retardation. These symptoms may lead clinicians to discount their relevance and thus disregard the possibility of a treatable depression. However, a physical symptom may be "caused" by a physical illness (e.g., cancer) or by a major depressive illness or both. It is important to *include* these symptoms in the initial diagnostic approach to depression in the medically ill, and exclude them *only if they are clearly and fully accounted for by the physical illness*. Although this "inclusive" approach might seem to result in the overdiagnosis of major depression; studies in stroke, Parkinson disease, hospitalized elderly, and traumatic brain injury indicate that the problem of overdiagnosis is quite low (around 2%) and the underdiagnosis of depression is more of a problem.

THE MEDICAL INTERVIEW

Build Trust by Responding to Distress

The medical interview holds the key to the assessment of major depression. Efficient assessment involves attention to data-gathering as well as rapport-building functions of the interview. Physicians should always be alert for nonverbal cues of depression: for example, a sad mood may be communicated by downcast eyes, slow speech, wrinkled brow, or tearful affect. When a depressed mood is detected or emotional distress is suspected, physicians should first respond empathically to this distress, by demonstrating a caring attitude, and using attentive silence or direct reflective and empathic statements, such as "I can see you're having some trouble," or "It sounds like you've been under a lot of stress lately," or "You seem pretty down right now." Responding directly to the patient's distress in this way builds trust and encourages the patient to more openly share his or her feelings that may underlie a depressive illness.

Use Direct, but Open-Ended Questioning

Use open-ended questions and facilitation techniques to provide patients with the opportunity to discuss the issues that may be troubling (see Chapter 1). In gathering data for assessment, physicians should focus on *anhedonia* (e.g., "What do you enjoy doing these days?") and *depressed mood* (e.g., "How has your mood been the last few weeks?" or "Have you been feeling sad, blue, or down in the dumps?"). These simple questions can effectively uncover an underlying depression in most patients, despite the fact that most depressed patients in the general medical setting initially present with chief complaints more related to physical and bodily symptoms (e.g., headache, fatigue, and insomnia).

Involve the Family

Optimal assessment and management of the depressed patient is enhanced by involvement of one or more significant other(s). A spouse, a partner, a parent, or others can help the physician gather useful information regarding the patient's mood, activities, behaviors, and history. In fact, because of stigma, denial, and other psychosocial barriers, other persons often provide much more accurate information regarding depressive illness than the self-report of the patient himself or herself.

The Patient Health Questionnaire: Screening, Assessment, Engagement, & Monitoring

The US Preventive Services Task Force (USPSTF) supports screening for depression "in clinical practices that have systems in place to assure accurate diagnosis, effective treatment, and careful follow-up." Although many tools to screen for depression are available, USPSTF recommends the use of a straightforward two-item ("yes/no") screener for major depression that is as effective as longer screening instruments. When administered verbally, clinicians can ask:

1. "Over the past 2 weeks, have you ever felt down, depressed, or hopeless?" and
2. "Over the past 2 weeks, have you felt little interest or pleasure in doing things?"

A positive answer to either of these two questions requires a full diagnostic assessment for major depression.

This screener has over 90% sensitivity but relatively low specificity (many false positives). Alternatively, many experts now advocate administration of the full PHQ-9 (Appendix 25-A) to "red flag" patients, that is, patients likely to be at high risk of major depression. "Red flag" patients generally include those with chronic medical illness (e.g., diabetes), and patients with persistent unexplained medical complaints. This one-step approach, combining screening and assessment, can simplify operational strategies.

The PHQ-9 is an assessment and severity tool that has been validated for use in general medical as well as specialty psychiatric settings. A score of 10 or more has been demonstrated to have 88% sensitivity and 88% specificity for the diagnosis of major depression. Furthermore, the tool can also be used effectively as a severity tool to track patients' symptom severity and improvement over time. The instrument and scoring key are in Appendices 25-A and 25-B. Pfizer holds the copyright for this tool, but it can be used in the public domain for clinical purposes or research. Readers are also referred to the web site of the MacArthur Foundation Initiative on Depression in Primary Care for materials related to the use of this instrument (www.depression-primarycare.org).

BARRIERS TO DIAGNOSIS

Patient Barriers: Somatic Presentations & Stigma

Patients in general medical practice with major depression typically present with physical complaints, such as pain (headache, backache), fatigue, insomnia, dizziness, or gastrointestinal (GI) problems. Many of these patients are willing to acknowledge feelings of depressed mood and to consider the possibility that biologically mediated depression may also cause or exacerbate their physical problems. There are many somatically preoccupied patients, however, who do not experience any depressed affect at all, and, without this self-appraisal of sadness, they are reluctant to consider the possibility that depression may contribute to their physical problems. In these patients, evaluating both general medical and psychiatric problems simultaneously saves time, expense, and frustration for both the physician and the patient. In addition, many patients and families (particularly in some cultures) are reluctant to accept the diagnosis of depression because of associated social stigma. Physicians can help overcome this barrier by understanding and explaining to patients and families that depression is a common and treatable illness, like other medical illnesses. They may explain that depression represents a chemical imbalance that can, like diabetes and other medical conditions, be corrected or managed with adequate treatment.

Clinician Barriers

Depression is often undetected or is not adequately treated in the medical setting. Some physicians avoid depression diagnoses because they harbor the same stigmatizing attitudes toward depression that many of their patients feel. In addition, inadequate knowledge and skill, lack of time, reluctance to "open up" new domains of emotional distress, and misaligned financial incentives all operate as barriers to physician recognition and treatment. However, early recognition of behavioral and psychiatric disorders is time efficient in the long run while minimizing the cost and risk of extended, unnecessary workups for nonspecific physical complaints.

SUICIDE

Suicide risk must be evaluated in all patients with symptoms of depression. It is one of the top 10 causes of death in all age groups, and one of the top 3 causes in young adults and teenagers. Risk factors for completed suicide include gender (elderly white males are at highest risk), alcoholism, psychosis, chronic physical illness, lack of social support, recent humiliation, and use of generally lethal methods (e.g., gun rather than overdose of pills). Increased risk of suicide has also been noted among depressed adolescents and among gay and lesbian patients. Explicit suicidal intent, hopelessness, and a well-formulated plan indicate relatively higher risk. Many patients who eventually commit suicide visit a primary care physician in the weeks before they take their lives.

Physicians are sometimes reluctant to explore suicidal ideation in the mistaken belief that asking about suicide may actually increase a patient's risk. To the contrary, assessment of suicidal tendencies usually reassures patients, reduces anxiety for both patient and provider, and facilitates partnership in suicide prevention.

The assessment of suicidal ideation is best approached gradually, with general questions like, "Do you sometimes feel that life is not worth living?" and then asking more specifically about a history of suicide attempts, any specific current plans, hopelessness, and any specific current intentions. Once a patient reveals suicidal ideation, the physician must consider psychiatric consultation and hospitalization. If outpatient management is considered, some experts suggest that physicians consider use of a "no suicide contract." The no suicide contract involves asking the patient to promise that he or she will contact the physician (or other appropriate caregiver) if there is a danger of losing control of a suicidal impulse. In using such a "contract," however, physicians need to realize that there is no convincing empirical evidence to support its validity. In fact, other experts specifically advise against its use, arguing that a mechanistic pursuit of obtaining a "contract" can functionally undermine an open relationship and provide physicians with a false sense of security. The main utility of the "contract" may be as tool to discuss the strength of the individual's suicidal ideas.

In all cases, when treating depression, physicians must evaluate suicidality at the initiation of treatment and throughout the treatment program.

Routine use of the PHQ-9 can aid in assessing suicide risk at the initiation of treatment and, of equal importance, can also aid in the recognition of any subsequent or treatment-emergent suicide risk. Because the risk of suicide sometimes increases within the first few weeks of treatment and can emerge at any point in the subsequent treatment, regular and routine use of the PHQ-9 can function as an efficient and effective suicide reassessment tool. The Columbia-Suicide Severity Rating Scale is a useful clinician-administered instrument (http://www.cssrs.columbia.edu/about_cssrs.html).

Van Gogh—Image of Depressed Man.

PHYSICAL EXAMINATION

There are no specific diagnostic signs of depression. A careful medical history and physical examination are required for the evaluation of depression at all ages, but especially in the elderly. Some medical "mimics" of depression (e.g., hypothyroidism and Cushing syndrome) present with classic physical signs.

LABORATORY STUDIES

No laboratory studies can be used to diagnose major depression reliably or specifically. A general laboratory screen (complete blood count, chemistry profile, urinalysis, TSH, and vitamin levels), however, may be useful in selected patients to rule out other conditions that may mimic or exacerbate depression. In treatment-resistant cases, or when indicated, brain imaging, an electroencephalogram (EEG) or lumbar puncture (LP) can be considered, but these studies are not part of the standard work up. Patients over the age 40 years usually require an electrocardiogram (ECG) to rule out conduction disturbances or bradycardia if treatment with a tricyclic antidepressant (TCA) or if citalopram at doses greater than 40 mg/day are being considered since those doses may be associated with prolonged QT intervals and arrhythmias

DIFFERENTIAL DIAGNOSIS

Mental Disorders

Other mental disorders often present with symptoms similar to depression; in addition, depression often presents in combination with other mental disorders. Thus, knowledge of other mental disorders common in medical practice is essential for adequate assessment and management of depression. In the presence of psychiatric comorbidity, effective treatment of depression may lead to improvement in the other condition as well. Modifications of treatment, however, may be necessary depending on the particular comorbidity present.

Major Depressive Disorder versus Bipolar Depression

One of the most important, yet difficult, differential diagnostic questions facing the physician is to distinguish MDD from bipolar depression (discussed earlier). The clinical signs and symptoms of the two disorders are identical and the differential diagnosis hinges on one and basically only one crucial historical question: *Did the patient ever experience clinical mania or hypomania?* The symptoms of a manic episode are listed in Table 25-2, the most common of which include an elated or irritable mood, racing thoughts, poor judgment in interpersonal, sexual, or financial situations, and excess energy. Criteria for hypomania are the same, but are less intense and not disruptive of normal functioning. To uncover a possible history of mania/hypomania, the physician should ask about any personal or family history of treatment of mania/hypomania/bipolar disorder and whether the patient has ever experienced any distinct period when he or she experienced racing thoughts, markedly decreased need for sleep, especially high energy or unusually poor judgment, out

Table 25-2. Criteria for manic episode.

A. A distinct period of abnormally and persistently elevated, expansive, or irritable mood, lasting at least 1 week (or any duration if hospitalization is necessary).

B. During the period of mood disturbance, three (or more) of the following symptoms have persisted (four if the mood is only irritable) and have been present to a significant degree:
  1. Inflated self-esteem or grandiosity
  2. Decreased need for sleep (e.g., feels rested after only 3 hours of sleep)
  3. More talkative than usual or pressure to keep talking
  4. Flight of ideas or subjective experience that thoughts are racing
  5. Distractibility (i.e., attention too easily drawn to unimportant or irrelevant external stimuli)
  6. Increase in goal-directed activity (either socially, at work or school, or sexually) or psychomotor agitation
  7. Excessive involvement in pleasurable activities that have a high potential for painful consequences (e.g., engaging in unrestrained buying sprees, sexual indiscretions, or foolish business investments)

The mood disturbance is sufficiently severe to cause marked impairment in occupational functioning or in usual social activities or relationships with others, or to necessitate hospitalization to prevent harm to self or others, or there are psychotic features.

of character to the patient's usual behavior. The Mood Disorders Questionnaire (MDQ) can be added to the physician's diagnostic armamentarium as a guide (Table 25-3), though its sensitivity and specificity are not high enough to rely on as a stand-alone tool. Even if there is no history of mania/hypomania, if the individual has a strong family history of bipolar disorder, the clinician must consider that at least one-third of bipolar patients have depression as their index mood episode. Such a history should help make the clinician alert to potential mood switches with antidepressant treatment. In addition, such patients may also be resistant to antidepressant strategies and require mood stabilizers instead.

Anxiety Disorders

Anxiety and depression commonly co-occur in medical patients. Most patients with depression suffer from anxiety symptoms or a formal anxiety disorder and most patients with an anxiety disorder have depressive symptoms or meet criteria for major depression. The most common anxiety disorders in medical outpatients are PTSD, generalized anxiety disorder (GAD), panic disorder (PD), and obsessive-compulsive disorder (OCD). Central features of these disorders include pervasive and disabling anxiety (e.g., GAD), discrete panic attacks (e.g., PD), or the presence of unreasonable, uncontrollable,

Table 25-3. The MDQ and scoring guide.

THE MOOD DISORDER QUESTIONNAIRE

Instructions: Please answer each question as best you can.

	YES	NO
1 Has there ever been a period of time when you were not your usual self and …		
… you felt so good or so hyper that other people thought you were not your normal self or you were so hyper that you got into trouble?	O	O
… you were so irritable that you shouted at people or started fights or arguments?	O	O
… you felt much more self-confident than usual?	O	O
… you got much less sleep than usual and found you didn't really miss it?	O	O
… you were much more talkative or spoke much faster than usual?	O	O
… thoughts raced through your head or you couldn't slow your mind down?	O	O
… you were so easily distracted by things around you that you had trouble concentrating or staying on track?	O	O
… you had much more energy than usual?	O	O
… you were much more active or did many more things than usual?	O	O
… you were much more social or outgoing than usual, for example, you telephoned friends in the middle of the night?	O	O
… you were much more interested in sex than usual?	O	O
… you did things that were unusual for you or that other people might have thought were excessive, foolish or risky?	O	O
… spending money got you or your family into trouble?	O	O
2 If you checked YES to more than one of the above, have several of these ever happened during the same period of time?	O	O
3 How much of a problem did any of these cause you—like being unable to work; having family, money or legal troubles; getting into arguments or fights? Please circle one response only.	O	O
No problem Minor problem Moderate problem Serious problem		
4 Have any of your blood relatives (i.e. children, siblings, parents, grandparents, aunts, uncles) had manic-depressive illness or bipolar disorder?	O	O
5 Has a health professional ever told you that you have manic-depressive illness or bipolar disorder?	O	O

Positive Screen (all three of the following criteria must be met) Questions 1: 7 of 13 positive (yes) responses + Question 2: positive (yes) response + Question 3: "moderate" or "serious" response

---

Source: Reprinted from Hirschfeld RM, Williams JB, Spitzer RL, et al. Development and validation of a screening instrument for bipolar spectrum disorder. The Mood Disorder Questionnaire. *Am J Psychiatry* 2000;157(11):1873-1875.

and repetitive behaviors (e.g., compulsions such as hand-washing or checking the stove) or the presence of intrusive, uncontrollable, and disturbing thoughts (e.g., sexual and violent obsessions in a patient who has no history or risk of such behaviors) (e.g., OCD). Treatment of the major depression by itself, however, often helps to resolve or improve these other coexisting conditions (see Chapter 26), especially since many antidepressant medications have proven safe and effective for treating some common anxiety disorders.

Somatic Symptom Disorders

Depression often presents with unexplained bodily complaints. It can therefore be challenging to differentiate between a depressive illness and somatic symptom disorder which includes previously used terms such as medically unexplained symptoms (see Chapter 28). Depressive disorders are highly treatable, but somatic symptom disorders can be more chronic and refractory to treatment. Somatic symptom disorders are usually best managed conservatively with a focus on improved functioning, whereas depression should be treated aggressively with the goal of complete recovery. Any of the somatic symptom disorders (formerly diagnosed as conversion, somatization, hypochondriasis, body dysmorphic disorder, and somatoform pain disorder) can present comorbidly with major depression. Approximately 50% of patients with persistent unexplained physical complaints suffer from depression. Effective treatment of major depression usually improves the severity, intensity, and functional impairment of a comorbid somatic symptom disorder.

Substance Abuse

Patients with alcohol dependence or other substance use disorders commonly present with major depression. Likewise, all patients diagnosed with depression should be screened for comorbid substance use disorders, particularly alcohol. Major depression even in the context of substance dependence deserves treatment in its own right, as long as the treatment plan attends to potential complications from continuing substance abuse. Furthermore, effective treatment of depression may help ameliorate the alcohol problem itself and does not generally lead to increased complications. Some patients will benefit from referral to a specialty mental health or substance abuse facility for treatment of their substance dependence and some severely ill patients will need treatment in settings with the capacity to treat "dual diagnosis" patients.

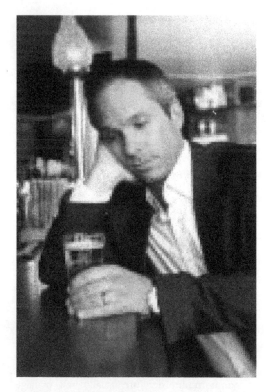

Personality Disorders

Personality disorders represent enduring character patterns that are deeply ingrained and are not generally amenable to alteration (see Chapter 29). They often complicate the diagnosis and management of mood disorders. Because patients with personality disorders can be difficult and demanding, physicians often try to minimize contact with them. Unfortunately, this may lead to avoidance of emotional issues and failure to diagnose depression. Effective treatment of major depression often improves functioning when the depression coexists with a personality disorder, even if the underlying personality disorder is itself not fundamentally changed.

Dementia

In its early stages, dementia can be often difficult to distinguish from depression. Depression often leads to reversible cognitive impairment in the form of decreased concentration, memory difficulties, impaired decision-making ability, difficulty planning and organizing, and difficulty getting started on tasks. These are also impairments that can result from an insidious and irreversible neurodegenerative process. Likewise, the effect of dementia on a person's functioning can lead to a depressed mood. When diagnostic uncertainty exists, because the cognitive impairments of MDD are reversible, clinicians should treat the depressive component (with both medication and counseling) and observe for changes in the patient's cognitive symptom cluster.

The term "pseudodementia" is used to describe treatable depression presenting with features of cognitive impairment. While it is useful for clinicians to understand that depression may be associated with cognitive impairment, clinicians should avoid use of this terminology. In actual practice, some patients for whom the concept of "pseudodementia" is considered may actually suffer from both conditions. Furthermore, late-onset depression (even reversible late-onset depression) is itself predictive of future dementia.

Depression due to General Medical Conditions or Medications

Approximately 10–15% of all depression is considered to be the direct physiologic result of a medical illness, such as hypothyroidism or hyperthyroidism, pancreatic cancer, Parkinson disease, or stroke (Table 25-4). Because there are no clear criteria to help guide clinicians in their evaluation, this diagnosis is ultimately made by clinical inference, considering the timing of the depression in relation to the physical illness. Limited data seem to indicate that standard treatments for major depression are effective in these cases.

Similarly, depression can be caused by exogenous medications (Table 25-5). Approximately 50% of patients treated with interferon develop a full major depressive episode and the history of previous depression or the presence of even mild current depressive symptoms can reliably predict the development of subsequent depression during treatment with interferon. Evidence now supports the prophylactic use of antidepressants before initiating interferon treatment, especially in patients with histories of depression. No medication has

Table 25-4. General medical conditions with high prevalence of depression.

Disease/Condition
Lewy Body disease
End-stage renal failure
Parkinson disease
Stroke
Cancer or AIDS
Chronic fatigue
Diabetes mellitus
Chronic pain
Heart disease
Chronic lung disease
Following CABG surgery

been noted to "cause" depression in all patients, so it is therefore crucial to carefully evaluate the patient's clinical history and link the onset of depressive symptoms to the initiation of new medications or changes in the current regimen as well as considering psychosocial stressors to obtain the clearest picture of depression causation.

TREATMENT

Use Communication Skills, PHQ-9 Scores, & the Family for Engagement

Building on the patient's trust, the working alliance, and the doctor–patient relationship, the physician should integrate his or her understanding of the patient's symptoms and life situation into a clear presentation of the diagnosis to engage the patient for collaborative management.

In addition, the process of the clinician's communication with a depressed patient should be informed by an appreciation of the patient's slower rate of cognitive processing. Information should be given in small chunks, allowing adequate attentive silence for the patient to assimilate and respond. In addition, the physician should

Table 25-5. Medications that can cause depression.

- Interferon
- Antihypertensives
- Hormones
- Anticonvulsants
- Steroids
- Digitalis
- Antiparkinsonian agents
- Antineoplastic agents

verify adequate assimilation of information by asking the patient to summarize what has just been communicated. The following statement would be appropriate:

"Doctors sometimes have a hard time communicating clearly with their patients. Just to be sure I have been able to make my thoughts clear to you, would you mind summarizing what we just went over."

By using the PHQ-9, practitioners can integrate these results into the engagement process. The first step is to check some of the symptoms with the patient to verify the validity of specific responses. After verifying that the actual score on the PHQ-9 appears to accurately capture the patient's symptoms, discuss the diagnosis and engage the patient for collaborative treatment planning. Because some patients may feel shame or embarrassment with a diagnosis of depression, it may be helpful for some patients to explain that major depression is a common *biological* disorder. Drawing a picture of a synapse and neurotransmitters also may be helpful for some.

A crucial part of the engagement process involves instilling hope that this painful illness is treatable. The treatment involves mobilizing patient resources and/or external resources such as medication and social support. Indicate that depressive symptoms can be relieved and note that "others may notice improvements in you before you notice the change yourself." When adverse life circumstances play a role in the cause of major depression, the physician can acknowledge the role played by the stressors, but must also help the patient understand that treatment of the depression can help him or her cope better with life's adversities.

The physician should attempt to involve the family or other support systems (however, defined) in treatment planning to help ensure adherence to the collaborative plans. Keep in mind, however, that family and/or friends may at times sabotage or undermine treatment and impede recovery. Approximately 40% of depressed patients suffer from some degree of discord in the relationship that contributes to illness onset and/or becomes a barrier to recovery. When discord is detected, it should be acknowledged and included in the overall treatment.

 CASE ILLUSTRATION

The following case illustrates many of the principles discussed earlier.

Mrs. Gladstone, a 45-year-old single woman presents complaining of abdominal pain and fatigue. The abdominal pain is similar to episodes in the past of irritable bowel syndrome and after a very brief history, the physician is convinced that conservative management with added fiber in the diet and anti-spasmodic medication is appropriate.

Within the first 5 minutes of the interview, however, her physician also noted that her affect was flat and that she spoke with long latencies. She also complained of having trouble sleeping, frequently awakening after 4 hours with inability to get back to sleep because of worries that she is not qualified for her new managerial position. Things are not going well at home either. Her husband is complaining that her work keeps her from her responsibilities to her adolescent children, to the household, and to him.

The physician then asked her to fill out the PHQ-9 (copies are in the examination room). After leaving the room for 2–3 minutes to return a phone call, the physician then returned and noted that the patient scored 16 on the PHQ-9, with significant symptoms including sleep problems, energy problems, low self-esteem, anhedonia, and sad mood. She did not endorse any suicidal ideation. Knowing that this score is associated with a high probability of moderate-to-severe major depression, the following dialogue represents one possible method for presenting the diagnosis and engaging the patient in treatment planning.

Physician: I see you answered positively to a lot of the questions on this form. I wonder what you think about the questions.

Mrs. Gladstone: I kind of surprised myself. I'm having trouble with almost everything on that form.

Physician: It seems like you're under a lot of stress.

Mrs. Gladstone: (Tearful) I am. When I go to bed, I dread the next day . . . I know I won't get enough rest and I get this sinking feeling I just can't do it—I'm not good at anything anymore—my work, my home, my marriage. And the stomach pain isn't going away.

Physician: I have some ideas for the stomach pain, but I wanted to check a few of your answers on this form before we come up with a plan for your stomach. It seems like you are feeling very sad almost all the time and there's no more fun in your life.

Mrs. Gladstone: (nods positively—with tears again). And I'm crying by myself a lot. I don't want the kids or my husband to see me.

Physician: It sounds like you're really struggling. The good news is that I think I know what is going on and I think I can help. Your score on this questionnaire is 16—which tells me you're probably suffering from depression—on top of everything else.

Mrs. Gladstone: Well, with the stress of the job, no sleep, the kid's constant whining, and my husband's criticism, who wouldn't be depressed?

Physician: You're right. A lot of people would get depressed with this kind of stress. But now you've got a depression that reflects a chemical imbalance in your brain. And the good news is that there's a lot we can do to help you feel better. If that makes sense to you, you and I can start talking about different ways we might begin to treat this problem and help you feel a lot better.

Treatment Goals: Defining Clinically Significant Improvement, Response, & Remission

A wide variety of biological and psychological therapies have been shown in randomized clinical trials to be effective for treatment of depression. The concept of "effectiveness," however, hinges on the demonstration of a "response" to treatment defined as "50% improvement in symptoms." A 50% improvement is important clinically, but this criterion is broad enough to leave significant residual symptoms unresolved. The concept of "remission," therefore, has been introduced to underscore the importance of helping the depressed patient reach full return of function and achieve relative absence of all depressive symptoms.

The following sections review broad treatment guidelines, psychotherapies, biological treatments, self-management support (SMS), and the need for objective monitoring of symptoms to help the patient attain full remission. Using the Case Illustration of Mrs. Gladstone, a 5-point decrease in her PHQ score from 16 to 11, would be considered a *clinically significant improvement* (the "minimally important clinical difference"). A decrease of 50%, from 16 to 8, would be considered a treatment "*response*," but the score of 8 reflects the persistence of residual symptoms of depression. Not until her PHQ score goes below 5, can Mrs. Gladstone be considered to be in *remission*.

General Treatment Guidelines: Close Monitoring, Persistence in Treatment Trials, & Chronic Reassessment

Research indicates a disappointingly low overall 50% response rate and a 33% remission rate for the first antidepressant a physician selects for the treatment of depression. Using logical strategies to switch or combine antidepressants after the first failure, about 70% of all patients will eventually respond to treatment. And we also know now that depression is a chronic disease. At least 50% of patients with a major depressive episode will have a second episode, and patients who have had two or more episodes of major depression have a 75–90% likelihood of recurrence.

These results suggest the following 7-point treatment program to encourage close monitoring, persistence of treatment trials, and chronic care for patients suffering from major depression. These points are all aligned with current evidence-based guidelines.

1. Use the PHQ-9 to help confirm the diagnosis and establish baseline severity.

2. For those treated with medication, patients should have an "early follow-up" contact, visit or phone call (1–3 weeks) to check on adherence to treatment, side effects, or potential change in symptoms for better or worse (e.g., emergent suicidality).

3. The first goal of treatment should be achieving a 5-point decrease in PHQ-9, which can be considered a clinically significant improvement. General target goal (which is very difficult to attain) should be achievement of a 5-point decrease in PHQ-9 score every month until a score below 5 is attained.

4. Patients should be evaluated with a repeat PHQ-9 once per month until remission is achieved (PHQ-9 <5). In general, the treatment approach should be modified if the patient does not show continuing improvement in PHQ-9 scores. (Modifications could include, for example, adding medication to psychotherapy or the converse, increasing the dose of a medication, switching medication, augmenting medication, considering couple therapy, reevaluating the diagnosis, and so on.)

5. Once patients reach remission, treatment should be continued (at the current dose of medication(s), or decreased frequency of psychotherapy) for at least 6–12 months.

6. For patients achieving remission with medications, evidence is clear that maintenance therapy requires the same dose of medication used for recovery. For patients achieving remission with psychotherapy, evidence is less clear, but there is some indication that intermittent "refresher" maintenance psychotherapy sessions can help prevent recurrences.

7. Patients with a history of depression should receive PHQ-9 "check-ups" every 6–12 months for the rest of their lives.

Choosing Initial Treatments: Respect Patient Preferences

Evidence-based treatment for depression includes antidepressant medication, several forms of psychotherapy, a combination of medication and psychotherapy and, in refractory cases, ECT. Electroconvulsive therapy (ECT) remains the single most efficacious treatment available for severe depression, and can be lifesaving.

Management of depressive illness, like any other chronic illness, should be collaborative. After providing basic education, physicians should offer patients realistic treatment options and respect patient preferences.

Patients tend to be more adherent to a treatment if they have selected it. Patients may need to be reminded that, even if they are pessimistic about treatment, such a perception is due to depression affecting their outlook. If they can stick with the treatment they have an excellent chance of responding to treatment. They should also be told that without treatment, they are likely to continue to suffer from depressive symptoms for a long time.

CASE ILLUSTRATION: MRS. GLADSTONE CONTINUED

Let's consider the way the physician and Mrs. Gladstone might collaboratively agree on a management strategy and self-management plan.

Physician: *OK, let's review the treatment options. The kind of depression you're struggling with responds well to antidepressant medication, counseling, or a combination of both medication and counseling. Often the combination works best, but if you are interested in either medication or counseling alone, that should work fine. Do you have any preferences?*

Mrs. Gladstone: *Well, I don't really like the idea of taking medication, but I have no time and no interest in psychobabble stuff. I'm OK with giving the medication a try, if you think it will help.*

Physician: *Great. That's fine. I'll get to the medication recommendation in another moment, but first I wonder if we could talk about some things you might want to do for yourself, to help manage your own illness.*

Mrs. Gladstone: *Sure, but I'm not sure what you mean.*

Physician: *Ok, let me explain. We have found that there are lots of things depressed patients can actually do themselves that can help them feel better … and I wonder if you would be interested in doing something specifically that might help your depression.*

Mrs. Gladstone: *Sure, why not. I don't have anything to lose—but I don't have any time for anything anymore.*

Physician: *Ok, let me tell you a little about some things that have worked for other depressed folks and then you can let me know if any one of them sounds like something you might want to do.*

Mrs. Gladstone: *OK.*

Physician: *Well, taking your medication regularly helps, of course. Getting some exercise helps. Planning a schedule and including things you enjoy are helpful. Getting together with friends and family helps. These are some of the things that have worked for others. Would you like to make a plan to do one of these, or perhaps something else you think might help?*

Mrs. Gladstone: *Well, I already said I'm going to take the medication. The other things sound great but*

I don't think I'm ready to do anything like that—I just don't have the time or energy for any of them. Can we start with the medication first—maybe later I'll think of something else I can do.

Physician: *Sure, that's fine. Let's see how the medication works for you. You will need to take it every day, once a day. Lots of people find it difficult to take their medication every day as prescribed. On a scale of 1 to 10, where 10 means you're sure you will take it every day, and 1 means you're not at all sure, how confident do you feel that you will actually take your medication every day.*

Mrs. Gladstone: *I want to get better. I am sure I'll take it—at least an 8 or 9.*

Individual Office Counseling by the Physician

Counseling by the primary care physician anchors all treatment modalities (pharmacotherapy, care management, psychotherapy) and provides the relational framework for continuity with the patient's other health care needs. Physician counseling provides the context for discussing the diagnosis, instilling hope for change, mobilizing the patient's self-management, and planning treatment. The time frame for such counseling can be a few minutes to an extended 30-minute visit.

Some physicians may want to engage in more specific counseling. The patient, however, should be notified that this interaction should not be considered formal psychotherapy, unless the practitioner has been adequately trained. Psychotherapeutic situations invariably arouse strong emotions in both patients and physicians. When complex interpersonal issues or strong feelings emerge during office counseling, the physician should seek supervision from a trained therapist or consultation from a colleague.

The acronym SPEAK was developed by one of the authors (JFC) to help physicians in counseling depressed patients (Table 25-6). The five components of **SPEAK** (**S**chedule, **P**leasurable activities, **E**xercise, **A**ssertiveness, and **K**ind thoughts about oneself) are grounded in core elements of evidence-based psychotherapies of depression including behavioral, interpersonal, and cognitive approaches. They provide a framework both for patient education and for ongoing supportive counseling by the physician. The SPEAK summary in Table 25-6 can be given to the patient as a handout to use as a component of *guided self-help* (see below).

Including the Patient's Partner

For patients in a significant relationship, including the partner in conjoint counseling can place the patient's symptoms and recovery within a relational context. Engaging the partner as an ally in the patient's self-management activities can increase adherence as well as external motivation in the context of a caring relationship. It can also help the partner understand the patient's symptoms as part of the illness being treated. In working with couples, practitioners can utilize some of the following interventions, all of which now have an emerging evidence base. Again, make it clear to patient and their partner that these interventions are not a substitute for therapy by a mental health specialist.

1. *Listen attentively* to the patient and their partner; discuss their current life stresses and emotional difficulties. Allowing straightforward "ventilation" can be therapeutic in itself and you will learn the extent to which discord in the relationship may be a factor in the depression. In addition, by expressing empathy to each partner, the physician can model appropriate interpersonal behavior for the discordant couple and build mutual support and trust.

2. *Straightforward education about the biological nature of depression* is a necessary component of all treatment, but in the context of discord in a couple it can help both partners view the depression in a more "forgiving" manner. In a common, but painful and maladaptive "dance," the discordant partner typically expresses a blaming attitude toward the depressed partner, which the patient accepts wholeheartedly because it resonates with his or her own highly negative cognitive self-appraisal. Similarly, an educated spouse is more likely to be able to view the depressed individual's depressive irritability as a symptom needing to be addressed, rather than a personal attack. By reframing the illness as an involuntary biological condition, the practitioner helps build the relationship and aids medication adherence (if antidepressants are part of the treatment plan).

3. *Encourage or facilitate joint problem solving.* Helping the depressed patient and their partner identify two or three troubling life problems they face and helping them develop a shared, concrete behavioral solution can help build their alliance and contribute to recovery. However, continuing or persistent discord may undermine treatment or recovery and should be referred for formal couples counseling.

When involving the partner in assessment or management of depression, it is essential to obtain informed consent first.

Psychotherapy

The psychotherapy strategies commonly used in treating depression include cognitive behavioral therapy (CBT), interpersonal therapy (IPT), psychodynamic therapy (PDT), problem-solving therapy (PST), hypnotherapy, and family therapy (including couple therapy). Some of

Table 25-6. SPEAK approach to physician counseling for depression.

S Schedule
P Pleasurable activities
E Exercise
A Assertiveness
K Kind thoughts about oneself

S Schedule:

Make a weekly schedule for yourself, with columns for each day of the week and rows for the hours of the day. Using a pencil (so you can make changes) make a plan for activities you will do each hour. Some of the times will already be structured for you, e.g., at work. Focus especially on the times that are currently unstructured. Start with things you know you usually do, e.g., eating meals, preparing meals. Include on the schedule time to do household chores and errands, but also include times for fun activities and exercise. Because temporarily you may not feel the motivation or desire to do any of these things, follow what the schedule says **whether or not you feel like doing it**. Sometimes you might feel like you are just going through the motions. When the time comes to switch to another activity, do so **whether or not you have completed the previous task**. You are making progress by putting in time on all these activities, not by getting through your "to do" list. Proceeding in this way will help you move out of depression by getting yourself moving through the day.

P Pleasurable activities:

Some of the items on your schedule should be activities that previously were fun for you before you became depressed. For the time being, you may feel you are just going through the motions in these activities. When we are depressed the part of the brain that allows us to feel pleasure is not functioning smoothly, so it is important to have a "jump start." You should plan something each day that would normally be fun and make yourself do it.

E Exercise:

Aerobic exercise increases oxygen and circulation to the brain and counteracts the hormonal changes caused by depression. It helps activate the natural pharmacy in your brain that will work with other parts of your treatment to help you come out of depression. Times for daily exercise should be included on your schedule. Running, swimming, bicycling, aerobic dancing, and walking are all forms of exercise that will help.

A Assertiveness:

This involves being **direct** with other people in your communication. Practice letting others know your feelings, needs, wants, opinions, and choices. This is more difficult when we are depressed, because we tend to doubt our own judgment. Or we might hold back because we are afraid others will think poorly of us. These thoughts are a product of depression, so it is necessary to act as if you were confident, even though inside you don't feel it. It takes more energy to hold in feelings than to express them. You might find that by stating clearly what you need or by saying "No" to what you don't want will help increase your energy and confidence. Read *Your Perfect Right* by Alberti and Emmons.

K Kind thoughts about yourself:

Since depression leads us to think self-punishing thoughts, it is very important to increase your awareness of when this is happening and to replace the negative thoughts with positive ones. Most of the time these negative thoughts are strongly held opinions that are not based on evidence. It is like carrying a negative, opinionated relative with you wherever you go. Once you become aware of this pattern of thoughts, begin to analyze them. You might write the most persistent negative thought on a 3 × 5 card. Then turn the card over and write three positive thoughts that you could replace it with. Carry this card with you and refer to it frequently. It takes about three positive statements to counteract the effect of one negative statement.

Source: Courtesy of John F. Christensen, PhD.

these therapies can be administered in individual or group sessions (CBT, IPT, and PST). In addition, some therapies can be offered via the Internet (real-time text messaging, email, or video conference) or by telephone. Psychotherapy is typically provided by a licensed mental health therapist (psychiatrist, clinical psychologist, clinical social worker, psychiatric nurse practitioner).

Cognitive behavioral therapy attempts to identify and challenge cognitive distortions (e.g., "I fail at everything") that are pessimistic or self-critical thoughts which contribute to and maintain the depressed mood. Once these negative cognitive patterns are identified, the patient learns to challenge them and to develop counter-messages that are more evidence based and positive. In addition, CBT teaches "behavioral activation" to counter the inertia of depression (e.g., engaging in pleasurable activities in the presence of anhedonia, or engaging in physical exercise in the absence of motivation). Evidence supports the effectiveness of CBT in treating depression, both as a single problem and as a comorbidity with somatic illnesses. Cognitive behavioral therapy combined with pharmacotherapy has higher effectiveness than CBT alone in treating older adults, particularly in patients with chronic, treatment-resistant depression.

There is also evidence that several variants of CBT, such as mindfulness-based cognitive therapy (MBCT) and cognitive behavioral analysis system of psychotherapy (CBASP) may be effective in the treatment of depression. Mindfulness-based cognitive therapy utilizes mindfulness meditation to teach patients to recognize and let go of ruminative thinking by enhancing "metacognitive awareness," which is a nonjudgmental observation of the passage of thoughts and feelings and how they are constructed. Patients undergoing this approach learn to experience negative thoughts and feelings as mental events, rather than as the self (see Chapter 7).

Within the domain of CBT, two methods of therapy have emerged in recent years with a promising evidence base for treatment of depression: Dialectical behavior therapy (DBT) and acceptance and commitment therapy (ACT). Dialectical behavior therapy was originally developed to treat the parasuicidal behavior of patients suffering from borderline personality disorder. The treatment is dialectical in that its goal is to synthesize the alternative principles of acceptance and change. Acceptance strategies are similar to the notion of unconditional positive regard in client-centered therapy. Change strategies have the objective of changing thoughts and overt behavior. Dialectical behavior therapy addresses four skill sets: mindfulness, interpersonal effectiveness, emotion regulation, and distress tolerance. Group DBT treatment has shown positive effects in reducing symptoms in patients with treatment-resistant depression.

Acceptance and commitment therapy conceptualizes psychopathology as stemming from unhealthy efforts to control emotions, thoughts, memories, and other private experiences and a lack of clarity about one's core values and the ability to act in accordance with them. The goal of ACT is to diminish the role of thought while encouraging the patient to embrace experience directly without suppression. At the same time it encourages behavior consistent with one's chosen values. Compared to traditional cognitive therapy, ACT has shown equal effectiveness in reducing symptoms of depression.

Interpersonal therapy focuses on one or more of several interpersonal situations that may relate to initiating or sustaining depression: interpersonal conflict, role transition, grief, or social skills deficits. Assertiveness training is one component of IPT that develops patients' capacity to be direct in communicating feelings, thoughts, and preferences in their current relationships. In the treatment of depression, IPT has been shown to be more effective than placebo and equivalent to medication in adults. In late life depression, medication was more effective. Overall, CBT and IPT have the broadest evidence base for effectiveness in treatment of depression.

Psychodynamic therapy focuses on interpersonal relationships and unconscious feelings, desires, strivings, and thoughts to treat symptom disorders. It involves using the therapeutic alliance to gain an understanding of the ways maladaptive defense mechanisms have developed and contribute to depression and then working through these mechanisms in an effort to build more adaptive and less punishing defense mechanisms. A meta-analysis of short-term dynamic psychotherapy (STDP) found that it had significant effects pre-to posttreatment for depressive symptoms and that these changes endured at 1-year follow-up. Although other forms of psychotherapy showed a greater effect immediately posttreatment, there were no differences at 1-year follow-up.

Problem-solving therapy teaches patients to break down larger life problems into smaller elements and to identify specific steps to address these elements. It has been shown to be as effective as antidepressant medication in the treatment of depressed primary care patients. Meta-analysis has shown a modest effect of PST on depression, with greater effects noted in group treatment with PST.

The evidence from many randomized clinical trials is that these psychotherapies are as effective as antidepressant medication (in mild-to-moderate MDD) in achieving a significant reduction of symptoms (over 50% response rate) after 10–16 weeks of treatment. Although the response to antidepressants is generally more in the first 4 weeks, response to psychotherapy catches up and by 12 weeks the efficacy of medication and psychotherapy are roughly similar. There is some reason to believe that antidepressant medication and psychotherapy of depression achieve their benefits through different neurobiological mechanisms, so it is not surprising that combination treatments (medication and psychotherapy) have generally been found to be more effective than either one alone. For individuals with severe depression, antidepressants are generally important mainstays of treatment and more effective than psychotherapy alone.

Cognitive behavioral therapy is generally considered the treatment of choice for depression in children and adolescents, though one medication (fluoxetine) is FDA approved for the treatment of child and adolescent depression. The clinical benefits of psychotherapy are usually seen in 8–12 weeks, and the duration of treatment is typically 6–16 sessions. Meta-analysis has shown that psychotherapy is moderately effective in the short run, especially for adolescents aged 12–18 years, but that after 6 months psychotherapy does not show enduring effects.

Guided self-help involves the patient working at home with a standardized psychological treatment, such as CBT, with guidance from a physician or mental health therapist, who provides initial support and occasional coaching. Therapist support can be face-to-face or

Table 25-7. Considerations for acute-phase treatment with psychotherapy alone.

- Less severe depression
- Prior response to psychotherapy
- Incomplete response to treatment with medication alone
- Chronic psychosocial problems
- Availability of trained, competent therapist
- Patient preference

via telephone or email. The standardized treatment can be in various formats—book, audio CD, video, or Internet. Remote psychotherapy via phone or Internet also has shown promise for the treatment of depression.

Considerations for choosing psychotherapy in the acute phase of treatment are shown in Table 25-7. Besides being an adjunct to medication for the treatment of depression, psychotherapy may also have a role in prophylactic maintenance therapy for the prevention or delay of future depressive episodes in patients susceptible to recurrences. For example, MBCT has been shown to reduce depressive relapse rates at levels similar to maintenance antidepressants in several randomized controlled trials. Psychotherapy can also be useful for women with major depression who want to become pregnant and bear a child in a medication-free condition or for other patients with major depression who must be medication free for limited periods. In mild-to-moderate depressions, psychotherapy alone may be as effective as psychotherapy combined with antidepressants.

Marital and Couple Therapy

As mentioned above, marital or couple therapy may be an appropriate choice of psychotherapy, especially when marital problems are entwined with depression. Marital therapy for depressed women who are also in troubled relationships can be effective in alleviating the depression as well as in decreasing the marital discord.

Marital therapy is no more or less effective than individual therapy, even when depression is associated with marital distress. Although individual therapy for depression can be effective in decreasing depressive symptoms even in the presence of marital discord, if the discord is not addressed relapse into depression is more likely. Moreover, it is useful for the physician to get some idea of what the patient believes caused the depression. If the patient believes that the marital discord caused the depression, then addressing the discord is even more important for the prevention of relapse.

Exercise & Physical Activity

Evidence from randomized clinical trials is inconclusive on the benefits of moderate exercise in the treatment of depression. In the Standard Medical Intervention and Long-term Exercise (SMILE) study, 16 weeks of aerobic exercise training was comparable to that of standard pharmacotherapy with sertraline and combined exercise and medication. In a 10-month continuation study, remitted subjects in the exercise group had significantly lower relapse rates than subjects in the medication group. A more recent meta-analysis of exercise compared with other therapies for depression found that exercise did not differ from CBT and antidepressant medication. When rigorous methodology was applied to these studies, the affect of exercise was only moderate.

Self-Help Books

For motivated, literate patients, self-help books that increase understanding of depression and provide guidance on self-management strategies can be an effective adjunct to treatment. For patients without access to psychotherapy, the use of self-help materials can be a helpful substitute. A meta-analysis of studies examining the use of self-help books in the United Kingdom found that one book, *Feeling Good*, had a large treatment effect compared to delayed treatment.

ANTIDEPRESSANT PHARMACOTHERAPY

Evidence demonstrates that antidepressant medications are effective for the treatment of major depression and dysthymia. There are no compelling data, however, to support the use of antidepressant medication for patients with adjustment disorders or other minor depressive disorders. The initial treatment of choice for most patients with an adjustment disorder or other minor depressive episode is "watchful waiting," which consists of physician support, office counseling, and close observation, with repeat assessment to document improvement, remission, lack of improvement, or possible transformation into major depression. Physicians can also support patient self-management goal setting and problem solving with Ultra-Brief Personal Action Planning (UB-PAP) (discussed earlier). Patients with minor depression who do not improve after 3–6 months of watchful waiting can be treated empirically with a trial of antidepressant medication or referred for psychotherapy.

Communicating With Patients About Medication

Patients initiating antidepressant medication for the first time sometimes are concerned about the stigma associated with their use. Some fear getting "hooked" on the medicine or that it will change their personality in some way. It is important to explain that antidepressants are nonaddictive medicines that can restore the natural balance of neurotransmitters and normalize neural pathways in the brain. It can be helpful to inform the patient about the possibility of experiencing some of the known side effects of the particular antidepressant and to refer to those side effects as an indicator of the drug's potency to achieve the desired results. Finally, it is important to build a realistic expectation about the tempo of therapeutic effectiveness by letting the patient know that even though the symptoms of depression may persist for a week or two after starting the antidepressant, the healing process has already begun.

Adherence to treatment has been shown to be enhanced when the physician–patient alliance is optimized, when the patient's attitudes toward and experience with treatment are thoroughly explored, and when the patient's opinion in treatment decisions is explicitly valued.

Pharmacotherapy Options

The cyclic antidepressants include the TCAs, SSRIs, serotonin norepinephrine reuptake inhibitors (SNRIs), and a noradrenaline and specific serotonin antagonist (NaSSa). The cyclic antidepressants are generally equally effective; however, due to the adverse effect profile of the TCAs, they have been supplanted by the SSRIs, SNRIs, and NaSSa agents. Nevertheless, TCAs are still commonly employed as second-line antidepressants in patients who do not respond to first-line agents and for augmentation therapy.

Antidepressants illicit immediate first-dose pharmacological effects on the catecholamine reuptake system; however, these agents only begin to provide some symptom improvement after 1–2 weeks of treatment. An adequate trial of an antidepressant requires a minimum of 4–6 weeks at appropriate doses. Cyclic antidepressant response rates approximate 50–70%; hence, physicians should expect that up to half of the patients they treat with the first antidepressant may not respond. Patients with no response or minimal response should be switched to another agent. Patients with partial response can be managed with augmenting agents. If the first SSRI trial fails, patients may be switched to another SSRI (e.g., bupropion, venlafaxine, mirtazapine, or a TCA). Of note, 25–50% of patients who fail to respond to the first trial of an SSRI will respond to a different SSRI on a second trial. A list of antidepressant side effects, mechanisms of action, and dosages is listed in Table 25-8.

Tricyclic Antidepressants

The TCAs have fallen out of favor predominantly because of their adverse effects and toxicity profile in the overdose setting. Common antimuscarinic effects include dry mouth, blurred vision, constipation, urinary retention, and sinus tachycardia; histamine receptor blockade effects include sedation, drowsiness, and weight gain; and alpha-1 receptor blockade effects include orthostatic hypotension and sedation. The

TCAs also possess quinidine-like effects, such as QRS and QTc prolongation, which can predispose to ventricular dysrhythmias and torsades de pointes—especially in the overdose setting, or in patients with preexisting cardiac disease. A TCA overdose is a medical emergency, with significant risk of lethality. Tricyclic antidepressants lower the seizure threshold, with the potential for refractory seizures in overdose. To minimize the risk of lethal overdose in patients with suicidal ideation, principles of prudent care suggest that only limited amounts of TCAs should be prescribed at any one time (e.g., 7–10 days supply, especially in higher doses). Secondary amines, such as desipramine and nortriptyline, are favored over tertiary amines, such as amitriptyline and imipramine, because of a lower propensity to induce antimuscarinic adverse effects, less orthostatic hypotension, and less sedation. The adverse effects of the TCAs are dose related, and can be minimized by starting patients on low doses, and titrating upward slowly. Though the newer antidepressants seem to be generally as effective as the TCAs for the broad category of major depression, these older agents may be more effective for the more severe depressive disorders and, especially depression with melancholic features.

Selective Serotonin Reuptake Inhibitors

There are five SSRIs approved for major depression in the United States—fluoxetine, paroxetine, sertraline, citalopram, and escitalopram. The SSRIs have replaced the TCAs as first-line agents for major depression because they are generally better tolerated and are not life-threatening in overdose. Selective serotonin reuptake inhibitors are virtually free of antimuscarinic, antihistaminic, and antiadrenergic side effects. All SSRIs are equally effective; therefore, choice of any particular SSRI is generally based on side effect profiles, pharmacokinetics, drug interactions, dosage forms, cost, formulary availability, and so on. Table 25-9 demonstrates comparative SSRI adverse effects. As a class, many SSRIs have also been shown to be effective for PD, GAD, OCD, social anxiety disorder, PTSD, premenstrual dysphoric disorder, and bulimia nervosa. Fluoxetine is the only SSRI with an FDA indication for the treatment of childhood or adolescent depression and fluoxetine paroxetine, and sertraline have FDA indications for the treatment of childhood and adolescent OCD. Vilazodone, a new SSRI, is also a partial agonist at the 5HT1A receptors and appears to have less sexual dysfunction and potential for weight gain. With the exception of fluoxetine and paroxetine, SSRIs show very little inhibition of liver isoenzyme systems. Because of a common SSRI discontinuation syndrome, marked by GI and autonomic signs and symptoms, physicians taking patients off these medications should taper them slowly. Withdrawal from paroxetine seems to be more problematic than other

Table 25-8. Commonly used antidepressants.

Drug	Usual Daily Oral Dose (mg)	Usual Daily Maximum Dose (mg)	Sedative Effects[*]	Anticholinergic Effects[*]	Cost per Unit	Cost for 30 Days Treatment Based on Maximum Dosage[†]
SSRIs						
Citalopram (Celexa)	20	40	<1	1	$2.53/40 mg	$75.90
Escitalopram (Lexapro)	10	20	<1	1	$5.02/20 mg	$150.60
Fluoxetine (Prozac, Sarafem)	5–40	80	<1	<1	$2.67/20 mg	$320.40
Fluvoxamine (Luvox)	100–300	300	1	<1	$2.64/100 mg	$237.60
Nefazodone (Serzone)	300–600	600	2	<1	$1.92/200 mg	$172.80
Paroxetine (Paxil)	20–30	50	1	1	$2.65/20 mg	$159.00
Sertraline (Zoloft)	50–150	200	<1	<1	$2.85/100 mg	$171.00
Vilazodone (Viibryd)	40	40	<1	<1	$4.74/20 mg	$147.20
Tricyclic and Clinically Similar Compounds						
Amitriptyline (Elavil)	150–250	300	4	4	$1.16/150 mg	$69.60
Amoxapine (Asendin)	150–200	400	2	2	$1.67/100 mg	$200.40
Clomipramine (Anafranil)	100	250	3	3	$1.40/75 mg	$149.70
Desipramine (Norpramin)	100–250	300	1	1	$1.50/100 mg	$135.00
Doxepin (Sinequan)	150–200	300	4	3	$1.15/100 mg	$103.50
Imipramine (Tofranil)	150–200	300	3	3	$1.22/50 mg	$219.60
Maprotiline (Ludiomil)	100–200	300	4	2	$1.60/75 mg	$192.00
Nortriptyline (Aventyl, Pamelor)	100–150	150	2	2	$1.46/50 mg	$131.40
Protriptyline (Vivactil)	15–40	60	1	3	$3.07/10 mg	$552.60
Monoamine Oxidase Inhibitors						
Phenelzine (Nardil)	45–60	90	...	...	$0.84/15 mg	$151.20
Selegiline transdermal (Emsam)	6 (skin patch)	12	...	...	$23.77/6 mg patch	$713.02
Tranylcypromine (Parnate)	20–30	50	...	...	$1.25/10 mg	$187.50

(Continued)

Table 25-8. Commonly used antidepressants. (Continued)

Drug	Usual Daily Oral Dose (mg)	Usual Daily Maximum Dose (mg)	Sedative Effects*	Anticholinergic Effects*	Cost per Unit	Cost for 30 Days Treatment Based on Maximum Dosage†
Other Compounds						
Bupropion SR (Wellbutrin SR)	300	400‡		<1	$3.59/200 mg	$215.40
Bupropion XL (Wellbutrin XL)	300§	450§		<1	$4.77/300 mg	$286.20
Desvenlafaxine (Pristiq)	50	100	1	<1	$5.41/100 mg	$162.30
Duloxetine (Cymbalta)	40	60	2	3	$6.65/60 mg	$199.50
Mirtazapine (Remeron)	15–45	45	4	2	$2.80/30 mg	$85.53
Trazodone (Desyrel)	100–300	400	4	<1	$0.73/100 mg	$87.60
Trimipramine (Surmontil)	75–200	200	4	4	$5.78/100 mg	$346.80
Venlafaxine XR (Effexor)	150–225	225	1	<1	$4.67/75 mg	$420.30

*4, strong effect; 1, weak effect.
†Average wholesale price (AWP, for AB-rated generic when available) for quantity listed. Source: *Red Book Online*, 2012, Thomson Reuters (Healthcare Inc.). AWP may not accurately represent the actual pharmacy cost because wide contractual variations exist among institutions.
‡200 mg twice daily.
§Wellbutrin XL is a once daily form of bupropion. Bupropion is still available as immediate release, and, if used, no single dose should exceed 150 mg.
SSRIs, serotonin selective reuptake inhibitors.
Source: From CMDT 2011.

SSRIs. Brief use of the long-acting SSRI fluoxetine (for several days) can be used to help "cover" SSRI withdrawal effects when discontinuing other SSRIs. In the overdose setting, SSRIs can cause dose-related toxicity, manifesting with nausea and vomiting, tremor, myoclonus, dysrhythmias, and seizures—plausibly all manifestations of the serotonin syndrome.

Gastrointestinal Adverse Effects

The SSRIs inhibit serotonin reuptake, thereby activating $5-HT_3$ receptors, which can cause nausea and vomiting in 10–15% of patients. Due to desensitization of the $5-HT_3$ receptors, tolerance to nausea and vomiting usually occurs within 1–2 weeks. Short-term use of cyproheptadine (5-HT3 receptor antagonist) may decrease uncomfortable nausea and vomiting. To minimize GI irritation, nausea, and vomiting, it is useful to administer the SSRIs with food. Dose-related diarrhea is also a common adverse effect of the SSRIs, with the possible exception of paroxetine which possesses mild-to-moderate anticholinergic effects and can cause constipation.

Weight Gain & Weight Loss

Both weight gain and weight loss have been reported with the SSRIs. The incidence of SSRI-induced weight gain greater than 5–10% of body weight can approach 25%,

Table 25-9. Comparative adverse effects of SSRIs.*

Drug	Nausea/GI Upset	Insomnia	Somnolence	Weight Gain	Sexual Dysfunction	Anticholinergic Effects
Fluoxetine	+++	++++	+	+	+++	0
Sertraline	+++	++	+	+	+++	0
Paroxetine	+++	++	++	+++	++++	+
Citalopram	+++	++	+	Unknown	+++	0
Escitalopram	+++	++	+	Unknown	+++	0

*0, none; +, minimal; ++, mild; +++, moderate; ++++, severe.

especially in females and, especially in patients using paroxetine (possibly due to its anticholinergic effects). Addition of bupropion may decrease SSRI-induced weight gain. Anorexia and weight loss have also been reported during early treatment, especially in overweight individuals with carbohydrate cravings, underweight depressed patients, bulimics, or patients using fluoxetine.

Syndrome of Inappropriate Antidiuretic Hormone Secretion

A clinically relevant and underappreciated adverse effect of the cyclic antidepressants is the syndrome of inappropriate antidiuretic hormone secretion (SIADH). Syndrome of inappropriate antidiuretic hormone secretion presents with serum hyponatremia and hypoosmolality, and urinary hypernatremia and hyperosmolality. This syndrome is caused by an excessive release of antidiuretic hormone, presenting with signs and symptoms such as nausea, vomiting, weakness, fatigue, confusion, and seizures. Syndrome of inappropriate antidiuretic hormone secretion has been reported with all antidepressants, and is reversible upon dose reduction or discontinuation. Management also includes fluid restriction and demeclocycline. Syndrome of inappropriate antidiuretic hormone secretion is more common in the context of tobacco use.

Bleeding Diatheses

Many physicians, including psychiatrists are still unaware of recent reports (mostly retrospective case-controlled studies) associating SSRIs with a plethora of bleeding diatheses including GI bleeding, epistaxis, petechiae, purpura, and ecchymosis. Approximately 95% of serotonin is stored in the platelets, and serotonin is one of many chemotactic factors responsible for platelet aggregation. SSRIs possess an aspirin-like effect and inhibit platelet aggregation, but the potency and duration of this effect is not yet well elucidated. When SSRIs are administered with nonsteroidal antiinflammatory drugs (NSAIDs), the risk of NSAID-induced gastropathy can increase significantly. Physicians should be cautious when prescribing an SSRI in patients with a history of GI bleeding and in patients who are already taking other antiplatelet medications. In the context of concurrent NSAIDs, aspirin, or other antiplatelet therapy, physicians should consider adding a proton pump inhibitor for prophylaxis of gastropathy.

Sexual Dysfunction

Decreased libido, orgasmic difficulties or anorgasmia, penile anesthesia, and erectile dysfunction (impotence) are very common adverse effects associated with the SSRIs in men and women. Sexual side effects occur in 25–75% of all patients, a higher prevalence than reported in package inserts because of underreporting

and the short duration of clinical trials. The only available cyclic antidepressants that are less likely to cause sexual dysfunction are bupropion and mirtazapine. Sexual dysfunction in males, especially erectile dysfunction has been successfully managed with phosphodiesterase type-5 antagonists, such as sildenafil, tadalafil, and vardenafil. Other medications such as bupropion, yohimbine, amantadine, buspirone, bethanechol, neostigmine, and *Ginkgo biloba* have all been utilized with mixed results, with no clear evidence of efficacy from randomized, placebo-controlled clinical trials. Some clinicians will attempt a *drug holiday*, and skip the dose of the SSRI 24 hours prior to sexual activity (not effective with fluoxetine because of its long half-life). Because sexual dysfunction has such a significant impact on quality of life, this problem may be the most common limiting factor in use of SSRIs.

Serotonin Syndrome

Poison control centers report over 27,000 toxic exposures to SSRIs annually, with 15% of these reporting a serotonin syndrome. The serotonin syndrome can occur in overdose or when two or more serotonergic agents are combined. Table 25-9 lists common serotonergic agents. The serotonin syndrome presents as a clinical triad of autonomic dysfunction (e.g., hyperthermia, labile blood pressure), neuromuscular dysfunction (e.g., clonus, hyperreflexia), and mental status changes (e.g., agitation, delirium). This spectrum of clinical findings can be mild and transient and include akathisia, tremor, and altered mental status; however, it can progress to life-threatening symptoms such as sustained clonus, muscular hypertonicity, and hyperthermia approaching 40°C. Severe serotonin syndrome is a medical emergency. Although it is important for physicians to be aware of the signs, symptoms, and risk factors for the serotonin syndrome, it is also important for physicians treating depression to understand that pharmacological combination and augmentation treatment strategies often include the cautious prescription of two or more medications with proserotonin effects. Bupropion does not have serotonin effects.

Venlafaxine

Venlafaxine is a bicyclic antidepressant, approved in 1994 as the first *dual-acting* antidepressant agent to inhibit the reuptake of both norepinephrine and serotonin. These agents are often referred to as SNRIs. At lower doses, venlafaxine exhibits relatively more serotoninergic activity; however, at doses above 150 mg daily the adrenergic and serotonergic effects become more balanced. Venlafaxine is also FDA approved for the management of generalized and social anxiety disorder and PD. The extended release form of the product (XR) has become preferred because it can be used once daily and has much lower propensity to cause nausea, vomiting, and increases in blood pressure (3% of patients on doses of 375 mg experience sustained elevation in blood pressure). Venlafaxine shows very low inhibition of liver isoenzyme systems and has much lower protein binding (about 30%) than most other antidepressants that are very highly protein bound. Discontinuation of venlafaxine is associated with an SSRI-like discontinuation syndrome, requiring gradual taper (or "covering" for withdrawal effects with fluoxetine). Desvenlafaxine is a newer preparation consisting of a metabolite of the desmethyl metabolite of venlafaxine. It offers simpler dosing at a starting dose of 50 mg that is the same as the full continuation dose. This is a modest advantage in that venlafaxine typically requires gradual increases in dosing to avoid GI side effects.

Duloxetine

Approved by the FDA in 2004, duloxetine is a bicyclic SNRI antidepressant indicated for MDD, GAD, and diabetic peripheral neuropathic pain, fibromyalgia, and chronic musculoskeletal pain. Duloxetine, like venlafaxine can produce modest increases in blood pressure, nausea, sweating, insomnia, dizziness, and sexual dysfunction. Duloxetine is metabolized by CYP-1A2 and -2D6, and is a -2D6 inhibitor. Of clinical importance, physicians should be aware that when duloxetine is administered with 1A2 inhibitors, such as fluvoxamine or ciprofloxacin, or 2D6 inhibitors, such as paroxetine, duloxetine serum concentrations can increase considerably. Duloxetine should not be used in patients with a creatinine clearance less than 30 mL/min due to significant accumulation of the parent (two-fold) and numerous metabolites (nine-fold). Duloxetine has been associated with hepatotoxicity; in controlled trials, 1% of the patients experienced elevations in liver enzyme tests three times the upper limit of normal. Duloxetine is best avoided in patients with a history of alcohol abuse or hepatic disease, and in patients receiving concomitant hepatotoxic agents.

Mirtazapine

Mirtazapine, a tetracyclic noradrenaline and specific serotonin antidepressant (an NaSSa agent), is a potent serotonin-2 (5-HT2), serotonin-3 (5-HT3), and central alpha-2-adrenergic receptor antagonist. Advantages of mirtazapine include the following: it is less likely to cause sexual dysfunction, may reduce sleep latency and prolong sleep duration, may have anxiolytic effects, is relatively devoid of alpha-1 blocking effects such as orthostatic hypotension, and may cause less GI adverse effects than the SSRIs. Mirtazapine is a potent appetite stimulant, causing substantial weight gain in many patients. This can be advantageous in patients who are cachectic and nutritionally deficient, such as debilitated elderly, and cancer and HIV patients. However, in obese, diabetic, and patients with cardiovascular diseases,

mirtazapine-induced weight gain is undesirable, and has been associated with deleterious effects on the lipoprotein profile (increased cholesterol and triglycerides). Patients should be warned about this side effect and often refuse to take it for this reason. Mirtazapine possesses significant antihistaminergic and minimal antimuscarinic effects, with the potential for considerable drowsiness, dry mouth, and constipation. Mirtazapine has a very low incidence of transient rise in liver enzymes (2%) and severe neutropenia or reversible agranulocytosis (0.1% incidence). It may be prudent for physicians to check white counts at initiation of the medication, semiannually, and with occurrence of infectious illnesses. Mirtazapine is unlikely to have clinically significant effects on the metabolism of other medications through liver enzyme systems.

Bupropion

The monocyclic antidepressant bupropion inhibits the reuptake of norepinephrine and dopamine into presynaptic neurons and is referred to as a norepinephrine dopamine reuptake inhibitor (NDRI). Bupropion does not inhibit serotonin reuptake and does not cause the serotonin syndrome. Bupropion is also indicated for smoking cessation under the trade name Zyban. Bupropion may enhance energy and motivation due to norepinephrine- and dopamine-induced activating effects. However, bupropion's activating effect can also cause agitation, irritability, aggression, vivid dreams, nightmares, and insomnia. Despite this pronorepinephrine and prodopamine effect, only 2% of patients on this medication demonstrate elevations in blood pressure. Bupropion may be used for sexual dysfunction, it may promote weight loss, and it has a lower propensity to induce mania in patients with a bipolar diathesis.

Bupropion is contraindicated in patients with seizure disorders, bulimia, anorexia, and alcohol withdrawal. Bupropion-induced seizure disorders are dose related, and total daily doses above 450 mg, or single doses above 150 mg of immediate-release dosage or 200 mg of the sustained-release dosage forms increase the risk of seizures and should be avoided. Up to 450 mg of the XL form of the medication can be prescribed once a day, which is a major advantage for improving adherence. Bupropion has been shown to inhibit selective liver isoenzyme systems.

Black Box Warning on Antidepressant-Induced Suicide Ideation in Children & Adolescents

In 2004, the FDA issued a "black box" warning that the use of antidepressant medication in children and adolescents may be associated with an increase in suicide ideation and suicide attempts. In 2007, the "black box" warning was expanded to include young adults up to the age of 24 years. In brief, the warning results from a pooled analysis of 4400 subjects in 24 placebo-controlled drug trials with nine different antidepressant medications in children and adolescents for treating depression or OCD. The study found prevalence rates of treatment-emergent suicidal thoughts or suicide attempts in 4% of all patients in the active medication group, compared to 2% of patients taking placebo (a statistically significant difference). *There were no completed suicides in any of the studies.* Similar pooled analyses in adults found no difference between active drug and placebo in studies totaling more than 50,000 patients. The black box recommends that when prescribing antidepressant medication in children, adolescents, and young adults, physicians should warn patients and families to report immediately any increase in agitation or thoughts of suicide, and physicians should monitor patients through regular and frequent follow-up visits.

Physicians should also be aware of some important general epidemiologic findings. In the decade before this warning was issued, suicide attempts and completed suicides decreased significantly in children and adolescents, somewhat paralleling the increased use of antidepressant medications in the population. Since 2004, however, use of these medications in children and adolescents has decreased by 25%, and of interest and concern, rates of suicide attempts and completions in children and adolescents have increased for the first time in over a decade. Furthermore, large observational studies have documented that the risk of a suicide attempt actually decreases after patients begin taking medication and that communities with higher rates of antidepressant use have, on average, lower rates of suicide.

Drug Interactions

Whenever prescribing a new medication, practitioners must consider the possibility of drug–drug interactions. In addition, the use of the new drug in combination with another drug the patient is already taking may create a new condition of potential risk (e.g., additive sedative risks or potential serotonin syndrome). Because antidepressants are in such common use, questions of potential antidepressant drug interactions become issues of daily importance to most physicians, especially in the medically ill or the elderly.

Physicians should routinely use an electronic database to check potential drug interactions whenever they prescribe a new medication. They should understand the basic principles of enzyme substrates and enzyme inhibitors to be able to better interpret the results they receive from such an electronic database check on drug interactions.

All antidepressant medications are metabolized by cytochrome P450 liver enzyme subsystems. That is, they are *substrates* for one or more major P450 isoenzyme systems 1A2, 2C9, 2C19, 2D6, and 3A4. While all antidepressants are metabolized in the liver, only some of the SSRIs are moderate inhibitors of either 2C19 (fluoxetine and sertraline) or 2D6 (fluoxetine and paroxetine). Fluoxetine and paroxetine, for example, are moderate 2D6 inhibitors. As such, these drugs inhibit the metabolism of drugs metabolized by the 2D6 subsystem, for example, several beta-blockers, some antipsychotic medications, most TCAs, some benzodiazepines, and the over-the-counter cough suppressant dextromethorphan. When dextromethorphan is combined with fluoxetine or paroxetine, its plasma levels can increase significantly, which could theoretically increase the likelihood of a serotonin syndrome. Also, some SSRIs may inhibit the hepatic 2D6-mediated conversion of several prodrug-like opioids into their active analgesic metabolites, such as codeine to morphine, oxycodone to oxymorphone, and hydrocodone to hydromorphone. Clinically, this inhibition could theoretically decrease the analgesic effect of the opiates listed above. Among the SSRIs, sertraline, citalopram, and escitalopram present the least inhibition of 2D6, while mirtazapine and venlafaxine also have little effect on 2D6.

Clinicians should evaluate the probability, outcome, and risk of drug–drug interactions prior to prescribing antidepressants. In most settings, an alternative agent that does not interact can be prescribed. When patients are receiving drugs that can interact with each other, patients should be counseled on the signs and symptoms of toxicity, and clinicians should heighten monitoring techniques. Patients should be advised that using only one pharmacy allows the pharmacist to maintain a complete, comprehensive, and accurate medication profile and improves the likelihood that the pharmacist will also detect potential problematic drug–drug interactions.

Pharmacogenomics

Pharmacogenomics refers to the interaction of multiple genes in determining drug response. For example, genetic polymorphisms in the serotonin transporter gene have been associated with differential SSRI response rates. Some individuals have been shown to have differential activity levels of 2C19 and 2D6 isoenzymes—some patients are "extensive" metabolizers (high activity) and some are "poor" metabolizers (low enzyme activity). Of interest to researchers is that the prevalence rates of "poor metabolizers" vary by ethnicity: 30% of Asians, 10% of African Americans, and 5% of whites are poor metabolizers. From a clinical perspective, given the same dose of drug, poor metabolizers are likely to have much higher blood levels of the medication than extensive metabolizers. Why some individuals are more sensitive to lower doses of medication and/or respond better to lower doses, may be secondary to this genetically determined rate of metabolism, though how to apply this information clinically has not been clearly established.

The FDA has licensed and accredited several laboratories to provide DNA testing as well as blood tests for determination of CYP-2C9, -2C19, -2D6, and -1A2 genotypes. Although these tests are currently available, they have not yet gained widespread acceptance. The next decade will probably witness great progress in pharmacogenomics, such that testing and genomic-based medication algorithms will become part of the routine practice of medicine.

Antidepressant Withdrawal

Abrupt withdrawal of SSRIs, usually within 24–48 hours may cause a *discontinuation syndrome* consisting of a constellation of somatic, neurologic, and psychological symptoms. These symptoms include GI complaints, headache, fever, malaise, vivid dreams, myalgias, paresthesias, "electric shock-like" sensations, worsened mood, irritability, anxiety, confusion, and forgetfulness. These symptoms can be extremely uncomfortable, even leading to emergency room visits, but they are not life threatening. The incidence of the SSRI *discontinuation syndrome* may be as high as 40%, but the most common and most severe withdrawal syndrome is most commonly associated with paroxetine, probably due to its short half-life (21 hours) and the absence of any active metabolites. All of the SSRIs except for fluoxetine can cause this syndrome. Fluoxetine is unlikely to cause the discontinuation syndrome because of its long half-life (4–14 days, plus its active metabolite norfluoxetine), and hence has a self-tapering discontinuation mechanism. Venlafaxine, duloxetine, trazodone, and mirtazapine have also been associated with the discontinuation syndrome. Treatment of the discontinuation syndrome consists of reinstituting the SSRI and taper more slowly, or substitute the SSRI with one or two doses of fluoxetine (10–20 mg). In summary, all known antidepressants, with the possible exception of fluoxetine and bupropion should be withdrawn very gradually to avoid the discontinuation syndrome.

Antidepressant "Tolerance"

Despite the absence of clear evidence, clinicians commonly observe a tolerance phenomenon or *poop-out syndrome* that may occur in 10–20% of patients who have successfully responded to antidepressant therapy and remain compliant. Possible mechanisms for this observed tachyphylaxis include adaptation of central nervous system receptors via upregulation and decreased receptor density, disease severity or exacerbation, loss of a placebo effect, unrecognized rapid cycling, accumulation of a less potent or competitively antagonistic metabolite, or drug interactions. Enzyme-inducing

medications, such as St. John wort, phenytoin, barbiturates, carbamazepine, oxcarbazepine, rifampin, and rifabutin, may increase the hepatic metabolism of non-CYP-2D6 substrate antidepressants, thus decreasing plasma levels. For example, phenobarbital has been associated with a 25% decrease in the area under the paroxetine serum concentration–time curve; St. John wort has been associated with a 22% decrease in the area under the serum concentration–time curve of amitriptyline and a 41% decrease in its metabolite nortriptyline; and phenobarbital can decrease the plasma levels of mirtazapine by 60%. Additionally, clinicians should be suspicious of a lack of compliance in all patients with the poop-out syndrome. Management of the poop-out syndrome includes increasing antidepressant doses, switching to an alternative agent, or adding augmentation therapy.

Augmentation Therapy

After an antidepressant at maximal doses has produced only a partial response, with persistent residual symptoms, experts usually recommend consideration of augmentation therapy, which consists of adding another agent to the antidepressant currently in use. Quantitative assessment with the PHQ-9 can help clinicians make decisions about when to initiate augmentation therapy.

Clinicians can use the following guideline.

When a depressed patient experiences a significant clinical improvement (as manifested by a drop in PHQ-9 score by 5 points or more), but *fails* to reach remission (PHQ <5) within a minimum of 1 month after the dose of the initial antidepressant is raised to its maximum, then consider augmentation therapy.

The only two augmentation agents with a substantial evidence base include lithium carbonate (300–1200 mg) and triiodothyronine (T3, 25–50 µg). More commonly used agents, however, include use of a second antidepressant from a different class (e.g., bupropion, venlafaxine, and mirtazapine), buspirone (a 5-HT1A receptor agonist, approved for GAD), pindolol (beta-blocker), atypical antipsychotics (e.g., aripiprazole and olanzapine are FDA approved for augmentation), and psychostimulants (e.g., methylphenidate, dextroamphetamine, and modafinil).

ANTIDEPRESSANTS IN THE ELDERLY & MEDICALLY ILL: SAFETY, EFFICACY, IMPACT ON MORBIDITY, MORTALITY, & COST

Are antidepressant medications effective in the medically ill and the elderly? There have been surprisingly few randomized-controlled trials supporting the safety and efficacy of antidepressant medication in the medically ill and elderly. However, a recent systematic review of studies in specific medical populations, such as post-MI, poststroke, cancer, diabetes, cancer, Alzheimer disease, as well as other recent studies in general medical populations and elderly medical populations, suggest the safety and efficacy of antidepressant medications in these populations. Physicians should be aware, however, that most studies suggest that concurrent general medical illness is associated with somewhat lower overall depression response and remission rates compared to patients without concurrent medical illness.

Of particular importance, the SADHART study (Sertraline Antidepressant Heart Attack Trial) documented the safety of SSRI use (sertraline) immediately after heart attack, even in patients with severe cardiac disease and in patients using multiple other medications. Other recent studies now also document the safety and effectiveness of citalopram and of mirtazepine for depression after heart attack.

For many of the reasons enumerated earlier, the SSRIs and other new agents have become the agents of choice in the elderly and in the medically ill. When tricyclic agents are used, however, the safer ones are nortriptyline and desipramine, which are preferred because of their relatively lower anticholinergic and antiadrenergic side effects. Because of their quinidine-like effects, however, all TCAs are relatively contraindicated in patients with unstable cardiac disease or with recent MI. In depressed patients with diabetes, use of TCAs, compared to SSRIs has been associated with impaired glycemic control. Because of this finding, as well as their other autonomic side effects (constipation, postural hypotension, and so on), use of tricyclic medications such as amitriptyline should be used only with caution in diabetics, including for the treatment of neuropathic pain. For treatment of painful diabetic neuropathy, physicians could consider the preferential use of nortriptyline (a metabolite of amitriptyline) or one of the SNRIs (duloxetine or venlafaxine).

Dosing strategies in the elderly and medically ill should adhere to the general well-known guideline "start low and go slow." Pharmacokinetically, these agents are metabolized more slowly, resulting in accumulation and toxicity. Increased pharmacodynamic effects in the elderly may result from lower albumin levels, leading to higher levels of unbound drug.

Because depression is associated with increased morbidity, mortality, and cost in patients with concurrent general medical illness, it is reasonable to ask whether improvement in depression in medical patients leads to improvements in these other domains. There are limited and somewhat conflicting data on these questions, but some recent and notable studies point to potential decreases in morbidity, mortality, and overall health care costs with adequate treatment of depression. The SADHART study showed a trend (but not statistically significant) toward decreased rate of incident severe cardiac events and death in the sertraline group compared to placebo. A naturalistic outcome report of patients in the Enhancing Recovery in Coronary Heart Disease (ENRICHD) psychotherapy study noted that depressed patients treated with SSRIs (at physician/patient discretion, outside of protocol) had a statistically significant decrease in cardiac morbidity and mortality compared with the depressed patients who did not receive this treatment. A 2-year study of the collaborative care of patients with both depression and diabetes has shown an overall decrease in total health costs (general medical and psychiatric) in patients successfully treated for depression.

Electroconvulsive Therapy

Electroconvulsive therapy is still the most effective means available for the treatment of refractory depression. It is the treatment of choice for patients with psychotic depression, depression refractory to pharmacotherapy, and for some patients who are acutely suicidal. Despite prejudices and fears about ECT, new methods of administration have proven it to be a safe and effective treatment. In fact, ECT can be safer than antidepressant medication in the elderly. Some short-term memory loss is common, but research indicates that this reverts to normal in most patients. In some cases, ECT can be lifesaving and should not be denied to patients because of poor understanding or unrealistic fear. Electroconvulsive therapy does not lead to permanent remission of depression in patients susceptible to recurrence. Thus, patients with recurrent depression who receive ECT should receive either prophylactic medication after a course of therapy (as an outpatient) or maintenance ECT.

Light Therapy

Light therapy has been used successfully in the treatment of seasonal affective disorder (SAD), a condition in which recurrent depressive episodes occur during autumn and winter alternating with nondepressive episodes during spring and summer. Phototherapy is based on the principle that the presentation of artificial light at a similar strength to natural sunlight will prevent the biological changes that mediate SAD during the winter.

Other Brain Stimulation Interventions

With increasing awareness of alterations in brain networks, a number of direct brain stimulation interventions have been explored recently. These include approaches such as repetitive transcranial magnetic stimulation (rTMS), deep brain stimulation, and magnetic seizure therapy. Of these, only rTMS has an FDA-approved device. Even that approval has a narrow indication of only being used in individuals who have failed to respond to one antidepressant. Whether rTMS will be proved to have broader utility remains to be evaluated. Although its mechanism is unclear, high frequency stimulation is delivered over the left dorsolateral prefrontal cortex. Deep brain stimulation is available on an experimental basis for refractory depression. It focuses on decreasing activation of Brodmann Area 25, in the subgenual cingulate gyrus. This intervention can have immediate effects, but is a neurosurgical procedure with attendant risks, so that its application appears limited. Magnetic seizure therapy is being researched as an alternative to ECT and shows preliminary promise.

COLLABORATIVE CARE MODELS OF DEPRESSION

A generation of randomized, controlled health services trials indicates that systematic implementation of a "collaborative care model," or "chronic illness care" (or "chronic disease management") model of health care for depressed medical outpatients improves key processes and outcomes of care such as detection of depression; adequacy of depression treatment; patient adherence with treatment; improved clinical outcomes as assessed by measures such as PHQ-9 scores; and improved patient satisfaction. Key components of most of these new models generally include use of structured tools for assessment and management; utilization of care managers to help educate patients, support self-management, coordinate care and ensure follow-up; use of formal evidence-based guidelines and decision support tools; and finally, integration of behavioral health specialists into the medical team for consultation and ongoing support.

WHEN TO REFER

The criteria for referral to a mental health specialist depend a great deal on the experience and expertise of the primary treating physician. Patients should be informed that consultation with a mental health specialist may be necessary if the depression does not fully remit. This can make referral at a later stage much more acceptable. Because partial remission is a common occurrence, physicians should make every effort to establish clear indications of predepression functioning, and if full return to baseline functioning does not occur, referral to a specialist should be made. A baseline pretreatment PHQ-9 should be obtained and repeated at regular intervals to insure that the patient is responding appropriately to treatment. Patients with persistently elevated PHQ-9 scores (20 or above) or whose scores are not reduced to at least 50% of pretreatment levels, should be evaluated by a mental health specialist. Other indications for referral include patients with active suicidality, bipolar disorder, or psychosis; for evaluation of

any patient in whom the diagnosis is in doubt; and for advice about pharmacological management of patients with treatment-resistant depression. The primary practitioner should communicate with the mental health specialist and provide the following information: the nature of the depressive symptoms; baseline premorbid functioning; baseline and follow-up PHQ-9 scores; other treatments, including medication, that have been tried previously or are concurrent; and patient understanding and expectations about psychotherapy. Communication should be maintained with the mental health therapist about whether therapy is completed, since failure to follow through on a referral and/or premature discontinuation of psychotherapy is even more common than failure to comply with pharmacotherapy.

CONCLUSIONS

Of all the psychiatric conditions relevant to the general physician, major depression is arguably the most common and most important. Major depression is common, serious, often disabling, and associated with increased morbidity and mortality in general medical conditions. It is often missed and often inadequately treated. Recognition and adequate treatment is associated with response and remission and can often be provided adequately in the general medical sector. Increased understanding of the biopsychosocial etiology of major depression, the biopsychosocial manifestations of major depression, and the biopsychosocial treatment of major depression holds great promise for improving outcomes in this debilitating condition.

SUGGESTED READINGS

Rihmer Z, Akiskal H. Do antidepressants threaten depressives? Toward a clinically judicious formulation of the antidepressant-suicide FDA advisory in light of declining national suicide statistics from many countries. *J Affect Discord* 2006;94:5–13.

Cheng-Ta L, et al. Association between antidepressant resistance in unipolar depression and subsequent bipolar disorder: cohort study. *Brit J Psychiatr* 2012;200:45–51.

Gartlehehner MD, Hansen RA, Morgan LC et al. Comparative benefits and harms of second-generation antidepressants for treating major depressive disorder. *Ann Intern Med* 2011;155: 772–782.

Gibbons RD, Hur K, Brown CH, Davis JM, Mann JJ. Benefits from antidepressant: synthesis of 6-week patient-level outcomes from double-blind placebo-controlled randomized trials of fluoxetine and venlafaxine. *Arch Gen Psychiatry* 2012; Jun;69(6):572-9. doi: 10.1001/archgenpsychiatry.2011.2044.

Hollon SD, Javrett RB, Nierenberg AA, Thase ME, Trivedi M, Rush AJ. Psychotherapy and medication in the treatment of adult and geriatric depression; which monotherapy or combined treatment? *J Clin Psychiatry* 2005;66:455–468.

Holtzheimer PE, et al. Subcallosal cingulate deep brain stimulation for treatment-resistant unipolar and bipolar depression. *Arch Gen Psychiatry* 2012;69:150–158.

Karg K, et al. The serotonin transporter promoter variant (5HTTLPR), stress, and depression meta-analysis revisited. *Arch Gen Psychiatry* 2011;69:444–454.

Leuchter AF, et al. Resting-state quantitative electroencephalography reveals increased neurophysiologic connectivity in depression. *PLoS* 2012;7:e32508.

Mann JJ. The medical management of depression. *N Engl J Med* 2005;353:1819–1834.

Rush AJ. STAR*D: what have we learned? *Am J Psychiatry* 2007;164:201–204.

PATIENT BIBLIOGRAPHY

Alberti RE, Emmons ML. *Your Perfect Right: Assertiveness and Equality in Your Life and Relationships,* 8th ed. Atascadero, CA: Impact Publishers, 2001.

Burns DD. *Feeling Good—The New Mood Therapy.* New York, NY: Avon Books, 1999.

Greenberger D, Padesky C. *Mind over Mood: Change How You Feel by Changing the Way You Think.* New York, NY: The Guilford Press, 1995.

Hayes SC, Smith S. *Get Out of Your Mind and into Your Life.* Oakland, CA: New Harbinger Press, 2005.

Williams M, Teasdale J, Segal Z, Kabat-Zinn J. *The Mindful Way through Depression: Freeing Yourself from Chronic Unhappiness.* New York, NY: Guilford Press, 2007.

WEB SITES

National Institute of Mental Health Depression Information Web site. http://www.nimh.nih.gov/health/topics/depression/index.shtml. Accessed February 2014.

The MacArthur Initiative on Depression and Primary Care Web site. http://www.depression-primarycare.org/. Accessed February 2014.

Appendix 25-A. Patient Health Questionnaire—PHQ-9.

Name _____ Physician _____ Date _____

Over the last 2 *weeks*, how often have you been bothered by any of the following problems?

	Not At All (0)	Several Days (1)	More Than Half the Days (2)	Nearly Every Day (3)
1. Feeling down, depressed, or hopeless?	☐	☐	☐	☐
2. Little interest or pleasure in doing things?	☐	☐	☐	☐
3. Trouble falling or staying asleep, or sleeping too much?	☐	☐	☐	☐
4. Feeling tired or having little energy?	☐	☐	☐	☐
5. Poor appetite or overeating?	☐	☐	☐	☐
6. Feeling bad about yourself—or that you are a failure or have let yourself or your family down?	☐	☐	☐	☐
7. Trouble concentrating on things, such as reading the newspaper or watching television?	☐	☐	☐	☐
8. Moving or speaking so slowly that other people could have noticed? Or the opposite—being so fidgety or restless that you have been moving around a lot more than usual?	☐	☐	☐	☐
9. Thoughts that you would be better off dead or of hurting yourself in some way?*	☐	☐	☐	☐

10. If you are experiencing any of the problems on this form, how *difficult* have these problems made it for you to do your work, take care of things at home, or get along with other people?

☐ Not difficult at all   ☐ Somewhat difficult   ☐ Very difficult   ☐ Extremely difficult

Office Use Only
Number of Symptoms: _____ _____ Severity Score: _____

If you have had thoughts that you would be better off dead or of hurting yourself in some way, please discuss this with your doctor, go to a hospital emergency room, or call 911.

Appendix 25-B. Scoring the PHQ-9.

How to Score the Patient Health Questionnaire (PHQ-9)

The PHQ-9 can assist in diagnosing depression, as well as planning and monitoring depression treatment. There are three steps to scoring the PHQ-9: Number of Depressive Symptoms, Severity Score, and Functional Assessment. The Number of Depressive Symptoms is used to aid in making the diagnosis of Depression. The PHQ-9 Severity Score and Functional Assessment are measured at initial assessment and regularly after treatment begins to determine the severity of depression and to evaluate patient progress.

Number of Depressive Symptoms (Diagnosis)

1. For questions 1–8, count the number of symptoms the patient checked as "More than half the days" or "Nearly every day."
   For question 9, count the question positive if the patient checks "Several days," "More than half the days," or "Nearly every day."
2. Use the following interpretation grid to diagnose depression subtypes:

0–2 PHQ symptoms   Not clinically depressed
3–4 PHQ symptoms*   Other depressive syndrome
5 or more PHQ symptoms*   Major depression

Severity Score

1. Assign a score to each response by the number value under the answer headings (Not at all = 0; Several days = 1; More than half the days = 2; and Nearly every day = 3).
2. Total the values for each response to obtain the severity score.
3. Use the following interpretation grid:

0–4   Not clinically depressed
5–9   Mild depression
10–14   Moderate depression
≥15   Severe depression

Functional Assessment

The final question on the PHQ-9 asks the patient how emotional difficulties or problems impact work, things at home, or relationships with other people and if this has caused difficulty for 2 years or more. Patient responses can be one of four: "Not difficult at all"; "Somewhat difficult"; "Very difficult"; or "Extremely difficult."

• If the patient selects one of the last two responses, "Very difficult" or "Extremely difficult," his or her functionality at work, at home, or in relationships with other people is significantly impaired.
• If the patient has had difficulty with these problems for 2 years or more, consider the diagnosis of dysthymia (chronic depression).

---

*PHQ-9 items #1 or #2 must be one of the symptoms checked.
PHQ-9 is adapted from PRIME-MD Today, developed by Spitzer, Williams, Kroenke, and colleagues. Copyright 1999, by Pfizer, Inc. All rights reserved. Reproduction permitted for the purposes of clinical care and research only.

Anxiety

Jason M. Satterfield, PhD & Mitchell D. Feldman, MD, MPhil

INTRODUCTION

Anxiety is a common, normal emotion; most people experience occasional trepidation, fear, nervousness, "jitters," or even panic. Mild anxiety may aid mental sharpness as uncertainty or pressure mounts. For some individuals, however, anxiety occurs as part of an anxiety disorder that is a prominent, persistent, and disruptive aspect of their daily lives. Among the general population in the United States, about 25% will experience an anxiety disorder at some time in their life, making anxiety more common than depressive disorders. At over $50 billion per year, the direct and indirect annual costs associated with anxiety disorders in the United States are similar to, and may even surpass, the economic burdens attributed to mood disorders.

The major anxiety disorders are shown in Table 26-1. They are often comorbid with depression and with one another (e.g., panic disorder [PD] and agoraphobia). Similar to depression, patients with an unrecognized anxiety disorder tend to present to general medical or specialist settings, rather than to the specialty mental health sector, as they generally complain of the prominent physical symptoms of the anxiety disorder rather than its emotional symptoms.

It is important to distinguish among the various anxiety disorders and identify possible comorbidities because of differences in treatment, complications, and prognoses. Although cross-cultural epidemiologic research has shown that anxiety disorders are present in all cultures, ethnicities, and age groups, providers also must be alert to a variety of common medical conditions and medication side effects that can have symptoms resembling an anxiety disorder (Table 26-2).

DIAGNOSIS

Office-based screening instruments can improve the detection of anxiety and other mental disorders, and can be used to evaluate treatment response. Several instruments have been developed to aid in recognition of an anxiety disorder. A two-question screener, the GAD-2 subscale of the GAD-7, has been found to perform well as a rapid screening tool for the most common anxiety disorders. The GAD-2 questions are as follows: *Over the last 2 weeks how often have you been bothered by the following problems: (1) Feeling nervous, anxious, or on edge; and (2) Not being able to stop or control worrying.* A single "yes" response to the anxiety screening questions has a sensitivity of 94% and a specificity of 53% when compared to more formal assessment by a mental health professional. Other clinically useful screening questions are listed in Table 26-3.

Early recognition of anxiety disorders can help identify patients suffering from treatable problems and provide the patient and the clinician with a formal diagnosis to better explain the patient's symptoms. It may also reduce patients' medical expenses and risk of iatrogenic complications by decreasing or eliminating unnecessary medical testing and referrals to specialists to evaluate unexplained physical and somatic symptoms, and various "treatment" trials of pharmacological agents.

Symptoms & Signs

Understanding the signs, symptoms, and epidemiologic features of the various anxiety disorders can help the physician make an accurate diagnosis and initiate timely, appropriate treatment while avoiding invasive or unnecessary testing.

Anxiety disorders typically manifest with *emotional symptoms* (e.g., fear and nervousness), *cognitive symptoms* (e.g., worry, a sense of doom, or derealization), and *physical symptoms* (e.g., muscular tension, tachycardia, dizziness, and insomnia). General medical practitioners must, therefore, decide how much diagnostic investigation is both feasible and necessary to rule out other important nonpsychiatric diseases. For example, when should a patient with palpitations undergo cardiac monitoring, thyroid function studies, evaluation for pheochromocytoma, or referral for cardiac catheterization? When does a patient with episodic nausea and abdominal pain require upper and lower endoscopy?

Edvard Munch (The Scream).

    CASE ILLUSTRATION 1

Gwen is a 28-year-old woman who was admitted for a "rule out" and evaluation of syncope after presenting to the emergency department (ED) with

Table 26-1. Anxiety disorders.

Anxiety Disorder	Prevalence in Primary Care (%)
Acute stress disorder	3–5
Agoraphobia	1–3
Generalized Anxiety Disorder	4–9
Obsessive Compulsive Disorder	1–2
Panic Disorder	1–6
Post-traumatic Stress Disorder	2–12
Social phobia	3–7
Specific phobia	8–13
Adjustment disorder with anxiety	4.5–9.2
Anxiety disorder due to a general medical condition	14–66
Substance-induced anxiety disorder	Unknown prevalence
Anxiety disorder not otherwise specified (NOS)	Unknown

Table 26-2. Selected medical conditions that can simulate an anxiety disorder.

- Cardiac
  Ischemic heart disease, mitral valve prolapse, arrhythmias
- Endocrine/metabolic
  Hyperthyroidism, hypoglycemia, pheochromocytoma, carcinoid
- Gynecologic
  Menopause, premenstrual syndrome
- Neurologic
  Transient ischemic attacks, seizure disorders
- Pharmacological
  Caffeine, alcohol, sympathomimetic agents, amphetamines, corticosteroids, theophylline, illicit drugs
- Respiratory
  Asthma, chronic obstructive pulmonary disease

shortness of breath, tachycardia, and a sensation that she is going to faint. The episodes started approximately 4 months ago, shortly after her husband was temporarily laid off from his job, and are not associated with activity. They have been increasing in frequency to where she is now experiencing as many as four episodes per week lasting approximately 5–10 minutes each. Gwen is fearful that she may faint while driving or when out with her child. She is also worried about her heart, as her mother had heart disease in her early fifties.

Gwen was monitored overnight and had several tests, including thyroid function studies and a Holter monitor. She was told those test results were all "normal" and to follow-up with her primary care provider who after reviewing the history and test results recognizes that the symptoms are consistent with panic disorder. Further historical details eliminate other medical or substance-related illness, or new use of caffeine or over-the-counter herbal or other remedies. The physician then reassures Gwen that her symptoms are not unusual and that 2–4% of all people suffer from PD. Sensing Gwen might be embarrassed by a psychological diagnosis, the doctor explains the nature of PD emphasizing its biological basis and asks her if she thinks the new onset of her symptoms are possibly related to her concerns regarding her family's financial security. To help Gwen learn more about PD, the doctor gives her a booklet and a web site address to read about self-managing her anxiety symptoms (see "Suggested Readings") and schedules a follow-up visit in 2 weeks to review this information and see how she is doing.

At their follow-up encounter, Gwen asks about medication for her panic symptoms as she has become worried about experiencing new attacks Her physician recommends a selective serotonin reuptake

Table 26-3. Suggested screening questions for anxiety.

Disorder	Question
Generalized anxiety disorder (GAD)	Would you describe yourself generally as a nervous person? Are you a worrier? Do you feel nervous or tense?
Panic disorder (PD)	Have you ever had a sudden attack of rapid heartbeat or rush of intense fear, anxiety, or nervousness? Did anything seem to trigger it?
Agoraphobia	Have you ever avoided important activities because you were afraid you would have a sudden attack like the one I just asked you about?
Social anxiety disorder	Some people have strong fears of being watched or evaluated by others. For example, some people do not want to eat, speak, or write in front of people for fear of embarrassing themselves. Is anything like this a problem for you?
Specific phobia	Some people have strong fears or phobias about things like heights, flying, bugs, or snakes? Do you have any strong fears or phobias?
Obsession	Some people are bothered by intrusive, silly, unpleasant, or horrible thoughts that keep repeating over and over. For example, some people have repeated thoughts of hurting someone they love even though they do not want to; that a loved one has been seriously hurt; that they will yell obscenities in public; or that they are contaminated by germs. Has anything like this troubled you?
Compulsion	Some people are bothered by doing something over and over that they cannot resist, even when they try. They might wash their hands every few minutes, or repeatedly check to see that the stove is off or the door is locked, or count things excessively. Has anything like this been a problem for you?
Acute stress disorder (ASD) and posttraumatic stress disorder (PTSD)	Have you ever seen or experienced a traumatic event when you thought your life was in danger? Have you ever seen someone else in grave danger? What happened?

inhibitor (SSRI), and advises that she use one-half of a tablet for the first week and then increase to a full tablet in 7–10 days. The doctor also advises Gwen that it may take 4–6 weeks before she notices any improvement from the medication, and recommends another follow-up visit in 2 weeks to see how she is feeling, review the self-help recommendations, and answer any new questions she may have. After a month on the medication Gwen's symptoms resolve and she returns to full function.

Differential Diagnosis

Symptoms resembling an anxiety disorder can be triggered by use of or intoxication from over-the-counter cold medications, caffeine, cocaine, theophylline preparations, amphetamines, and marijuana or withdrawal from alcohol, benzodiazepines, barbiturates, sedative–hypnotic agents, and other central nervous system (CNS) depressants. These conditions are commonly referred to as "substance-induced anxiety disorder" (Table 26-2). Therefore, the astute clinician must review the patient's list of medications and inquire about the use of over-the-counter medications including "herbal supplements" and performance-enhancing

preparations (anabolic steroids), legal (alcohol, tobacco, and caffeine) and illegal substances (cocaine).

Many medical conditions also have symptoms resembling those of anxiety (Table 26-2). Some are relatively common and obvious to practitioners (arrhythmias and asthma) and others are less so (insulinoma, pheochromocytoma, and carcinoid). Anxiety symptoms may also develop as a consequence of a medical condition. Examples include patients who experience anxiety symptoms following a myocardial infarction or following a pulmonary embolism. Clues to help sort medical from psychiatric patient presentations to guide diagnostic testing, if any, include patient age and gender, past medical and psychiatric history, family history, and social history, Indeed, people who have been in excellent physical health and develop new-onset anxiety symptoms after the age of 50 years are more likely to have medical etiologies explaining their anxiety symptoms than those under the age of 25 years who have presented previously to several physicians and undergone extensive medical testing for evaluation of multiple unexplained somatic symptoms.

Etiology

The development of anxiety disorders involves multiple factors, including biological abnormalities, past and present psychological stressors, maladaptive cognitions, and environmentally conditioned behaviors. Abnormalities in the CNS associated with anxiety disorders relate to the gamma-aminobutyric acid (GABA) receptor as well as to the locus ceruleus. Animal studies have shown that stimulation of the locus ceruleus produces hyperarousal states similar to those seen in anxious humans. Gamma-aminobutyric acid is an inhibitory neurotransmitter found throughout most of the CNS. It may decrease anxiety by inhibiting locus ceruleus activity and modulating the reticular activating system, another area of the brainstem thought to affect alertness and fear. Benzodiazepines, a class of medications commonly used to treat anxiety, bind to specific sites on the GABA receptor. When the benzodiazepine molecule binds the GABA receptor, the effect of GABA on the GABA receptor is enhanced, reducing anxiety. Two other neurotransmitters, serotonin and norepinephrine, are also under investigation based on therapeutic responses to medications that affect these systems (e.g., SSRIs and serotonin norepinephrine reuptake inhibitors [SNRIs]). Poor regulation of the adrenergic system is also suspected as beta-adrenergic agonists induce symptoms of panic and alpha-adrenergic agonists decrease symptoms of anxiety.

Genetic factors also likely play a role in anxiety disorders, as evidenced by twin studies showing a higher concordance for PD and obsessive-compulsive disorder (OCD) among monozygotic twins than among dizygotic twins.

Cognitive behavioral therapy (CBT) holds that behavior is driven by underlying beliefs or *cognitions*. Patients with anxiety typically overestimate danger or threats and underestimate their ability to effectively cope. These patients subsequently feel "stressed" or anxious and select avoidant or other maladaptive coping strategies.

Conditioned learning may also play a pivotal role in the development of anxiety disorders and the resulting avoidance often seriously compounds patients' anxiety-related functional impairment. For example, patients may notice some unusual autonomic arousal or physical sensation while driving a car. They may misinterpret this initially random and benign sensation as a life-threatening event (e.g., "I'm having a heart attack!"), which further intensifies the autonomic response, fuels the misinterpretation, and snowballs into a full-blown panic attack. They may learn to associate the physical sensation and the subsequent attack with the act of driving and feel heightened anxiety—fueled by catastrophic thinking—when they drive or anticipate driving. Initially, the association between driving and panic is coincidental (driving is not the event provoking the initial sensation or the panic attack). Eventually, however, a patient may completely stop driving for fear that another panic attack will occur. This conditioned learning between driving and panic may gradually become so strong that driving becomes a precipitant of panic attacks. Thus, the driver mistakenly becomes conditioned to fear driving.

Traumatic, highly stressful, and catastrophic life events are also key factors leading to anxiety disorders, particularly PTSD. Posttraumatic stress disorder and adjustment disorder with anxiety are examples of disorders in which these events play a specific causal role. Other research suggests that childhood trauma, sexual assault, battle exposure, and terrorism can predispose individuals to develop hyperactive physiologic responses to everyday stressors, placing them at greater risk for developing anxiety and other mood disorders.

SPECIFIC DISORDERS

Panic Attacks

A panic attack is characterized by a discrete period of intense fear accompanied by the abrupt onset of several cognitive and somatic symptoms. Cognitive symptoms may include but are not limited to racing thoughts, preoccupation with health concerns, catastrophic misinterpretation of somatic symptoms, or believing one is going insane. Somatic symptoms may include a choking sensation, racing heartbeat, sweating, "jelly" legs, nausea, shaking, chest pain, numbness, or feeling detached or unreal. Frightening physical symptoms are commonly prominent and scare many patients into seeking urgent medical care. Primary care providers can usually be reassuring, as panic attacks are often infrequent, self-limited, and not related to any serious mental or physical disorder. Panic attacks are categorized as follows:

- Unexpected (untriggered or uncued);
- Situationally bound (always environmentally or psychologically cued); or
- Situationally predisposed (sometimes, but not invariably, cued).

Panic attacks can be comorbid with a number of other anxiety disorders including social and specific phobias, OCD, and PTSD. The presence and type of a panic trigger help clinicians make a correct diagnosis. Uncued panic attacks are characteristic of PD, whereas cued attacks suggest other psychiatric conditions such as the following:

- Social phobia (attack triggered by fear of embarrassment in social situations);
- Specific phobia (fear of places or things);
- OCD (triggered by exposure to the object of an obsession, such as contamination); or
- PTSD (triggered by an event resembling the original trauma).

Panic attacks are quite common; most people experience a subclinical or limited-symptom attack at some time. Only about 9% of the general population ever experiences a full-blown panic attack.

Panic Disorder

DIAGNOSIS

Panic disorder is diagnosed when panic attacks are uncued and recurrent and are followed by a month or more of persistent fear of another attack or avoidance of situations because of fear of having another attack. Lifetime prevalence in the community is 2–4%, and about 3–8% of patients who present to primary care physicians meet current criteria. Panic disorder is approximately twice as common in women as among men. Community-based studies also reveal that suicide attempts are more common among patients with PD than among patients with major depression.

Panic disorder is a potentially debilitating disease with major complications. It leads to agoraphobia, a fear of being in a place or a situation where escape or rescue might be difficult if another attack occurs, in 30–50% of cases, most often within 6 months of the first panic attack. This fear may cause many patients to avoid important activities of daily living, such as shopping or using public transportation. Patients who develop PD as adolescents often develop depressive disorders in early adulthood.

MANAGEMENT

Effective treatment exists for many of the anxiety disorders and has proved to be effective in clinical trials at reducing anxiety symptoms and in improving health-related quality of life and employment patterns. Appropriate treatment may also reduce substance use among patients who self-medicate with alcohol, benzodiazepines, or other substances in an effort to ameliorate their symptoms.

Initial management of the anxiety disorders begins with providing the patient with a clear understanding of the problem. This tends to ease anxiety, increase the strength of the therapeutic alliance, and the subsequent likelihood that the patient will adhere with the treatment plan. It may be helpful to emphasize the biological nature of PD, as most patients find it reassuring and destigmatizing to know that they have a recognized, treatable biological syndrome that typically has a good prognosis. Patients should also be referred to self-help books, support groups, and cognitive behavioral resources, which are widely available (see "Suggested Readings").

In tailoring the treatment of PD to the patient, several factors should be weighed, including the degree of avoidance present, the severity of physical manifestations, and the comorbidity of other psychiatric disorders. The clinician must balance patient education and supportive counseling with patients' beliefs about the cause of their symptoms. For example, if the physical symptoms are attributed to a cardiac problem, correcting this misinterpretation and emphasizing the biological basis of PD may help the patient accept the diagnosis and thus improve adherence to treatment. The primary physician has a vital role to play in many of the treatments, such as patient education, advice to avoid possible triggering substances (such as caffeine and cold medicines), supportive counseling, and initial pharmacotherapy, which can appropriately be incorporated into routine office visits.

Patients with PD often focus on the somatic symptoms of the disorder, thus presenting to medical settings with chest pain, dizziness, abdominal concerns, and other unexplained complaints. Iatrogenesis and unnecessary medical costs can and often do result from unnecessary procedures and treatments. The dilemma for clinicians, therefore, is to decide whether and how extensively to evaluate the patient's specific symptoms.

One clinical strategy is to evaluate conservatively those symptoms that are potentially catastrophic, involve objective findings, or present as a classic constellation of symptoms. While the investigation is proceeding, the patient can be treated for PD and the symptoms periodically reassessed. Effective pharmacological treatment can reduce the cognitive and physical symptoms of panic and lessen the patient's belief that the problem is caused by an undiscovered medical condition.

Medications used to treat PD include antidepressants, most commonly SSRIs and SNRIs, but tricyclic antidepressants (TCAs) and monoamine oxidase inhibitors (MAOIs) can also be used. Benzodiazepines (alprazolam, clonazepam) relieve symptoms rapidly, usually within the first week of treatment, and they have a relatively wide therapeutic index. Their main disadvantages are their potential for misuse and dependence, a high incidence of rebound panic attacks when the medication is discontinued, and interference with exposure-based CBT. In contrast, SSRIs, SNRIs, and TCAs are not associated with dependence and may have a synergistic effect with CBT, but generally take 3–4 weeks or longer before reaching maximum effectiveness. In addition, some antidepressants may exacerbate symptoms of anxiety during the first 1–2 weeks of administration.

A benzodiazepine can also be used in combination with either an SSRI or an SNRI (to avoid a "serotonin syndrome," SSRIs and SNRIs should not be used in combination). Given the availability of several potential first-line agents believed to be of similar efficacy (Table 26-4), the clinician is advised to first inquire about past personal and family experience with pharmacotherapy, side effects, brand preference, and insurance formulary restrictions before suggesting a particular medication.

Table 26-4. Preferred anxiolytic medications for use in medical outpatients.

Generic Name	Class	Starting Dosage	Step-up Dose	Target Dose	Top Dose/day	Comment
First-line Agent						
Citalopram	SSRI	10 mg qd	10–20 mg/qd	20–40 mg/day	40 mg	Possibly fewer cytochrome P450 drug interactions
Duloxetine	SNRI	20 mg qd	20 mg/day	30 mg bid or 60 mg qd	60 mg bid	FDA-approved for depression
Escitalopram	SSRI	5 mg qd	5–10 mg qd	10–20 mg/day	20 mg	Enantiomer of citalopram; possibly fewer cytochrome P450 drug interactions; FDA-approved for GAD
Fluoxetine	SSRI	10 mg qd	10 mg/day	20–40 mg/day	80 mg	Most activating of SSRI class; slower onset of action; FDA-approved for depression, PD, OCD, and bulimia
Paroxetine	SSRI	10 mg qd	10–20 mg/day	40 mg/day	40 mg	FDA-approved for depression, PD, GAD, PTSD, OCD, social anxiety; slightly sedating
Sertraline	SSRI	25 mg qd	25 mg/day	100 mg/day	200 mg	FDA-approved for depression, PD, OCD, PTSD, social anxiety
Venlafaxine XR	SNRI	37.5 mg qd	37.5 mg qd	75–150 mg qd	225 mg	FDA-approved for depression, PD, GAD. Social anxiety; may increase blood pressure at higher doses
Second-line Agent						
Fluvoxamine	SSRI	50 mg qd	50 mg bid	50 mg bid	300 mg	FDA-approved for OCD, social anxiety (extended release)
Bupropion SR	NDRI	100 mg/day	50 mg bid	150 mg bid	450 mg	FDA-approved for depression; favored if comorbid depression; may induce seizures at higher doses in seizure-prone individuals
Nefazodone	SARI	100 mg bid	50 mg bid	150 mg bid	600 mg	Sedation prominent at start; FDA-approved for depression; possible hepatotoxicity
Alprazolam	BZD	0.25 mg bid–tid	0.25 mg bid	0.25 mg prn	4 mg	Short onset and duration of action; FDA-approved for anxiety and PD
Lorazepam	BZD	0.5 mg tid–qid	0.5 mg qd	1.0 mg tid	10 mg	Short onset and duration of action; FDA-approved for anxiety
Clonazapine	BZD	0.5 mg bid	0.5 mg qd	1.0 mg bid	4 mg	Longer onset and duration of action; FDA-approved for PD and anxiety
Third-line Agent						
Buspirone	Other	5 mg tid	5 mg qd	20–30 mg bid	60 mg	Moderate efficacy compared to SSRIs; no antidepressant effect; FDA-approved for GAD only
Mirtazapine	NaSSA	15mg qhs	7.5–15 mg qd	45–60 mg qd	60 mg	Approved for treatment of depression. Commonly used for comorbid depression and anxiety; common adjunct with other antidepressants; inverse relationship between dose and sedation

Abbreviations: BZD, benzodiazepine; NDRI, norepinephrine and dopamine reuptake inhibitor; SARI, serotonin agonist and reuptake inhibitor.

A common practice is to initiate treatment with a low daily dose of a generically available SSRI (e.g., escitalopram, 5 mg orally each day), titrating the dose slowly upward to 20 mg daily over 1–2 weeks as tolerated until symptom relief or the maximum dosage is attained, whichever arrives first. If the panic symptoms are particularly troublesome or if they worsen in the initial week of therapy, a benzodiazepine such as alprazolam or clonazepam can be added for more rapid control of symptoms and then tapered off and discontinued when the SSRI or SNRI commences effect. As with treatment of major depression, to avoid symptom relapse experts currently recommend that anxiolytic pharmacotherapy be continued for a minimum of 9–12 months, and longer if the symptoms are particularly disabling or recurrent, or per patient preference and ability to tolerate relapse.

Adjunctive cognitive behavioral interventions (e.g., relaxation training, challenging catastrophic thinking, and gradual exposures) can treat both the physical manifestations and avoidance behaviors and substantially decrease the likelihood of symptom relapse following discontinuation of pharmacotherapy. Patients should be helped to gradually face the situations and activities they feared and fully experience the physical sensations they once believed indicated a serious medical problem. For example, the patient in Case Illustration 1 would be encouraged to drive, shop, and manage other tasks outside her home while experiencing and eventually managing her shortness of breath, racing heartbeat, and sensation of fainting. If patients are at first overwhelmed by the prospect of doing this, they can first initiate exposure mentally, using relaxation techniques and guided imagery. The patient should be instructed to imagine a frightening but tolerable aspect of the activity (in this case, driving) while doing a relaxation exercise and to repeatedly visualize successfully coping with the activity. In some cases, it may be necessary to enlist the assistance of a cognitive behavioral therapist who can design and manage successive "exposure" exercises for overly frightened patients. Cognitive behavioral therapy and antidepressant medications have been found equally efficacious with combined CBT and antidepressants showing a modest advantage.

Phobias

DIAGNOSIS

Specific phobias and social anxiety disorder (formerly known as social phobia) are characterized by episodic anxiety in response to specific precipitants. Stimuli for specific phobias include places, things, or events, such as airplane flights, heights, insects, snakes, or rodents. Affected individuals are aware that their fears are exaggerated or unreasonable; nonetheless, when exposed to the precipitant, patients experience intense, excessive fear subsequently leading to avoidance behaviors. Specific phobias are perhaps the most common but least disabling of the various anxiety disorders. Although many individuals have at least one, most experience only minor related dysfunction, and therefore seldom seek medical care. Indeed, when care is sought, the diagnosis is usually evident from the history and requires no further testing.

Social anxiety disorder involves excessive fear of embarrassment, failure, or humiliation before others. Social anxiety disorder is classified into one of the two subtypes—nongeneralized and generalized. The more common nongeneralized subtype may be manifested as a fear of speaking, performing, eating, or writing in public. Less often, it presents as a generalized type of anxiety that disables the patient in a wide range of social situations. Its physical symptoms include blushing, profuse sweating, trembling, nausea, and difficulty talking. Marked anticipatory anxiety can also cause avoidance behaviors that significantly disrupt patients' functioning.

CASE ILLUSTRATION 2

Charlie, a man in his mid-thirties, presents to his primary care provider complaining of severe palpitations, sweating, and tremulousness. The symptoms occur when he is waiting in the customs line. As he approaches the front of the line, fear of evaluation and fear of talking with the customs official intensifies until the symptoms occur. Sometimes he flees to the end of the long line before he feels ready to face the customs official. Charlie realizes this cycle is silly and laughs anxiously as he describes it. This symptom is a major problem for him because his occupation is writing travel books. He has begun avoiding travel and is increasingly worried about his ability to meet writing deadlines and to continue working. A conservative medical workup is unrevealing, and the primary care provider makes the diagnosis of specific social anxiety disorder, prescribing a trial of alprazolam to be used a short time before standing in the customs line. Charlie is also given a self-help book and a tape on relaxation techniques and the use of guided imagery as a way of visualizing success in the customs line. Charlie uses these treatment approaches successfully on his next trip and realizes that the problem is controllable. He incorporates them into his routine work schedule, and within 2 months has returned to full occupational functioning.

MANAGEMENT

Treatment of specific phobias and social anxiety disorder almost always involves some form of CBT, such as systematic desensitization, in which the patient is gradually exposed to the feared object or situation. Generally accepted pharmacotherapy guidelines have not been established for specific phobias. As noted in Case Illustration 2, patients with phobia and specific social anxiety disorder are often prescribed short-acting benzodiazepines (or beta-blockers) to be taken prior to an anticipated exposure to the phobic stimulus. Benzodiazepines are often given for exposures to infrequent events that have no complex performance requirements (e.g., traveling by commercial airplane). Patients should be informed of the risk of anterograde amnesia, or blackouts, associated with some of these drugs. Sertraline, paroxetine, fluvoxamine (extended release), and venlafaxine have all been Food and Drug Administration (FDA)-approved for the treatment of social anxiety disorder. Therapeutic effects typically occur within 2–6 weeks but may take up to 12 weeks. Although less data are presently available, the other SSRI and SNRI medications may be similarly effective at treating this disorder.

Obsessive-Compulsive Disorder

DIAGNOSIS

Patients with OCD experience regular, intrusive, anxiety-provoking thoughts—called obsessions—or are driven to repeatedly perform seemingly unnecessary or bizarre rituals—called compulsions. Aggression, sex, and religion are common obsessional themes. Compulsions may involve mental tasks, such as counting or praying, or they may involve physical rituals, such as repeated hand-washing or checking the state of an object. In patients with both obsessions and compulsions, the ritualized compulsions are usually performed to control the anxiety generated by the obsessive thoughts (e.g., obsessive fear about germs is eased by compulsive hand-washing). Although patients' level of insight is typically high—they generally experience obsessions and compulsions as intrusive, upsetting, and silly—such insight may diminish acutely when they are faced with the focus of an obsession. They may also become so preoccupied with their obsessions and compulsions that they become extremely anxious, slow, and disabled. In one instance, a patient wrung her hands so constantly she could not cook, work, or sleep. Another washed his hands every 10–15 minutes, which interfered significantly with his normal business and social activities.

Until the introduction of effective pharmacotherapies for OCD, the disorder was markedly underrecognized in both primary care and psychiatric practice.

About 1–3% of the general population develops OCD during their lives. The disorder has been found to have a distinct biological component, a finding supported by the efficacy of biological therapies that selectively inhibit the reuptake of serotonin at CNS neurosynapses, and twin studies that show a significantly higher percentage of monozygotic twins with diagnostic concordance than dizygotic twins. Additionally, there is a distinct and reciprocal association between OCD and Tourette syndrome, a neurologic disorder involving persistent motor and verbal tics.

MANAGEMENT

Psychotherapy for OCD often involves a form of CBT called "exposure with response prevention" in which the patient is exposed to the anxiety-provoking obsessions or situation but does not engage in the subsequent compulsions or other maladaptive strategies to manage the anxiety. Patients are taught alternate ways of coping with the anxiety including diaphragmatic breathing and progressive muscle relaxation. The cognitive behavioral therapist may also guide the patient in identifying faulty beliefs and assist the patient in testing those beliefs. The belief, "something terrible will happen if I don't check my lock a hundred times a day," is first rationally examined, then a behavioral test of that belief is collaboratively designed and executed—much as a scientist would design and run a test for any hypothesis.

Selective serotonin reuptake inhibitors inhibit presynaptic reuptake of serotonin and are effective in treating OCD. In addition, clomipramine, the only TCA with this quality, is also effective. Selective serotonin reuptake inhibitors have the advantages of ease of dosing and low toxicity in overdose. FDA-approved SSRIs for treatment of OCD include fluoxetine (Prozac), fluvoxamine (Luvox), paroxetine (Paxil), citalopram (Celexa), escitalopram (Lexapro), and sertraline (Zoloft). The dual SNRIs (venlafaxine and duloxetine) may also have efficacy in OCD. However, neither has yet been FDA-approved specifically for treatment of OCD. A recent meta-analysis recommends antipsychotic (haloperidol and risperidone) augmentation of SSRIs for treatment-refractory OCD.

Posttraumatic Stress Disorder & Acute Stress Disorder

DIAGNOSIS

Posttraumatic stress disorder (PTSD) and acute stress disorder (ASD) are the common mental sequelae of catastrophic trauma. Acute stress disorder involves symptoms that occur within the first month after trauma. Posttraumatic stress disorder is essentially the same syndrome, but beginning or persisting beyond a month. Severe trauma of either ASD or PTSD entails exposure to actual or threatened death, serious injury or sexual violation. Patients subsequently develop a mix of flashbacks, nightmares, persistent avoidance of stimuli resembling (concretely or symbolically) the precipitating event, numbing of general responsiveness (restricted range of affect, feelings of interpersonal estrangement, anhedonia), and persistent signs and symptoms of physiologic arousal. Secondary depression, panic attacks, substance abuse, unexplained physical symptoms, and aggressive behavior may also be present.

Epidemiologic studies suggest that about one-third of the population suffers some trauma, placing them at risk for PTSD, and one-fourth of those at risk will develop PTSD, usually within 1 year following exposure to the event, although on occasion, it may develop years after the event. While men experience more lifetime trauma, women in the general population are more likely to develop PTSD. Women have a 10% lifetime prevalence of PTSD, double that of men. The prevalence of PTSD is considerably higher among certain groups including 18% among professional firefighters, 34% in adolescent survivors of motor vehicle crashes, 48% in female rape victims, and 67% in former prisoners of war.

CASE ILLUSTRATION 3

Jacques was a successful accountant with no psychiatric history until he had mitral valve surgery at the age of 42 years. Subsequently, he became totally dysfunctional, losing jobs and clients. He now also suffers flashbacks about the postoperative period of pain and confusion. Jacques gradually became depressed, and his obnoxious, angry behavior alienated both friends and providers.

Jacques' primary care physician noted a change in his demeanor during a conversation at a routine follow-up visit to monitor his chronic anticoagulation therapy for his replacement valve. The physician asked Jacques how work was going for him since his return following surgery. Then Jacques began to disclose his personal fears and perceived failures triggered by the traumatic brush with serious illness and fear of a stroke caused by his replacement valve. His doctor then helped Jacques recognize the role of the surgical trauma event in his life and explained the potential for improvement with psychotherapy and pharmacotherapy for his symptoms. Jacques subsequently accepted referral to an established multidisciplinary treatment program for PTSD.

MANAGEMENT

Treatment of PTSD typically begins with a detailed evaluation and development of a treatment plan to meet the unique needs of the survivor. This is best accomplished with a multidisciplinary team that may include the primary care physician, a mental health professional, an addiction specialist, a social worker, and possibly community-based referral resources such as theme counseling groups (e.g., veterans groups and abuse-survivor groups). PTSD-specific treatment typically begins after the patient has been safely removed from the crisis situation. If the patient is still being exposed to trauma (e.g., ongoing domestic violence), or is severely depressed, experiencing extreme panic, suicidal, or is in need of drug or alcohol detoxification, then it is important to address these issues as a part of initial treatment.

It is generally helpful to label the problem as PTSD and thus legitimize the manifestations, as patients often blame themselves or others. Thus, the physician might say to the patient, "The kinds of feelings, thoughts, and problems you're having are not unusual—in fact they're fairly common among people who have gone through a catastrophe." Support groups of persons who have suffered similar trauma help patients feel understood and normalize their symptoms as they share their experiences and solve problems together. Cognitive-behavioral therapy is the nonpharmacological treatment of choice for PTSD where patients are taught behavioral skills to manage their autonomic hyperarousal, and then are guided through repeated and desensitizing retellings of their traumatic experience.

Pharmacotherapy can reduce the anxiety, depression, and insomnia often experienced by patients with PTSD. Although no particular drug has emerged as a definitive treatment for PTSD and its associated flashbacks and nightmares, currently, only sertraline and paroxetine have been FDA-approved for the treatment of PTSD. Initial trials of venlafaxine have shown promising results. Benzodiazepines have also been used to treat the anxiety, hyperarousal, and insomnia of PTSD. However, early and prolonged use of benzodiazepines to treat ASD may actually be associated with a higher rate of subsequent PTSD. Thus, it is recommended that benzodiazepines be reserved for time-limited treatment of extreme arousal, insomnia, and anxiety.

Generalized Anxiety Disorder

DIAGNOSIS

Generalized anxiety disorder (GAD) consists of almost constant, nonepisodic worry and anxiety that affects patients for more than 6 months and interferes with normal functioning. The worry and anxiety are difficult for the patient to control and are associated with edginess or restlessness, easy fatigability, difficulty concentrating, irritability, muscle tension, or sleep disturbance. Worries typically involve multiple domains and may include concern about routine life circumstances, with the magnitude of worry being out of proportion to the severity of the situation. Symptoms must not be due to the physiologic effects of a medical problem, such as hyperthyroidism or abuse of a medication or drug. Patients with GAD usually complain of feeling "up-tight" or constantly nervous. Physical symptoms such as muscle aches, twitching, trembling, sweating, dry mouth, headaches, gastrointestinal symptoms, urinary frequency, and exaggerated startle often accompany the disorder and are often the patient's presenting complaint.

General anxiety disorder has a lifetime prevalence of 4–6%, and two-thirds of those affected are women. The disorder tends to have a chronic, fluctuating course that worsens under stress. Approximately half of all cases are comorbid with depression.

MANAGEMENT

Short-term supportive psychotherapy can be helpful. Many patients with GAD have focal life conflicts or stressors for which psychotherapy may be helpful. Basic primary care strategies include empathic listening; encouragement; and assisting patients to identify problems, discuss possible solutions, and solve the problem. Cognitive behavioral techniques can be used to help patients examine the catastrophic beliefs that underlie their unrealistic worries. Biofeedback and relaxation techniques are useful for improving patient control over muscle tension and other physiologic signs of anxiety.

Several SSRIs and benzodiazepines, venlafaxine, and the nonbenzodiazepine anxiolytic buspirone are all FDA-approved for treatment of GAD. Benzodiazepine therapy at doses lower than those required for PD is usually rapidly effective with few adverse effects. Sedation is the most common side effect but diminishes over time. Tolerance to therapeutic effects is minimal. Minimum effective doses should be used, but care must be taken not to undertreat patients out of fear of making them drug dependent. As with benzodiazepine treatment for other anxiety disorders, rebound symptoms of anxiety are the rule as medication is discontinued. Often a lengthy (a month or more) taper is required.

Buspirone is a nonsedating medication specifically indicated for patients with GAD. It alleviates the symptoms of this anxiety disorder but like the SSRIs and venlafaxine has a similarly slow onset of action to reach efficacy. Unlike these other medications, buspirone also requires twice daily dosing, which may adversely affect patient adherence. Importantly, it only has moderate efficacy compared with the SSRIs, and it lacks an antidepressant effect placing it at a disadvantage for patients with comorbid depression.

Adjustment Disorder With Anxiety

DIAGNOSIS

Adjustment disorder with anxiety should be considered in patients who are responding with maladaptive anxiety to a recent situational stressor but who do not meet the criteria for another mental disorder. The stressor may be a medical event (e.g., surgery, hospitalization, onset of an illness), but most often is a personal crisis such as a divorce, financial problems, or a job change. Symptoms usually begin within 2 months of the onset of the stressor and significantly impair social or occupational functioning. If symptoms persist for more than 6 months, then another diagnosis, such as GAD, is usually more appropriate. Sleeplessness and the physiologic aspects of anxiety predominate, and the patient may seek care for somatic complaints. Eliciting the history of the stressful life event and ascertaining the relationship of symptoms to that event help to establish this diagnosis.

MANAGEMENT

The fundamental management of adjustment disorder with anxious mood is supportive counseling, in which the patient discusses the stressful event and the provider helps the patient actively identify and solve problems and/or find ways to more effectively manage the stress (e.g., more effectively access social supports or engage in pleasant activities). Patients with adjustment disorder are generally well cared for by a primary care physician who has learned the details of the precipitating event and can incorporate brief supportive strategies into the office visit. Structured relaxation exercises and stress management or other support groups may also be helpful. Sometimes a brief trial of benzodiazepine (less than 3 weeks) can help improve patient coping by reducing the debilitating stress-related symptoms (e.g., insomnia or overwhelming fear). Referral to mental health professionals may help if patients do not respond quickly, are severely incapacitated, show a repetitive pattern of maladaptive coping, or specifically request a therapist.

Many studies suggest that there is a substantial group of primary care patients who present with relatively minor complaints of anxiety and depression. Although they do not satisfy criteria for a mental disorder, they do experience associated poor functioning. Often psychosocial stressors or chronic medical problems exacerbate the emotional symptoms. Generally speaking, effective management should emphasize supportive psychosocial rather than pharmacological interventions.

MANAGEMENT OF ANXIETY: GENERAL PRINCIPLES

Several general principles pertaining to the primary care treatment of anxiety disorders are worthy of note.

Psychosocial Therapies

Primary care providers should not underestimate the importance of basic supportive measures that can easily be performed in the general medical setting. The relationship between the doctor and patient usually plays a pivotal role for anxious patients in need of reassurance. Patient–provider trust is especially important for anxious patients, enhancing timely and accurate history taking, physical examination, diagnosis, and treatment adherence.

Symptoms of anxiety are extremely distressing to patients, who often fear that occult disease is causing their symptoms. Clinicians must try to view the symptoms through the eyes and perceptions of the affected patient—what seems trivial to a provider may be overwhelming for the patient. Listening to patients, expressing empathy for their feelings and concerns, and providing information about anxiety disorders are crucial ways to improve patient rapport (see Chapters 1 and 2) and should be routine in the course of care.

Equipping patients with basic information about anxiety disorders is essential ("bibliotherapy"). Patients with anxiety are common in medical settings so hospitals and clinics should be prepared and knowledgeable with patient education resources such as brochures, and relevant web sites to enable patients to find high-quality information. Most patients find such explanations and self-management strategies from appropriate lay publications reassuring. A number of well-validated and available psychosocial treatments can be recommended (Table 26-5).

Pharmacotherapy

Pharmacological treatment (Table 26-4) is appropriate when the patient's symptoms are severe enough to significantly interfere with functioning and the benefits of medication outweigh the risks for a given patient. The treatment must be carefully individualized, based on the patient's prior experiences with pharmacotherapy—if any, such as family experiences, brand name preference, insurance formulary restrictions, symptom severity, complicating medical or substance-abuse problems,

vulnerability to various side effects, and willingness to collaborate in a psychopharmacological approach to treatment.

When medications are prescribed, it is important to recognize, track, and document specific target symptoms. We generally recommend treatment with a generically available SSRI or SNRI for treatment-naïve patients unless there is a compelling reason to use a branded medication as no medication within these classes have been proved to be more effective than another. The medication should be initiated at half the typical starting dosage for unipolar major depression, and then titrated upward at 1–3 week intervals so as to minimize both the target symptoms and bothersome side effects. Lower starting dosages are recommended for those aged 60 years and older, because these drugs have longer half-lives in this age group, accumulation can easily occur, and sensitivity to unwanted cognitive and other toxic effects is greater. In addition, for this age group we recommend against use of TCAs to avoid the potential for cardiac side effects, and benzodiazepines to avert cognitive and physical impairment (e.g., falls).

It is critically important to speak to the patient by telephone or in the office within 1–2 weeks and then again approximately every 2–4 weeks after the start of pharmacotherapy until symptoms remit. The purpose of these follow-up contacts are to: (1) promote medication adherence; (2) monitor for potential side effects; (3) assess for emerging suicidality; (4) monitor treatment response; and (5) answer any new questions or concerns the patient may have. Following complete symptoms remission, patients should be seen or contacted every few months over the first year of treatment.

Although monotherapy is almost always preferable to medication combinations, a common exception is prescribing both ongoing antidepressants and 2–4 weeks of minor tranquilizers for patients with PD. This strategy achieves rapid reduction of symptoms, avoids the intensification of anxiety sometimes seen in early antidepressant treatment of anxiety disorders, and allows discontinuation of benzodiazepines before dependence occurs. If patients are being referred to

Table 26-5. Nonpharmacological management of anxiety disorders.

Type of Treatment	Description	Indication
Education	Provides basic information and reassurance	Appropriate in all disorders Lay publications useful
Cognitive behavioral therapy (e.g., systematic desensitization)	Gradually increases exposure to feared stimulus using relaxation techniques Helps patient reorganize way of thinking about symptoms	Useful in all disorders Particularly effective for PD and OCD
Relaxation techniques	Uses muscle relaxation therapy, including hypnosis, biofeedback, meditation	Particularly useful in PDs, GAD, adjustment disorder with anxious mood

CBT, a benzodiazepine taper, typically a reduction by 25% of the daily dose every week, and discontinuation are recommended. Benzodiazepines should seldom be used in patients with a history of substance abuse.

INDICATIONS FOR REFERRAL

Multiple randomized, controlled trials have shown that pharmacotherapy and/or CBT are effective treatments for most anxiety disorders. Patients should be considered for referral to a mental health professional under the following circumstances:

1. The patient has suicidal or homicidal thoughts or plans or exhibits intended suicidal or homicidal behavior.
2. The treatment does not lead to improvement in the patient's symptoms within the expected time frame.
3. Diagnostic uncertainty. It is particularly important to differentiate patients who have bipolar disorder, alcohol abuse/dependence, or personality disorders from those with an anxiety disorder. Mental health consultation is appropriate if the primary care doctor is uncertain and the distinction has therapeutic implications.
4. Comorbid substance abuse is suspected.
5. The provider has questions about appropriate administration or tapering of benzodiazepines and questions regarding possible dependence.
6. The patient has an especially complicated set of ongoing psychosocial stressors whose resolution requires greater time and expertise than can be provided in primary care.
7. When a multidisciplinary or more specialized treatment approach is indicated. Such conditions include, but are not limited to ASD, PTSD, and desensitization therapy for specific or social phobia.

In some circumstances, the primary care physician may be uncertain about whether a patient has another medical illness and believes a specialist is necessary to consider that possibility. It is helpful to select a specialist who understands anxiety disorders and will work with the referring physician to explain the nature of the specific anxiety disorder to the patient. It is imperative that the specialist brings a conservative approach to diagnostic studies, an understanding of the many physical manifestations of anxiety, and a respectful approach to treatment of the anxiety-disordered patient.

The accurate and prompt diagnosis of anxiety disorders can prevent unnecessary diagnostic testing, specialty referral, and iatrogenic harm. The primary care physician who is knowledgeable and skilled in the diagnosis and management of anxiety disorders can make an important contribution to the quality of patient care and to the appropriate use of health resources, particularly in the managed care environment. Nevertheless, delivery for appropriate care can be difficult in typical practice settings. To overcome patient, physician, and system barriers to provision of guideline-based treatment and provide sustained patient follow-up, "collaborative care" models have been developed and subsequently proved to be effective at improving clinical outcomes for panic and GAD. They typically involve a nurse or other allied health professional who follows an evidence-based protocol under the direction of a primary care physician with specialty back-up when necessary, who has the time to educate the patient about his or her disorder, provide monitor use of pharmacotherapy, and impart self-management skills either in person or via telephone. Still, more clinical trials are necessary to examine the effectiveness of this strategy at improving clinical outcomes for other anxiety disorders.

SUGGESTED READINGS

Baldwin D, Woods R, Lawson R, Taylor D. Efficacy of drug treatments for generalised anxiety disorders: systematic review and meta-analysis. *BMJ* 2011;342:d1199. doi:10.1136/bmj.d1199.

Hicks D, Cummings T, Epstein SA. An approach to the patient with anxiety. *Med Clin North Am* 2010;94:1127–1139.

Kroenke K, Spitzer RL, Williams JBW, et al. Anxiety disorders in primary care: prevalence, impairment, comorbidity, and detection. *Ann Intern Med* 2007;146:317–325.

Roy-Byrne P, Craske MG, Sullivan G, et al. Delivery of evidence-based treatment for multiple anxiety disorders in primary care: a randomized controlled trial. *JAMA* 2010;303:1921–1928.

PATIENT BIBLIOGRAPHY (REFERENCE BOOKS FOR PATIENTS)

Bourne EJ. *The Anxiety and Phobia Workbook,* 4th ed. Oakland, CA: New Harbinger Press, 2005.

Craske MG, Barlow DH. *Mastery of Your Anxiety and Worry,* 2nd ed. New York, NY: Oxford University Press, 2006.

Davis M, McKay M, Eshelman ER. *The Relaxation and Stress Reduction Workbook,* 5th ed. Oakland, CA: New Harbinger Press, 2000.

Foa E, Wilson R. *Stop Obsessing! How to Overcome Your Obsessions and Compulsions.* New York, NY: Bantam, 2001.

Zuercher-White E. *An End to Panic: Breakthrough Techniques for Overcoming Panic Disorder,* 2nd ed. Oakland, CA: New Harbinger Press, 1998.

WEB SITES

Anxiety Disorders Association of America Web site. http://www.adaa.org. Accessed October 2012.

Cognitive Behavioral Therapy Web site. http://www.abct.org/Home/. Accessed October 2012.

Consumer Nonprofit Web site. http://www.freedomfromfear.org. Accessed October 2012.

National Institute of Mental Health Web site. http://www.nimh.nih.gov/health/topics/anxiety-disorders/index.shtml. Accessed October 2012.

Attention Deficit Hyperactivity Disorder

27

H. Russell Searight, PhD, MPH & Cheyenne Shinabarger, MS

Attention deficit hyperactivity disorder (AD/HD) is a condition typically first evident in early childhood. Symptoms include deficits in attention, concentration, and short-term memory. Behaviorally, children with AD/HD are overly active (as if "driven by a motor") and unable to remain seated, highly distractible, and impulsive. Concerns about AD/HD often initially arise during kindergarten or first grade, since these deficits significantly impair academic performance and are disruptive in a typical classroom. However, AD/HD is increasingly viewed as a lifelong condition with functional impairment extending throughout adulthood.

Recent data suggest a 6–8% prevalence rate. To date, the majority of epidemiologic studies have been conducted in North America and Europe. However, available data suggest that the condition has similar prevalence rates in Asia, Africa, and Latin America with a pooled worldwide rate of 5.3%. However, there is also considerable variability in prevalence rates that may reflect differing diagnostic practices, differing definitions of the condition, or both. A recent US study by the Centers for Disease Control reported state-based prevalence rates ranging from 5.6% (Nevada) to 15.6% (North Carolina). AD/HD disproportionately affects males with a sex ratio between 3:1 and 9:1, with more conservative figures in clinic rather than community samples. Lower socioeconomic status (SES) has been associated with increased AD/HD rates in international studies.

There are two essential clusters of AD/HD symptoms: inattention and hyperactivity/impulsivity. Symptoms of AD/HD include either **inattention** (failing to give attention to detail, problems maintaining attention, not appearing to listen when spoken to directly, failure to follow through on instructions and to complete schoolwork or other tasks, problems with organization, avoiding activities requiring sustained concentration, losing important items, being easily distracted, and forgetfulness), or **hyperactivity/impulsivity** (fidgeting, inability to remain seated, inappropriate running and climbing, difficulty playing quietly, acting as if "driven by a motor," excessive talking, blurting out answers before questions are finished, difficulty taking turns, and intruding upon others' activities and/or conversations), or of both clusters. Children must have at least six symptoms from either (or both) the inattention group of criteria and the hyperactivity and impulsivity criteria, whereas older adolescents and adults (over the age of 17 years) must present with five. Most symptoms should have been present before the age of 12 years.

CASE ILLUSTRATION 1: PRESCHOOL CHILD

Four-and-a-half year old Ronnie has been dismissed from three preschools during the past 9 months. Ronnie's mother brings a teacher's note chronicling Ronnie's recent behavior:

- *2/25 = "Ran out of classroom and was on his way out of the building before I stopped him."*
- *2/28 = "Threw all of the students' coats on the floor . . . won't listen when he's told to hang them up."*
- *3/2 = "Would not sit through story time. Threw milk cartons during lunch time."*

In your examination room, Ronnie is lying across your stool face down yelling, "I'm flying," while pushing off from the walls with his feet. His mother, appearing exhausted, makes a few half-hearted attempts to get Ronnie to settle down but quickly gives up saying, "You see doctor, this is what it's like."

Although there are no precise longitudinal figures, AD/HD is increasingly accepted as a lifelong condition for many, if not most, patients. Development, however, does affect the symptom picture. Research indicates that at around the age of 9 years, hyperactivity and impulsivity begin to become less pronounced, whereas inattention and other cognitive deficits persist, with hyperactivity being replaced by restlessness and fidgeting.

With children referred in preschool or the early grades, there is typically a high level of parental distress and urgency. Hyperactivity may take the form of an inability to remain seated for more than 5 minutes at school or during family meals. Even when seated, the child may be swinging their legs, rocking, or picking up nearby objects. By the time they reach first grade, children may also have a number of scars on their legs, arms, and head, and can provide a number of stories about jumping off the garage roof, rear-ending a car with their bicycle, and running into countless pieces of furniture. Among older adolescents and adults, household chores may be initiated but not completed, bills are forgotten, sitting through a movie or presentation is extremely difficult, and others complain about the patient's frequent conversational interruptions. The phrase "as if driven by a motor" captures the quality of the child's activity level. Although the child, with adult urging, may sit relatively still for 2–3 minutes, they will begin moving around as if they cannot stop themselves. The hyperactive/impulsive behavior is not experienced as under the patient's control—particularly among younger children.

CASE ILLUSTRATION 2: EARLY ELEMENTARY SCHOOL CHILD

Christopher is a 7-year-old boy and first grader, who is accompanied by both parents. They bring several notes that the teacher has sent to them since school began several months ago. They also bring samples of Christopher's schoolwork. The teacher's notes describe situations in which Chris got up from his seat to sharpen his pencil 20 times in the course of a day, was repeatedly told to stop playing with the girl's hair who sits in front of him, and continued to yell out answers to the teacher's questions before she finished speaking. Christopher's parents say that he is not learning to read or spell because he is easily distracted and cannot follow the lessons. At home, they describe mealtime as a "hit and run" experience where Chris eats while alternately sitting and standing at the table for no more than 10 minutes, during which he frequently knocks over his milk. Christopher's mother says she no longer takes him shopping

because he runs off from her in the store and she is afraid he will get lost.

Impaired attention and concentration, distractibility, and short-term memory deficits are often misattributed to "laziness," poor motivation, or "not caring" rather than a central nervous system disorder. Parents frequently complain about having to tell their child "a hundred times" to do something before the request "seems to register." Multistep directions are particularly challenging for those of all ages with AD/HD. A mother tells her teenaged son to go upstairs and get his new pants to be hemmed, the sewing kit, and a piece of chalk. Fifteen minutes later, when he has not appeared, his mother goes upstairs to find him. He is in his room, trying on a shirt with his new pants in his hand, having forgotten what he was asked to do.

CASE ILLUSTRATION 3: MIDDLE ELEMENTARY SCHOOL CHILD

Miranda, a 9-year-old fourth grader, is seen because of poor grades. Her teacher describes Miranda as "spacey" with difficulty concentrating, paying attention, and remembering. However, she and Miranda's mother both describe Miranda as a "sweet, sensitive, and helpful girl" without any disruptive behavior. A Vanderbilt Scale confirms this picture. The teacher's version includes a comment that Miranda may have to repeat the grade unless her academic performance improves.

At school, inattention and poor concentration impair academic performance. Much of school success is still based on memorization. To encode material into longer-term memory for a test, it is necessary to pay attention to relevant information, relate it to existing knowledge, and rehearse in short-term memory. When this process is disrupted, retaining information from textbooks and classroom presentations is extremely challenging. In elementary school, a typical didactic process is that the teacher will present a lesson (e.g., steps involved in long division, identifying adverbs) with several examples of the concept and then students will individually work on exercises applying that particular concept. In the later elementary years through college, there is much greater emphasis on reading and retaining what is read. College students with untreated AD/HD often report that despite rereading material multiple times, they cannot remember it.

CASE ILLUSTRATION 4: ADOLESCENT

Josh, a 15-year-old, is brought in by his father for a drug test. Yesterday, Josh was suspended from school after a baggie of marijuana was found in his locker. He readily admitted smoking it several times a week for the past 6 months to "help calm me down." Josh was diagnosed with AD/HD-mixed type at the age of 7 years and responded well to stimulant pharmaco-therapy until about a year ago. At that time, Josh's grades declined—largely because of missing assignments—and he has had several detentions because of being late to class. His father describes his son as increasingly fidgety, disorganized, and forgetful. During the seventh grade, Josh said he felt embarrassed about going to the school nurse's office for his second methylphenidate dose. Josh was switched from short-acting methylphenidate to an extended-release formulation that he only took once, in the morning, before school. When asked about how he was tolerating the current medication, Josh responded: "I don't like taking that stuff; it doesn't do anything for me. My friends don't have to take it." Josh's father adds, "Now that I think about it, we have at least two extra bottles full of pills at home. I don't think Josh is taking it every day."

CASE ILLUSTRATION 5: ADULT

Jim, a 35-year-old man, comes to see you after a particularly poor performance evaluation at work. Jim is an auto salesman who was recently promoted to manager of a small group of junior sales people. On his evaluation, Jim's supervisor describes Jim as " . . . scattered, unable to set priorities; starts projects but doesn't finish them; paperwork late or lost." His supervisors describe him as a "nice guy" but "it's hard to know what he wants; he contradicts himself a lot."

At home, Jim's wife took over the family's schedule after Jim forgot several important dates, including her birthday. Many mornings, he dashes around the house looking for misplaced car keys. Jim's wife has also become the primary disciplinarian of their two children because Jim had difficulty being consistent and following through with consequences.

Jim describes having a hard time getting through high school: "I did really badly on tests; I just couldn't memorize." Even in elementary school, "I was sent to the principal's office for being the class clown." College was a greater challenge. Jim had to repeat several classes and required an extra three semesters to graduate.

Among adults with AD/HD, work and family are affected by inattention and poor short-term memory. Birthdays and anniversaries are forgotten, as are commitments to attend children's school activities. Multiple auto accidents are also common. At work, projects may be initiated but remain uncompleted. Phone calls, coworkers, and e-mail all pose distractions that make it particularly difficult to get back "on track."

Up to 80% of adolescents diagnosed with AD/HD continue to exhibit symptoms with a comparable adult rate of approximately 60%. Even when they no longer meet formal AD/HD diagnostic criteria, deficits are often present along with comorbid conditions, such as oppositional defiant disorder (ODD) or conduct disorder (CD) in adolescence and substance abuse, mood disorders and antisocial personality in adulthood. Among those adults with childhood histories that appear to remit, other psychiatric conditions are likely to emerge. Although findings have been mixed, there are indications that stimulant treatment during childhood reduces the likelihood of grade retention in school as well as the later development of comorbid psychiatric conditions, such as mood and anxiety disorders in adulthood.

ETIOLOGY

Heritability for AD/HD is approximately 0.76. Adoption studies further support the strong role of genetics in the condition. Recent molecular genetic studies have attempted to locate specific neurotransmitter receptor sites. Specifically, genes coding for dopaminergic (*DAT1*, *DRD4*, and *DRD5*), serotonergic (*5HTT* and *HTR1B*), and axonal growth and synaptic activity (*SNAP-25*) have been implicated. These neurogenetic findings are generally consistent with the action of stimulant drugs that block the dopamine transporter. However, it is likely that there is considerable heterogeneity for AD/HD with different genetic combinations associated with the same phenotype.

Certain environmental exposures, although not specific to AD/HD, have been associated with increased prevalence. Lead exposure appears to be associated with hyperactivity and cognitive difficulties; however, most AD/HD children do not have elevated lead and, conversely, most children with elevated lead do not develop AD/HD. Pregnancy and delivery complications, including toxemia, maternal age, fetal postmaturity, low birth weight, long duration of labor, fetal distress, hemorrhage, and prematurity are all AD/HD risk factors.

Alcohol use and maternal smoking during pregnancy also elevate AD/HD risk. It is likely that these factors, both directly and indirectly, are associated with subtle central nervous system damage in regions associated with the condition.

Several subtle structural brain anomalies have been associated with AD/HD. The subcortical structures involved include pathways involving the thalamus. Additional neural circuits involving the frontal lobe, basal ganglia, and central cerebellum have been implicated. There are suggestions that stimulant treatment is associated with fewer structural abnormalities and greater cerebral brain volume as compared with that of untreated AD/HD children and adolescents. Reduced dopaminergic activity in the frontal brain region has been conceptually linked to core deficits of disinhibition and poor self-monitoring.

THE CLINICAL HISTORY

In obtaining a clinical history, there are several essential features regardless of age. First, the symptoms must be persistent and evident in at least two settings. Typically, parents report that hyperactivity was first evident at the age of 3–4 years. Inattention may not be apparent until a child is in elementary school. In many instances, when evaluating AD/HD-inattentive type, the child's difficulties may not be apparent in school for several years—until the child is at the age of 9 or 10 years. A recent onset of hyperactivity and inattention in an older child, adolescent, or adult is generally inconsistent with AD/HD, and other diagnostic possibilities should be considered. In adults, a high percentage of those presenting to primary care providers do not have an established childhood diagnosis of AD/HD. However, it is suggested that when the age of onset is moved upward to age 12 years as established by the DSM-5, a majority of patients will be captured.

Among children, AD/HD symptoms are almost always evident in school. If a parent reports that inattention and/or hyperactivity are only demonstrated at home, an AD/HD diagnosis is unlikely. The physician's office cannot be used as one of the two environmental settings. The diagnosis cannot be ruled out from a parental report that the child can focus on video games for hours at a time. The constantly changing visual and auditory feedback unique to video games often engages the child with AD/HD.

Eliciting specific behavioral examples is important—particularly in evaluating hyperactivity/impulsivity. Parents and, at times, teachers often conceptually group all externalizing behavior under AD/HD. Significant, repeated aggression and/or property destruction, talking back, theft, lying, or refusal to do schoolwork are not core AD/HD symptoms. These behaviors suggest

Table 27-1. Process of AD/HD evaluation.

1. What are the symptoms?
   - Are they core AD/HD symptoms?
   - In self-diagnosed patients, are there other problems that the patient is misattributing to AD/HD?
2. How long have symptoms been present?
   - Must be present consistently since before age of 12 years.
3. Do the symptoms impair daily functioning?
   - If symptoms do not, is there a plausible explanation?
4. Use rating scales.
5. Screen mental status in office.
6. Do symptoms seem to be better explained by another condition? If yes, treat that condition and reassess at later date.
7. If information is generally consistent with AD/HD diagnosis, initiate treatment.
8. If information is ambiguous, there is a complicated differential diagnosis or significant comorbidities, refer to psychologist or psychiatrist for further assessment.

other diagnoses (CD or ODD) instead of, or possibly comorbid with, AD/HD.

Similarly, children with poor academic performance may be seen because school personnel and/or parents attribute a child's poor grades to AD/HD. Because of budgetary issues and the large number of children with learning and/or behavioral problems, adequate special education services are often not readily available. School personnel, hoping that if there is a problem it can be managed without additional educational resources, may encourage parents to seek an AD/HD evaluation (Table 27-1). Reviewing academic testing, report cards, schoolwork samples, as well as the developmental history may suggest a learning disability. Again, learning disabilities are frequently comorbid, with reading disorders the most common.

MENTAL STATUS TESTING

Although detailed neuropsychological assessments are beyond the scope of the typical primary care setting, there are several cognitive tasks that, when used along with other information, may be helpful. Attention and immediate memory may be assessed by saying a sentence (in the case of preschool children) or string of random numbers and asking the patient to repeat them. A task assessing concentration requires the patient to say the numbers immediately afterward but in reverse order. Words can also be used as the auditory stimulus with the request to spell them forward and backward. Vigilance may be evaluated by asking the patient to tap their finger every time they hear the letter "A." The examiner then says a string of random letters and frequently, yet at unexpected intervals, says "A." The ability to recall four words after a 5- to 10-minute delay tests short-term memory.

MEDICAL TESTING

There is no agreed upon set of laboratory tests to aid in diagnosing AD/HD. In geographic regions with high levels of lead exposure, lead levels should be obtained since elevations have been associated with hyperactivity. Since hyperthyroidism may present with inattention, decreased recent memory, and increased motor activity, thyroid function tests are occasionally obtained—particularly with adults.

Obstructive sleep apnea is associated with impaired attention and concentration. A sleep study should be considered when other indications are present (loud snoring, brief breathing cessation, and so on).

RATING SCALES & CHECKLISTS

Children with attention deficit hyperactivity disorder do not reliably report their own symptoms. While recognizing that they often get into trouble with their parents ("My parents often yell at me, but I don't know why"), children with AD/HD typically do not recognize their hyperactivity, impulsivity, inattention, or distractibility.

Because parents, teachers, and spouses rather than patients often notice symptoms, standardized behavioral ratings should be obtained. Although these scales vary somewhat according to the instrument's developer and, more importantly, the age group to which they are applied, most instruments share basic properties. All require judgment about symptom frequency. The cognitive or behavioral symptoms must be nearly always present (observable everyday) to be considered positive. The scales may simply list the DSM symptoms or they may be intermingled with ODD or CD symptoms, as well as academic problems. The Conners Rating Scales-Revised (CRS-R) includes forms for parents, teachers, and a self-report version for adolescents. The 26- to 28-item CRS-R short forms assess oppositional and conduct disordered behavior, cognitive difficulties, hyperactivity, as well as include a Global AD/HD Index. The Conners Scales have a large reference population for interpreting scores. The Vanderbilt Scale also includes pediatric mood disorder symptoms, as well as a section for teachers and parents to rate the level of impairment created by the symptoms.

Since the classroom places demands on attention, concentration, organizational skills, and impulse inhibition, teacher ratings should always be obtained, if possible. Maternal child behavior ratings have been found to be strongly influenced by the mother's level of emotional distress. Depressed mothers rate their children as having more behavioral problems.

Adult rating scales demonstrate greater heterogeneity, reflecting the greater emphasis placed on cognitive DSM-5 symptoms and more subtle forms of hyperactivity among older AD/HD patients. Distinct conceptual adult AD/HD models are also reflected in these scales. For example, the frequently used Brown Adult AD/HD Rating Scale emphasizes activation deficits—the ability to initiate and self-direct activities—as a core deficit. The Wender Utah Rating Scale (WURS) asks the adult to retrospectively rate behaviors exhibited in childhood. Although frequently cited, recent research suggests that the WURS may not be specific to adult AD/HD and may reflect current personality dysfunction. The Conners Adult ADHD Rating Scale (CAARS) assesses current symptoms. The CAARS is a self-report measure but can be completed by a collateral informant such as a spouse or parent. The Adult Self-Report Scale-V1.1 is a brief screening tool that can help primary care providers identify adult patients at risk for having AD/HD. Finally, the Adult ADHD Investigator Symptom Rating Scale (AISRS) uses a clinician-administered instrument covering the diagnostic criteria for AD/HD but with adult versions of symptoms.

TREATMENT

Pharmacotherapy

STIMULANTS

Stimulant medications, specifically methylphenidate and amphetamine-based formulations, are the mainstays of AD/HD therapy. Their mode of action appears to be blocking of dopamine transporters. Historically, the most commonly prescribed treatment has been immediate-release methylphenidate given two to three times per day in doses of 5–20 mg. Methylphenidate typically begins working in 30–60 minutes, with effects peaking at 1–2 hours and an overall duration of 2–5 hours. The somewhat longer-acting D,L-amphetamine salts (Adderall) are equally effective in treating core AD/HD symptoms and are an alternative for patients who do not respond to methylphenidate.

In the past decade, the major pharmacotherapeutic innovation has been in the delivery systems for these two stimulants. Whereas the initial mode of release was immediate, more recent long-acting stimulants in a continuous-release (CR) form permit once-a-day dosing. Medications such as lisdexamphetamine dimesylate (Vyvanse) as well as methylphenidate (Concerta), dexmethylphenidate (Focalin-XR) and amphetamine preparations (Adderall XR) are examples of "second-generation" CR delivery systems. Delivery systems also include a transdermal patch (Daytrana) and more recently, an extended-release oral suspension (Quillivant). These medications are typically taken once, and on occasion twice, per day.

Stimulants' adverse effects include appetite suppression, insomnia, and weight loss. Less common side effects include headaches and nervousness. Ritalin "rebound" is frequently experienced when the stimulant wears off and is characterized by fatigue and irritability. In some patients, irritability is less pronounced with longer-acting stimulants. Side effects occurring within 2 hours of ingestion are probably best addressed by reducing the dose. The stimulants, particularly amphetamine and methylphenidate, have some cardiovascular risk, prompting the Drug, Safety and Risk Management Advisory Committee of the Food and Drug Administration (FDA) to issue a black box warning for these medications.

Stimulant therapies appear to be less effective with preschool children with AD/HD. Up to a third of these younger patients demonstrate pronounced side effects with methylphenidate, leading to a higher discontinuation rate compared with school-aged children.

NONSTIMULANT MEDICATIONS

Nonstimulants are second-line therapies to be considered under certain circumstances such as: difficulty with stimulant side effects, comorbid conditions such as Tourette syndrome or seizure disorders, concerns about stimulant abuse, or parents philosophically opposed to stimulant use.

Atomoxetine (Straterra), a norepinephrine reuptake inhibitor, has demonstrated efficacy relative to a placebo in reducing AD/HD symptoms. As a nonstimulant, atomoxetine is not associated with growth suppression, tics, or insomnia. It is also not a Schedule II drug and less tightly regulated. Adverse effects may include nausea, vomiting, weight loss, and sleep problems. After reports of serious liver damage, the FDA required a written warning that it should be discontinued when jaundice is present or there is laboratory evidence of liver disease. Atomoxetine does not demonstrate any abuse potential and is unscheduled. Its peak efficacy develops over 2–6 weeks. It is initiated at a dose of 0.5 mg/kg/day and then increased to 1.2 mg/kg/day in 2 weeks. There do not appear to be drug interactions between the stimulants and atomoxetine—a factor suggesting that the combination may be particularly helpful in treating refractory cases. Because atomoxetine is an antidepressant, it has the standard black box warning about risk of suicide accompanying antidepressant medication, including the possibility of increased suicidal ideation. To date, suicide risk has not been a significant clinical concern with atomoxetine.

Extended-release guanfacine in 1-, 2-, 3-, and 4-mg doses (INTUNIV) is marketed both as monotherapy as well as adjunctive treatment in conjunction with a stimulant. A timed-release clonidine preparation (KAPVAY) has also received FDA approval for a similar indication. The alpha-2 agonists have been helpful with comorbid conduct disturbance, particularly when angry outbursts and aggression are present. In addition, they may reduce motor tics that may accompany stimulant treatment and also may reduce headaches and "jitteriness" that are common stimulant side effects. Patients should be closely monitored for hypotension and sedation.

Atomoxetine, clonidine, and guanfacine all appear to be less effective in reducing AD/HD symptoms than stimulants.

Other antidepressants, such as bupropion and tricyclic agents, have demonstrated some efficacy with AD/HD in open-label studies. Presently, these agents are more commonly used with adult rather than childhood AD/HD. The TCAs have associated cardiovascular risk, and children as well as adult patients with preexisting cardiac disease should generally avoid these medications. Bupropion should be avoided in patients with seizure histories as well as in patients with eating disorders.

Once pharmacotherapy has been titrated to optimal effectiveness, patients' comorbid conditions and residual difficulties are often more apparent. Learning disabilities, social skills deficits, and in adult patients, communication and organizational skills may become a treatment focus.

Nonpharmacological Treatment

Psychoeducational approaches for parents of AD/HD children may be beneficial for increased medication adherence, as well as decreasing school and family stress. Key components include: (1) an explanation of AD/HD's etiology as a biologically based condition; (2) reassurance to parents that they are not at fault or responsible for AD/HD; (3) distinguishing between impulsive, uncontrollable behavior and volitional acts; (4) explaining the role of pharmacotherapy—specifically, the type of symptoms addressed and not treated by medication; (5) description of common medication side effects; and (6) discussing the likelihood that medication doses may be changed and that trying different agents may be necessary before achieving optimal symptom control.

Encouraging parents to communicate frequently with their child's teacher helps identify problems early, before they have significant academic consequences. If possible, a daily note to home system should be established between the school and parents.

At home, high levels of structure and predictability will make AD/HD more manageable. Bedtimes, meals, and homework should ideally occur at preplanned times that rarely vary from day to day. Encouraging children to lay out all material needed for the next day, including wardrobe, will make mornings run more smoothly. Older children should keep their desk or homework completion area free of distracting clutter, whereas younger children should pick up all of their play items before moving to another activity.

For children with AD/HD alone, the addition of behavior therapy to stimulant medication does not appear to add further benefit. However, for the high proportion of AD/HD children with comorbid CD or ODD, behavioral intervention is strongly indicated. Key elements of parent training include: (1) specifying no more than two to three target behaviors to address at one time; (2) establishing positive reinforcement for appropriately prosocial behavior; (3) developing a reasonable time frame and frequency of target behavior so that the child will realistically receive early positive reinforcement; (4) responding to inappropriate behavior through ignoring or time out; and (5) clear communication of requests and expectations.

An educational approach with demonstrated efficacy for adult AD/HD is meta-cognitive therapy emphasizing effective self-management, including time awareness, breaking down larger tasks into manageable parts, self-reward, and disputing depressionogenic thoughts.

In addition, adults with AD/HD benefit from making frequent lists, using planners and calendars, as well as smartphones, to help organize activities and remember important events and deadlines. For those employed in office settings, going into work early before most coworkers arrive will allow task completion without interruption.

Adult AD/HD can wreak havoc on intimate relationships. In many instances, marriage counseling may be valuable for addressing effects of long-standing forgetfulness and the inability to actively listen and be psychologically present to one's spouse or partner. For the spouse without AD/HD, it is important to recognize that this pattern of neglect does not indicate a lack of loving concern but is a by-product of the condition that can be improved.

A number of complementary and alternative therapies have been promoted for both childhood and adult AD/HD. There is some suggestion that omega-3 oils and a variant on biofeedback called neurofeedback may have some efficacy. However, the limited number of studies coupled with research design issues do not permit recommendation of these treatments.

CONCLUSIONS: THE COST OF AD/HD

In addition to health care expenditures, AD/HD has economic, legal, and social costs. Youth with AD/HD have more outpatient physician office visits—even exceeding those for children and adolescents with asthma. Adults with AD/HD as well as parents of children with the condition have greater health care costs, more lost workdays, and greater job turnover. Rates of accidental poisoning, as well as injuries, are also higher among children with AD/HD. In addition to greater health care utilization, the high comorbidity of AD/HD with learning disabilities leads to more costly special education services.

By adolescence, there is also a marked rise in comorbidity. Conduct Disorder, when together with AD/HD, is particularly pronounced and contributes to property damage, theft, and harm to others. High school is particularly challenging for youth with AD/HD. Approximately one-third of adolescents with AD/HD do not complete high school; a disproportionate number are expelled compared with non-AD/HD teens. The high drop-out rate may, in part, reflect the fact that by high school nearly half of AD/HD adolescents have repeated at least one grade. A significant percentage of AD/HD teens are having sexual intercourse by the age of 15 years and with multiple partners, reflecting the brevity of their relationships.

By the time adulthood is reached, AD/HD has adversely impacted most significant life arenas. In the workplace, AD/HD adults change jobs and are fired at a rate two to three times greater than those without the condition. These outcomes likely stem from reduced productivity as well as increased work-related accidental injuries and illness-related absences. Annual medical costs are two to three times higher.

Adults with AD/HD have three times as many sexual partners and are significantly more likely to have unplanned pregnancies, as well as to contract a sexually transmitted disease. A disproportionate number of parents with AD/HD no longer have custody of their children. Auto accident rates are disturbingly high with approximately 20% of AD/HD adults having had 12 or more traffic citations. Nearly one-third have had three or more crashes. While there is often concern among parents whether treatment with a stimulant medication will increase the risk of later psychiatric and behavioral problems, the opposite appears to be the case. Several longitudinal studies have found that when compared with those not treated with stimulant medication, adolescents and young adults with AD/HD who had stimulant treatment as children were less likely to develop mood and anxiety disorders and to perform better academically.

SUGGESTED READINGS

Akinbami LJ, Liu X, Pastor PN, Reuben CA. Attention deficit hyperactivity disorder among children aged 5-17 years in the United States, 1998-2009. *NCHS Data Brief* 2011;70.

Barkley RA. *Attention Deficit Hyperactivity Disorder: A Handbook for Diagnosis and Treatment*, 3rd ed. New York, NY: Guilford Press, 2005.

Conners CK. *Attention Deficit Hyperactivity Disorder: The Latest Assessment and Treatment Strategies.* Philadelphia: Jones & Bartlett, 2006.

Correll CU, Kratochvil CJ, March JS. Developments in pediatric psychopharmacology: focus on stimulants, antidepressants, and antipsychotics. *J Clin Psychiatry* 2011;72:655–670.

Kessler RC, Adler L, Ames M, et al. The World Health Organization adult ADHD self-report scale (ASRS): a short screening scale for use in the general population. *Psychol Med* 2005;35:245–256.

Searight HR, Robertson K, Smith T, Perkins S. Searight BK. Complementary and alternative therapies for pediatric attention deficit hyperactivity disorder: a descriptive review. *ISRN Psychiatry* 2012;2012:804127. doi:10.5402/2012/804127.

Searight HR, Evans SL, Gafford J. Attention deficit hyperactivity disorder. In: Mengel MB, Schwiebert LP, eds. *Family Medicine: Ambulatory Care and Prevention,* 5th ed. New York, NY: Appleton and Lange, 2009.

Solanto MV, Marks DJ, Wasserstein J, et al. Efficacy of meta-cognitive therapy for adult ADHD. *Am J Psychiatry* 2010;167: 958–968.

Spencer TJ, Adler LA, Qiao M, et al. Validation of the Adult ADHD Investigator Symptom Rating Scale (AISRS). *J Atten Dis* 2010;14:57–68.

Somatic Symptom Disorders

J. Jewel Shim, MD & Stuart J. Eisendrath, MD

INTRODUCTION

CASE ILLUSTRATION 1

Ms. A, a 57-year-old woman, makes an appointment with a new clinician. She presents with a 10-year history of multiple, unexplained symptoms. She has seen many physicians over the past decade, including several primary care physicians and numerous subspecialists. Her principal complaints today include abdominal pain, chest pain, headache, palpitations, fatigue, and intermittent dizziness. She brings a thick stack of records from some of her prior physicians. These records include multiple laboratory tests and diagnostic procedures, none of which has identified any cause for her symptoms.

Clinician: How can I help you today, Ms. A?

Patient (sighing): I don't know. A friend of mine saw you a few months ago and said you were very good. I hope you can help me. I've had these problems for years now, and no one seems to be able to figure them out. Maybe you can. I know there's something wrong. I've been so sick.

Clinician: Why don't you tell me about your symptoms?

Patient: Well, it all began about 10 years ago. . . .

Clinicians are taught that patients will present with symptoms (subjective complaints) and signs (objective findings) that suggest the presence of a pathophysiological process. They are trained to recognize these presentations and to diagnose the underlying disease so that they may institute the appropriate treatment. Satisfaction for the care provider arises from the ability to perform these tasks proficiently and see the patient benefit. Patients typically come to the clinician's office seeking an explanation for and relief from their symptoms. Difficulties arise in the relationship when the patient presents with symptoms and the clinician can find no disease to explain them. Symptoms that lack discernible physical pathology have been referred to variously as medically unexplained, functional, or somatization.

The term *somatization* (as used in this chapter) refers to the experience and reporting of physical symptoms that cause distress but that lack a corresponding level of tissue damage or pathology and are linked to psychosocial stress. In contrast to this broad and inclusive view of the process, psychiatrists have developed strict diagnostic criteria that define several distinct disorders, which are collectively referred to as the somatic symptom and related disorders. As such, clinicians should be careful to distinguish between somatization, as defined above, and somatization disorder, which is one type of somatic symptom disorder. In general, these latter conditions are chronic and reflect an enduring way for the affected individuals to cope with psychosocial stressors. However, it is much more common in the primary care setting to encounter patients who have somatization symptoms but do not meet the full criteria for a psychiatric diagnosis. In many individuals, the somatization might be a transient phenomenon during a particularly stressful period such as divorce proceedings, consisting of an exaggeration of common physical symptoms such as headache. In other patients, the process may be more persistent and the symptoms may be disabling. The latter group of patients can be particularly difficult for clinicians. Although their symptoms are suggestive of an underlying medical or neurologic condition, no such etiology is discovered upon appropriate diagnostic evaluation. Some patients do find reassurance in the provider's statements that no medical cause for their symptoms has been found. Other patients may become upset and accuse the clinician of not believing them or of being incompetent. Some patients insist on continued diagnostic testing or referral to specialists. Further, the symptoms do not respond to standard medical treatments; this therapeutic failure can lead to requests for more testing, referrals, or different treatment regimens. The combination of increasing demands made by patients and their lack of response to treatment can be very frustrating for the clinician.

HISTORICAL CONCEPTS

The existence of medically unexplained symptoms has been recognized throughout the history of medicine. Each historical period has described syndromes composed of such symptoms. The scientific knowledge and theories of the time have shaped the etiologies proposed for these disorders. The treatments advocated by medical practitioners were directed at attempting to correct the abnormality assumed to cause the illness. Each of these syndromes shared the recognition by medical authorities of the time that the illness lacked the demonstrable, pathologically defined tissue changes that characterize most medical conditions.

Before the Renaissance, medical theories were based on limited understanding of anatomy or physiology and, as a result, seem quite primitive to modern practitioners. Diseases lacking an apparent cause were believed to result from gross disturbances in the function and behavior of bodily organs. For example, hysteria, an earlier conceptualization of somatization, was attributed to a "wandering uterus" as early as 1900 BC. The treatments for hysteria flowed from this conceptual model and included the application of ointments to the labia or manipulation of the uterus to return it to its "natural" position. It was not until after the Renaissance that medical practitioners began to implicate disturbances of the nervous system in the genesis of medically unexplained symptoms. However, despite this change in the understanding of these disorders, the treatments utilized by clinicians did not become significantly more advanced. For instance, some practitioners in the latter half of the seventeenth century advocated hitting patients who had symptoms of hysteria with a stick.

By the end of the seventeenth century, and continuing into the eighteenth century, clinicians increasingly recognized the role psychological factors played in the origin and maintenance of somatic symptoms. For example, Thomas Sydenham attributed conditions such as pain, convulsions, and diarrhea to a disordered mind. More importantly, the treatments for these symptoms were beginning to reflect this appreciation. Medical authorities no longer focused exclusively on somatic therapies in the care of afflicted individuals. Instead, practitioners were encouraged to inquire about and demonstrate an active interest in their patients' mental state and welfare. Further, clinicians recognized the need to attempt to promote optimism about recovery in their patients.

In the nineteenth century, there was awareness that despite many advances in the understanding of pathology, patients suffering from somatization syndromes lacked discernible anatomic abnormalities. As a result, the medically unexplained disorders were attributed to a subtle or "functional" pathological disturbance. This explanatory model of illness was associated with a return to predominantly somatic interventions for treating the symptoms. However, some practitioners maintained that psychological treatments were important for managing these patients. These clinicians also recognized that unless the therapy was delivered in a way that was consistent with the patients' belief that their illness had a physical etiology, the intervention would be rejected. Paul Briquet, in his seminal *Treatise on Hysteria* (1859) described the in-depth study of over 400 patients with "hysteria" during a 10-year period and emphasized that the treatment of such patients addresses social and environmental problems.

At the turn of the twentieth century, an exclusively psychological model for these disorders was developed. The idea of a functional pathological lesion of the nervous system was replaced with the concept of psychogenesis (i.e., the somatization symptoms arose from the mind). Somatization was viewed as the means by which unconscious mental conflicts could be manifested in the form of physical symptoms. As a result, mental health practitioners became responsible for the diagnosis and treatment of these disorders. However, the idea of physical complaints originating from the mind was also associated with implications that the symptoms were not "real." Further, many patients were not convinced of the value of this interpretation of illness.

Medically unexplained syndromes have persisted as clinical problems for practitioners. Patients often present with many symptoms that are not associated with abnormalities demonstrable by physical examination or laboratory or radiological studies. The symptoms are often clustered together as syndromes with a variety of proposed etiologies including environmental exposures, infections (e.g., *Candida*, Epstein–Barr virus), or multiple chemical sensitivity. In addition, the broad range of advocacy and educational groups that try to promote various agendas with regard to the disorders can make the evaluation of these syndromes difficult.

CASE ILLUSTRATION 2

Mr. B is a 32-year-old man who presented to his primary care physician with complaints about being tired, weak, and nauseated. He also complained about intermittent abdominal and chest pain as well as a feeling of "dizziness." He noted that he lived in an old building and was worried he had been exposed to lead or some other toxin. His physical examination and laboratory values were all normal. However, he was not relieved by these results and his complaints persisted. He began to phone frequently with questions about chronic Candida infections, postviral syndromes, and multiple chemical sensitivity syndromes. His physician would discuss each process with him and continued to perform appropriate medical evaluations of Mr. B's symptoms. The patient began to research his symptoms on the Internet. He was convinced that he suffered from sensitivity to multiple compounds in his home and became involved in a number of "online" support groups. He resisted other explanations for his symptoms and gradually became dissatisfied with his primary care physician and chose to seek care from "experts" on his disorder.

ETIOLOGY

Somatization can be understood from a number of different perspectives, each of which proposes a cause for the symptoms. However, because the precise cause of these symptoms is not known, none of the following theories are fully explanatory. Rather, each view of somatization provides practitioners with insight into the genesis of these symptoms and suggests possible treatments as well. Unfortunately, each model is able to explain the symptoms of only a select group of patients. A more comprehensive understanding of patients comes from incorporating more than one perspective.

Neurobiological

According to the neurobiological perspective, somatization symptoms result from dysfunction in the neuroendocrine systems responsible for processing peripheral sensory and central emotional information. As a result, the affected individual misinterprets normal bodily sensations or emotional signals as indicating a dangerous somatic process. The mechanism is unknown by which dysfunction in the nervous or endocrine systems results in the preoccupation with somatic symptoms. There is growing evidence of the role of such abnormalities in these disorders. For example, researchers have recently suggested that hypocortisolism plays a role in posttraumatic stress disorder, fibromyalgia, chronic fatigue syndrome, and some chronic pain disorders. Although hypocortisolism has been found in groups of individuals with the above diagnoses, the relationship between a deficiency of cortisol and the production of these symptoms is not well understood. Additional research has examined the inability of individuals with somatization symptoms to habituate to novel stimuli. Individuals with somatization syndrome reported higher levels of tension in novel situations and were less likely to habituate to the situation over time. In addition, the affected individuals had a slower return to baseline heart rate upon leaving stressful situations. These studies suggest a relationship between physiologic mechanisms involved in adapting to novel or stressful stimuli and the apparently psychological symptoms of individuals with somatic symptom disorders.

Psychodynamic

According to psychodynamic theory, somatic symptoms arise solely from the mind. They are believed to represent the outward expression of underlying, internal psychological conflicts. Studies have demonstrated that individuals with somatization have higher rates of prior emotional and physical abuse, depression, and anxiety than nonaffected populations. It is hypothesized that abuse places individuals at risk for the types of internal conflicts that result in somatic symptom disorders. For example, women who have suffered sexual abuse in childhood have increased rates of chronic pelvic pain when compared with those without a history of abuse. Depression and anxiety may be both a product and cause of these internal conflicts. Patients with somatic symptom disorders may be less able to correctly interpret emotional arousal and instead identify these signals as physical symptoms. This is further supported by studies that demonstrate a link between alexithymia, or the inability to identify and verbally describe emotions and feelings in oneself or others, and somatic symptom disorders. Other findings suggest that childhood trauma in women is associated with higher levels of somatization, mediated by the development of insecure attachment. Attachment theory predicts how individuals' interactions in interpersonal relationships are influenced by early experiences with caregivers. A four-category model has been proposed, which describes four different types of attachment: *secure, preoccupied, dismissive,* and *fearful*. In particular, research examining the role of attachment style and its link to somatization and subsequent health care utilization has found that patients with *preoccupied* attachment, where the individual tends to idealize others, is less self-reliant and needs more reassurance; and *fearful* attachment, where the individual may be less trusting of others as well as less self-reliant, are more likely to be high in somatic symptom reporting and are higher users of medical resources.

CASE ILLUSTRATION 3

Mrs. G is a 51-year-old woman who had suffered from abdominal pain and progressive loss of function over the last 1 ½ years. She had failed conservative management and was admitted to the hospital for an exploratory laparotomy. However, there were no organic findings to explain her symptoms. Psychiatric consultation was requested to evaluate for a psychological component to her pain. At evaluation, Mrs. G denied any psychological stressors, but her husband shared that around the time of the onset of her symptoms, Mrs. G's mother, with whom she is very close, had moved out of state to care for another daughter who had become ill. Mrs. G was referred for psychotherapy to explore this perceived loss and to explore alternatives for support. Over the course of this treatment, Mrs. G's abdominal pain resolved.

Cognitive Behavioral

According to cognitive behavioral theorists, in somatic symptom disorders, symptoms arise from incorrect beliefs about bodily sensations, for example, the belief that mild gastroesophageal reflux (or panic symptoms) represents myocardial ischemia. These misinterpretations, in turn, result in certain maladaptive behaviors, such as going from one emergency room to another seeking evaluation of the symptom and reassurance that the heart is functioning normally. These symptoms are reinforced by factors in the individual's environment such as the responses of other people to the perceived illness. For instance, the affected individual may be excused from work or social obligations. As an example of this process, some researchers proposed that learning about a disease may lead certain individuals to attribute previously overlooked symptoms to the illness. The affected person seeks out confirmatory evidence of additional symptoms that both reinforce the belief in the illness and amplify the somatic symptoms. The person's self-validating review of symptoms may be augmented by contact with advocacy or educational groups that promote awareness of the disease. The processing of bodily information gradually becomes colored by the belief that the person has a disease, and this can result in the affected individual embracing the sick role.

 CASE ILLUSTRATION 4

Mr. C is a 53-year-old man who worked as a manual laborer. He had always been in good health. One day, while lifting a particularly heavy item, he experienced pain on the right side of his chest. A colleague said that his father had a similar experience and died of a heart attack shortly thereafter. Mr. C became focused on the idea that he has heart disease, and began visiting a number of emergency rooms, primary care physicians, and cardiologists. His evaluations were always completely negative.

However, his concern has persisted and he now presents to a new clinician.

Clinician: How may I help you Mr. C?

Patient: Doc, I know that I have a problem with my heart.

Clinician: What are your symptoms?

Patient: Well, I sometimes feel like I am more out of breath and if I lift heavy things I can feel some pain in the muscle over my chest. Other times, I start to breathe fast and my fingers get tingly. I've watched programs on TV and they say those are the things that can mean I have angina. I've stopped working because I don't want to stress myself out and have a heart attack.

Sociocultural

According to the sociocultural perspective, individuals learn to express disease and distress in culturally sanctioned ways. In any culture, the expression of certain bodily symptoms and illness behaviors are encouraged whereas others are discouraged. Although somatization is a universal process, an individual's culture can affect the manner in which somatic representations of emotional distress are utilized. Further, this theory maintains that because the patient and the clinician are often from different backgrounds, the cultural interaction between the clinician and the patient is important. This interaction often determines how the patient's symptoms are experienced, interpreted, and reported. The clinician's task in these meetings is to correctly recognize which of the patient's somatic complaints represent cultural idioms of emotional distress. Mistakes in this assessment can lead to misdiagnosis, unnecessary medical treatment, or evaluation, frustration on the part of the provider when the patient does not respond as expected, and patient dissatisfaction.

A DIFFERENT PARADIGM

Although the theoretical models discussed above have evidence to support them and have been used as the basis for treatment in cases of somatization, there is another way to conceptualize somatization and the associated disorders. This view begins with the clinician abandoning the either–or categories of "physical" and "psychological." This dichotomous framework leads to interactions in which the patient can feel that the clinician is rejecting them and the reality of their symptoms by concluding, "The doctor's saying it's all in my head." Instead, the provider adopts a more comprehensive view of disease based on the *biopsychosocial* model of illness that includes key elements from other explanatory models.

In this paradigm, all illnesses are understood to have biological, psychological, and sociocultural dimensions.

Although the western medical model focuses on the biological aspects of disease, it often ignores the psychological and sociocultural facets of the patient's experience. In addition, this model, often very effective for understanding and treating acute disease processes, may fail to explain much of the complexity of chronic illness. For example, pain researchers have found that psychological factors are more important than physical factors in predicting future disability. Such research has led to the development of new treatment paradigms that recognize the interplay between the biological disease process and the psychosocial impact of symptoms. Treatment is focused on both relieving the biomedical symptoms and modifying the thoughts, feelings, and behaviors associated with the pain and disability.

Using the more comprehensive biopsychosocial model, illness can be understood as occurring along a spectrum with disorders characterized by predominantly somatic problems at one end and disorders with predominantly psychological or social manifestations at the other. Therefore, evaluation of patients should routinely include inquiries into both the physical and psychosocial dimensions of their illness. With this biopsychosocial framework, the somatic symptom disorders are seen as arising when the patient neglects the psychosocial components of his/her illness and focuses on viewing the problem solely from a somatic perspective. For example, an individual with a history of chronic pelvic pain who has undergone multiple thorough evaluations with no identified anatomic etiology but who insists on repeating the workup rather than discussing psychosocial facets of the symptoms may be experiencing somatization. According to this model, symptom amplification, a phenomenon seen commonly in somatization, may arise when the experience of these symptoms is modified by psychosocial factors. This is illustrated in Figure 28-1, where these factors are represented by a psychosocial lens, which alters the "image" of the stimulus (somatic symptoms), resulting in a magnified image (effect), or increased experience of these symptoms. Somatization itself is not a single entity. Like most illnesses it can be understood to have a continuum of expression. At one end is the transient, stress-related exaggeration of common physical symptoms and at the other are the serious, persistent complaints that leave the patient disabled.

> **Patient:** I don't know. Maybe I am crazy . . . that's what everyone else seems to think.
> **Clinician:** Let me assure you that you're not crazy. I hear your concern. Why don't we talk about this a little bit?
> **Patient:** Well, a friend of mine had a disease called Cushing's. Do you think I might have that?

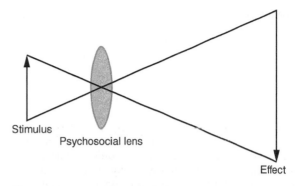

Figure 28-1. Symptom amplification.

> **Clinician:** That's a good question. There are a great many diseases that can present with symptoms like yours. I want you to know that as I've listened to you and examined you, I've tried to think of rare diseases. I don't believe any of them are very likely, especially since you've had your symptoms for so long. I do want to be honest with you, though. There's no way to be absolutely certain. There are so many different diseases that it would be impossible to get tested for all of them. Let's get a few laboratory tests done, though. If they're normal, let's not do any more tests, but I'll keep an open mind as to these possibilities as we get to know each other during the course of the next few months. If you develop symptoms later that suggest one of these rare diseases to me, I'll certainly order more tests. How does that sound to you?
> **Patient:** Okay, that sounds like it could work.
> **Clinician:** Are there other things going on that add stress to your life?
> **Patient:** Now that you mention it, there are some stressful things going on. . .

In this brief dialogue, the practitioner acknowledges uncertainty while communicating a sense of honesty and trustworthiness. By reinforcing the continuity of the relationship and the willingness to entertain different possibilities in the future, the provider helps the patient feel cared for without the need for multiple, and most likely unnecessary, diagnostic tests. Moreover, the clinician has helped the patient to entertain the idea of a connection between psychosocial and somatic factors in illness.

PREVALENCE

Somatization is frequently encountered in primary care clinics with estimates of prevalence between 25% and 75%. Other studies have found that somatic symptom disorders can be diagnosed in up to 22% of patients in primary care outpatient clinics. One study found an absence of organic cause in 80% of primary care visits scheduled for the evaluation of common symptoms such as dizziness, chest pain, and fatigue. Similarly, studies of medical inpatients have found that between 20% and 40% of these individuals have evidence of a coexisting mental disorder. Epidemiologic studies have demonstrated that 25–35% of the patients in primary care settings will meet criteria for a recognized psychiatric disorder, most commonly anxiety or depression. In addition, research has shown that 50–80% of patients who have an anxiety or depressive disorder initially present to health care providers with physical symptoms. A recent study found that somatic symptom disorders were the most common psychiatric diagnoses in a population of medical inpatients.

Worldwide, medically unexplained symptoms are more common in females and individuals of lower socioeconomic status. In the United States, there is higher prevalence among Latinos. While rates of somatization disorder are relatively low (0.1% in the United States, 0.8% in Germany), these numbers increase as the inclusion criteria for somatic symptom disorders are broadened, ranging from 22% to 80% in some European countries. Although studies have demonstrated there is no systematic pattern of cultures which are more or less likely to have somatization, it appears that patients who lack an ongoing relationship with a stable provider are more likely to have a greater number of somatization symptoms. In other words, the "culture" of the clinician–patient encounter also has significant impact on the presence of somatization. Overall these results indicate that the phenomenon of somatization, as well as more rigorously defined somatic symptom and related disorders, is very common among patients presenting for medical services.

IMPACT AND OUTCOMES

Somatization is not only common but it is also an expensive problem. One study estimated that patients with somatic symptom disorders generate medical costs nine times those of the average medical patient. Other work has calculated total annual health care costs attributable to somatization in the United States to be over $250 billion, even after adjusting for comorbid psychiatric disorders. In addition, these patients often require a great deal of time and attention but frequently do not respond to the prescribed treatment. This can eventually lead to frustration for the practitioner and even feelings of incompetence or inadequacy. A patient's seemingly unending complaints can lead to feelings of anger at the individual or dread when his/her name appears on the appointment list. Thus, patients with somatization symptoms not only tax the health care system by disproportionately utilizing limited resources, but also burden health care providers who can feel overwhelmed by the needs of these individuals.

Research has consistently demonstrated that individuals with somatization have worse outcomes in regard to health status, physical functioning, and psychological well-being than those patients who do not manifest these symptoms. Patients with somatization symptoms have ongoing difficulties not only with their somatic complaints and concerns about physical illness, but also with emotional and social impairment and reduced quality of life. It is important to accurately diagnose these individuals so that appropriate management can be instituted.

DIFFERENTIAL DIAGNOSIS

Patients with somatic symptoms should be evaluated for a biomedical etiology that could explain the presenting complaints. The nature of the evaluation will depend on the patients' medical history, presenting symptoms, and age. In evaluating patients, it is important to remember that the onset of multiple physical symptoms late in life is almost always due to a general medical condition; somatic symptom disorders generally start decades earlier.

The new classification of "somatic symptom and related disorders" is based on the common feature of prominent somatic symptoms and related significant distress and functional impairment. In addition, the somatic complaints in these disorders are produced unconsciously and are not under the voluntary control of the patient (Table 28-1). A number of functional syndromes have also been identified, such as irritable bowel syndrome, fibromyalgia, chronic fatigue syndrome, and noncardiac chest pain. These disorders may fall under the "other specified somatic symptom and related disorder" diagnosis.

Criticism of the taxonomy and nomenclature of what were previously called the somatoform disorders suggested that the various disorders in this category were quite disparate, had limited validity, and the diagnoses did little to inform an effective treatment approach. Moreover, the term "somatoform" was felt to be pejorative; the absence of a clear medical etiology did not rightly categorize the cause as psychological. This "either or" approach also set up an unintended mind-body dualism. Ultimately patients were made to feel their symptoms were not "real" and overlooked their very real experience of physical symptoms. For this reason, attempts were made to revise the criteria for these disorders in the most recent edition of the Diagnostic and Statistical Manual for Mental Disorders (DSM-V). A further problem was that a considerable number of patients who presented for care with medically unexplained symptoms did not meet criteria for the somatoform disorders (10-15% prevalence in primary care).

Several psychiatric disorders have been associated with somatic symptoms and should be considered when

Table 28-1. Somatic symptom and related disorders.

Somatic symptom disorder: Includes disorders previously known as Somatization disorder, Hypochondriasis, and Pain disorder. The focus of this disorder is distress about one or more somatic symptoms which can lead to persistent thoughts about the symptoms, an accompanying high level of anxiety, and excessive time and energy devoted to these symptoms in the form of recurrent thoughts and multiple, repeated visits to health care providers for evaluation and work up.

Illness anxiety disorder: Encompasses similar criteria to Hypochondriasis. The focus of this disorder is preoccupation with or fear of having or acquiring a serious illness, without corresponding significant somatic symptoms. It is differentiated from Somatic symptom disorder by the absence of somatic symptoms.

Conversion disorder (Functional neurological symptom disorder): Characterized by the presence of one or more symptoms of altered voluntary motor or sensory function. An important criterion is that clinical findings clearly do not support and are incompatible with a neurological or medical etiology for the symptoms. For example, there is a lack of internal consistency within the examination such as when physical signs elicited via one method are not replicated when tested in a different manner.

Psychological factors affecting other medical conditions: The key feature of this disorder is the presence of one or more psychological or behavioral factors that have negative impact on an existing medical symptom or condition by either influencing the course of the medical condition, interfering with its treatment, influencing the underlying pathophysiology of the medical condition, causing or exacerbating symptoms, or necessitating medical intervention. The factors themselves may also pose well-established health risks. Factors can include poor adherence, denial of illness, maladaptive coping styles and interpersonal interactions, and psychological distress.

Factitious disorder: Previously not included in this category of disorders. It is characterized by the conscious feigning of physical or psychological signs or symptoms or the purposeful induction of injury or disease. This disorder is contrasted to malingering in that there is no clear external reward associated with the production or feigning of these symptoms.

Other specified somatic symptom and related disorder: This disorder includes all presentations in which symptoms characteristic of a somatic symptom disorder predominate but do not meet full criteria for a specific diagnosis Pseudocyesis, the false belief of being pregnant that may be associated with some objective signs and symptoms of pregnancy is included in this category.

Unspecified somatic symptom and related disorder: Symptoms characteristic of a somatic symptom disorder are present but do not meet full criteria for a specific diagnosis. This is differentiated from other unspecified somatic symptom and related disorder by the presence of significant unusual symptoms with insufficient information to make a more specific diagnosis.

---

evaluating a patient who has physical complaints. For example, anxiety in the form of panic attacks often involves symptoms in multiple organ systems, such as palpitations, nausea, shortness of breath, and tingling in the extremities. Unlike symptoms of somatic symptom disorders, however, the symptoms of a panic attack have an abrupt onset and are limited to the episode. A careful history can often elicit this time course and prove to be helpful in making the diagnosis. Patients with generalized anxiety disorder may also present with multiple somatic complaints, such as fatigue and muscle tension. Excessive worrying about multiple domains in life is the key feature of this disorder and helps to separate it from the somatic symptom disorders. Depressed patients often present to medical practitioners with unexplained physical symptoms, especially headache, pain, and gastrointestinal problems. Whereas the somatic symptoms of the somatic symptom and related disorders tend to be chronic, the physical complaints in depression exist only in the presence of the mood symptoms. In such cases, the depression and the somatic complaints resolve contemporaneously. Studies have demonstrated a high level of comorbidity between depression and somatic symptom disorders, so clinically both disorders may be present.

Patients with obsessive-compulsive disorder whose beliefs focus on bodily functions or organs can appear to be suffering from a somatic symptom disorder. The key to diagnosis is a careful history about the presence of the obsessions and compulsions. Patients with psychotic disorders, such as schizophrenia, may also present with multiple somatic complaints. In contrast to the concerns in the somatic symptom disorders, psychotic symptoms tend to be bizarre or completely irrational (e.g., "My insides are rotting" or "I have pain from the dinosaur eggs in my stomach"). It is important to remember, however, that the patients may have both a diagnosable mental disorder as well as a somatic symptom disorder. Conversely, patients with clear medical conditions may simultaneously qualify for a diagnosis of a somatic symptom and related disorder.

In contrast to the psychiatric disorders described above, there are conditions in which the individual's symptoms are consciously produced. Factitious disorder is included in the category of somatic symptom and related disorders. It is diagnosed when the clinician determines that the symptoms are consciously or voluntarily induced or exaggerated. However, in these individuals there is no discernible external incentive, such

Table 28-2. Abnormal illness-affirming states.

	Symptom Production	Motivation
Malingering	conscious	conscious
Factitious disorder	conscious	unconscious
Somatic symptom disorder	unconscious	unconscious
Illness anxiety disorder	unconscious	unconscious
Conversion disorder (Functional Neurological symptom disorder)	unconscious	unconscious
Other specified somatic symptom and related disorder	unconscious	unconscious
Unspecified somatic symptom and related Disorder	unconscious	unconscious

Source: Adapted, with permission, from Eisendrath SJ, Lichtmacher J. Psychiatric Disorders. In *Current Medical Diagnosis and Treatment* 2007, S. McPhee et al (ed); Appleton and Lange, 2006.

as financial compensation, to produce the symptoms. The patient's primary goal is to assume the sick role. Malingering, on the other hand, is diagnosed when the clinician determines that the individual has consciously produced the symptoms for clear external gain, such as obtaining a monetary award, acquiring drugs, or avoiding a noxious situation such as military duty or incarceration. Malingering is not considered a mental disorder (Table 28-2).

EVALUATION

Most patients do not meet criteria for a formal diagnosis of a somatic symptom disorder, yet somatization is quite frequent. As these patients present overwhelmingly to primary care settings (not mental health providers), it is useful for medical clinicians to have a systematic method of elucidating the presence of somatic symptoms without a clear medical basis by first excluding the presence of organic disease.

A stepwise, evidence-based approach is invaluable to the evaluation of patients with suspected somatization. This framework can help the clinician avoid unnecessary and costly diagnostic procedures or referrals to specialists. In addition, it can spare the patient potential iatrogenic complications from any of the evaluation procedures. As with all of medicine, the first step in evaluating the patient with multiple somatic complaints is a detailed and thorough history of the presenting problem. The clinician should, of course, include review of pertinent medical records in the history-gathering phase of the evaluation. The practitioner should then perform appropriate physical and neurologic examinations. The provider may then consider what tests are indicated to confirm the diagnosis or rule out a predominantly biomedical disease based on the information obtained. The urge to order a wide variety of tests should be resisted. Instead, a rational determination of the patient's needs is more helpful in clarifying the treatment plan. Obtaining an informal consultation from a colleague can be useful in appropriately evaluating these individuals.

Once the provider determines that the patient's physical symptoms are not explained by any underlying pathological abnormalities, the focus can turn to more predominantly psychological disorders. The assessment of psychiatric disorders can be accomplished through the use of a careful clinical interview, a semi-structured interview tool, or by referral to a mental health clinician. The clinical interview can be helpful in establishing the presence of psychiatric illness as well as in communicating to the patient that the clinician is taking an active interest in the individual's life. Instruments such as the self-administered Patient Health Questionnaire (PHQ), which are designed for use in primary care settings, can help the provider diagnose somatic symptom disorders as well as depression, anxiety, eating disorders, and substance abuse. Such instruments have the advantages of rapid administration and established validity. The PHQ-15 is a subscale of the PHQ that assesses somatic symptoms, and can be used to monitor symptom severity as well as symptom improvement. Such instruments are useful as many patients decline referral to a mental health specialist as an option because they fear that their complaints are being dismissed. Above all, when evaluating a patient the clinician should recognize and articulate the interplay between the physical and psychosocial realms.

Clinician: Today I would like to talk about how you are doing.

Patient: Well, my chest has been hurting again and I have been really worn down.

Clinician: (after several pertinent questions about the symptoms) It sounds like this is the same pain you've had before, although I do understand that it's a little worse. I wonder if there is anything else that has changed in your life recently besides the intensity of the pain?

Patient: Nothing . . . really. Well my wife and I are arguing about the mortgage again.

Clinician: Oh, I remember that's been a problem before when you've been having pain.

Patient: Yeah. I just get tired of her nagging and the stress of barely making ends meet.

Clinician: I think it's possible that the stress you've been under may be taking its toll on your body and your sense of well-being.

TREATMENT

The following treatment strategies are not specific to a certain somatic symptom disorder diagnosis. In most cases, it is less important to make a specific psychiatric diagnosis of a somatic symptom disorder than it is to recognize that the patient's symptoms represent somatization. However, if a psychiatric disorder such as anxiety, depression, or psychosis is present, specific treatments for the identified disorder should be utilized.

Treatments Designed for Primary Care Providers

A management plan with an emphasis on nonsomatic interventions is a useful treatment approach for somatization and the somatic symptom disorders. Patients with somatization symptoms most often present to the primary care setting and are resistant to psychiatric referrals. Techniques are required that are effective, acceptable to primary care clinicians, and useful in busy primary care settings. Finally, the intervention must be congruent with patients' beliefs about the nature of their illness so that they are willing to engage in the treatment.

The most important aspect of managing patients with somatization is the development of a stable, empathic, trusting relationship. Although it is not easy to form such a relationship with these individuals, establishing a therapeutic alliance is critical to both diagnosis and treatment. It can be helpful to remember that patients with somatization are reacting in the best and, without treatment, only way available to them. Before considering specific therapies for these individuals, it is useful to consider basic techniques for interacting with them.

The practitioner should never challenge the reality of the patient's physical symptoms. Somatization is an unconscious process, and therefore the somatic complaints are very real to the patient. Further, because most of the symptoms are subjective in nature, there is no means to verify or dispute them. It can be helpful to explicitly acknowledge and validate the patient's suffering to bolster the therapeutic relationship.

Clinician: I can see how much you've suffered with all of these symptoms.
Patient: You're the only one who seems to understand that.

Medical providers should avoid trying to convince the patient that the symptoms are psychological in origin. They should also avoid the use of psychological labels (e.g., depression, anxiety). Instead, they should try to use easily understandable and mutually acceptable language to discuss symptoms. Each appointment should begin with a discussion of the somatic complaint. The provider can then use descriptive physiologic explanations, which are more acceptable to these individuals, to describe the symptoms (e.g., "abnormally tense muscles in your neck go into painful spasm"). It is important to note that although such descriptors imply a physiologic component to the symptoms, they do not provide an etiology. Over time (often months or years), the patient and clinician may begin to explore possible explanations for the symptoms that integrate somatic and psychosocial aspects of the problem.

Patient: I just don't get why my neck keeps getting spasms.
Clinician: I have noticed that sometimes you mention this happening after your supervisor criticizes you. Sometimes our muscles react to emotions like anger or stress by tightening up. When this becomes extreme, they can spasm.
Patient: You know that makes some sense. When he comes around I can feel myself grit my teeth and begin to feel stiff.

Another management suggestion is to have the provider evaluate the patient in an appropriate manner to rule out somatic causes of their symptoms. Once somatization is identified, the clinician continues to schedule the individual for brief, regularly spaced intervals. These visits are time contingent; patients need not have new symptoms to be able to meet regularly with their medical practitioner. These visits allow for an initial brief check-in regarding the somatic symptoms followed by discussions of events in the patient's life and the patient's emotional well-being and relationships. The clinician can adopt a conservative approach toward new treatments or diagnostic workups when the patient presents with new or worsening symptoms. The goal is to focus patients on behaviors that promote well-being and help them discuss the psychosocial aspects of their life and illness. Patients are redirected from pursuing new therapies or evaluations for their symptoms. At the same time, they are shown that the provider is taking an active interest in their problems. Moreover, patients learn that they will receive this care and attention even without new symptoms or exacerbations of existing symptoms. The clinician may also ask patients when they want to return for the next visit. This provides them with a sense of control, and over time many patients will suggest lengthening the interval between appointments.

Establishing appropriate goals is also important when working with these patients. These disorders, like any chronic disease, are often not curable. However, clinicians often hope that another medication will relieve the symptoms or that one more diagnostic procedure will elucidate the cause of the patient's problem. However, these beliefs can lead to disappointment for both the patient and the clinician. Rather than aiming for complete resolution of the symptoms, it is better to set more realistic goals. For the primary care practitioner, these might include reducing the number of phone calls and visits with new symptoms, the number of requests for medications or referrals to specialists, and the number of emergency room visits. For patients, these goals might include an increased sense of control in their lives, improved social functioning, better coping with day-to-day symptoms, and overall enhanced functioning.

> **Clinician:** Today I would like to talk about what we should expect from each other in this relationship. From your perspective, I suspect that the best thing I could do would be to figure out what's causing these symptoms and make them go away completely. Given all of your years of suffering and the many doctors you've seen and the limited success of treatments so far, it might be more realistic for us not to focus so much on pursuing a cure but to look at how to improve how you feel and maximize your functioning. What do you think?
>
> **Patient:** Well, of course I was hoping that you could find a cure. So—does this mean that you can't help me?
>
> **Clinician:** No, I didn't mean to imply that. I do think I can help. First, I'd like to work on helping you learn to cope more effectively with your symptoms. We could also work to improve how you function from day to day. Whether or not we are immediately successful, I'm committed to helping you in the best way I can.

A novel treatment for somatic symptom disorders involves the use of a "written self-disclosure protocol." This therapy involves having the patient periodically write in a journal format. The clinician convinces the patient to spend 20 minutes one time per week at home writing about distressing experiences in his/her life. The patients do the writing outside of the office visit. They are specifically encouraged to think about experiences involving relationships with others. The patients are also instructed to write about how these experiences have affected them in the past and how they may continue to affect them in the future. The journal may be shared with others if the patient wishes, but it does not have to be shared to have a benefit. This technique has been found to be acceptable by both patients and providers. It has also been found to be helpful, as well as time- and cost-effective. Studies of this management

strategy have demonstrated decreases in health care utilization.

Another method for treating patients with somatization symptoms in the primary care setting is designed to help general practitioners teach these patients to reattribute and relate physical symptoms to psychosocial problems. The clinician is encouraged to take a history of the patient's illness, including related physical, mood, and social factors. The clinician then broadens the view of the problem and the necessary treatment by reframing the complaint using the biopsychosocial information provided by the patient. The practitioner then links the patient's distress and the physical complaint using a coherent explanation of how psychosocial factors can give rise to and contribute to physical symptoms. This intervention model has been found to be both clinically and cost-effective.

Despite all of these interventions, it may be necessary to refer the patient to a mental health specialist. Many individuals with somatization will resist such a referral. Although this reluctance on the patient's part can be frustrating, the primary care provider should remember that many of these patients have experienced such a referral as the first step in the termination of the relationship with a health care provider. The primary care clinician can address this concern by making a follow-up appointment with the patient prior to the referral. Once the continuity of the relationship is ensured, the referral can be discussed. Further, a consultation model in which the patient is asked to see the mental health provider for one or a few visits to "advise and help the primary care provider do a better job" is often more acceptable to patients than a referral for ongoing treatment. The consultation can be useful in confirming a diagnosis or in providing advice on the use of psychotropic medications.

> **Clinician:** I'd like to see you in a month. In the meantime, I'd like you to consider seeing Dr. R, the psychiatrist we've talked about. I know that you don't think that your chest pain is caused by your depression. But we've both agreed to try to treat the depression. I still don't know if we've found the right antidepressant, and I'd really value Dr. R's opinion. What do you think?

Psychotherapy

Cognitive behavioral therapy (CBT) has been studied as a means of addressing the medically unexplained somatic symptoms. This treatment is based on the theory that incorrect beliefs about bodily functioning underlie these symptoms or produce much of the dysfunction. The first task in therapy is to identify these beliefs and behaviors. Next, the patient is encouraged to challenge the beliefs and is taught to formulate more accurate ideas about bodily functioning. This change is paired with adoption of more appropriate behaviors. An analysis of randomized trials of specific treatments for patients with somatic symptom disorders indicated that CBT had the strongest and most consistent evidence of effectiveness. A subsequent review of intervention studies in patients with somatic symptom disorders, functional somatic symptoms, somatization, or medically unexplained symptoms corroborated this finding. Furthermore, a growing body of evidence supports the benefit of mindfulness-based cognitive therapy in treating associated stress, depression, and anxiety in patients with multiple somatic complaints, as well as in patients with medically unexplained symptoms. However, although early results of these studies are promising, there is a need for larger, controlled trials. Overall, this research suggests that CBT approaches are effective in patients with somatic symptom and other related disorders.

Psychodynamic psychotherapy is based on the assumption that the individual is experiencing internal emotional conflicts and that the associated emotions cannot be identified or expressed. As a result, the conflict is manifested through somatic symptoms. The therapy focuses on attempting to uncover and resolve these conflicts by having the patient identify associated emotions and express them openly in the therapy sessions. As the patient does this work, the somatic symptoms become unnecessary and remit. A meta-analysis of short-term therapy for somatic symptom disorders found benefits for subjects in multiple areas, including physical symptom reduction, improvement in social and occupational functioning and psychological symptoms as well as decreases in health care utilization. Unfortunately, many patients with somatization may not be enthusiastic about exploring unconscious conflicts. In general, the psychodynamic psychotherapy is a longer-term, time-intensive approach that requires a referral to a specialist and a significant commitment from the patient.

In family-oriented approaches to therapy, therapists must integrate the biological and psychosocial aspects of the patient's illness. The care provider must collaborate with the patient and the patient's family in treating the illness. Further, the clinician must demonstrate true interest in and curiosity about the patient's symptoms, family, relationships, and life. These therapies attempt to help the patients and their families break down the distinction between physical and psychological and move their thinking from "either–or" (e.g., it is either a physical problem or a mental problem) to "both–and" (e.g., the problem has both physical and mental facets). Relational therapists argue that effective therapy involves validating the illness, involving the family, working closely with the health care team, and enhancing the patient's curiosity about symptoms. They also emphasize demonstrating interest in the patient's somatic symptoms, helping the patient to see the relationship between the somatic symptoms and psychosocial stressors, and using physical interventions (e.g., biofeedback and relaxation techniques) to form an alliance with the patient to deal with the illness.

Medication

Data on the efficacy of using medications to treat somatic symptom disorders is limited; to date there are few randomized, controlled studies. However, there have been several small, open studies demonstrating the effectiveness of fluoxetine, sertraline, escitalopram, venlafaxine, and mirtazapine in reducing somatic complaints, depressive symptoms, and improving overall assessment of health. Other studies have found similar results with agents that enhance serotonergic transmission in the treatment of patients with body dysmorphic disorder. There is also evidence that St. John's Wort is effective in treating somatic symptom disorders, with reduction in somatization symptoms and improvement in patients' self-assessments of health. However, information on the long-term effectiveness of such treatments is yet to be elucidated. Moreover, investigations into the benefits of treatment of comorbid anxiety and depression have yielded mixed results depending on the specific somatic condition, with less success in patients with chronic pain and fibromyalgia.

A summary of recommendations for managing patients with somatization symptoms is found in Table 28-3.

Table 28-3. Management of somatization.

Interventions
1. Take a detailed history, perform a physical examination, and order appropriate diagnostic studies.
2. Screen individuals with multiple somatic complaints for psychiatric disorders.
3. Integrate the patient's physical and psychosocial concerns by inquiring not only about somatic symptoms but also about other events in the person's life.
4. Develop an empathic relationship.
5. Never challenge the validity of the patient's somatic symptoms.
6. Do not utilize psychological labels for the patient's symptoms.
7. Schedule the patient for appointments at regular intervals.
8. Establish realistic expectations.
9. Care for yourself.

Source: Adapted with permission from Eisendrath SJ, Lichtmacher J. Psychiatric Disorders. In *Current Medical Diagnosis and Treatment* 2007, S. McPhee et al (ed); Appleton and Lange, 2006.

CLINICIAN–PATIENT RELATIONSHIP

Caring for individuals with somatic symptom disorders is difficult. Patients present with symptoms suggestive of a medical or neurologic illness and require an appropriate evaluation. However, at the completion of the evaluation the clinician is faced with an individual who, by definition, does not have a physical condition or who has a condition that cannot account for the level of symptoms or disability experienced. In contrast, the patient views the symptoms as somatic and strenuously resists the idea that the symptoms have a psychological component. As a result, neither party is satisfied with the interaction.

Why is dealing with patients who experience somatic symptom disorders so difficult? One theory is that clinicians use terminology that was developed to promote communication with other health care providers. It is not meant to provide the patient with an explanation of or validation of their illness experience. Health providers focus on understanding the pathophysiology of disease in a scientific manner. Laypersons have different explanatory models of disease, and therefore when they present to the clinician's office they may already have a theory about the origin of their symptoms. In the case of patients with somatization, this theory involves a physical cause. In contrast, the practitioner may feel that a physical cause for the symptoms is less likely than a psychological etiology. As a result, the patient and clinician possess models of illness that are not only competing but also conflicting. To work effectively with the patient, the provider must reconcile these theories.

> **Patient:** So you think I have "depression"? How is that causing me to be tired all the time? I don't understand how you can say that. I don't cry and I don't feel sad.
>
> **Clinician:** Depression is not just feeling sad. It is a medical illness, just like diabetes or epilepsy. It is caused by an imbalance in the chemicals in the brain that help the brain cells communicate with each other. When those chemicals, or transmitters, are out of balance the brain does not function correctly and people develop symptoms such as fatigue, sadness, changes in sleep and appetite, and changes in their ability to concentrate.
>
> **Patient:** Well what can be done?
>
> **Clinician:** The good news is there are a number of treatments. Medications can be very helpful by directly affecting the balance of the transmitters. Other treatments involve working with someone to help you train your brain to function better without medications.

It seems, then, that working with these patients is difficult because they do not share the clinician's explanatory models and they resist giving up their own ideas about their illness. When providers are able to explain the patient's symptoms in a way that provides a holistic and empowering perspective, they are viewed as a positive and helpful influence. As a result, the patient is satisfied, an alliance is formed to address the symptoms in a collaborative manner, and the practitioner may feel more positive about the patient.

Research has also focused on the reasons clinicians experience certain patients as difficult. Patients who are rated as difficult by health providers have twice the prevalence of psychiatric disorders (see Chapter 4). Further, the presence of more physical symptoms, both those judged to result from medical causes and those judged to be related to a somatic symptom disorder, contributes to the sense that the patient is difficult. In addition, clinicians expect physical symptoms to be associated with medical diagnoses, and the lack of such an association leads to frustration over the "vagueness" of the symptoms and their own inability to make a diagnosis. The practitioner may feel that the patient is consciously faking symptoms. However, patients may have reasons, conscious or unconscious, for holding onto the symptoms. The assumption of the sick role may confer some benefits, through changes in social and family systems that are difficult for the provider to discern or understand. Clinicians should attempt to understand the role that the symptoms play in the patient's family and social systems to gain insight into why the symptoms persist despite the lack of a somatic etiology.

CARING FOR THE CLINICIAN

The care of patients with somatization can be a draining experience, and the clinician must take care to avoid burnout (see Chapter 6). The patient's seemingly unending physical concerns, resistance to recommended treatments, and complaints that the clinician is not doing enough can easily overwhelm the provider. The practitioner needs to remember that these are chronic disorders. As a consequence, it can be helpful to set reasonable goals for treatment such as "care and not cure." Clinicians must understand that they can provide support and effective treatment but that the patient will likely have some residual symptoms. The practitioner should feel comfortable setting limits with their somatizing patients. Once the clinician and patient have committed to regular follow-up appointments, it is appropriate to set limits on calls and drop-in visits. For example, the patient can be asked to reserve all but emergency complaints for the regular visits. If the patient calls between scheduled sessions, the discussion should be limited to ascertaining that there is no emergency. If there is none, then the patient can be gently urged to defer further discussion until the next visit.

Outside of work, practitioners should take time for exercise, family, friends, and other interests. They may also wish to discuss difficult cases with colleagues to manage the powerful feelings these patients can elicit. In this way, they can maintain a healthy lifestyle and balance in their life. Clinicians must keep in mind that the illness belongs to the patient and not to them. They must not allow the patient's frustration or demands make them forget this. The combination of empathic listening, conservative (but appropriate) evaluation, and gentle limit setting can not only benefit these patients, but also improve the primary care provider's satisfaction with these relationships.

ACKNOWLEDGMENT

The authors wish to thank Won Kim for his assistance in preparing this chapter.

SUGGESTED READINGS

Abbas A, Kisely S, Kroenke K. Short-term psychodynamic psychotherapy for somatic disorders. *Psychother Psychosom* 2009;78:265–274. PMID: 19602915.

Allen LA, Woolfolk RL, Escobar JI, Gara MA, Hamer RM. Cognitive-behavioral therapy for somatization disorder: a randomized controlled trial. *Arch Intern Med* 2006;166:512. PMID: 16864762.

Creed, FH, Davies I, Jackson J. The epidemiology of multiple somatic symptoms. *J Psychosom Res* 2012:72;311–317. PMID: 22405227.

Duddu V, Isaac MK, Chaturvedi SK. Somatization, somatosensory amplification, attribution styles and illness behaviour: a review. *Int Rev Psychiatry* 2006;18:25. PMID: 16451877.

Kirmayer LJ, Sartorius, NS. Cultural models and somatic syndromes. *Psychosom Med* 2007;69:832–840. PMID: 18040090.

Kroenke K. Efficacy of treatment for somatoform disorders: a review of randomized controlled trials. *Psychosom Med* 2007;69:881–888. PMID: 18040099.

Kroenke K, Spitzer RL, Williams JB. The PHQ-15: validity of a new measure for evaluating the severity of somatic symptoms. *Psychosom Med* 2002;64:258. PMID: 11914441.

Rizzo M, Creed F, Goldberg D, Meader N, Pilling S. A systematic review of non-pharmacological treatments for depression in people with chronic physical health problems. *J Psychosom Res* 2011:71;18–27. PMID: 21665008.

Sumithipala A. What is the evidence for the efficacy of treatments for somatoform disorders? A critical review of previous intervention studies. *Psychosom Med* 2007;69:889–900. PMID: 18040100.

Somatic Symptom and Related Disorders. *Diagnostic and Statistical Manual of Mental Disorders,* Fifth Edition. Arlington, VA, American Psychiatric Association, 2013.

Sharma MH, Manjula M. Behavioural and psychological management of somatic symptom disorders: An overview. *Int Rev Psychiatry* 2013;25:116–124. PMID: 23383673.

Someshekar B, Jainer A, Wuntakal B. Psychopharmacotherapy of somatic symptoms disorders. *Int Rev Psychiatry* 2013;25:107–115. PMID: 23383672.

Personality Disorders

29

John Q. Young, MD, MPP

INTRODUCTION

Patients with a personality disorder are common in medical practice; yet, establishing and maintaining a therapeutic alliance with such patients can be challenging for clinicians. Complications associated with patients with comorbid personality disorders are myriad, including suboptimal utilization of medical care (over-and under-use), difficulty adhering to treatment plans, providing a history embedded with distortions, and problematic relationships with clinicians. In addition, these patients are more likely to be hospitalized. An understanding of personality disorders allows physicians to anticipate the challenging interpersonal and behavioral problems that can arise in working with these patients and can help physicians work through the negative emotions that these patients may arouse. This facilitates the development and implementation of appropriate treatment plans, improved alliance between patient and clinician, and better outcomes.

The American Psychiatric Association (APA) defines a personality disorder as: *an enduring pattern of inner experience and behavior that deviates markedly from the expectations of the individual's culture, is pervasive and inflexible, has an onset in adolescence or early adulthood, is stable over time, and leads to distress or impairment.* People suffering from personality disorders have dysfunctional beliefs about self and others. These dysfunctional beliefs and patterns of relating impair their capacity to establish and maintain intimate relationships, function at work, and experience pleasure in life. These patients have difficulty negotiating complex situations and coping with stress and anxiety. The sick role and the demands of medical care can be particularly problematic for them. The stress of illness is often extreme and sets into motion defensive and inflexible emotional processes, cognitions, and behaviors—with negative consequences for their medical treatment. In addition, these patients' difficulties in relating to others typically manifest in the doctor–patient relationship. They may be quite demanding or disrespectful of the needs of others,

or the need to trust or confide in others may trigger so much anxiety that they avoid building relationships.

Personality theorists have long debated how best to understand and classify personality disorders. The debate has centered on two models. The **categorical model**, adopted by the APA, views personality disorders as entities that are distinct from one another—that is, classified in separate categories—and also distinct from normalcy. This model blends more easily with traditional medical diagnosis than does the **dimensional model**, which views personality disorders as entities that overlap each other and that are not distinct from normalcy, so that the maladaptive traits of patients with personality disorders represent normal traits that are exaggerated. The APA's *Diagnostic and Statistical Manual 5* (DSM-5), uses a categorical model but discusses the use of a dimensional framework in a new provisional section.

DIAGNOSTIC CLASSIFICATION OF PERSONALITY DISORDERS

DSM-5 groups personality disorders into three clusters based on descriptive similarities. Cluster A includes paranoid, schizoid, and schizotypal personality disorders—individuals who often appear odd or eccentric; cluster B includes antisocial, borderline, histrionic, and narcissistic personality disorders—individuals who often appear dramatic, emotional, or erratic; and cluster C includes avoidant, dependent, and obsessive–compulsive personality disorders—individuals who often appear anxious or fearful. Given the unique nature of any individual personality, a patient can exhibit traits of two or more personality disorders, or meet the full diagnostic criteria for more than one disorder. Hence, co-occurrence is very common. National survey data suggest that approximately 15% of the general population have at least one personality disorder. Table 29-1 indicates the prevalence of each personality disorder within the general US population. It is important to remember that the prevalence is higher in medical patients.

Table 29-1. DSM-5 personality disorders and their prevalence.

Cluster	Personality Disorder	Discriminating Feature	Prevalence in General Population (%)
A: Odd or eccentric	Paranoid	Suspicious	4
	Schizoid	Socially indifferent	3.1
	Schizotypal	Eccentric	3
	Antisocial	Disagreeable	3.6
B: Dramatic, emotional, or erratic	Borderline	Unstable	2
	Histrionic	Attention seeking	1.8
	Narcissistic	Self-centered	0.5
C: Anxious or fearful	Avoidant	Inhibited	2.4
	Dependent	Submissive	0.49
	Obsessive-compulsive	Perfectionistic	7.9

Diagnosing a personality disorder can be difficult. To make an accurate diagnosis, it is usually necessary for the physician to get to know the patient over time, to learn how the patient reacts and relates to people in other situations, and to obtain collateral information from family and friends. Clinicians should attend to three key issues.

First, it is important to differentiate a true personality disorder from personality traits that become exaggerated under stress. The stress of illness often causes a patient to behave in maladaptive ways; because of this, many patients, at one time or another, seem to have a personality disorder. Patients who do not suffer from a true personality disorder, however, are usually capable of more adaptive functioning. The maladaptive behavior itself is less "enduring" and "engrained" and more situational and modifiable. In these cases, the physician can successfully intervene by supporting and strengthening these patients' own natural coping skills.

Second, it is also important to differentiate personality disorders from disorders such as major depression or generalized anxiety disorder. For example, patients with panic disorder may—out of sheer terror—become extremely dependent on their physician. If their panic disorder is diagnosed and treated, they may reveal an underlying independent and self-sufficient personality. Similarly, a patient's grandiosity and arrogance may stem largely from a bipolar mania rather than a narcissistic personality disorder. When patients who do have a personality disorder are evaluated, looking for episodic and/or comorbid psychiatric disorders is particularly important as the latter are more frequent and difficult to treat if patients actually have a personality disorder. Treating an episode of major depression in a patient with borderline personality disorder, however, can alleviate suffering and lead to better coping with illness.

Third, it is important to distinguish personality disorders from personality changes caused by general medical conditions, such as traumatic brain injury, stroke, epilepsy, or endocrine disorders. Patients with one of these problems may exhibit many of the characteristics of a personality disorder. These behaviors can be distinguished from a true personality disorder, however, in that they typically represent a change from baseline personality characteristics. Medical conditions such as these may also exacerbate preexisting personality traits (e.g., obsessive mannerisms). Treatment of the underlying medical problem may bring about reversal of the personality changes.

Finally, personality disorder diagnoses, like other mental disorder diagnoses, are often misunderstood and may serve to stigmatize the patient. These diagnoses should therefore be made carefully, deferred in cases of uncertainty, and noted in medical records and correspondence only when their notation is likely to be helpful in enhancing patient care.

Doctor–Patient Relationship Issues

The primary care provider may find many challenges in working with patients with personality disorders. Personality disorders often significantly impair the quality of interpersonal relationships. Because the doctor–patient relationship requires effective communication about important health issues of a personal nature, tensions and at times overt conflict may develop between patients with personality disorders and their providers. These tensions may also affect other members of the health care team and may be especially pronounced in the context of acute illness or crisis situations. In fact, the first diagnostic clues suggesting personality dysfunction or disorder may appear as difficulties in the doctor–patient relationship.

For patients with personality disorders, physical illness can cause exaggerated degrees of emotional distress, not always expressed to the provider. Although some patients do tell their providers about their emotional distress, others may instead manifest distress as noncompliance with the agreed-upon plan of evaluation or treatment or as changed, unexpected, or undesirable behavior (as judged by the physician) toward the physician.

In response to patients' actions or statements, physicians may have a significant emotional reaction to the patients and may change their behavior toward them. Even when they experience no subjective distress from a medical condition or the doctor–patient relationship, patients with personality dysfunction may have such aberrant expectations of others that their statements or behaviors are troubling or burdensome to the physician. Physicians must be aware of their own emotional responses to such patients so as to avoid reacting inappropriately. Physicians who deny their negative feelings toward patients may fail to recognize a personality disorder or other psychiatric diagnosis, or fail to address the diagnostic and treatment needs of the patient with the necessary compassion, rigor, and thoroughness. When clinicians recognize and deal with their negative feelings, they are better able to make thoughtful and appropriate responses to these patients' symptoms and behavior, minimizing the emotional strain for both patient and doctor and optimizing the quality of the medical outcome.

Appreciating the unique vulnerabilities associated with each personality disorder can aid in identifying problematic behaviors and can help to maintain the necessary degree of cooperation and collaboration, even when the patient has significant personality dysfunction. Table 29-2 outlines typical responses to illness by patients with each of the most common personality disorders, details troublesome reactions by physicians, and suggests strategies to avoid further problems with these challenging patients.

Management of Patients with Personality Disorders

In most cases, a stable therapeutic alliance with patients who have personality disorders can be maintained by implementing the behavioral strategies suggested in the following sections. Sometimes other factors must also be addressed. As mentioned earlier, comorbid diagnoses must be treated (e.g., depression or anxiety disorders). Pharmacotherapy and psychotherapy are often more complex for patients with comorbid disorders. This is particularly evident when patients with personality disorders have concurrent substance-abuse problems or psychotic symptoms (e.g., hallucinations, delusions, and paranoid ideation). In such cases, mental health consultation can be particularly helpful.

When a provider feels unable to continue productive work with a patient with a personality disorder, it may be appropriate to transfer the patient to another clinician. Although such transfers of care may be both necessary and helpful, they require consideration of the impact of the transfer on the well-being of the patient. Patients with certain personality disorders may experience such transfers as rejection or abandonment, perceptions that may exacerbate their emotional distress and potentially disrupt their medical treatment. Prior consultation with a mental health provider can be useful in determining whether such a transfer might be helpful and can aid in carrying it out smoothly.

The remainder of this chapter discusses the 10 personality disorders as they manifest in the medical setting, and, for each, presents management recommendations.

PARANOID PERSONALITY DISORDER

Symptoms & Signs

Patients with paranoid personality disorder have a long-standing pattern of distrust and suspiciousness. They perceive the behavior and motives of others as malevolent in nature and expect others, in many situations, to disappoint or take advantage of them. They are reluctant to confide in others and can be preoccupied with unwarranted doubts about the loyalty or trustworthiness of friends and associates. They may perceive seemingly benign or innocuous statements or behavior by others as threatening, insulting, or hurtful. To defend against their perceived vulnerability, they usually adopt a rigid, distanced, or guarded position. In general, persons with this personality structure find intimate relationships undesirable and difficult, which often leave them without any significant social supports.

Differential Diagnosis

Long-standing psychotic symptoms, such as delusions and hallucinations, suggest a diagnosis of paranoid delusional disorder or paranoid schizophrenia. Although persons with paranoid personality disorder usually do not have frank paranoid delusions, at times of extreme stress they may develop such symptoms for brief periods. Paranoid ideation may also be associated with medical causes or with alcohol or substance abuse or withdrawal.

Illness Experience & Illness Behavior

Illness is difficult for individuals with paranoid personality disorder because illness makes them more dependent, and, hence, more vulnerable. Communicating personal information to the physician may challenge the self-protective, rigid way they approach social interactions.

Table 29-2. Common personality disorders and typical manifestations.

Personality Disorder	Paranoid	Schizoid	Schizotypal	Antisocial	Borderline
Prominent features of disorder	Distrust and suspiciousness of others, such that their motives are interpreted as malevolent	Pattern of detachment from social relationships and a restricted range of emotional expression	Odd beliefs, inappropriate affect, perceptual distortions, and desire for social isolation	Disregard for and violation of the rights of others, beginning in adolescence	Pattern of instability in interpersonal relationships, self-image and affects, and marked impulsivity
Patient's experience of illness	Heightened sense of fear and vulnerability	Threat to personal integrity; increased anxiety because illness forces interaction with others	May have odd interpretations of illness, increased anxiety because of interactions with others, may become overtly psychotic	Sense of fear may be masked by increased hostility or entitled stance	Terrifying fantasies about illness; feels either completely well or deathly ill
Problematic behavior in the medical care setting	Fear that physician or others may harm them; Misinterpretation of innocuous or even helpful behaviors; Increased likelihood of argument or conflict with staff	May delay seeking care until symptoms become severe, out of fear of interacting with others; May appear detached and unappreciative of help	May delay care because of odd and magical beliefs about symptoms, may not recognize symptoms as a sign of illness; May appear odd and eccentric and paranoid toward others	Irresponsible, impulsive, or dangerous health behavior, without regard for consequences to self or others; Angry, deceitful, or manipulative behavior	Mistrust of physicians and delay in seeking treatment; Intense fear of rejection and abandonment; Abrupt shifts from idealizing to devaluing caregivers; splitting; Self-destructive threats and acts
Common problematic reactions to patient by caregiver	Defensive, argumentative, or angry response that "confirms" patient's suspicions; Ignoring the patient's suspicious or angry stance	Overzealous attempts to connect with patient; Frustration at feeling unappreciated	Frustration about patient's misinterpretation of illness; Not wanting to connect with an odd and eccentric patient	Succumbing to patient's manipulation; Angry, punitive reaction when manipulation is discovered	Succumbing to patient's idealization and splitting; Getting too close to patient causing overstimulation; Despair at patient's self-destructive behaviors; Temptation to punish patient angrily

(Continued)

Table 29-2. Common personality disorders and typical manifestations. (Continued)

Personality Disorder	Histrionic	Narcissistic	Avoidant	Dependent	Obsessive-Compulsive
Helpful management strategies by caregiver	Attend to and be empathic toward patient fears, even when irrational in appearance. Carefully detail care plan for patient with advance information about risks of procedures/treatments. Maintain patient's independence when possible and optimize the patient's control. Not overly friendly, but professional, objective stance	Appreciate need for privacy and maintain a low-key approach. Focus on technical elements of treatment; these are better tolerated. Encourage patient to maintain daily routines. Do not become overly personally involved or too zealous in trying to provide social supports	Try not to be turned off by patient's odd appearance. Try to educate patient about the illness and its treatment. Do not become overly involved in trying to provide social support	Carefully, respectfully investigate patient's concerns and motives. Communicate directly; avoid punitive reactions to patient. Set clear limits in context of medically indicated interventions	Don't get too close to patient. Schedule frequent periodic check-ups. Provide clear, nontechnical answers to questions to counter scary fantasies. Tolerate periodic angry outbursts, but set limits. Be aware of patient's potential for self-destructive behavior. Discuss feelings with coworkers and schedule multidisciplinary team meetings
Prominent features of disorder	Pattern of excessive attention seeking and emotionality	Pervasive pattern of grandiosity, need for admiration, and lack of empathy for others	Pattern of social inhibition because of fears of being rejected or humiliated by others	Pervasive and excessive need to be taken care of that leads to submissive and clinging behavior, and fears of separation	Pattern of preoccupation with orderliness, perfectionism, control
Patient's experience of illness	Threatened sense of attractiveness and self-esteem	Illness may increase anxiety related to doubts about personal adequacy and disrupts image of self as resilient and superior	Illness may heighten sense of inadequacy and worsen low self-esteem	Fear that illness will lead to abandonment and helplessness	Fear of losing control over bodily functions and over emotions generated by illness; feelings of shame and vulnerability

Problematic behavior in the medical care setting	Overly dramatic, attention-seeking behavior, with tendency to draw caregiver into excessively familiar relationship Inadequate focus on symptoms and their management, with over emphasis on feeling states May provide answers they believe physician wants to hear Tendency to somatize	Demanding, entitled attitude Excessive praise toward caregiver may turn to devaluation, in effort to maintain sense of superiority Denial of illness or minimization of symptoms	May not be forthcoming about symptom severity, may easily agree with physician out of fear of not being liked	Dramatic and urgent demands for medical attention Angry outbursts at physician if not responded to Patient may contribute to prolong illness or encourage medical procedures in order to get attention May abuse substances and medications	Anger about disruption of routines Repetitive questions and excessive attention to detail Fear of relinquishing control to health care team
Common problematic reactions to patient by caregiver	Performing excessive workup (when patient is dramatic) or inadequate workup (when patient is vague) Allowing too much emotional closeness, thereby losing objectivity Frustration with patient's dramatic or vague presentation	Outright rejection of patient's demands, resulting in patient distancing self from caregiver Excessive submission to patient's grandiose stance	Feeling overly concerned for the patient, taking on a paternalistic role that may increase patient's sense of inadequacy May feel angry and betrayed by patient if the patient's symptoms turn out to be more extensive than initially reported	Inability to set limits to availability, thus leading to burnout Hostile rejection of patient	Impatience and cutting answers short Attempts to control treatment planning
Helpful management strategies by caregiver	Show respectful and professional concern for feelings, with emphasis on objective issues Avoid excessive familiarity	Generous validation of patient's concerns, with attentive but factual response to questions Allow patients to maintain sense of competence by rechanneling their "skills" to deal with illness, obviating need for devaluation of caregivers Present treatment recommendations in the context of their right to the best care	Provide reassurance, validate patient's concerns Encourage reporting of symptoms and concerns	Provide reassurance and schedule frequent periodic check-ups Be consistently available but provide firm realistic limits to availability Enlist other members of the health care team in providing support for patient Help patient obtain outside support systems Avoid hostile rejection of patient	Thorough history taking and careful diagnostic workups are reassuring Give clear and thorough explanation of diagnosis and treatment options Do not overemphasize uncertainties about treatments Avoid vague and impressionistic explanations Treat patient as an equal partner; encourage self-monitoring and allow patient participation in treatment

Patients may experience a heightened sense of vulnerability and fear of harm by the physician. In their fearful state, they may perceive innocuous or even overtly helpful behavior as threatening. They may then question or challenge the physician about the content of an intervention or the motives behind it. This can lead to conflict and argument between patient and doctor or to the patient disengaging from care.

THE DOCTOR–PATIENT RELATIONSHIP

Physicians confronted with such a paranoid stance may react in ways that exacerbate the situation. If they feel that their intentions are inappropriately suspect they might argue with the patient or become defensive, perhaps using an angry tone. This kind of reaction may frighten the patient and may be perceived as confirmation of the patient's suspicion. Although such a response should be avoided, ignoring the patient's distrustful or angry behavior can also be problematic; the patient's concerns, however irrational, may increase if not addressed.

Specific Management Strategies

It is essential to address the patient's concerns and fears empathically, however irrational they seem. Although the physician may see the patient's concern as unrealistic, to the patient the fear is real. Dismissing these patients' concerns or calling them paranoid will not address their emotional needs and may instead create distance in the doctor–patient relationship. A professional, "matter-of-fact" or objective stance is most reassuring to these patients. Excessive friendliness or reassurance may be misinterpreted and may intensify their paranoia. It is important to give these patients detailed information about their proposed treatment plan, allowing them to feel they are in control of the treatment and can make independent decisions. Provide factual information about risks associated with the treatment, whenever possible, before any major procedures or changes in treatment.

CASE ILLUSTRATION 1

Simon, a 42-year-old, single, male parking lot attendant, presents to the urgent care clinic complaining of 3 months of tension headaches and fatigue in the context of what he calls "job stress." The only notable finding in the physical examination is a mild elevation of blood pressure. The physician also observes that Simon seems angry and anxious. When asked about his job stress, Simon reveals anxieties about not being able to trust two new coworkers, along with fears that his supervisors are conspiring to dismiss him from his job. He also mentions, hesitantly, that he had not sought evaluation of his headaches sooner because he worried that the physician would dismiss his fears as unfounded or "crazy." Additional social history reveals difficulty with close relationships and recurrent problems adjusting to changes in the workplace.

The physician listens in a nonjudgmental and empathic manner. He responds with scientific curiosity asking specific and thorough questions in order to define the nature of the complaint. An over-the-counter analgesic for the headaches and buspirone for anxiety and agitation are prescribed after a discussion of the likely diagnosis and the pros and cons of each treatment option. The physician plans follow-up measurements of the blood pressure and suggests that Simon see a psychiatrist for further evaluation of his very stressful job situation.

Simon feels that his concerns have been taken seriously. He finds the referral to a psychiatrist acceptable because it has been proposed in a way that offers support and does not dismiss his fears as pathological. The physician's matter-of-fact responses to Simon's somatic complaints help increase the patient's trust in the physician.

SCHIZOID PERSONALITY DISORDER

Symptoms & Signs

Individuals with schizoid personality disorder remain detached from social relationships and exhibit a restricted range of emotional expression in their interactions with others, often appearing cold or indifferent. Because patients with this disorder find emotions, intimacy, and conflict threatening, they tend to isolate themselves and avoid close or sexual relationships. They prefer dealing with technical or abstract concepts rather than people, and so they may devote their time to pursuits such as mathematical games. Work can be problematic if it involves interactions with others, but many individuals can perform quite well if they work with some degree of independence.

Differential Diagnosis

Patients with schizoid personality disorder do not exhibit prolonged psychotic symptoms. They may, however, suffer a brief psychotic decompensation during times of extreme stress. In addition, schizoid personality disorder may in some cases precede the development of psychotic conditions, such as schizophrenia or delusional disorder. It can also coexist with schizotypal, paranoid, or avoidant personality disorders.

Illness Experience & Illness Behavior

Illness can be especially stressful for these patients because it gives rise to strong emotions with which they are not prepared to cope. The necessity of interacting with caregivers when ill, often around quite intimate issues, forces them to do the very thing they systematically avoid. They may therefore delay seeking care until their symptoms become more serious. When they finally present for medical attention, they may appear indifferent or detached as a way of protecting themselves from overwhelming emotion. They may show little facial expression and may not respond in kind to caregivers' empathic nods or comments—which may make establishing a therapeutic relationship difficult.

The Doctor–Patient Relationship

Because these patients often appear cold or indifferent, physicians may consider them as unappreciative of help. They may also be puzzled or frustrated by their patients' delay in seeking medical care and their apparent passivity in the face of illness. As a result, caregivers may make overzealous attempts to connect with patients by trying to be especially empathic, a tactic that may instead frighten them away. On the other hand, providers may themselves draw back and lose their enthusiasm for helping patients who seem so unappreciative or uninvolved in their own treatment.

Specific Management Strategies

Understanding that individuals with schizoid personality disorder have difficulty tolerating emotions and intimate interactions is important. Physicians should appreciate their patients' need for privacy and should maintain a low-key approach, avoiding attempts to reach out by becoming too close or by insisting on providing social support. It is helpful to focus on the more technical aspects of treatment, as these are better tolerated, and encourage patients to maintain daily routines. Caregivers should remain available and provide steady but unobtrusive help.

CASE ILLUSTRATION 2

Ben, a 44-year-old computer programmer, is admitted to the University hospital for evaluation of nausea, anorexia, and a 30-lb weight loss occurring over the previous several months. When asked by the admitting resident why he had not sought treatment before, Ben states that he has always been healthy and thought he would probably regain the lost weight.

Throughout the interview, Ben makes poor eye contact and gives brief answers to questions. He appears to dislike being interviewed by both a medical student and a resident. He becomes more uncomfortable when asked questions about his personal life and how he likes spending his time. Ben states that he usually keeps to himself, with the exception of visiting his sister about once a month. He spends much of his time programming and playing with his computer.

Ben appears visibly anxious when the resident recommends a consultation by the gastroenterology service. He asks whether this is truly necessary. The resident emphasizes the importance of this consultation, and Ben seems to calm down a bit when the conversation focuses more on the possible tests that might be done to evaluate his symptoms, thereby distracting his attention from his concerns about having to see yet another doctor. The resident later explains to the medical student that it is important to minimize the number of doctors Ben sees over time and to avoid an overfriendly style, which might frighten him.

SCHIZOTYPAL PERSONALITY DISORDER

Symptoms & Signs

Patients with schizotypal personality disorder behave in an odd and eccentric manner, are socially inept and isolated, and experience cognitive or perceptual distortions. Their distortions include magical thinking, odd beliefs, ideas of reference, bodily illusions, or telepathic and clairvoyant experiences. These beliefs and distortions are inconsistent with subcultural norms, occur frequently, and are an important and pervasive core component of the patient's experience. The patient's enduring psychotic-like symptoms may worsen under stress. Patients often dress in an odd and peculiar fashion and their affect is often inappropriate; for example, they may laugh inappropriately during the visit while talking about their problems.

These patients are socially isolated and usually have few or no close friends. Their social isolation stems from their odd behavior as well as from their persistent social anxiety due to suspiciousness or paranoia toward others.

Differential Diagnosis

Schizotypal personality disorder shares the symptom of suspiciousness and paranoia with paranoid personality disorder and that of social isolation with schizoid personality disorder. However, the latter two disorders do not present with odd and peculiar mannerisms and behaviors and also lack cognitive or perceptual distortions.

The differential diagnosis includes schizophrenia. Although patients with schizotypal personality disorder lack signs and symptoms of overt psychosis, the disorder is considered a schizophrenia-spectrum disorder. This means that it may be related to schizophrenia. Family studies show an increased risk of schizophrenia in relatives of patients with schizotypal personality disorder and an increased risk of schizotypal personality disorder in families of patients with schizophrenia.

Illness Experience & Illness Behavior

Patients with schizotypal personality disorder may present late in the course of their illness because they may have odd interpretations of their illness and may, therefore, not recognize the serious nature of their symptoms. Also, like patients with schizoid personality disorder, they do not like to interact with and seek the company of others. Illness forces them to interact with health care providers and their support staff, something they may not be prepared to do. This may lead to increased paranoid ideation or overt psychotic symptoms.

THE DOCTOR–PATIENT RELATIONSHIP

These patients' eccentric appearance may cause the clinician to be hesitant in approaching them. Odd and weird interpretations of illness may lead to misunderstandings between patient and clinician. It may be challenging for the physician to improve these patients' understanding of their problems.

Specific Management Strategies

Clinicians should try to overcome their apprehension about treating these patients, often caused by their eccentric appearance. It is helpful to find out what these patients think about their symptoms and to help them obtain a better understanding of their illness. At the same time, the physician should not get overly involved in trying to increase their patients' social support or exposure to others. Knowing that patients with schizotypal personality disorder desire social isolation is important. Occasionally, assessing decision-making capacity can be complicated by odd or magical beliefs associated with the illness. Consultation can be helpful.

CASE ILLUSTRATION 3

Donna, a 35-year-old single female, has developed a cough, high fever, and chills and her family noticed that she started to look ill. She was brought to the emergency room by her mother. She is oddly dressed in a long and colorful country-style wraparound shirt with military-type boots. Her hair is unkempt and pinned up with a number of different hairpins. During the interview, Donna laughs in a silly manner while discussing her problem with the physician and the nurse. She says that she does not like to see a doctor because she prefers to walk in the woods by herself and communicate with the birds and insects.

The physician focuses on the patient's presenting symptoms and explains to her that she may suffer from pneumonia. He explains to her in simple terms what pneumonia is and that she needs sputum cultures and a chest X-ray to confirm the diagnosis.

While Donna has her chest X-ray taken, the physician and the nurse discuss how the health care team should help the patient understand her symptoms as well as the rationale for her medical workup and treatment. The physician also recommends focusing on the patient's problems and respecting her need for distance from others.

ANTISOCIAL PERSONALITY DISORDER

Symptoms & Signs

Persons with antisocial personality disorder demonstrate a disregard for others and behavior that violates others' rights. The diagnosis can be made only in persons over the age of 18 years, and it requires a history of conduct disorder prior to that age. Characteristics include lack of conformity to social norms and laws, using lies or other deceitfulness for personal gain, and impulsiveness and irresponsibility in many settings. These individuals may be threatening, manipulative, or harmful to others, and they are generally not remorseful. Their tendencies toward aggressive behavior may not be immediately evident, but contact with collateral sources frequently reveals a criminal record. These character traits affect relations with both strangers and family alike, as persons with antisocial personality disorder may engage in inconsiderate, angry, or harmful behaviors. These individuals may present themselves in a superficially grandiose manner, and they can also initially appear somewhat charismatic, until others recognize their charm as manipulative.

Differential Diagnosis

Antisocial personality disorder can overlap significantly with other personality disorder traits, most commonly narcissistic, histrionic, or borderline personality disorder. Because substance abuse is a frequent comorbid diagnosis, it is important to distinguish between the problems when making the diagnosis.

Illness Experience & Illness Behavior

To mask the fear that illness may cause, patients with antisocial personality disorder may unconsciously adopt an excessively self-assured, entitled, or hostile stance. Irresponsible, impulsive, or dangerous health behavior may help these patients deny their vulnerability to illness. This behavior can occur without regard for medical consequences, and many patients show blatant disregard for the health care personnel and resources from which they have benefited. Patients may assume a privileged, self-deserving stance and can become antagonistic if they fail to obtain the desired response. They may attempt to manipulate their physician, malingering to obtain things such as drugs or inappropriate disability benefits. This behavior can be an embellishment of a real illness, or it can occur when they are not ill.

THE DOCTOR–PATIENT RELATIONSHIP

Because these patients often behave in ways that are noncompliant, ungracious, or dishonest, they are frequently irritating to health care providers. Physicians may become angry with these individuals or reject them if they see that the treatments in which they have invested their knowledge and time have not been followed, or if they discover these patients have manipulated them.

Specific Management Strategies

Managing manipulative patients can be particularly challenging. If the patient successfully manipulates the physician, the outcome is usually detrimental to the patient's overall health (broadly defined). On the other hand, although recognizing the manipulative behavior may avert a detrimental health outcome, the physician's confrontation can alienate the patient. The more authoritarian the physician's stance, the more likely it is that the patient will become oppositional, reducing the possibility for development of an effective therapeutic alliance.

The key here is to maintain an objective, thorough, nonauthoritarian, and respectful approach to investigating the patient's presenting complaints. If the patient's presentation or motives are suspicious, the provider should gather corroborating data from collateral sources (other providers or family members) when needed. Such behavior by the physician can cause the patient to become hostile, with additional deterioration in the doctor–patient relationship. If confrontation or disagreement is necessary, it is essential to avoid humiliating the patient while identifying the attempted manipulation. Communication should be direct and factual with these patients, based on what is medically indicated, and clear limits should be set on the diagnostic or treatment plan.

 CASE ILLUSTRATION 4

On returning from vacation, the doctor's first patient is Randy, an angry 42-year-old man, well known to her for his problems with long-standing recurrent low back pain. Although his back pain is generally well controlled with back exercises and as needed nonsteroidal analgesics, Randy frequently takes long motorcycle trips with friends, during which he does not exercise or take his analgesics. While the physician was away, Randy went on a motorcycle tour and had a recurrence of acute back pain. He then telephoned the clinic and became angry and abusive toward the on-call nurse practitioner, who would not submit to his demands for narcotics.

The physician, who has seen similar behavior from Randy in the past, listens carefully to his story, acknowledges his anger, and reflects empathically on how painful his back must be. She inquires, nonjudgmentally, about the reasons for his failure to exercise. She then explains the benefits of a more preventive approach–using exercise and avoiding pain-inducing behaviors–compared with the long-term risks of relying on narcotics and failing to exercise. Finally, she offers him referral to a physical therapist for a review of the exercise plan, along with a refill of his nonsteroidal analgesic, emphasizing her view that this would offer the best long-term outcome. With some bitterness, Randy acknowledges the benefits of the physician's recommendations and agrees to try to follow through with them.

In dealing with Randy, the physician uses her past experience with him as a guide. Randy's self-destructive behavior, hostility, and disregard for others are met with clear limit setting by the physician, who responds in a calm and nonpunitive manner, emphasizing her concern for the patient's long-term well-being.

BORDERLINE PERSONALITY DISORDER

Symptoms & Signs

Patients with borderline personality disorder exhibit instability in their self-image, their affect, and their relationships with others. They can be quite impulsive and may engage in self-destructive behaviors, such as substance abuse, self-mutilation, and suicide attempts. These behaviors reflect a deep sense of emptiness and an intense fear of abandonment by others. On the other hand, patients with borderline personality disorder are also often fearful of closeness. They experience many contradictory emotions and feelings that are not integrated into a stable sense of who they are and that may be associated with rapid shifts in mood. This instability can cause frequent changes in goals and values. These patients usually have difficulty differentiating reality from fantasy and tend toward all-or-nothing thinking in their view of themselves and others, alternating between overidealization and devaluation.

Differential Diagnosis

Some patients with borderline personality disorder may suffer brief psychotic episodes when under stress. They may, for example, become very anxious or experience auditory hallucinations. The brief duration and specific association with stressors distinguishes these episodes from psychotic disorders. In addition, patients with borderline personality disorder also often suffer from a concurrent mood disorder, such as major depression or bipolar disorder, which should, of course, be treated. Other personality disorders (e.g., histrionic or narcissistic) may co-occur or be confused with borderline personality disorder.

Illness Experience & Illness Behavior

Patients with borderline personality disorder have difficulty distinguishing reality from fantasy, and they may have terrifying fantasies about illness. The complex and contradictory feelings engendered in response to illness can feel intolerable to these patients, so they may try to cope by pretending that they are completely well and denying the presence of illness. Alternatively, they may become convinced that they are deathly ill, even when suffering from a mild illness. Having felt wounded in earlier relationships, individuals with borderline personality disorder mistrust and fear caregivers. In an attempt to cope with their simultaneous intense wish for, and fear of, closeness, they tend to conceptualize caregivers as all good or all bad—a mechanism called "splitting." To complicate things further, these conceptualizations are not stable. Even an overidealized caregiver can abruptly be devalued if a borderline patient becomes angry and disappointed or feels abandoned. In addition, patients with borderline personality disorder may respond to feeling overwhelmed by engaging in impulsive and self-destructive acts, such as self-mutilation, substance abuse, and suicide attempts. They may also be noncompliant with treatment in order to test the limits of the clinician's availability, devalue the clinician, or even to remain ill and thus maintain an ongoing relationship with the caregiver.

THE DOCTOR–PATIENT RELATIONSHIP

A common mistake clinicians make in treating patients with borderline personality disorder is getting too emotionally close or over-involved in meeting their needs. This occurs when clinicians feel intensely drawn to help patients through their suffering and spend a great deal of time with them. This usually causes overstimulation of the patient's emotions, leading to initial idealization of the clinician and then increased instability and acting out. It should be noted that the patient's emotional behavior can cloud the clinician's judgment, causing the clinician to succumb to the patient's idealization and splitting. The idealization lasts only so long; the clinician will inevitably disappoint the patient. The borderline patient's self-destructive or often provocative behaviors can then cause despair and helplessness in caregivers. Caregivers may also feel tempted to punish the patient, for example, by becoming uncharacteristically inflexible or even verbally hostile or by withholding needed (e.g., pain) medication or care (e.g., more frequent visits).

Specific Management Strategies

While providing basic support and reassurance, clinicians should be careful not to become emotionally over-involved with the borderline patient. It is appropriate to counter the patient's frightening fantasies about illness and "overwhelming neediness" by scheduling frequent periodic check-ups and providing clear, nontechnical answers to questions. Caregivers may have to tolerate periodic angry outbursts, but it is appropriate to set firm limits on both the patient's disruptive behavior and on the caregiver's response. When a multidisciplinary team of clinicians is involved, meetings of all providers should be arranged, to allow them to vent their feelings about the patient and to reach consensus on a treatment plan. It is helpful to select a small number of caregivers to interact with the patient directly and to present the same clear and consistent plan. This approach often prevents splitting. Finally, it is essential to remain aware of these patients' potential for self-destructive and/or overly demanding behavior and not to retaliate by displaying anger at them when setting limits or even punishing them (e.g., not responding).

 CASE ILLUSTRATION 5

A primary care resident expresses concern about her patient Amanda to her clinic's attending physician. She is scheduled to leave the clinic in 3 months and believes that Amanda will find transferring to a new doctor difficult.

Amanda is a 35-year-old temporary clerical worker with a long-standing history of migraine headaches. She often delays taking medication until her migraine headaches become severe, and then calls the resident, complaining of unbearable pain, sometimes stating that the pain is so intolerable that she wishes to die. She sometimes comes to the clinic without a scheduled appointment, demanding to be seen right away. On the other hand, she often misses regularly scheduled appointments. During her visits, she expresses a fear of becoming homeless; she house-sits at other people's homes but does not have a stable place of her own.

The resident asks for a psychiatric consultation to help her work with Amanda. She is particularly concerned about Amanda's periodic statements that she wishes to die.

Following the psychiatrist's recommendations, the resident continues to schedule regular, brief follow-up appointments, and encourages Amanda to keep these appointments. She explains that this is not a walk-in clinic, and that Amanda will have to seek treatment for acute pain in the emergency room. She also reminds Amanda that taking medication early will likely keep the headache from becoming very intense.

Other helpful interventions include providing increased support to Amanda by referring her to a psychotherapist and asking the team social worker to assist her in finding a stable residence. It is also important to monitor Amanda for suicidal ideation. If she expresses a wish to die, the resident assesses her suicidal ideation and intent. One afternoon, Amanda drops in at the clinic expressing suicidal ideation, and a nurse practitioner calls for an urgent psychiatric consultation. After talking to the psychiatrist, Amanda gradually calms down and denies any suicidal intent; however, she refuses a referral for ongoing psychiatric treatment.

Over time, Amanda continues to miss some appointments, and occasionally becomes demanding or complains bitterly about the resident to the nurse practitioner. When both the resident and the nurse practitioner, however, firmly and supportively continue to reiterate their treatment plan—to meet with the doctor for regular appointments, to treat migraines early, and to go to the emergency room for acute pain—Amanda's unpredictable visits and non-compliance diminish. Periodic meetings between the resident and the nurse practitioner help them both present the same coherent plan to Amanda, thus minimizing splitting.

In planning ahead for her departure from the clinic, the resident and the attending physician discuss some helpful strategies to facilitate this transition, such as introducing the new resident to Amanda ahead of time and involving the nurse practitioner-who is staying at the clinic—in the process.

In this case, regular meetings of all the involved clinicians and staff (e.g., trainees, the attending physician, consultants, receptionist, and the nurse practitioner) allow them to present the same coherent plan to the patient, minimize the splitting, and reduce the patient's anxiety and unpredictable behavior. This approach successfully combines increased support and limit setting.

HISTRIONIC PERSONALITY DISORDER

Symptoms & Signs

Histrionic personality disorder is marked by excessive attention seeking and emotionalism. These patients may present with dramatic, theatrical shows of feeling, or they may dress or behave in a sexually provocative fashion in an unconscious effort to engage others and draw attention to themselves. The emotions they express may be shallow and inconsistent, but the patients may still believe that the sharing of those feelings creates a special closeness (which they often exaggerate) with the physician. These patients have a tendency to prefer subjective and intuitive impressions to objective, linear, logical thinking. They often have somatic complaints, with impressive—but inconsistent—presentations.

Differential Diagnosis

Histrionic personality disorder may be difficult to distinguish from narcissistic or borderline personality disorder, and patients in each of these categories may exhibit traits common to patients in the others. Patients with histrionic personality disorder are deeply affected by perceived frailties in relationship bonds, as are patients with borderline personality disorder. The latter, however, display less emotional stability and are more impulsive and self-destructive. Patients with histrionic personality disorder may crave attention—as patients with narcissistic personality disorder crave admiration—but the former tend to be less grandiose, arrogant, and self-absorbed.

Illness Experience & Illness Behavior

Medical illness represents a particular threat to the emotional well-being of patients with histrionic personality disorder, who derive much of their sense of self-worth and personal desirability from their sense of physical attractiveness. To reduce the fear of being deemed less desirable by others, these patients may attempt to bolster their physical appearance or embellish their abilities.

As a result, patients of either gender may engage in flirtatious or seductive behavior. When they feel weak and vulnerable, they may express their emotions with more intensity, in an attempt to strengthen their bond with the physician. In addition, because these patients focus on feelings, rather than on carefully observed physical symptoms, they may present with a collection of loosely connected somatic complaints. Their descriptions of the symptoms may reflect their desire to capture the physician's interest.

THE DOCTOR–PATIENT RELATIONSHIP

In working with the histrionic patient, the physician may be drawn in by the patient's dramatic and somewhat dependent style, become overly involved, and perhaps embark on an excessive workup. As the physician becomes increasingly engaged by the patient's style, the patient may then become anxious, distant, or noncompliant, puzzling and frustrating the physician. Alternatively, the physician may instead pursue too cursory an evaluation, because of a lack of objective information, or out of frustration with the patient's emotional and vague style.

Specific Management Strategies

Because the patient with histrionic personality disorder has a vague and global emotional (rather than a precise, logical) style and may display contrasting behaviors—that range from excessive anxiety about potentially minor symptoms to inappropriate indifference about significant medical problems—it is essential that the physician maintain an objective stance. The physician must offer a supportive and logical approach to the patient's problems. This requires being both sensitive to the patient's emotional concerns and sufficiently distanced to avoid any degree of closeness that the patient might misperceive as intimate or sexual.

CASE ILLUSTRATION 6

Rita is 38-year-old, single, unemployed actress with lupus. She is excessively friendly and flirtatious with her 45-year-old male physician, calling him frequently with questions about her medical problems and dressing somewhat seductively for office visits. During these visits she asks for examinations of a variety of somatic complaints. Over time, the physician becomes increasingly uncomfortable. Finally, Rita complains that she would like more time to discuss her problems at each office visit, and asks the physician if he thinks her problems "deserve more time."

After reflecting on the chronicity of this pattern of behavior, the physician responds that Rita's medical problems are significant and deserving of attention. He states that he intends to evaluate each of them

carefully, allocating time on the basis of his impression of their medical necessity. He also says that he understands that she would like more time to discuss her concerns, but that as a busy doctor he cannot make additional time available to her. He suggests, gently, that if he cannot provide adequate emotional support to her, he could refer her to a local clinic's health psychologist. Although she is rather disappointed, Rita is able to accept this limit setting and continues to work with this doctor.

This approach is successful because the physician shows positive regard for the patient and her problems—while clearly setting the limits of the doctor–patient relationship.

NARCISSISTIC PERSONALITY DISORDER

Symptoms & Signs

Narcissistic personality disorder is characterized by a long-standing pattern of grandiosity, with a need for praise and admiration that stands out in contrast to a lack of sensitivity to the feelings of others. These persons may have an exaggerated sense of self-importance and social status and require excessive admiration. They may be driven toward attaining an idealized position in terms of social, personal, romantic, or career accomplishment. In this regard, they may be envious and potentially devaluing of others whose accomplishments they perceive as exceeding their own. Beneath the grandiosity and devaluation exists an underlying view of self as inferior or inadequate. To avoid these beliefs and their associated painful effects, patients seek to convince self and others of their "specialness" or "unusual talent."

Differential Diagnosis

Narcissistic personality disorder may be difficult to distinguish from borderline, antisocial, histrionic, or obsessive-compulsive personality disorders, and in many cases it may overlap with these disorders. When the differentiation is unclear, identifying a high degree of grandiosity and a need for admiration can help clarify the diagnosis. In contrast to persons with borderline personality disorder, persons with narcissistic personality disorder have a more stable self-image and display less impulsiveness and sensitivity to relationship losses. In addition, persons with narcissistic personality disorder are generally less aggressive and deceitful than are persons with antisocial personality disorder, who also display evidence of childhood conduct disorder. Persons with histrionic personality disorder, in contrast, may be relatively more dramatic and emotional than those with narcissistic personality disorder. Although persons with narcissistic personality disorder, like those with obsessive-compulsive personality disorder, may be perfectionists, the former often have a higher self-assessment of their accomplishments.

Clinicians must be careful not to misdiagnose a person with transient hypomanic or manic grandiosity as having narcissistic personality disorder. Similarly, it is important to distinguish between narcissistic personality disorder and transient substance-related personality changes (e.g., from central nervous system stimulants) or personality changes caused by a general medical condition.

Illness Experience & Illness Behavior

Health problems are a particular blow to patients with narcissistic personality disorder. Illness threatens these patients' unconscious attempts to maintain an intrapsychic and external image of untarnished well-being, resiliency, and superiority. Medical problems and physical limitations may disrupt this image, threaten their public personas, and leave them fearing disruption of their (unrealistically unchallengeable) sense of self. In an attempt to defend against this threat, patients may minimize the significance of symptoms or deny the presence of the illness. More commonly, as patients try to recapture their admired, idealized status, they may demand special treatment, second opinions, or transfer of care to more "senior" or "well-known" clinicians. These patients may devalue, criticize, or question the behavior or credentials of the treating physician, or they may fail to comply with treatment recommendations.

THE DOCTOR–PATIENT RELATIONSHIP

Narcissistic patients' arrogant and grandiose behavior, combined with demands for special treatment, can be extremely irritating to physicians. Reactions to these patients can take many forms. Sometimes, in an attempt to avoid conflict, physicians submit to the demands. With particularly critical patients, providers may feel frustration, resentment, and even anger. Alternatively, they may feel devalued and question their own competence. Frustration may be especially great if the physician expends special energy on behalf of a charismatic or demanding patient, only to later become the butt of unfair criticism. Physicians may reject or avoid the patient, withhold treatment, or respond in an angry manner—responses that can harm both the patient and the doctor–patient relationship.

Specific Management Strategies

The most effective strategy for dealing with narcissistic patients is to be respectful and nonconfrontational about their sense of specialness and entitlement and to help them use their self-perceived talents in the service of their treatment. If narcissistic patients feel vulnerable and threatened by the illness, they are more likely to criticize and devalue the physician. Thus, physicians should not take this devaluation personally, and instead understand it as the patients' attempt to cope with their own intense insecurity. Providers can appeal to the patients' narcissism by explaining that they chose a particular course of action because they believe it represents the best possible care—a course of action they feel the patients deserve. Physicians can further support the patients by validating their concerns about the illness and pointing to their patients' ability to respond competently to its challenges. This approach helps the patients feel more secure and able, allowing them to ally confidently with—rather than defensively attack—their physicians.

   CASE ILLUSTRATION 7

Maggie, a 44-year-old married female lawyer who is quite prominent in the community, is an unusually demanding patient. She becomes very angry with her male physician, whom she accuses of not responding adequately to her complaints about menopausal symptoms. In fact, the physician has done all the necessary laboratory tests, has conferred extensively with the patient's gynecologist, and has answered numerous phone calls by the patient over a period of several months.

The physician, aware of Maggie's long-standing sense of entitlement and her extreme sensitivity to slights, responds by reviewing her concerns, discussing the treatment plan and rationale, and encouraging her to discuss some of her emotional reactions to this unexpectedly early menopause. He then emphasizes the special consideration he has put into her evaluation and treatment plan. He arranges more frequent office visits and tells Maggie that he predicts a relatively good response to treatment, given her active involvement in her own care.

This response is reassuring to the patient, because it validates her concerns and satisfies her narcissistic feelings of entitlement.

AVOIDANT PERSONALITY DISORDER

Symptoms & Signs

Patients with avoidant personality disorder have a long-standing pattern of excessive anxiety in social situations and in intimate relationships, and extreme hypersensitivity to what other people think about them. These patients desire relationships but avoid them because of fears of being rejected, humiliated, or embarrassed. If they do engage in social situations or relationships, they are constantly preoccupied with being rejected, criticized, and not being liked by others. As a result, these patients have low self-esteem, feel socially inept, have feelings of inferiority, and are shy and inhibited.

Differential Diagnosis

Patients with schizoid personality disorder also avoid social situations and relationships but they do desire social isolation. In contrast, patients with avoidant personality disorder strongly desire relationships but avoid them because of anxiety and fears of rejection and humiliation.

Avoidant personality disorder should be distinguished from social phobia. Whereas patients with avoidant personality disorder try to avoid social interactions in general, patients with social phobia usually have more specific concerns related to social performance, such as saying something inappropriate to unfamiliar people at a social gathering.

Illness Experience & Illness Behavior

Illness provokes anxiety and increases feelings of ineptness in patients with avoidant personality disorder. Patients may delay care or not be forthcoming about their problems out of fear of not being liked or being rejected by the caregiver. They may blame their physical discomfort on themselves and may actually not ask for appropriate pain relief. Because these patients feel that they may not deserve attention by their physician, they may be reluctant to undergo necessary medical procedures.

The Doctor–Patient Relationship

Physicians treating patients with avoidant personality disorder may initially not realize the full extent of their patients' symptoms. Because these patients are shy and easily agreeable to what their physicians propose, physicians may be prone to take a more paternalistic stance with them. If they discover later that the patient's symptoms are more severe than initially reported, clinicians may react with concern or feel betrayed by the patient for withholding information and for their passive attitude.

Specific Management Strategies

Patients with avoidant personality disorder need reassurance and permission to express their distress and concerns in a nonjudgmental environment. It is helpful for health care providers to explain that they are interested in knowing about the patient's problems.

CASE ILLUSTRATION 8

Michael, a 45-year-old single office clerk, presents 45 minutes early for his annual check-up with his primary care physician. While signing in at the reception desk, he asks whether he has arrived on time for his appointment.

The physician finds a marked rash over the patient's elbows upon physical examination. The patient has a known history of psoriasis. Michael's face turns red out of embarrassment. He starts to explain that he applied the cream that his physician prescribed for him last year but that he ran out of the prescription some time ago. When asked why he did not call the physician's office for a refill, Michael states that he felt that he should not bother his physician for just a rash.

The physician expresses concern about the patient's rash. He writes a new prescription and asks Michael to call his office for a refill once he finishes the prescription. The doctor explains to the patient that he does not feel bothered by the patient's phone calls and that communication between patient and doctor is necessary to ensure appropriate medical care. He again requests that Michael call him for any refills or problems in the future.

This reassuring and supportive approach encourages the patient to communicate with his physician and not hold back out of fear of being rejected.

DEPENDENT PERSONALITY DISORDER

Symptoms & Signs

Patients with dependent personality disorder have a pervasive and excessive need to be taken care of. They experience intense fear of separation and abandonment and feel great discomfort when they are alone. This leads to submissive and clinging behavior in their interpersonal relationships. These patients have difficulty making independent decisions without a great deal of advice and reassurance, and they are afraid of disagreeing with others.

Differential Diagnosis

It is important to distinguish dependent personality disorder from the dependency that arises from panic disorder, mood disorders, or agoraphobia. Patients suffering from medical illnesses may also become very dependent on others, without having this disorder. Dependent personality disorder can sometimes be confused with other personality disorders, and dependent personality traits may be the result of chronic substance abuse.

Illness Experience & Illness Behavior

Patients with dependent personality disorder fear that illness will lead to both helplessness and abandonment by others. In their interactions with caregivers, they may become very needy and make dramatic demands for urgent medical attention. If the response is not what they wish, they may display angry outbursts at the physician. They may also blame their physical discomfort on others, including their physician. In addition, they may use addictive substances or overuse medications in a desperate attempt to obtain immediate relief from their suffering. Because receiving medical care may fulfill their wishes for attention from others, some dependent patients may unconsciously contribute to prolonging their illness, or—in some extreme cases— they may encourage unnecessary medical procedures.

THE DOCTOR–PATIENT RELATIONSHIP

Clinicians treating patients with dependent personality disorder may initially react with aversion to their patients' clingy and demanding behavior. Alternatively, clinicians may find it difficult to set limits on their availability and may try to provide reassurance by attempting to meet every demand, which ultimately leads to burnout or feelings of inadequacy. Eventually, caregivers may react in a hostile fashion and openly reject these patients.

Specific Management Strategies

Effective ways to provide reassurance to dependent patients and allay their fear of being abandoned include scheduling frequent periodic check-ups and being consistently available. It is nonetheless important to provide firm, realistic limits to this availability early in treatment or as soon as the patient's dependent traits become apparent. To prevent burnout, enlist other members of the health care team in providing support for the patient. In addition, physicians should help these patients find outside support systems to lessen fears of abandonment. They must also be alert to the patients' potential contribution to prolonging their illness or to their possible abuse of substances or medications.

CASE ILLUSTRATION 9

Terry, a 50-year-old divorced secretary, repeatedly presents to her primary care physician complaining of various somatic symptoms, including dizziness, headaches, blurred vision, and leg pains. Repeated workups of her symptoms are negative, and her evaluation for major depression is negative. Further inquiry into Terry's life reveals that after her divorce 6 years ago, her daughter became the focus of her life. Even though her history of occasional somatic symptoms goes back to her teenage years, there had been no appreciable change until 2 years ago, when her daughter got married and left her home.

Terry makes frequent phone calls to her doctor. She usually sounds nervous, expresses concern about some new symptom, and asks for medication. The doctor decides to schedule regular follow-up appointments to address Terry's concerns. Terry often complains during office visits that there is not enough time to evaluate all her symptoms and laments that her daughter no longer has much time for her. Her doctor listens in a supportive manner and acknowledges that the available appointment time is limited, explaining how he will ultimately address all the complaints. He also emphasizes the importance of continuing to meet for regular appointments. In addition, the doctor acknowledges Terry's increased sense of isolation after her daughter's marriage and evaluates her for possible major depression. He further suggests a referral to the clinic's social worker as a means of helping her pursue a volunteer activity and increase her social interactions.

This approach usually helps diminish the patient's anxiety and decreases the frequency of phone calls. If the patient's distress does not improve with such interventions, a referral for psychotherapy and evaluation for a possible underlying anxiety disorder are indicated.

OBSESSIVE-COMPULSIVE PERSONALITY DISORDER

Symptoms & Signs

Individuals with obsessive-compulsive personality disorder are preoccupied with orderliness, perfectionism, and control. They are excessively concerned with details and rules, tend to be overly moralistic, and are usually focused on work to the exclusion of leisure. They find it difficult to adapt themselves to others and instead insist that others follow their plans. Their general inflexibility and restricted emotional expression betray an underlying fear of losing control. Because they can be indecisive, they feel distressed when faced with the need to make decisions.

Differential Diagnosis

Obsessive-compulsive disorder (see Chapter 26) is distinguished from obsessive-compulsive personality disorder by the presence of actual obsessions (repetitive intrusive thoughts) and compulsions. Sometimes, however, both disorders coexist in one patient, and obsessive-compulsive personality disorder can also be confused with other personality disorders.

Illness Experience & Illness Behavior

Illness is threatening to persons with obsessive-compulsive personality disorder because it generates an intense fear of losing control over bodily functions and emotions. Patients may experience extremely unsettling feelings of shame and vulnerability. They may also feel anger at the disruption of their usual daily routines by medical appointments and treatments. They may fear having to relinquish control to health care providers. In the physician's office, their intense anxiety tends to drive them to ask repetitive questions and to pay excessive attention to detail.

THE DOCTOR–PATIENT RELATIONSHIP

Caregivers may react to patients with obsessive-compulsive personality disorder by becoming impatient at their repetitive questions, cutting their answers short. They may feel their competence challenged by their patients' insistence on knowing every single detail and reason for choosing a particular treatment. Clinicians may also inadvertently attempt to control treatment planning rather than making it a joint effort, without realizing how important it is for these patients to remain in control.

Specific Management Strategies

Helpful strategies in working with patients with obsessive-compulsive personality disorder include taking a comprehensive history, performing a careful diagnostic workup, giving patients a clear and thorough explanation of their diagnosis and treatment options, and providing and explaining laboratory test results. It is important not to overemphasize uncertainties about treatments or the patient's possible response to treatment. Patients find it reassuring when clinicians cite literature reports and avoid vague and inexact impressionistic explanations. It is helpful to treat these patients as equal partners, encourage self-monitoring, allow their participation in treatment, and give them recognition for their clear reasoning and high standards.

 CASE ILLUSTRATION 10

Sam, a 42-year-old biochemist, requests an appointment with his primary care physician for evaluation of an uncomfortable lump in his left groin. The physician is familiar with Sam's mild nervousness during routine medical check-ups and his tendency to ask detailed questions about his health. After a physical examination, the doctor diagnoses an inguinal hernia and recommends a surgical consultation for further evaluation and possible surgery. Sam, in his usual formal and somewhat restricted manner—but this time appearing visibly more anxious—repeatedly asks several questions about surgical repair, whether the literature discusses any alternative treatments, and what guidelines physicians follow to recommend one treatment over another. He then asks questions about the risks of general anesthesia and whether this procedure can be performed under local anesthesia.

When the physician tries to reassure him that this is a routine procedure, Sam asks him whether he is sure of his diagnosis; he also asks him to list the criteria he used in diagnosing the inguinal hernia. Sam also talks at length about his responsibilities at work and expresses concern that surgery might disrupt ongoing projects at his laboratory, as several people depend on him for regular supervision. He also wants to know how long his doctor has known the recommended surgeon, and whether they have worked together in the past.

Reassurance is essential here. The doctor explains that the surgeon is both trustworthy and well known to him. He praises Sam for his thoroughness and initiative in finding out about treatment alternatives before making a decision. He answers basic questions in a precise manner and defers some questions to the surgeon, explaining that these will be better answered by a specialist. He reassures Sam that he will not wait for a written report but will personally contact the surgeon after the consultation to discuss treatment options. The physician also suggests a follow-up appointment to help Sam with his decision.

Although Sam continues to express concern that the surgery will disrupt his work, his anxiety decreases somewhat after the physician takes his concerns seriously. His questions are answered precisely, and the physician further suggests an article in the literature that he can read to learn more about the treatment of inguinal hernias.

TREATMENT OF PERSONALITY DISORDERS

Effective psychopharmacological treatment does not exist for a given personality disorder. Nevertheless, pharmacotherapy plays an important role. Medication can be beneficial in targeting symptom clusters within the disorder and in treating other comorbid disorders, such as major depression, bipolar affective disorder, substance abuse, posttraumatic stress disorder, panic disorder, social anxiety, and obsessive–compulsive disorder.

Symptoms such as paranoid ideation and suspiciousness in patients with cluster A disorders (paranoid, schizoid, and schizotypal personality disorder) may improve with low-dose antipsychotic treatment (e.g., haloperidol, risperidone, olanzapine, ziprasidone, quetiapine, and aripiprazole). In case of overt psychotic symptoms, a psychiatric consultation and treatment with an antipsychotic medication should be considered.

Patients with cluster B disorders (antisocial, borderline, histrionic, and narcissistic personality disorder), who often appear dramatic and emotional, should be evaluated for prominent mood symptoms and the coexistence of an Axis I disorder, especially mood, anxiety, and substance-abuse disorders.

Patients with prominent depressive symptoms should be treated with selective serotonin reuptake inhibitors (SSRIs) or other antidepressants, such as fluoxetine, sertraline, paroxetine, citalopram, and escitalopram. Patients with prominent mood swings, irritability, or impulsive behaviors may be candidates for treatment with a mood stabilizer (e.g., valproate or lithium) or a second-generation antipsychotic. However, a psychiatric consultation is recommended for this type of treatment. Medications have been most extensively used in patients with borderline personality disorder. Borderline patients with more affective dysregulation can be considered for treatment with an antidepressant, mood stabilizer, and/or low-dose antipsychotic medication. Antipsychotics can also be considered in borderline patients with dissociative or psychotic symptoms.

Anxiety and fear are the most dominant symptoms of patients with cluster C disorders (avoidant, dependent, and obsessive-compulsive personality disorder). Symptoms in these patients may improve by treatment with an SSRI. Time-limited symptomatic treatment with a benzodiazepine might be considered.

In addition to psychopharmacological treatments, patients may be referred for various psychosocial and psychotherapeutic treatments, including dialectical behavioral therapy for borderline personality disorder, cognitive behavioral therapy, and psychodynamic therapies.

SUGGESTED READINGS

Fogel BS. Personality disorders in the medical setting. In: Stoudemire A, Fogel BS, eds. *Psychiatric Care of the Medical Patient*. New York, NY: Oxford University Press, 2000.

Gabbard GO. Psychotherapy of personality disorders. *J Psychother Pract Res* 2000;9:1–6.

Geringer ES, Stern TA. Coping with medical illness: the impact of personality types. *Psychosomatics* 1986;27:251–261.

Giesen-Bloo J, van Dyck R, Spinhoven P, et al. Outpatient psychotherapy for borderline personality disorder: randomized trial of schema-focused therapy vs transference-focused psychotherapy. *Arch Gen Psychiatry* 2006;63:649–658. [Erratum in: *Arch Gen Psychiatry* 2006;63:1008.]

Grant BF, Hasin DS, Stinson FS, et al. Prevalence, correlates, and disability of personality disorders in the United States: results from the national epidemiologic survey on alcohol and related conditions. *J Clin Psychiatry* 2004;65:948–958.

Gross R, Olfson M, Gameroff M, et al. Borderline personality disorder in primary care. *Arch Intern Med* 2002;162:53–60.

Gunderson JD. Borderline Personality Disorder. *A Clinical Guide*. Washington, DC: American Psychiatric Publishing, 2001.

Linehan MM, Comtois KA, Murray AM, et al. Two-year randomized controlled trial and follow-up of dialectical behavior therapy vs therapy by experts for suicidal behaviors and borderline personality disorder. *Arch Gen Psychiatry* 2006;63:757–766.

Markovitz PJ. Related articles, links: recent trends in the pharmacotherapy of personality disorders. *J Personal Disord* 2004;18: 90–101.

Marmar C. Personality disorders. In: Goldman H, ed. *Review of General Psychiatry*. New York, NY: McGraw-Hill, 2000.

Svraki DM, Cloninger RC. Personality disorders. In: Saddock B, Saddock V, eds. *Comprehensive Textbook of Psychiatry*. Philadelphia, PA: Lippincott Williams & Wilkins, 2005.

Dementia & Delirium

30

Anna Chodos, MD, MPH; Bree Johnston, MD, MPH;
& Kristine Yaffe, MD

INTRODUCTION

Dementia is a common disorder with a prevalence that doubles every 5 years after the age of 60 years, thereby affecting up to 45% of those aged 85 years and older. Dementia is defined as an acquired, persistent, and usually progressive impairment in intellectual function, with compromise in multiple cognitive domains, at least one of which is memory. The deficits must represent a significant decline in function, and must be severe enough to interfere with work or social life for the diagnosis to be formally applied. As the disorder progresses, individuals with dementia often fail to recognize family members, are unable to express themselves clearly and meaningfully, and often undergo dramatic personality changes. Table 30-1 lists some of the more common causes of dementia.

Despite the high prevalence of dementia, the diagnosis is often missed by clinicians, particularly in the early stages. The primary care practitioner can play an important role in diagnosing and treating dementia. An early diagnosis can offer the opportunity to involve patients in meaningful advance care planning while they are still able to express their preferences clearly. In addition, potentially treatable causes, though rare, are more likely to be partially or fully reversed if diagnosed early. Later in the disease, the practitioner can work with other team members to manage difficult behaviors, ensure that the patient is as comfortable and safe as possible, recognize when referral for specialist care is needed, educate caregivers about the condition, and support caregivers in coping with their situations to the best of their abilities. Furthermore, with several pharmacological treatments available for dementing illnesses, it has become more important for physicians to be proficient in diagnosing specific subtypes of dementia and knowing what therapies may (or may not) be helpful for that syndrome.

TYPES OF DEMENTIA

Alzheimer Disease

Alzheimer disease (AD) is the most common form of dementia, accounting for about 60–70% of the cases. The age of onset varies considerably, but most commonly symptoms arise after the age of 70 years. Incidence of the disease increases with age. Women may be at a slightly higher risk of developing the disorder than men. The rare patient with early onset of AD (before the age of 60 years) may have a genetic disorder with an autosomal dominant pattern of inheritance, so a thorough family history is important in these cases.

Alzheimer disease usually follows a slow, but progressive and insidious, course (Table 30-2). Life expectancy following the appearance of the disorder ranges from 3 to 15 years, but considerable variation may occur, and survival of up to 20 years has been reported. Memory deficits are prominent in all dementias, but especially so in AD. Typically, short-term episodic memory problems are the first and most obvious manifestation of the disorder. Alzheimer disease affects both the encoding and retrieval of new information to a profound degree, such that these patients do not appear to benefit from cueing and prompting of memory. For example, a patient asked to remember the words "piano," "carrot," and "green" may not be helped by hints such as "musical instrument," "vegetable," or "color." Although diagnostic certainty is less than 100% without pathological examination, careful clinical and neuropsychological evaluation results in a reliable diagnosis of the disease in most instances. A computed tomography (CT) or magnetic resonance imaging (MRI) scan often shows cerebral atrophy and hippocampal volume loss; the electroencephalogram (EEG) may show diffuse slowing.

Table 30-1. Common causes of dementia.

- Alzheimer disease (AD)
- Vascular disease (multiple infarcts and other cerebrovascular disease)
- Dementia with Lewy Bodies (DLB)
- Frontotemporal dementia (FTD)
- Parkinson disease
- Metabolic and potentially reversible disease (e.g., chronic vitamin B_{12} deficiency, hypothyroidism)
- HIV/AIDS
- Neurodegenerative disorders (e.g., Huntington chorea, progressive supranuclear palsy)

CASE ILLUSTRATION 1

Gertrude is 74 years old. She is brought by her family to a medical clinic for evaluation. Since the death of her husband 2 years ago, Gertrude has become increasingly absentminded, withdrawn, and sedentary. Her family assumed at first that she was grieving and would eventually readjust. Gertrude's condition, however, has continued to deteriorate. Now she is confused and disoriented and has difficulty recognizing family members. Her general physical examination is normal, but her mental status examination reveals multiple deficits. For example, given three words to remember, she is unable to recall any of them after several minutes. She cannot give the correct month and year and thinks she is in the city where she had lived many years ago. Asked to repeat several sentences, she makes a number of verbal slips. When she is given a geometric design to copy, her drawing is distorted and unrecognizable. Her laboratory examinations are normal, a CT scan of the head shows mild cerebral atrophy, and no other potential explanations for her deficits are found. A diagnosis of AD is eventually made.

In retrospect, her family recalls that Gertrude had been having some mild difficulties in memory and functioning prior to her husband's death and had been dependent on him for helping her to manage things. Recognition of Gertrude's emerging dementia had been made more difficult by her grief and possible depression after her husband's death.

The physician spends some time with family members discussing the nature of Gertrude's condition and options for future care. She inquires about immediate concerns such as agitation and other behavioral disturbances, none of which is currently present. The physician then refers the family to a social worker specializing in geriatric issues and indicates the availability of groups such as the Family

Table 30-2. Stages of Alzheimer Disease.

Stage	General Change	Specific Change
Early	Patients show relatively subtle changes in memory, along with declining clarity of thought and ability to perform everyday tasks. These changes may go largely unnoticed by the patient and significant others. Patients typically retain some ability to compensate for the cognitive changes.	• Mild memory problems such as missed appointments, failure to pay bills. • Occasional mild and transitory confusion and disorientation. • A "slowed-down" quality to thinking, personality, and lifestyle. • An increase in personal rigidity and intolerance of changes. • Social isolation, loss of interest in usual activities. • Possible increase in restlessness and impulsivity.
Middle	Cognitive deficits become more prominent during this stage and the loss of functioning becomes obvious to others.	• Severe memory impairment. • Frank and persistent confusion and disorientation. • Aphasia, apraxia, and visuospatial disturbances. • Serious difficulties in the ability to manage everyday activities. • Agitation, simple paranoia, other delusions.
Late	In the third, and terminal, stage of the disorder, the patient becomes very inactive, is extremely withdrawn, and loses nearly all ability to engage in purposeful activities.	• Profound loss of short- and long-term memory. • Severe confusion and disorientation. • Bladder and bowel incontinence. • Patient eventually is bedridden and nonresponsive. • Primitive reflexes such as grasping, rooting, and sucking are present. • Seizures. • Signs of gross neurologic impairment, such as hemiplegia, tremor, pronounced rigidity. • Bodily wasting despite adequate nourishment weeks to months prior to death.

Note: The signs and symptoms of dementia include the progressive loss of cognitive abilities, especially memory, and a decline in everyday functioning. Dementia is generally a deteriorating condition, and its progression is best described in terms of several stages. The stages outlined above are based on the most common form of dementia, AD.

Caregiver Alliance for education and support. She also advises Gertrude not to drive, and, in accordance with the law in her state, notifies the health department of the new diagnosis of dementia. Finally, the physician initiates a trial of donepezil, which is associated with no obvious benefits at 3 months, according to the family. The physician and family elect to continue treatment for another 3 months and reevaluate the treatment at that time.

Dementia with Lewy Bodies

Dementia with Lewy Bodies (DLB) is reported to be the second most common cause of dementia in autopsy studies, accounting for 15–30% of the cases. It is defined by the presence of cognitive impairment, parkinsonism, prominent (often bizarre) hallucinations or other psychotic symptoms, and fluctuations in alertness, although patients may not have all of these symptoms. Patients with DLB are often intolerant of traditional antipsychotic medications, and their use can induce severe parkinsonism or even death. At least one randomized-controlled trial suggests that cholinesterase inhibitors may be useful in treating the disorder.

Vascular Dementia

Previously known as multi-infarct dementia, vascular dementia is characterized by the development of cognitive impairment in association with single or multiple areas of infarction and/or subcortical ischemia. Not surprisingly, the risk factors for vascular dementia are identical to the risk factors for cerebrovascular disease, including smoking, hypertension, diabetes mellitus, coronary artery disease (CAD), and previous history of stroke. A patchy and inconsistent pattern of deficits may be seen initially, with relative preservation of some cognitive areas. Because vascular dementia can result from insults to a variety of cortical or subcortical areas, the neuropsychological profile of patients with vascular dementia can be quite varied.

Focal neurologic signs are more common in vascular dementia than in AD, and lateralized motor and sensory findings may be seen. CT and MRI scans frequently reveal multiple areas of infarction in the brain, often with diffuse subcortical white matter changes. Later in the course of the disorder, atrophy from loss of brain tissue may be seen.

A number of diagnostic criteria for vascular dementia have been proposed, but none are sensitive or specific enough to rule the diagnosis in or out with certainty. Many elders show diffuse white matter changes on brain imaging, and yet are cognitively intact. Other demented elders, who were thought by their clinicians to have vascular dementia because of cognitive decline following cerebral infarcts, are subsequently found to have Alzheimer's pathology at autopsy in addition to the known infarcts. Such individuals, with elements of both AD and vascular dementia, are considered to have mixed dementia. In short, current diagnostic instruments and criteria are often inadequate for clinicians confidently to employ or reject the "vascular dementia" label.

Other Causes

Frontotemporal dementias (FTDs) are a group of disorders characterized by personality change (e.g., apathy or socially inappropriate behavior), hyperorality, and cognitive decline especially involving language and executive function. Frontotemporal dementia tends to affect individuals at a younger age than AD, with many persons receiving the diagnosis in their 50s or 60s. Imaging studies may show marked atrophy in frontal and temporal lobes.

Advanced Parkinson disease commonly results in dementia. These patients frequently display mental sluggishness and a general lack of spontaneity. Language functions (compared with those of AD patients) are relatively preserved.

Chronic alcohol abuse can result in serious cognitive deficits if drinking is severe and prolonged, although it is not clear whether the dementing process occurs in the absence of coexisting thiamine deficiency. Severe head trauma can also result in permanent cognitive impairment, which might be viewed as static dementia.

Human immunodeficiency virus (HIV)-1-associated dementia (HAD) is caused by the direct infection of the brain by the HIV-1 virus. It is associated with late-stage AIDS and is generally seen in individuals whose T-cell count has fallen below 200. Features of this form of dementia are summarized in Table 30-3. HIV-1-associated dementia is discussed further in Chapter 36. Creutzfeldt–Jacob disease is a rare infectious cause that should be suspected when a nonelderly person develops a rapidly dementing illness associated with other neurologic deficits such as myoclonus.

Table 30-3. Signs and symptoms of advanced HIV-associated dementia.

- Impaired attention and difficulty learning new information
- Slow, soft, and impoverished speech
- Ataxia, decreased manual dexterity, and motor slowness
- Poor judgment
- Flat and unspontaneous facial expression with fixed gaze
- Personality changes that may include apathy or increased impulsivity

Table 30-4. Treatable syndromes that impair cognition.

Hydrocephalus	Chronic subdural hematoma
Metabolic disorders: hypercalcemia, hyper- and hypoglycemia, hyper- and hyponatremia, hyperuricemia	CNS infection (meningitis, encephalitis, abscess)
Myxedema	Medication side effects or toxicity
Hepatic encephalopathy	Vitamin deficiencies: B_{12}, thiamine, niacin
Depression	Delirium
Status epilepticus	CNS malignancy

Reversible Conditions

A number of medical conditions can result in cognitive impairment. These may be treatable, but full or partial reversal of dementia is relatively rare, even with appropriate treatment. However, because dementia is such a devastating diagnosis, assessing the patient for these conditions is an important part of the dementia workup. Fully or partially reversible dementia syndromes are usually the result of depression, medication, or a toxic or metabolic disorder. The most common types of primary and secondary treatable syndromes are listed in Table 30-4.

Differential Diagnosis

Persons suspected of having dementia are encountered in a number of medical settings. For example, a patient who presents to the emergency department with confusion, disorientation, and hallucinations should be evaluated for delirium (e.g., from infection, metabolic derangement, or use of or withdrawal from medications or recreational substances) and psychotic disorders. An older adult with a history of recent bereavement, withdrawal, and increased forgetfulness may indeed be demented, or may be suffering from cognitive deficits related to major depression. Other problems that initially may be confused with dementia include sensory deficits (severe visual or hearing impairment), aphasia, developmental disability, and low levels of literacy or education.

Normal Aging

As people age, some degree of decline in cognitive functioning is common. The presence of mild memory impairment among older adults has been reported to occur among a very wide range (11–96%) of participants in various research studies. Normal aging often brings minor word-finding difficulties, slowed memory retrieval, and some changes in the speed and efficiency of thought. These changes, however, typically do not cause significant problems in everyday functioning or produce confusion or disorientation, which are signs of impaired cognition (see Chapter 14).

Mild Cognitive Impairment

Mild cognitive impairment (MCI) is an increasingly recognized condition in which a patient complains of memory problems, demonstrates mild deficits (most commonly in short-term memory) on formal testing, but does not meet criteria for dementia. Dementia will develop in roughly 10% of people with MCI each year. Amnestic MCI, in which the deficit is primarily episodic memory, is more likely to progress to AD than nonamnestic MCI, which may be more pathophysiologically heterogeneous. At the time of this writing, no medication intended for the treatment of MCI has been approved by the FDA. Acetylcholinesterase inhibitors have shown mixed results in clinical trials. Any potentially reversible conditions, including depression, hearing loss, or B_{12} deficiency, should be addressed in patients with MCI. They also should be advised to complete advance care planning and followed with serial clinical evaluation at least every 6 months.

New Diagnostic Criteria for Alzheimer Disease and Mild Cognitive Impairment

Research suggests that AD pathophysiology begins many years and possibly decades prior to the clinical expression of the disease. In an attempt to identify a preclinical phase of AD and to improve the accuracy of the diagnosis of AD and MCI, several working groups have suggested new guidelines and diagnostic criteria. Many of these incorporate biomarker measures (either from neuroimaging or cerebrospinal fluid) as these may provide direct evidence of the underlying pathophysiology associated with AD. How these new guidelines will be incorporated into clinical practice is uncertain. In particular, the concept of a preclinical phase of AD will require much greater research and public health policy guidelines.

Dementia versus Delirium

 CASE ILLUSTRATION 2

George is an 80-year-old man who is admitted through the emergency department with a fracture of the femoral neck. He undergoes an open reduction and internal fixation. On the second postoperative day, he develops agitation, pulls out his IV, and

is restrained. Physical examination reveals an elderly man who is inattentive, moaning, and seeming to drift in and out of the conversation. The consultant notes that the patient was given 50 mg of diphenhydramine as a "sleeper" the night before, and he now appears to have a distended bladder. Placement of a Foley catheter, around-the-clock treatment with opioids, low-dose haloperidol, and having family members at his bedside, all seem to help calm him down. Over the next 3 days, he receives no further diphenhydramine, his pain improves, his catheter is removed, and his mental status clears somewhat, but not to his baseline level.

The family says that George had very mild dementia, but seemed to be functioning well at home prior to his hip fracture. Following hospital discharge, he goes to a nursing home for short-term rehabilitation, but he never seems to regain his former level of cognition or functioning. He lives in a nursing home for the remaining years of his life. He dies of apparent aspiration pneumonia after a period of progressive functional and cognitive decline.

Delirium is a state of cognitive impairment that is acute in onset and associated with fluctuations in mental status and behavior, inattention, disorganized thinking, and an altered level of consciousness. Because dementia is a significant risk factor for delirium, the two syndromes are closely linked (Table 30-5). It is not uncommon for delirious patients to be incorrectly labeled as demented by an inpatient team with no prior knowledge of the patient. Optimized communication between inpatient and outpatient teams, good baseline mental status testing on elderly outpatients, and/or collateral information from family and friends, can often be critical in trying to determine how likely it is that the delirious patient will "clear" enough to be able to live independently following hospital discharge. Unfortunately, some patients, like George, never return to their prior level of functioning following an episode of delirium.

Delirium is usually caused by toxic and metabolic derangements or infections. In determining the cause, a clinician should consider reviewing the medication record (looking for recent changes); checking blood cell counts, electrolytes, renal function, glucose, calcium, and urinalysis; and reviewing a chest film and electrocardiogram. In general, workup does not need to include neuroimaging or lumbar puncture unless routine labs or medication review is unrevealing, or focal neurologic deficits or fever are present.

Most studies have suggested that prevention of delirium is more effective than treatment. Preventive strategies include avoiding anticholinergic medications (like diphenhydramine); treating pain adequately; promoting normal sleep patterns; keeping patients active, stimulated, socially connected, and oriented during the day; making certain vision and hearing aids are available; promoting adequate hydration; and avoiding unnecessary tubes and catheters. Established delirium, if disruptive to care, is probably best treated with low-dose haloperidol, 0.5 mg once or twice daily. If the delirium is related to alcohol or benzodiazepine withdrawal, benzodiazepines are the treatment of choice.

Dementia versus Depression

Especially among older adults, symptoms of depression may masquerade as dementia (Table 30-6) making it difficult to distinguish between "true" dementia and the dementia syndrome of depression (DSD, formerly called "pseudodementia"). It has become increasingly apparent that depressed patients who present with cognitive impairment are much more likely to go on to develop true dementia within a few years. Formal neuropsychological testing and/or an empiric trial of antidepressant medication may provide the best means of distinguishing between dementia and DSD.

Dementia versus Psychotic Disorders

The symptoms of psychotic disorders, such as schizophrenia or bipolar disorder, may resemble the disorganization, confusion, delusions, and agitation that sometimes accompany dementia. The typical presence of more consistent and systematized delusions and the increased likelihood of previous psychosis and a family psychiatric history among individuals with nondementia-related psychotic disorders are important in making this differentiation.

Table 30-5. Delirium versus dementia: signs and symptoms.

Delirium	Dementia
• Rapid onset; short duration	• Insidious onset; progressive deterioration
• May show heightened autonomic arousal	• No impairment in autonomic arousal
• Clouded consciousness or gross confusion	• Alertness retained in early stages
• Prominent waxing and waning	• Consistently impaired mentation except in late-stage dementia
• Often restless, agitated, hypervigilant, or lethargic	• Agitation less prominent; varies with stress
• Gross perceptual distortions and hallucinations common	• If psychotic, usually vague paranoid ideas

Table 30-6. Differentiating between dementia and dementia syndrome of depression.

	Dementia	DSD
History		
	• Slow, insidious onset	• Rapid onset
	• Precipitating event not necessarily present	• Recent stress, loss
		• Previous depression
	• Family complains of problem	• Patient complains of problem
		• Multiple somatic complaints
Evaluation		
	• Often indifferent or anxious	• Sad, withdrawn, hopeless
	• Willing to put forth good effort on mental status examination	• Little motivation, poor effort on mental status examination
	• Excuses or denies deficits	• Complains of deficits
	• Psychotic symptoms usually not with depressive content	• If psychotic, has depressive quality

SCREENING FOR DEMENTIA

There is currently no consensus on whether older persons should be screened for dementia. At present, early detection and treatment does not improve outcomes, but that may change if disease-modifying treatments become available in the future. Despite the lack of data, the authors of this chapter still support screening for cognitive impairment in older adults because early detection can allow patients to participate in advance care planning for finances and health care. We favor the Mini-Cog (a three-item recall and clock draw test) as a screening test because it is a sensitive and easy to administer tool. When a patient fails this simple screen, following up with a standardized instrument is warranted.

DIAGNOSTIC WORKUP

A dementia workup should include a careful history (Table 30-7) and physical, neurologic, and mental

Table 30-7. Dementia workup: history.

- Time course and nature of symptoms and functional decline
- Slow and insidious versus more sudden/dramatic changes
- Current ability to function
- Accompanying mood or personality changes
- Presence or absence of confusion, agitation, and disorientation
- Psychotic symptoms
- Complicating factors, such as alcohol or substance abuse

status examinations. In many cases, additional tests and procedures may be helpful; these are discussed later.

HISTORY

A complete history should be elicited from both patients and their families. In many cases, it is helpful to ask both about the same topics. Although many demented individuals are unreliable historians, they may be able to provide much useful information, including symptoms of which family members are not aware. In addition, patients' abilities to provide a coherent and organized account of their complaints and recent history can often tell you much about their conditions.

A complete social and family history that includes native language; family history of dementia; and educational, marital, and employment background can also be useful. An educational and occupational history, for example, may provide information about a patient's previous level of functioning. A quality of vagueness in patients' reports or inconsistency in the information supplied may suggest less blatant memory deficits. Particular attention should be paid to patients' accounts of more recent events. Individuals with mild or moderate dementia often show intact recall for older, overlearned information (e.g., family, education, and work), but cannot provide accurate information about the immediate past.

Ask patients about their regular activities, appetite, and sleep habits, as well as any physical or cognitive complaints. Information about their mood can be gained not only by inquiring directly, but also by asking about things that they enjoy and look forward to, any worries or concerns they may have, and their plans for the future.

Family members may be able to supply a more complete and balanced impression of the patient's symptoms, behavioral changes, and level of functioning. Individuals with dementia typically lack insight into their cognitive problems and minimize or deny any difficulties. In fact, it is the family that most frequently raises concerns about the patient. Because family members may feel more comfortable discussing their observations away from the presence of the patient, they should be interviewed separately. It is especially important to inquire about both current and potential safety issues, such as driving (Table 30-8).

Physical & Neurologic Examinations

In addition to a routine physical examination, a complete neurologic examination should be done, although the results of the latter are generally unremarkable in cases of early AD. Parkinsonian signs may be apparent during the later course of many dementing illnesses. Individuals with a developing vascular dementia may show focal signs on the neurologic examination.

Table 30-8. Dementia workup: potential safety issues.

- Ambulation and balance
- Dizziness
- Ability to live independently
  Leaving stove or running water unattended
  Wandering behavior
  Confusion/agitation
  Ability to manage finances
- Ability to drive
- Level of supervision available

The Mental Status Examination

Because cognitive impairment is the hallmark of dementia, it is necessary to add additional screening items to the traditional mental status examination. Several brief dementia-screening instruments offer the advantages of both a structured format and a scoring system. These instruments must be used with caution, however, for the reasons discussed here.

The Mini-Mental State Examination (MMSE)© has been the most commonly used dementia-screening instrument (Table 30-9). It takes about 5 minutes to administer and samples a wide range of functions, including orientation, immediate and delayed memory, concentration, basic language and reading functions, and visual construction abilities. Patients are asked to count backward by 7, write a sentence, follow concrete directions, and copy geometric figures. A maximum score of 30 is possible; a score lower than 24 (some clinicians recommend 27) is suspicious for dementia.

The Montreal Cognitive Assessment (MOCA) is currently being used in many settings because it is more sensitive than the MMSE for the detection of MCI and has a less restrictive copyright agreement. The web site www.mocatest.org contains MOCA forms in 37 languages, instructions for administration and scoring, and normative data for the examination. Other brief dementia-screening instruments include the Mini-Cog, the Blessed Dementia Scale Neurobehavioral Cognitive Status Examination, and the SLUMS (St. Louis University Mental State Exam). Functional scales such as the FAST (Functional Assessment Staging) can be useful in determining what site of care may be most appropriate for a patient with dementia, including when hospice might be appropriate.

Other Tests

The American Academy of Neurology recommends that structural neuroimaging (with noncontrast CT or MRI) be employed in the initial evaluation of most

Table 30-9. Dementia workup: MMSE.

Function	Question or Task	Maximum Score
Orientation	What is the year, season, date, day, month? (5 points) Where are we: state, county, town, hospital, floor? (5 points)	10
Registration	Name three objects and ask the patient to repeat the names of the objects (each correct response = 1 point). Repeat the names of the three objects until the patient learns them.	3
Attention and calculation	Ask the patient to recite serial 7s backward from 100. Stop the patient after five responses (each correct response = 1 point).	5
Recall	Ask the patient to repeat the names of the three objects learned above (each correct response = 1 point).	3
Language	Show the patient two common objects, for example, a pencil and watch, and ask the patient to identify them (2 points). Ask the patient to repeat "no ifs, ands, or buts" (1 point). Instruct the patient to follow the three-stage command: "take a paper in your right hand, fold it in half, and put it on the floor" (3 points). Ask the patient to read and obey the following: "close your eyes" (1 point). Instruct the patient to write a sentence (1 point). Ask the patient to copy a design (1 point).	9

Source: Reprinted, with permission, from Folstein MF, Folstein SE, McHugh PR. "Mini-Mental State": a practical method for grading the cognitive state of patients for the clinician. *J Psychiatr Res* 1975;12:189–198.

patients with dementia, as some 5% of such patients have been found to have important but clinically unexpected structural lesions. We believe that in cases of long-standing dementia that is consistent with AD, there may be instances when the burdens of neuroimaging outweigh the benefits, particularly in a patient who becomes agitated in unfamiliar settings. An EEG is

Table 30-10. Dementia workup: recommended laboratory tests.*

Complete blood count	Calcium
Thyroid studies	Albumin
Blood urea nitrogen	Vitamin B$_{12}$
Creatinine	Electrolytes

*Consider: liver function, rapid plasma reagin, HIV serology, glucose, medication serum levels, toxicology screens, folate, urinalysis, and lumbar puncture.

Table 30-11. Overall principles of dementia management.

- Periodically assess safety and self-care function
- Assess caregiver each visit
- Address advance directives early
- Educate patient and caregivers about dementing condition
- Refer to Alzheimer's Association and supportive community organizations
- Treat secondary disorders (anxiety, depression)
- "Fine-tune" comorbid illnesses (e.g., congestive heart failure)
- Consider a trial of cholinesterase inhibitors for mild-to-moderate AD
- Consider a trial of memantine for moderate-to-severe AD

helpful if the differential diagnosis includes status epilepticus or postictal confusion. On the other hand, the major dementing disorders, especially early in their course, do not generate characteristic EEG patterns, and a normal EEG cannot be taken as definitive evidence of the absence of brain pathology.

Lumbar punctures are indicated when there is a question of an infectious process or when a rapidly progressing condition is present. In rare instances, brain biopsy may be employed to aid in diagnosis. Table 30-10 suggests other recommended laboratory tests.

Neuropsychological Testing

Neuropsychological testing involves the use of psychometric tests designed to detect and characterize a wide variety of cognitive problems. The testing requires the patient to be able to attend for a minimum of 20–30 minutes; some patients may be too agitated, withdrawn, or resistant to comply. Consider referring a patient for neuropsychological testing in the following circumstances:

- When the reported deficits are subtle or equivocal and the impairment is mild.
- When the differential diagnosis is difficult to resolve (e.g., distinguishing between dementia and depression).
- When a baseline is needed to measure the degree of cognitive deterioration over time.
- When a greater understanding of the patient's everyday level of functioning, limitations, potential safety issues, and the appropriate level of supervision is needed.
- When deficits or competency issues must be documented, such as in conservatorship proceedings.
- To monitor effects of treatment.

TREATMENT & MANAGEMENT ISSUES

Treatment of dementia consists of identifying and addressing a treatable basis for the underlying condition (if one exists), treating symptoms of the cognitive deficits, treating secondary disorders such as anxiety or depression, educating patients and their families as to the nature of the condition, and assisting caregivers with safety and management issues. Table 30-11 summarizes overall principles of dementia management.

BEHAVIORAL ISSUES

Management of patients with dementia involves matters of self-care, safety, and communication. Individuals with dementia are characteristically disorganized, forgetful, and inefficient in many of their activities making it difficult and unsafe for them to function independently. Complicating this, they may be impulsive, have limited insight into their abilities, and fail to learn from experience.

Neuropsychiatric symptoms are common and almost all persons with dementia will experience them at some point during the course of their illness (97% in one series of patients with dementia followed over 5 years). Providers should inquire about them with patients and caregivers at each visit. Specifically, they may be labile and unstable, irritable, or anxious; they may be fearful, easily frustrated, or apathetic and withdrawn. They may wander at night or endorse paranoid thoughts or delusions. Because of circadian rhythm disturbances, patients with AD may tend to be awake and wandering during the night, leading to sleep deprivation in caregivers.

These traits create special problems in managing and caring for patients with dementia, and many interactions with family and caregivers therefore focus on day-to-day management issues and behavioral problems. The following sections provide some general guidelines for addressing these issues. It is useful in many situations to refer patients and their families to groups that can provide counseling, home evaluations, and case management. (In some instances, there may be no more important knowledge for the primary doctor than familiarity with the capabilities of local support agencies.)

In general, nonpharmacological strategies for behavior management should be attempted first, and if unsuccessful, medication trials may be indicated. In practice, many distressing symptoms, such as agitation, prompt providers to try medications concurrently.

SELF-CARE

This area includes dressing, grooming, and hygiene. The best approach is to provide sufficient structure and guidance so that the patient can manage, while allowing some preservation of independence and choice. Individuals with MCI often get by with prompts and reminders. For individuals with more severe impairment, caregivers should offer a limited choice of clothing, food, or activities; use signs or pictures to identify important objects and locations; and emphasize routine and predictability. Breaking down complex and potentially overwhelming activities such as bathing into simple one-step tasks may keep these activities manageable well into the course of the illness. The caregiver may need to modify clothing, for example, by incorporating sweatshirts to avoid buttons, and using shoes with Velcro closures rather than laces. Incontinence often develops. Protective garments in clothing and timed toileting, for example, having the patient go every 2 hours while awake, may prevent frequent accidents.

SAFETY ISSUES

Individuals with dementia are at increased risk for accidents because of their problems with attention, perception, and judgment. They are also at increased risk of abuse, including physical, emotional, and financial.

To assess risk of accidents, ask caregivers and patients about conditions at home, how often the patient is left alone, and whether he/she wanders, cooks, or self-administers medications (see Table 30-8). Where safety is unclear, more detailed information can be provided by an early home safety evaluation, often done by an occupational therapist.

The following guidelines are designed to minimize the risk of household accidents:

- Carefully supervise use of medications.
- Keep the home relatively free of clutter and keep passageways clear.
- Install railings and other safety equipment, such as shower chairs and tub rails.
- Use a night-light where necessary.
- Remove stove and oven controls if necessary.
- Use safety gates or install keyless locks on exterior doors if wandering is a problem.
- Make sure patients wear medical and personal identification bracelets. Registering the patient in the Safe

Return program via the Alzheimer's Association is a common way to obtain identification bracelets or necklaces. (Access at http://www.alz.org/safetycenter/we_can_help_safety_medicalert_safereturn.asp)

Another important safety issue concerns driving and dementia. Deficits in attention, reaction time, visual spatial abilities, and judgment typically impair the ability of individuals with marked cognitive deficits to operate a motor vehicle safely. Individuals with advanced dementia who continue to operate a car seriously endanger others as well as themselves. Unfortunately, patients with dementia may insist on driving because of their lack of insight into their problems, and caregivers may be reluctant to press the issue. Because driving is symbolic of independence, this often becomes an emotional issue for everyone involved.

Confidentiality must be weighed against issues of competency, safety of the public, and the duty to warn. Legal requirements vary considerably between states. For example, in California, physicians are required by law to report patients with a diagnosis of AD or other related dementias. In the case of accident or injury, physicians who have failed to make such a report may be legally liable. Clinicians should inform themselves of the legal requirements in their own state regarding this issue.

Advance care planning should be addressed as early as possible. Evidence has shown that patients are more likely to have their care preferences followed at the end of life with these in place, and routine documentation of these preferences helps that occur. Similarly, referral to social workers and specialized legal agencies can help ensure that the patient has adequate financial and personal protections legally and medically. It may be helpful to know of legal resources for patients and families in the local community.

COMMUNICATION

Individuals with cognitive impairment may have specific deficits in language comprehension and expression similar to the various forms of aphasia that occur in stroke patients. More common may be a generalized difficulty in communication secondary to a short attention span, memory problems, or confusion. Some guidelines for communicating with the cognitively impaired are presented in Table 30-12.

Another factor affecting communication may be hearing or vision impairment, which is highly prevalent and often minimized by the patient. Therefore, we recommend asking about vision loss and referring to an ophthalmologist for full evaluation if there is any suspicion for vision loss. Hearing loss compounds cognitive difficulty profoundly. When speaking with someone with dementia, portable amplifiers, called "pocket talkers," help ensure that the person can hear the conversation.

Table 30-12. Tips for communicating with the cognitively impaired.

- Make sure you have patients' attention when you speak with them. Keep distractions, such as television, radio, or other conversations, to a minimum by meeting with patients in a quiet place.
- Keep communications brief, simple, and concrete. Break more complex information down into smaller pieces.
- Give patients several options to choose among, or phrase questions in multiple-choice format.
- Have patients paraphrase back the information to make sure they have understood what was said.

These can be kept in the clinic for regular use. Trying a pocket talker, even if the patient denies significant hearing impairment, often reveals undercorrected hearing loss and improves communication tremendously.

Drug Therapy

Cholinesterase inhibitors may confer mild benefits for patients with AD, vascular dementia, and DLB. These benefits, on average, are not clinically significant for cognition and are modest for global assessments; however, this class is approved by the FDA for mild-to-moderate AD. Anecdotal evidence suggests that a subgroup of patients may achieve clinically important improvements. The decision to initiate therapy with an acetylcholinesterase inhibitor should be based on evaluation of benefits and risks associated with an individual patient. A beneficial effect, that is, improvement or stabilization of target symptoms, would generally be expected within 6 months of initiation of therapy. Evidence is insufficient to determine the optimal timing or duration of therapy. Side effects of acetylcholinesterase inhibitors include nausea, anorexia, diarrhea, weight loss, syncope, and urinary frequency. An ECG should be checked after dose increases to monitor for bradycardia. Starting doses, respectively, of donepezil, galantamine, and rivastigmine, are 5 mg orally once daily, 4 mg orally twice daily, and 1.5 mg orally twice daily. The doses are increased gradually as tolerated.

Memantine, an *N*-methyl-D-aspartate (NMDA) antagonist, may be helpful in patients with moderate-to-severe AD or vascular dementia, with or without concomitant use of an acetylcholinesterase inhibitor. Clinical trials have shown a statistically significant, but most likely not a clinically significant, improvement on standard tests of cognition. Some studies have also demonstrated improvements in behavior and quality of life with use of memantine. The starting dose is 5 mg daily; the dose may be increased by 5 mg in weekly intervals up to a maximum of 20 mg per day. Table 30-13 shows medications commonly used for AD and their recommended doses.

Table 30-13. Drug therapy for AD.

Drug	Initial Regimen	Dose Escalation
Donepezil	5 mg orally every day	10 mg orally every day after 4–6 weeks
Rivastigmine	1.5 mg orally twice a day	Adjust every 2 weeks to 3 mg orally twice a day, then 4.5 mg orally twice a day, maximum 6 mg orally twice a day
Galantamine	4 mg orally twice a day	Adjust every 4 weeks to 8 mg orally twice a day, maximum 12 mg orally twice a day
Memantine	5 mg daily	Increase to 5 mg bid after 1 week, increase by 5 mg weekly until maximum 10 mg bid

BEHAVIORAL INTERVENTIONS AND MEDICATION FOR SEVERE BEHAVIORAL AND PSYCHIATRIC SYMPTOMS

Because of limited efficacy of many medications and higher risk of complications, nonpharmacological approaches should be attempted first before psychotropic medications.

Nonpsychotic agitation deserves careful evaluation before a drug is prescribed. New agitation may represent delirium, undertreated pain, depression, a distended bladder, or fecal impaction. If these disorders are not contributing and if nonpharmacological approaches are inadequate, an empiric trial of analgesics such as acetaminophen, an antidepressant medication, or a mood stabilizer may be worthwhile. However, any empiric trial should be time limited, and consultation with a geriatric psychiatrist is recommended in recalcitrant cases if at all possible.

When behaviors are severe and may lead to harm for the patient and caregiver, medications may be indicated. There is no clear consensus about pharmacological approaches to treatment of behavioral problems in patients who have not benefited from nonpharmacological therapies. The target symptoms—depression, anxiety, psychosis, mood lability, or pain—may suggest which class of medications might be most helpful in a given patient. Patients with depressive symptoms may show improvement with antidepressant therapy. In general, benzodiazepines should be avoided, especially for more than brief periods, as they have significant potential for causing sedation, confusion, ataxia, and falls.

Despite the lack of strong evidence, antipsychotic medications are commonly used as first-line agents for the treatment of behavioral disturbances, largely because of the lack of alternatives. The newer atypical antipsychotic agents (e.g., risperidone, olanzapine, quetiapine, aripiprazole, clozapine, and ziprasidone) may be better tolerated than older agents (e.g., haloperidol), but confer an excess risk of stroke, weight gain, and hyperglycemia. Both typical and atypical antipsychotics are associated with an increased risk of death compared with placebo when used to treat elderly demented patients with behavioral disturbances. When the choice is made to use these agents, patients and caregivers should be carefully warned of the risks. It is prudent to check an ECG prior to beginning antipsychotic therapy, and to seriously consider other alternatives when a patient is found to have a prolonged QTc. Starting and target dosages should be much lower than those used in schizophrenia (e.g., haloperidol, 0.5–2 mg orally; risperidone, 0.25–2 mg orally). Federal regulations require that if antipsychotic agents are used in treatment of a nursing home patient, drug reduction efforts must be made at least every 6 months. If the problem continues, consider another agent or obtain consultation with a psychiatrist, preferably one specializing in geriatric psychiatry.

Randomized controlled trials suggest that donepezil has no benefit when used to treat agitation in AD. However, if a medication such as a cholinesterase inhibitor or memantine is being considered for cognition, it is reasonable to see if it has an impact on behavior, as well. If at all possible, we recommend delaying the prescription of a second agent (e.g., antipsychotic or other psychoactive medication) until the impact of the cognitive agent medication can be evaluated.

Caregiver involvement is essential to managing neuropsychiatric symptoms without medications. Common strategies for behavioral problems are maintaining and promoting adequate daytime physical and social activity, avoiding confrontational approaches by redirecting questions or topics of conversation, and consistently using reassuring and calming responses to a patient's behaviors instead of anger or frustration. Guides and informational material may be a very useful resource for caregivers and can be easily downloaded from web sites such as www.indydiscoverynetwork.org or www.caregiver.org.

Caregivers

Caring for cognitively impaired individuals is often exhausting and stressful, especially in the presence of neuropsychiatric symptoms. Primary care providers should ensure that caregivers also attend to their own needs and guard against fatigue and burnout. Caregiver-specific inventories can be administered, such as the Revised Memory and Behavior Problems Checklist, to quantify the patient's behaviors and assess the caregiver's emotional burden. A number of support services, such as the Family Caregiver Alliance (http://www.caregiver. org), offer education, support groups, and information about resources. Specialized case management and home consultation services can also be very helpful in assessing patient and family needs and locating additional services. Respite-care and day-activity programs may be invaluable in allowing stressed families and caregivers time off and providing needed stimulation and increased structure for the patient. Many experienced clinicians often assess stressed caregivers at each clinic visit.

Nursing Home Placement

In the management of demented patients, the issue often arises as to whether the patient can continue to be managed at home. This is an area fraught with strong feelings on the part of patient and caregiver alike, and it is often difficult to make objective decisions. Major predictors of nursing home placement include the presence of behavioral problems, dementia severity, and extent of caregiver burden. Some important considerations related to nursing home admission are as follows:

- Can the necessary level of supervision and care required by the patient be realistically and dependably supplied at home? Such issues as wandering and the potential for neglect and abuse should be considered here.
- Is sufficient assistance available to caregivers for them to continue to care for the patient without becoming overstressed and burned out?
- What financial resources are available for the patient's care?

All things being equal, many patients and caregivers prefer to remain in their own home. In many cases, however, doing so creates other significant problems, and however desirable this goal, it must be carefully weighed against issues of safety and practical limitations. In the advanced stage of dementia, when the patient becomes mute, bedbound, and incontinent, very often the services of a skilled nursing facility are required to ensure that the patient receives proper care. Nursing facilities should be chosen carefully; obviously, cost must be considered, but the quality of care must also be investigated. Information about both complaints and compliance with state regulations can be found through government agencies, advocacy groups, published reviews, and organizations (e.g., geriatric care programs) that frequently place patients in such facilities. Although definitive data are lacking, some studies suggest that Alzheimer's special care units reduce behavioral disturbances and use of restraints. Some patients do better in structured environments such as Alzheimer's special care units or Alzheimer's day care programs than in less structured home settings.

Dementia is a terminal disease, and in late stages the patient may become bedbound, unable to recognize family, and have difficulty swallowing. In these instances, hospice care is often appropriate (see Chapter 40).

SUMMARY

Dementia is an increasingly common syndrome characterized by a progressive loss of cognition and functioning. Given the aging of the population, it is essential that clinicians become comfortable with diagnosis, counseling, community and specialist referral, and treatment. Early diagnosis may allow for identification of (unfortunately rare) reversible causes, improved symptom management, and planning for the future.

When patients present with cognitive complaints, the clinician must consider differential diagnoses including dementia, delirium, depression, and psychosis. Diagnostic workup includes a careful history from patient and family, physical examination, mental status examination, laboratory work, brain imaging, and on occasion, referral for neuropsychological testing or other specialized assessment.

Treatment and management consist of ruling out treatable conditions, treating secondary disorders such as anxiety or depression, providing information to patients and families, and assisting caregivers with safety and management issues. Use of medications may modestly slow the rate of cognitive decline or help with management of severe psychiatric symptoms, but interventions also consist of adjusting the environment to make the patient as comfortable and safe as possible and providing support for caregivers.

Taking care of demented patients and their caregivers can be extremely rewarding. Further, with abundant research efforts under way, there is reason to be optimistic that improved methods of preventing and treating dementing disorders are just over the horizon.

ACKNOWLEDGMENTS

David M. Pope, PhD and Alicia Boccellari, PhD, were authors of the first edition version of this chapter, and William Lyons, MD was author of the second edition version of this chapter.

SUGGESTED READINGS

Albert MS, et al. The diagnosis of mild cognitive impairment due to Alzheimer's disease: recommendations from the National Institute on Aging-Alzheimer's Association workgroups on diagnostic guidelines for Alzheimer's disease. *Alzheimers Dement* 2011;7:270–279. PMID: 21514249.

Borson S, Scanlan JM, Chen P, et al. The Mini-Cog as a screen for dementia: validation in a population-based sample. *J Am Geriatr Soc* 2003;51:1451–1454. PMID: 14511167.

Boustani M, Sachs GA, Alder CA, et al. Implementing innovative models of dementia care: the Healthy Aging Brain Center. *Aging Ment Health* 2011;15:13–22.

Etters L, Goodall D, Harrison BE. Caregiver burden among dementia patient caregivers: a review of the literature. *J Am Acad Nurse Pract* 2008;20:423–428.

Finley RR. Alzheimer's disease and dementia in the 21ˢᵗ century. A changing paradigm. *The Rx Consultant* March, 2008;17: no. 3.

Howard RJ, Juszczak E, Ballard CG, et al. Donepezil for the treatment of agitation in Alzheimer's disease. *N Engl J Med* 2007;357:1382–1392.

McKeith I, Del Ser T, Spano PF, et al. Efficacy of rivastigmine in dementia with Lewy bodies: a randomized, double blind, placebo controlled international study. *Lancet* 2000;356: 2031–2036. PMID: 1145488.

McKhann GM, et al. The diagnosis of dementia due to Alzheimer's disease: recommendations from the National Institute on Aging-Alzheimer's Association workgroups on diagnostic guidelines for Alzheimer's disease. *Alzheimers Dement* 2011;7:263–269. Epub April 21, 2011. PMID: 21514250.

Modrego PJ, Ferrandez J. Depression in patients with mild cognitive impairment increases the risk of developing dementia of Alzheimer type: a prospective cohort study. *Arch Neurol* 2004;61:1290–1293. PMID: 15313849.

Petersen RC. Clinical practice. Mild cognitive impairment. *N Engl J Med* 2011;364:2227–2234. PMID: 21651394.

Reisberg B, Doody R, Stoffler A, et al. Memantine in moderate-to-severe Alzheimer's disease. *N Engl J Med* 2003;348: 1333–1341. PMID: 12672860.

Silveira MJ, Kim SY, Langa KM. Advance directives and outcomes of surrogate decision making before death. *N Engl J Med* 2010;362:1211–1218.

WEB SITES

Alzheimer's Association. http://www.alz.org. Accessed July 2013.

Alzheimer's Disease Education and Referral Center. http://www.alzheimers.org. Accessed July 2013.

American Geriatrics Society. http://www.americangeriatrics.org. Accessed July 2013.

Assessment instruments for dementia and related disorders available at Society for Hospital Medicine. http://www.hospitalmedicine.org/geriresource/toolbox. Accessed July 2013.

Blessed Dementia Scale. http://www.strokecenter.org/wp-content/uploads/2011/08/blessed_dementia.pdf. Accessed July 2013.

Brain Injury Association of America. http://www.biausa.org. Accessed July 2013.

Eldercare Locator (nationwide toll-free service helps older adults and caregivers to fine local services for seniors). http://www.eldercare.gov. Accessed July 2013.

Family Caregiver Alliance. http://www.caregiver.org. Accessed July 2013.

Gerontological Society of America. http://www.geron.org. Accessed July 2013.

Indianapolis Discovery Network for Dementia. http://www.indydiscoverynetwork.org. Accessed July 2013.

Mini-mental state exam. http://www.minimental.com. Accessed July 2013.

Montreal Cognitive Assessment: http://www.mocatest.org. Accessed July 2013.

Revised Memory and Behavior Problems Checklist. http://www.alz.org/national/documents/c_assess-revisedmemoryandbehcheck.pdf Accessed July 2013.

Sleep Disorders

David Claman, MD; Karli Singer, BS, & Clifford M. Singer, MD

INTRODUCTION

Thirty-five percent of adults experience sleep-related symptoms over the course of a year, making them among the most common symptoms seen in medical practice. Ten to fifteen percent of adults suffer chronic insomnia and account for the largest proportion of patients seeing health care providers for sleep-related problems. Insomnia increases risk for other chronic diseases, including hypertension, diabetes, depression, and dementia. Daytime sleepiness impairs work performance and increases the risk of industrial and motor vehicle accidents. Sleep loss due to sleep-related breathing problems leads to profound sleepiness and life-threatening cardiovascular and pulmonary diseases. Sleep deprivation is known to increase risk for depression and dementia. Sleep medications themselves carry morbidity such as falls, daytime anxiety, and worsened sleep apnea. In this chapter, we review normal sleep, disorders of both sleep and wakefulness, and a logical clinical approach to these disorders.

SLEEP THROUGH THE LIFE CYCLE

Sleep has a structure, or architecture, that consists of nonrapid eye movement (non-REM) and REM sleep cycles. The wake electroencephalogram (EEG) contains low-voltage, high-frequency waveforms that become dominated by alpha waveforms (8–12 cps) as a person becomes drowsy. There are four stages of non-REM sleep. Stage 1 is defined by the disappearance of the alpha pattern, the appearance of slower theta waveforms (2–7 cps) along with slow, rolling eye movements. Stage 2 is defined by the appearance of low-frequency, high-amplitude discharges (K complexes) and brief high frequency (12–14 cps), variable-amplitude discharges (sleep spindles) on a background of theta waveforms similar to stage 1. The majority of sleep time is spent in stage 2 non-REM. The emergence of slow waves (high-amplitude, low-frequency [0.5–2 cps] delta waveforms) heralds stage 3 sleep, when they make up at least 20%

of sleep time, and stage 4 sleep when they comprise more than 50% of sleep time. These two stages are known as the "deep stages" of sleep, because they are associated with high-arousal thresholds. REM sleep is a distinct state of sleep characterized by wake pattern EEG, skeletal muscle paralysis, and rapid, conjugate eye movements. The central nervous system (CNS) is predominantly active during REM sleep, and this is when a majority of dreams occur.

With the initiation of sleep, the healthy adult will descend through the non-REM stages within 45–60 minutes before beginning the first REM cycle, which tends to be brief. As the night progresses, less time is spent in slow-wave sleep, and REM cycle duration increases, eventually comprising 20–25% of total sleep time. The non-REM/REM cycle typically lasts 90–110 minutes, with about four complete cycles per night.

The timing and duration of sleep are controlled by many factors. Although most adults have some control over when they go to bed and when they get up, they have less control over how much sleep they need, and the quality of the sleep they get. Although stimulants such as caffeine and habituation to a state of chronic fatigue can help people cope with inadequate sleep, they must ultimately pay the price of diminished energy and mental efficiency. Individual sleep requirements vary; although most people need 6–9 hours of sleep per night, the human range is thought to be from 3 to 12 hours. Children generally need more sleep than adults, but after adolescence, daily sleep requirement remains fairly stable until late life. In old age, sleep need may increase or decrease, but the most dramatic changes are in sleep quality and duration. There is a gradual reduction in the amount of time spent in deep sleep as we age, plus a tendency to have more awakenings at night and more naps during the day.

The body clock (hypothalamic suprachiasmatic nucleus or SCN), functions as the circadian pacemaker. It superimposes a rhythm of sleepiness and alertness to days and nights and determines whether a person is a night owl, morning lark, or somewhere in between. The light–dark cycle and nightly rhythm of melatonin secretion by the pineal gland act synergistically to keep the body clock synchronized with the day–night cycle, allowing alertness during the day and sleepiness at night for people who are entrained to a conventional diurnal schedule. The interaction of the SCN, melatonin cycle, and exposure to dawn and dusk time cues determines how well a person adapts to changes in sleep schedule in order to accommodate travel across time zones, seasonal changes in photoperiod, or work and social schedules that keep people active during the night. Blindness imposes special challenges in adaptation of sleep to the light–dark cycle. Consequently, sleep complaints are common among visually impaired people.

Yawning is a phenomenon that has intrigued humans for decades. Yawning is thought to be an arousal mechanism that provides signals to the diencephalon to remain awake. It may also serve a social function. "Contagious" yawning is seen in most mammalian species and most commonly occurs between individuals that are closely related to each other or engaged in collaborative activity.

Childhood

Newborns typically spend about 70% of each day asleep, with more time in REM than older children and adults. A circadian pattern of wake and sleep does not usually develop until 1–2 months of age, and rhythmic melatonin secretion is identified at 12 weeks. Sleeping through the night is one of the first maturational milestones, and this development is of great interest to parents. Children's sleep is initially polyphasic, with day as well as night sleep. There are decreasing amounts of daytime napping until the child is 4 or 5 years. From the age of 5 to 10 years, children are usually consummate nocturnal sleepers with few arousals. Total sleep time gradually decreases throughout childhood, but for hormonal and psychosocial reasons the amount and quality of sleep drops sharply with puberty.

Daytime restlessness, including the full spectrum of attention deficit hyperactivity disorder (AD/HD), should prompt consideration of obstructive sleep apnea (OSA) syndrome, often due to enlarged tonsils and adenoids in children (see Chapter 27). There is ongoing debate over household arrangements for children's sleep. Some anthropologists point out that isolating a newborn in a separate bedroom is unique to western cultures and that co-sleeping with infants is more natural and may be beneficial. Recent studies have linked bed sharing with Sudden Infant Death Syndrome (SIDS), however, and the current recommendation of the American Academy of Pediatrics is to place infants in a separate sleeping area in the same room with the parent.

Adolescence and Young Adulthood

Adolescents are generally able to maintain the high sleep efficiency of childhood, with few nighttime arousals and little daytime sleepiness. In practice, adolescents frequently become more night-oriented, staying up late to do homework, work part-time jobs, chat with friends via text or phone, using Internet social media sites or socializing away from home. Many adolescents and young adults develop strong tendencies to being "night owls" (see Delayed Sleep Phase Disorder in the "Chronobiological" section of this chapter). Getting up for school may become an extreme challenge for some, and overall sleep deprivation with daytime sleepiness (especially in the morning) is endemic in high schools. Also, high prevalence rates of mood and anxiety disorders and the normal emotional highs and lows of this period of life make transient insomnia more common, with difficulty falling asleep, staying asleep or both. Early experiences with various substances affecting sleep, such as caffeine, nicotine, alcohol, marijuana, hallucinogens, and stimulants also can be strong factors. Serious mental illness such as schizophrenia or bipolar spectrum mood disorders start to express themselves with significant prevalence in adolescence and young adulthood, sometimes expressed with sleep or wake disorders. Physical illnesses producing inflammation, pain, endocrine, and metabolic imbalances can all impact sleep and need to be considered in clinical assessment. Excessive daytime sleepiness at this age is usually due to sleep deprivation, but substance abuse and narcolepsy need to be considered. People may suffer for many years with narcolepsy before the diagnosis is made. It should be considered in anyone with spells of sleepiness off and on during the day, especially if a very brief nap is very helpful for an hour or two.

Middle Adulthood and Old Age

Sleep tends to be lighter as people age, with more frequent awakenings and the near disappearance of deep or slow-wave sleep. Sleep timing may "phase advance" with earlier bedtimes and early morning awakenings. Whereas younger insomniacs typically struggle with sleep onset, older people with insomnia may just as likely complain of sleep maintenance problems due to this tendency toward phase-advanced sleep–wake cycle. More frequent daytime napping, either through boredom or need, is very common in older adults. This, along with decreased daytime physical activity, further erodes nighttime sleep efficiency. Frequent nocturia and esophageal reflux can make a bad situation worse with regard to sleep. Clinical sleep disorders also increase with age. Obstructive sleep apnea, periodic leg movements, restless legs syndrome (RLS), depression, anxiety, alcohol, and pain all affect the restorative qualities of sleep. Little wonder, then, that insomnia becomes more prevalent in midlife, especially in women and people with multiple chronic diseases.

CLINICAL SLEEP DISORDERS

Sleep disorders are generally grouped into three categories: disorders of initiating and maintaining sleep (insomnia); disorders of excessive daytime sleepiness (hypersomnia); and abnormal sleep behaviors (parasomnia) (Table 31-1).

Every review of systems should include screening patients for daytime sleepiness and nighttime sleep problems. Four basic questions give clinicians a head start in diagnosing sleep disorders and determining whether they warrant treatment:

- *How are you sleeping?*
- *How much sleep do you get in a typical night?*
- *How much sleep do you typically need to feel your best?*
- *Do you feel alert during the day?*

Follow-up questions should sharpen the differential diagnosis of specific disorders of either sleep or wakefulness. In both pediatrics and geriatrics, it is often the parent, spouse, or caregiver who notices a problem. With children, ascertain whether the parent or caregiver is knowledgeable about normal sleep patterns for children. If the behavior is outside of the norm, then further questioning is necessary for diagnosis.

The sleep–wake cycle is a complex electrophysiologic process consisting of alternating periods of wakefulness, REM sleep, and non-REM sleep. Each of these periods has a characteristic EEG, peripheral muscle, and autonomic nervous system pattern that can be documented by polysomnographic (PSG) recording in hospital and clinic-based sleep laboratories or in the home, using technologies that allow for unattended in-home recordings. PSG allows clinicians to make specific diagnoses based on electrophysiologic monitoring of EEG, electrooculogram, electromyogram, nasal airflow, ear oximetry, and electrocardiogram.

Insomnia: Insufficient and Nonrestorative Sleep

TRANSIENT AND CHRONIC INSOMNIA

Insomnia is one of the most common complaints in primary care practice. It is diagnosed when there is either insufficient or nonrestorative sleep. It is essentially a subjective diagnosis although more objective means of assessment will be discussed later in the chapter. Certainly one of the first tasks is to confirm deficient sleep quantity or quality relative to normal sleep requirement for that person. Sleep requirement is best defined by how much sleep a person needs to be alert through the day, with perhaps a brief dip in alertness midday. Sleep requirement is genetically determined and also influenced by age, activity, and health. Eight hours is the adult mean sleep requirement with a range of 6–9 hours for most people. There can also be seasonal variation at high latitudes. Nonrestorative sleep diagnoses (e.g., sleep apnea, periodic leg movements, pain, depression, nightmares, etc.) should be pursued when there is adequate sleep time but poor daytime function.

It is best to think of insomnia as a symptom rather than a diagnosis. Many factors combine to produce insomnia, which often occurs when a delicate balance is tipped; for example, a constitutionally light sleeper may be fine until he or she enters a period of stress or uses a medication that has alerting effects. It may be necessary to deal with several causative factors concurrently to restore a natural sleep cycle.

Insomnia is often described as initial insomnia (trouble falling asleep), and middle or terminal insomnia (trouble staying asleep or early awakening). Insomnia may be transient (self-limited) or chronic (persistent or relapsing). Transient insomnia can evolve into chronic insomnia through a number of factors.

Transient insomnia caused by stress, environment (cold, noise, new baby), acute illness, or pain is easy to identify and usually needs no special intervention other than addressing the underlying problem. A brief course of sedative–hypnotic medication is occasionally warranted and may reduce the risk of developing long-term insomnia. Travel across time zones can cause a mismatch between the body clock and the day–night cycle, resulting in transient insomnia known as "jet lag." Combined with fatigue from travel, jet lag can ruin the first few days of a trip. Shift workers may experience the same phenomenon and can suffer severe health and social consequences because of it.

Table 31-1. The sleepless patient: disorders of initiating and maintaining sleep.

Category	Disorder
Insomnia	Transient and chronic insomnia, chronobiological insomnia, comorbid insomnia (secondary to RLS, periodic leg movements, mood and anxiety disorders, alcohol and drugs, and medical disorders affecting sleep)
Hypersomnia	Sleep apnea syndrome, narcolepsy, idiopathic CNS hypersomnolence, delirium, advanced dementia, and traumatic brain injury
Parasomnia	Pavor nocturnus (sleep terrors), nightmares, somnambulism (sleepwalking), and REM behavior disorder

Table 31-2. Cognitive behavioral treatment for insomnia.

Essential Cognitive Technique	Essential Behavioral Change
1. Talk about the frustration of not falling asleep and put this into perspective to facilitate a calm acceptance that will reduce frustration.	1. *Bed or sleep restriction*: time in bed limited to period of time the person can sleep; gradually increasing as sleep duration increases.
2. Education about the reality of insomnia as a potentially chronic or recurrent condition that may require behavioral adaptations.	2. *Stimulus control*: go to bed only when sleepy, use bedroom only for sleep and sex, out of bed if awake more than 30 minutes, remove stress and clutter from bedroom, no TV, reading, or eating in bed.
3. Teach technique of suppressing thoughts: mindful practice of putting disturbing thoughts aside while trying to rest.	3. *Improved sleep hygiene*: no caffeine, alcohol, or nicotine late for better sleep, mild-to-moderate exercise in the afternoon, naps OK if short (30–40 minutes) and not late afternoon.

Persistent or chronic insomnia accounts for 40–88% of patients who present with a primary complaint of insomnia. Chronic insomnia is a diagnosis of exclusion, and must be differentiated from the many other causes of long-term sleep disruption. Chronic insomnia may be due to persistence of the stress that initially caused transient insomnia. Occasionally, the insomnia continues even when the precipitating factors have resolved, presumably through a process of operant conditioning to an arousal state incompatible with sustained, restful sleep. "Conditioned" or learned insomnia may persist secondary to poor sleep hygiene, such as erratic sleep schedules, alcohol, caffeine, nicotine, work on finances, nighttime television or Internet and other habits that can prevent achieving the peaceful state of mind that is important to overcome sleep resistance. Growing frustration with failed attempts to sleep increases the psychophysiologic arousal that is the underlying cause of sleeplessness. In fact, this type of insomnia, developing over time in association with stress, worry, and frustration over sleep, is often called "psychophysiologic" insomnia. People with this type of insomnia show high levels of physiologic stress markers (hormonal, autonomic, and cognitive). Despite severe sleep deprivation and pent up sleep drive, the arousal mechanisms of the stress response create too much sleep resistance to be overcome. Occasionally, this psychophysiologic arousal may be seen early in life in a form of "primary insomnia" due to intrinsic biological variation in either sleep drive (reduced) or stress response (increased). In contrast to people with transient insomnia and sleep deprivation, patients with the psychophysiologic and primary forms of chronic insomnia report inability to nap.

As a model psychosomatic illness, chronic insomnia requires a holistic approach that can include use of medication as well as cognitive strategies to reduce anxiety and changes to improve sleep hygiene (Table 31-2). Short-term use of sedative–hypnotic medications is appropriate to break the cycle of anxiety, arousal, and insomnia (see "Medical Treatment," below). In some patients, the symptoms suggest another disorder that can be targeted separately (depression, RLS, pain, etc.).

CHRONOBIOLOGICAL DISORDERS

 CASE ILLUSTRATION 1

Greg is a 27-year-old man who presents with a complaint of insomnia. He describes having trouble getting up in the morning. He is chronically late for work and his job is in jeopardy. No matter what time he goes to bed, Greg cannot fall asleep until about 2:00 A.M. and then sleeps through the alarm set for 7:00 A.M. His wife has given up trying to wake him, and although he has arranged for an answering service to call him, the ringing telephone does not awaken him either. He is often tired and sleepy during the day, but in the evening gets his "second wind" just as his wife goes to bed. He craves weekends and vacations when he sleeps until noon and feels alert the rest of the day.

The keys to Greg's diagnosis of delayed sleep phase syndrome are his very strong drive to stay up late and sleep late, a relative inability to adjust to a conventional sleep schedule and normal sleep when able to sleep on his internal biological schedule. Adjusting his sleep–wake schedule will take discipline but can improve his health, marriage, and career. The strategic use of low-dose melatonin in the early evening, bright light exposure in the early morning, and resisting the temptations of late night activities will be necessary.

Many cases of both transient and chronic insomnia are due to underlying chronobiological or circadian rhythm disturbances. If there is a mismatch between a person's attempts to sleep and their endogenous circadian rhythm for sleep, insomnia may result. The circadian rhythm of the sleep–wake cycle is driven by the hypothalamic circadian pacemaker or "body clock." Disturbances in the circadian timing of sleep may be transient, as in jet lag and shift work syndromes, or chronic, as in delayed sleep phase syndrome (DSPS), advanced sleep phase syndrome, and free-running sleep syndrome. The last is most common in blind persons, who lack the critical input of the light–dark cycle in regulating circadian rhythms. Diagnosis of chronobiological disorders is based on the understanding that except for its timing, sleep is normal in these conditions.

In DSPS, patients are "obligate" night owls, staying up late into the night through varying proportions of choice and biological drive. Patients with this condition struggle to awaken in the morning for school or work. They tend to have more energy as the day progresses and may "come alive" in the evening. Attempts to fall asleep before midnight can result in hours of tossing and turning. Sleep efficiency is usually normal when they are free to choose their own bedtimes. The condition is common in young people but can persist into middle adulthood and even old age, although it does tend to moderate with time. Adults with DSPS typically migrate to jobs in which they can work swing or night shifts, or keep totally flexible hours. They may have particular difficulty flying east across time zones, as they are relatively resistant to circadian "phase advance." Most "night owls" have flexibility in their circadian pacemaker and can adapt to earlier sleep hours with effort. Those with true DSPS cannot adjust to conventional hours at all, or only with great effort and treatment.

Children and adolescents with DSPS may be thought of as "lazy" because of how difficult it is for them to get out of bed in the morning and their tendency to "sleep in" on weekends. When school is in session, Sunday night bedtime and Monday morning awakenings are particularly challenging. With a late sleep-onset, the child has trouble waking up Monday mornings and this starts the week off "on the wrong side of the bed." This may lead to disruptive behavior, hyperactivity, distractibility, failure to attend, and learning problems in school. Parents and teachers must recognize that DSPS is not a behavioral problem but a circadian rhythm disorder that can improve with proper treatment. A phase shift approach by the whole family of consistent bed times 7 days a week is very helpful. Practicing good sleep hygiene, bright light therapy and melatonin have been shown to be effective (see "Treatment for Insomnia").

Other forms of chronobiological sleep disorders are seen in practice. Shift workers often try to live on a conventional schedule to spend days off with friends or family. This can result in failure to adapt to either day or night and leads to poor sleep, poor energy, and chronically elevated risk for chronic illness and premature death. Scheduled exposure to bright light and melatonin can accelerate adaptation to shift work schedules.

Many blind individuals also have problems maintaining synchronicity between sleep and the day–night cycle. Lacking photic input to the circadian pacemaker via the retinohypothalamic tract, blind individuals can have an internal sleep propensity rhythm that is chronically out of phase with the day–night cycle, leading to frequent bouts of insomnia. Chronobiological insomnia from "free-running" circadian rhythms in blind patients is treatable with properly timed melatonin administration, but this and other chronobiological disorders should be treated in consultation with a sleep disorder specialist.

NEUROPSYCHIATRIC DISORDERS

 CASE ILLUSTRATION 2

Francine is a 47-year-old woman complaining of anxiety. She feels restless and fidgety during the day, but she is also tired. She cries easily and has trouble concentrating, making decisions, and getting things done. Although quite fatigued, it can take her an hour to fall asleep. When sleep finally comes, it is restless and interrupted by many awakenings, filled with worried thoughts. She has experienced similar symptoms before but this time they are more persistent, having lasted more than 2 months.

Francine's diagnosis is likely to be major depression, presenting with prominent symptoms of anxiety and insomnia. Medical or neurologic disease presenting with comorbid depression also needs to be considered, but Francine is at an age of higher risk for depression in women. If depression is the primary disorder, disease education, emotional support, and antidepressant medication are indicated. Short-term CBT can be very helpful both for the depression as well as the insomnia. Short-term use (several days to weeks) of a sedative–hypnotic can be offered if a less-sedating antidepressant is chosen as the primary agent.

Sleep disturbances are among the most common symptoms of mental illnesses, particularly mood and anxiety disorders. Depression should always be considered in patients complaining of frequent nighttime awakenings and early morning arousal, particularly when those arousals are accompanied by anxiety and worry. On the other hand, many depressed patients complain of hypersomnia with fatigue and difficulty getting going in the morning. This symptom is especially characteristic of seasonal affective disorder (SAD) and so-called atypical depression. Both are common in young and middle-aged adults. Depressed patients find the sleep changes of their mood disorder very distressing, in contrast to manic patients. Bipolar patients in manic or less severe hypomanic states, typically experience less sleep drive and will enjoy their round-the-clock energy even as it impairs their judgment and physical health (see Chapter 25).

Sedating antidepressant medications (e.g., mirtazapine) may help with the insomnia secondary to depression, but can also lead to daytime sedation. Trazodone and the more sedating tricyclic antidepressants (TCAs)—e.g., doxepin, amitriptyline, and nortriptyline—may be considered. The TCAs combine moderate-to-severe sedation with effective antidepressant activity but must be used with caution due to overdose toxicity and anticholinergic effects. Serotonin reuptake inhibitors (either SSRIs or SNRIs) generally will not improve sleep immediately, and can even increase leg movements and arousals. A brief course of a sedative–hypnotic agent for help with sleep is a comforting strategy for some patients. The sleep medication can be tapered and discontinued as the depression and secondary insomnia improve.

Anxiety disorders can also present with initial and middle insomnia (see Chapter 26). Nightmares, particularly in posttraumatic stress disorder (PTSD), frequently complicate the picture. Antidepressant medications, prazosin, and clonidine have been reported to be helpful with the sleep-related symptoms. Bereavement is usually accompanied by anxiety and insomnia. Short-term use of sedative–hypnotic medications may help patients who struggle to get through long nights.

Attention deficit disorder (ADD) and AD/HD may be associated with disturbances in REM sleep as well as frequent myoclonic or periodic movements throughout the night. Insomnia is common; many patients with the condition report difficulty controlling racing thoughts and restlessness day or night. Snoring and obstructive apneas are frequently present in children who have mild symptoms of ADD–AD/HD. In these cases, the cognitive and behavioral syndrome of ADD–AD/HD can improve with treatment of the sleep-related breathing disorder by tonsillectomy or dental appliances.

Traumatic brain injuries and stroke impair alertness more often than sleep, but disruption of circadian rhythms with daytime sleep and nighttime awakenings are common. Neurodegenerative diseases such as Alzheimer disease (AD) and Parkinson disease (PD) disrupt sleep. Alzheimer disease can erode normal diurnal sleep–wake patterns, resulting in long nighttime awakenings and increased daytime sleep. This can be stressful for caregivers, who must be vigilant during these nocturnal wanderings. Sleep disruption is among the most stressful aspects of caring for a person with dementia at home. Severe insomnia can develop in some patients with AD, with little sleep day or night.

Others may sleep all the time, creating a form of chronic delirium as the disease progresses into late stages. Structured daytime activity can help reduce daytime sleepiness, especially if boredom appears to be one of the contributing factors. Antihistamines and benzodiazepines should be avoided given the risk for confusion and paradoxical excitement. Cautious use of melatonin, trazodone, or quetiapine may be helpful, although the data are limited. However, given how stressful sleep disruption is for families and patients, trials of sleep-promoting medications at low doses can be justified.

Parkinson Disease patients can also have severe sleep problems. Akinesia causes physical discomfort over pressure points that normally would be relieved by tossing and turning in sleep. Medications used to treat PD can also impair sleep. Furthermore, the neurodegenerative and neurotransmitter changes caused by the disease adversely affect sleep quality. Dementia with Lewy Bodies, a disease related to PD, is associated both with impaired nighttime sleep, poor daytime alertness, and increased motor activity during REM sleep (see "REM Behavior Disorder," below).

ALCOHOL AND DRUGS

Alcohol has variable influence on sleep patterns, but it generally impairs both alertness and sleep. Like other sedatives, alcohol suppresses slow-wave sleep, making sleep lighter. With its short half-life, alcohol also tends to produce a rebound arousal in the second half of the night and can reduce total sleep time.

Other drugs can affect sleep. Amphetamines and cocaine cause marked reduction in sleep during acute intoxication and profound hypersomnia during the withdrawal phase. Opiates have acute tranquilizing effects and improve sleep when nighttime pain contributes to insomnia. Caffeine causes longer sleep latency (time needed to fall asleep) and increased wakefulness during the night. Some people do not perceive the effects of caffeine on sleep even when they are documented on sleep EEG; others are very aware of these effects. Caffeine can even affect sleep when ingested several hours before bedtime.

Both prescription and over-the-counter (OTC) sedative–hypnotic medications can contribute to rebound insomnia when doses are missed. Medication with short half-lives can lead to rebound insomnia in the second half of the night, whereas drugs with long half-lives can cause daytime sedation. Although they are common geriatric problems, memory impairment and unexplained falls should cue the physician to consider alcohol or sedative–hypnotic abuse in elderly patients. For example, the antihistamine diphenhydramine, a component of many OTC sleep-promoting products, has potent anticholinergic effects and can cause mild cognitive impairment and, rarely, frank delirium in older people.

Education about the effects of these substances on sleep may motivate patients to reduce their intake. Patients with more severe dependency and abuse problems need referral to specific treatment programs for chemical dependency (see Chapter 24).

MEDICAL DISORDERS

Cardiac and pulmonary diseases, dyspepsia, inflammatory bowel diseases, and nocturia may all contribute to insomnia. Gastroesophageal reflux disease (GERD) is an extremely common cause of nighttime awakening. Limiting nighttime meals and eating no later than 2 hours before bedtime can be helpful. Acquired immunodeficiency syndrome (AIDS) has been associated with daytime sleepiness, decreased total slow-wave sleep with alpha wave intrusions, increasing arousals, and frequent nightmares. The high comorbidity of major depression in patients with many chronic diseases should lead the clinician to consider using sedating antidepressants to improve sleep in this population.

Acute illness may cause diffuse cerebral dysfunction in the frail elderly. The resulting delirium is almost always accompanied by disruption of sleep and alertness. Medications can also cause insomnia and daytime drowsiness. Bronchodilators, activating antidepressants, and steroids, for example, often interfere with sleep, whereas many psychotropic medications, opioid analgesics, and clonidine can cause daytime drowsiness.

Pain and rheumatological disorders deserve special mention. Pain perception tends to be greater at night, and more time in bed may increase certain types of musculoskeletal pain. One of the classic medical syndromes affecting sleep is fibromyalgia syndrome (FMS), a condition characterized by nonrestorative sleep; patients complain of feeling tired despite sleep duration in the normal range. In overnight PSG recordings, the EEG of fibromyalgia patients reveals alpha wave intrusions into stages 2, 3, and 4 of non-REM sleep. This alpha–delta sleep may signify cortical arousals that impair sleep continuity. Sleep may be additionally fragmented in FMS patients by RLS (20% of patients) and OSA (5% of patients). Fibromyalgia syndrome patients have decreased slow wave and REM sleep duration. In addition to nonrestorative sleep, FMS is characterized by widespread muscle pain, focal tender points, and chronic fatigue. The common complaint of patients with fibromyalgia is the restless sleep pattern that blunts their daytime energy and vigor. In studies with normal human adult subjects, it has been shown that sleep deprivation lowers the pain threshold. Investigators have documented increases in generalized body pain, back pain, abdominal pain, and a heightened hyperalgesic state the following day after a night of disrupted sleep. Improved sleep can produce significant remission in pain.

RESTLESS LEGS SYNDROME

Restless legs syndrome (RLS) comes on with rest and produces an irresistible need to move, stretch, or rub the lower extremities. Severe dysesthesia may occur, which can variably be described as "creepy-crawling sensations," aching, tension, tingling, or prickling. The restless need to move makes it difficult to fall asleep, so the most common symptom of RLS is insomnia, particularly at sleep onset. The vast majority (80–90%) of people with RLS also have periodic limb movements during sleep, potentially causing further sleep disruption. Beyond sleep initiation, RLS can also interfere with any sedentary activity, such as plane travel, driving, theaters and concerts, deskwork, video media, and reading.

Restless legs syndrome is common, affecting 3–10% of the population (prevalence varies with ethnicity), and may be even more common as an intermittent cause of symptoms. In women it sometimes first appears during pregnancy, but in both genders it can run in families and worsen with age. It is especially common in patients with renal failure and PD. Many physicians do not think to ask about this symptom and hence fail to recognize it as a cause of discomfort and insomnia.

Diagnosis of RLS is based on four essential criteria: (1) an urge to move; (2) onset or exacerbation with rest; (3) relief with movement; and (4) nighttime onset or worsening of symptoms. The differential diagnosis includes neuropathy, nocturnal leg cramps, and akathisia induced by dopamine antagonists. Restless legs syndrome can be exacerbated by drugs and medications, especially caffeine, alcohol, and antidepressants. Iron appears to play an important role in RLS. Reduced iron levels, particularly in the substantia nigra, can contribute to worsening symptoms. This mechanism may contribute to the higher prevalence of RLS in women, since menstrual blood loss and pregnancy can worsen iron deficiency. It is recommended that ferritin and transferrin saturation be measured in all RLS patients. If the ferritin is less than 50 mcg/L, iron supplementation for 3 months is recommended with a goal of raising ferritin above 100 mcg/L.

The first-line treatment of RLS involves the use of the newer nonergotamine dopamine agonists (e.g., pramipexole and ropinirole). Dopamine precursor treatment levadopa/carbidopa is effective as well, but more frequently causes "rebound" or "augmentation" effects, with a tendency for the symptoms to develop earlier in the day. Benzodiazepines (clonazepam) and anticonvulsants (gabapentin) are second-line agents. Combination therapy can be effective for more severe symptoms, and opiates can also be considered in refractory cases. The syndrome is so distressful for some of its sufferers that there is a national support group and newsletter (see website www.rls.org).

PERIODIC LIMB MOVEMENTS OF SLEEP

Periodic limb movements of sleep (PLMS) are repetitive myoclonic movements of the extremities, most commonly in the legs, that occur every 5–90 seconds over many hours; they are more common in, but not limited to, the first half of the night. The movements can be associated with brief EEG arousals and potentially cause nonrestorative sleep and daytime somnolence (although larger studies have failed to show a consistent association with excessive daytime sleepiness). Prevalence estimates range from 5% in people aged 30–50 years, to 29% in those aged 50–65 years, and 44% in those over the age of 65 years. PLMS are often seen in metabolic and neurodegenerative diseases. Periodic limb movements of sleep should be distinguished from nocturnal leg cramps, which are painful, prolonged involuntary contractions of the muscles of the lower legs. Antidepressants, lithium carbonate, and withdrawal from benzodiazepines and alcohol can induce or worsen PLMS. It is often asymptomatic, but in severe cases patients may have sleep-onset insomnia, nonrestorative sleep, or frequent arousals during the night from more robust myoclonic movements. Not infrequently, the bed partner is the one complaining about the jerking leg movements at night.

Whereas RLS is primarily a clinical diagnosis based on patient-reported symptoms, PLMS are best documented by PSG in the home or sleep laboratory. PLMS are treated similarly to RLS. Dopaminergic agents are the treatment of choice, since they reduce the frequency of leg kicking, but rebound of symptoms in the second half of the night or during the following day can complicate treatment. Sedative–hypnotics can improve sleep continuity in PLMS patients, but do not reduce the number of leg movements. Opiates, such as a bedtime dose of codeine, work well in PLMS (as in RLS), but should be reserved for patients with severe symptoms.

TREATMENT OF INSOMNIA

Reframing the Psychosocial Context of Sleep Disturbance

Sleep problems in children and adolescents usually affect the rest of the family, causing sleep loss in parents and siblings who may in some respects suffer as much as the patient. Because misinformation and inappropriate blaming may confound the problem, the disturbed sleep of such patients needs to be addressed as a problem for the whole family.

Modifying family routines may be helpful. Good sleep hygiene, including well-maintained bedtime rituals such as bathing, storytelling, and rocking a small child can facilitate the winding-down process that is an important prelude to sleep. Occasionally, a child becomes overly dependent on a particular routine (e.g., repeated drinks of water every time he or she wakes up) and the parents must set limits. After an expected period of protest, most children relinquish the need for unnecessary attention. These benign disruptions must be differentiated from the more serious panic that some children experience with separation. For this latter kind of anxiety, parental access through the night may be necessary, at least for some time.

In adolescence, sleep is often shortened at both ends by social demands. In the evening, there is homework, socializing, school athletic events, and family life. In the morning, high school schedules often begin quite early, sometimes preceded by an even earlier bus ride. For many teenagers, the morning includes a formidable grooming ritual. Add to this the increasing tendency for teenagers to take part-time jobs after school, and the result is an epidemic of chronic sleep deprivation that is of increasing societal concern. Weekend sleeping-in may recover some of the lost sleep, but it tends to produce a phase delay that reinforces the tendency to stay up late during the week. In one experiment, high school students increased their IQ scores by 20 points after a week in which they systematically extended their sleep time.

In counseling teenagers, some flexibility and compromise are usually most effective. Adding naps during the day may improve alertness. A warning about the dangers of driving while sleepy, intoxicated, or both is important. Chronobiological interventions, such as light therapy, may be needed to counteract extremely delayed sleep. Outside the office, informed physicians may be able to influence public policy to help alleviate the problem, such as adopting sensible work rules for teens and scheduling school activities at reasonable hours.

Adults are not immune to the effects of social and occupational demands on sleep. Many working adults become progressively more sleep deprived as the workweek progresses. Educating patients about appropriate sleep hygiene and cognitive measures helps them regain some sense of control over their symptoms of fatigue (see Table 31-2). New knowledge of the health consequences of sleep deprivation can help motivate people to prioritize sleep as an important health behavior.

Persons with more persistent insomnia or those who appear to have severe emotional distress (as a result or cause of the sleep disturbance) may warrant evaluation by a mental health specialist.

As they do in children, sleep disorders in adults can affect family members. Partners and caregivers of patients with severe sleep disorders may need both emotional support and education about the nature of the sleep disturbance. Understanding the problem can help them to support the patient in following treatment recommendations.

Cognitive Behavioral Therapy

There is now ample evidence that cognitive behavioral therapy (CBT) for primary insomnia, especially over the long term, is at least as effective as sleep medication. The basic approach is to counsel patients to change critical beliefs that induce anxiety around falling asleep and to motivate them to change bedtime behaviors that may be perpetuating insomnia. The basic approach is to motivate patients to practice cognitive skills that will help minimize the worry and frustration that induces the physiologic stress response and impedes sleep. With time, patients can learn to suppress intrusive, unwanted thoughts and activate calming ones. Certain audio books or meditation CDs can help this practice. The "behavioral" component of CBT is the application of sleep hygiene measures. The National Sleep Foundation web site (www.sleepfoundation.org) has many helpful suggestions for people interested in improving sleep hygiene.

Medical Treatment

Insomnia has a good prognosis acutely, but can become chronic and recurrent. Acute insomnia can be treated with sedative–hypnotic drugs in conjunction with a sleep-hygiene program to maximize efficacy and reduce the dosage and duration of treatment (Table 31-3). These medications should not be used in pregnancy. People with secondary insomnia from depression, pain, substance abuse, medications, or circadian rhythm disorders are at risk for chronic insomnia if the acute symptoms do not resolve, and may need specific sleep therapies in addition to treating the underlying cause of sleeplessness.

BENZODIAZEPINES

All benzodiazepines have sleep-promoting effects, although only five are currently marketed as sedative–hypnotics. These drugs work well for short-term treatment of insomnia; tolerance and dependence can develop quickly in some patients. However, some patients, especially those with an anxiety component to

their insomnia, may benefit from long-term use. Benzodiazepines alter sleep structure, reducing both REM and slow-wave sleep, but the clinical significance of this is unknown. They are generally safe for younger adults, even in overdose, although combining them with alcohol and other depressants can produce potentially catastrophic synergistic effects. In older individuals, the safety profile is less benign; amnesia, ataxia, confusion, and worsening sleep apnea may develop.

Choosing one benzodiazepine over another for a specific patient is partly based on drug half-life, and this will require prioritizing goals. Short-acting drugs such as triazolam are useful for the treatment of sleep-onset insomnia, but many individuals will have rebound insomnia in the second half of the night or anxiety the following day. Longer-acting drugs may work better for middle-of-the-night insomnia, but some persons will have morning "hangover" effects. Longer-acting drugs can be particularly troublesome in the elderly, as drug accumulation will lead to ataxia, confusion, and daytime sedation. Temazepam and estazolam are intermediate in half-life and represent reasonable compromises for patients with sleep maintenance insomnia who get hangover effects from the longer-acting drugs.

These drugs should not be prescribed for patients with sleep apnea, severe respiratory disease, gait and balance problems, or alcohol abuse. Doses should be kept low in elderly patients and those with hepatic insufficiency. Rebound insomnia can complicate withdrawal from these drugs, causing patients to return to their use.

BENZODIAZEPINE RECEPTOR AGONISTS

These drugs are structurally unrelated to benzodiazepines, but share some characteristics with them due to the fact that they have agonist activity at more sleep-specific benzodiazepine receptors (GABAα). They have varying half-lives (eszopiclone and zolpidem, 1.4–3.8 hours; zaleplon, 1.0 hours), so they are most suitable for patients with sleep-onset or initial sleep maintenance problems. These medications preserve natural

Table 31-3. Sedative hypnotic medications.

	Trade Name	Type	Half-life (hours)	Dosing Range (mg)
Temazepam	Restoril	Benzodiazepine	8–15	7.5–30
Triazolam	Halcion	Benzodiazepine	2–5	0.125–0.25
Zolpidem	Ambien	Benzodiazepine agonist	3	5–10
Zolpidem CR	Ambien CR	Benzodiazepine agonist	3	6.25–12.5
Zaleplon	Sonata	Benzodiazepine agonist	1	5–10
Eszopiclone	Lunesta	Benzodiazepine agonist	5–7	1–3
Ramelteon	Rozerem	Melatonin agonist	2–5	8

sleep architecture, which provides at least a theoretical advantage over benzodiazepines. Precautions similar to benzodiazepines apply to these medications in terms of dependency, abuse, and adverse effects. Eszopiclone (Lunesta) and zolpidem in continuous-release formulation (Ambien CR) have been shown to retain efficacy over 6 months, and are the only benzodiazepine or benzodiazepine receptor agonists that are FDA-approved for chronic insomnia (see Table 31-3).

MELATONIN AGONIST

Ramelteon (rozerem) is a potent melatonin agonist that is the first nonscheduled, prescription sedative–hypnotic. It has the capacity to shorten sleep latency in people with sleep-onset insomnia, but does not help people stay asleep. It has no potential for abuse, tolerance, or physical dependency, and does not cause ataxia, confusion, or worsen sleep-related breathing disorders. In the clinical trials, the drug was associated with an increase in prolactin in a few subjects. Ramelteon is prescribed at 8 mg before bedtime. Higher doses have not been shown to improve response, but there is some evidence that the response improves over several weeks. Combining ramelteon with CBT or sleep hygiene measures seems a benign and potentially effective long-term strategy for many insomnia patients.

SEDATING ANTIDEPRESSANTS

Many clinicians use sedating antidepressants such as trazodone, mirtazapine, doxepin, and amitriptyline for long-term treatment of insomnia, especially when chronic pain, depression, or anxiety are comorbid conditions. Theoretical advantages over benzodiazepines include less cognitive impairment, more slow-wave sleep and treatment of underlying depression if present. Tolerance to the sedating effects of these drugs develops in some patients. Side effects are numerous, and special care must be taken in elderly patients, especially with amitriptyline, because of its potent anticholinergic effects. There are data indicating efficacy of doxepin and mirtazepine at very low doses (under 10 mg) that may enhance sleep while minimizing side effects.

ANTIHISTAMINES

Diphenhydramine is sedating and is found in many OTC preparations. It is generally safe and effective for short-term use, although tolerance develops very quickly after nightly ingestion. Diphenhydramine has some anticholinergic properties and can cause confusion and urinary retention in elderly persons.

COMPLEMENTARY AND ALTERNATIVE MEDICINES

The pineal hormone melatonin, sold in this country as a food supplement, has sleep-promoting effects in some people. Melatonin is the best studied of the food supplements and OTC remedies for insomnia and is commonly available at health food stores and pharmacies. Patients should be cautioned that melatonin remains an experimental drug and a naturally occurring hormone with potential neuroendocrine, immunologic, and reproductive effects, although it appears to be quite safe with short-term administration. Results from placebo-controlled trials of melatonin for insomnia in various populations suggest it has only modest efficacy, though some individuals respond quite well. Moreover, when taken at the correct point in the circadian cycle, melatonin can be an effective remedy for jet lag and can help people adapt to shift work. Commercial preparations may contain 0.5–5 mg of melatonin per capsule (sometimes in combination with vitamins). The most effective dose is unknown, and may vary from person to person.

CHRONOBIOLOGICAL THERAPIES

Sleep–wake cycle disorders can be treated with scheduled exposure to bright natural or artificial light. Patients with advanced sleep phase syndrome need to have a corrective phase delay with exposure to bright light in the evening. Bright light exposure must be carefully timed so that the circadian pacemaker is phase shifted to move sleep propensity to later hours, allowing these patients to be more alert in the evening. For the more common DSPS, patients need to force themselves awake by receiving appropriately timed light exposure, which should begin around the time they want to wake up. The first few days are very difficult, but after several mornings of 30-minute light exposure, patients can begin falling asleep before midnight and wake up for morning classes or work. For safety and efficacy, patients should use special fixtures marketed to treat SAD ("SAD lights"). Light fixtures are available from numerous commercial vendors.

Melatonin may achieve this same goal with greater convenience, although probably with less robustness and with opposite timing. For example, people with DSPS who want to advance the timing of their sleep might take synthetic melatonin (0.5–1 mg) in the evening at 9:00 or 10:00 P.M.—hours before their own phase-delayed melatonin secretion begins and more synchronous with the timing of melatonin onset in people with earlier sleep—to reset their body clock to the desired phase position. Ramelteon can be effective when used in this same way. These treatments may also be of value in helping shift workers, time zone travelers and persons with visual impairments adapt to a new sleep–wake schedule. Shift workers should be counseled to try to maintain their workweek sleep schedule on their days off work, although this can be difficult because of family and social demands. Some cases may require referral to a sleep specialist.

The Sleepy Patient: Disorders of Excessive Somnolence

Patients are more likely to complain about insomnia than about excessive daytime sleepiness. They may complain of fatigue or feeling tired, but sleepiness per se may not be acknowledged without specific inquiry by the clinician. Two questions that should be included in every sleep-related "review of systems" are:

- *Do you struggle to stay awake while driving, reading, watching television and movies, or listening to lectures during daytime hours?*
- *Do you feel tired, fatigued, and lacking in energy during the day, especially in the morning?*

If the answer is "yes" to either question, follow-up questions should determine if the problem is inadequate nighttime sleep, drowsiness from medications, narcolepsy, or sleep-related breathing problems. The Epworth Sleepiness Scale (see Table 31-4) is a validated instrument used to assess pathological sleepiness in patients. It is a questionnaire that scores a patient's tendency to fall asleep in eight hypothetical situations on a 0–3 scale, with zero scored for "not at all likely to doze" and three for "extremely likely to doze" in each situation. A cumulative score above 10 suggests the need for referral to a sleep disorders specialist. A discussion of driving or operating machinery while sleepy should also be initiated. Excessive daytime sleepiness requires a thoughtful diagnostic approach.

Sleep-Related Breathing Problems

OBSTRUCTIVE SLEEP APNEA SYNDROME AND SNORING

CASE ILLUSTRATION 3

Jim is 64 years old and visits his primary care physician for a follow-up of his hypertension treatment. His wife has accompanied him to the office to ask whether there is any medical explanation for her husband's fatigue. Close questioning reveals that the fatigue predates the antihypertensive medication and is not clearly attributable to the drug. The tiredness is accompanied by true sleepiness; Jim can fall asleep anytime during the day while reading or driving. He scores 12 on the Epworth Sleepiness Scale, indicating significant daytime sleepiness. He minimizes the problem, yet acknowledges having trouble with memory and concentration. He falls asleep easily after getting into bed at night, but his wife describes him as a restless sleeper who snores loudly.

As a late middle-aged man with hypertension and daytime sleepiness, Jim needs to be referred to a sleep laboratory to rule out OSA, which would be the overwhelmingly most likely diagnosis in a sleepy middle-aged man. Although more common in men, the incidence of OSA increases in middle-aged women, especially with higher body mass indices. Fatigue, rather than sleepiness, is more likely to be the chief complaint in women with OSA.

Obstructive sleep apnea (OSA) is increasingly recognized as a common, important, and treatable disease. Originally thought of as a relatively rare disturbance in severely obese patients with the classic "Pickwickian Syndrome" of somnolence, hypoventilation, and polycythemia, OSA is now known to represent a range of upper airway narrowing in sleep. Epidemiologic studies in middle-aged adults show a prevalence of 2% of women and 4% of men, but these estimates are likely very low, especially given recent trends in increased body weight.

Obstructive sleep apnea is a significant cause of fatigue, daytime somnolence, and cardiovascular morbidity in adults. Nighttime symptoms of OSA include loud snoring (often beginning early in adulthood and worsening with age and increased weight), apnea witnessed by the sleeping partner, snorting or gagging sounds, restlessness, night sweats, and abrupt awakenings with a feeling of choking. Electroencephalogram arousals triggered by the apneic episodes cause interrupted sleep quality, excessive daytime sleepiness, and subjective fatigue. There is also mounting evidence of objective deficits in cognitive processing, attention, and executive functions. Although less common, insomnia may be the presenting complaint. Patients are often unaware of the severity of the sleep disruption and may attribute their sleepiness to some other cause, such as working too hard. The degree of sleepiness is variable, but is a key symptom. Questions about dozing while reading or watching television, nodding off at the wheel, or poor concentration need to be posed directly to patients. Assessment with a standardized scale measuring daytime sleepiness such as the Epworth Sleepiness Scale may be helpful (Table 31-4).

Cardiovascular morbidity and mortality has now been strongly associated with severe OSA (Apnea Hypopnea Index [AHI] > 30). Cardiovascular manifestations of OSA include hypertension, heart failure, stroke, and possibly myocardial infarction. Although not a randomized trial, in the long-term observational study from Spain, continuous positive airway pressure (CPAP) treatment reduced the incidence of cardiovascular events, thus strengthening the rationale for CPAP treatment, particularly in severe OSA.

Diagnosis of OSA begins with a clinical assessment, but a sleep study is necessary to confirm the diagnosis

Table 31-4. Epworth Sleepiness Scale

How often are you likely to doze off or fall asleep in the following situations, in contrast to feeling just tired? This refers to your usual way of life in recent times. Even if you have not done some of these things recently, try to work out how they would have affected you. Use the following scale to choose the *most appropriate number* for each situation:	
0 = would *never* doze	
1 = *slight* chance of dozing	
2 = *moderate* chance of dozing	
3 = *high* chance of dozing	
Sitting and reading	_____
Watching TV	_____
Sitting, inactive in a public place (e.g., a theater or a meeting)	_____
As a passenger in a car for an hour without a break	_____
Lying down to rest in the afternoon when circumstances permit	_____
Sitting and talking to someone	_____
Sitting quietly after lunch without alcohol	_____
In a car, while stopped for a few minutes in traffic	_____
TOTAL	_____

Source: From MW Johns. *Sleep* 1991;14:540.

and severity of OSA. A formal PSG in a sleep laboratory remains the gold standard for diagnosis, but less-detailed home testing using portable technology that does not require a sleep technician to be in attendance can provide diagnostic information in some cases. When PSG in the sleep laboratory confirms the diagnosis of OSA, there is an opportunity for the patient to try CPAP treatment with a supervised mask fitting by an experienced sleep technologist. If the diagnosis is made with a home-based study, it is still best if they come to the sleep laboratory for PSG-monitored CPAP mask fitting and pressure titration.

Treatment options should be individualized depending on the severity of OSA, and also patient symptoms and comorbidities. Initial treatments to reduce OSA include weight loss, avoidance of sedating medications or alcohol near bedtime, and appliances to prevent back sleeping (tennis balls sewn in the back of nightshirt are an inexpensive option). Continuous positive airway pressure (with either mask or nasal pillows) remains the most common and effective treatment for improving sleep quality, reducing daytime symptoms, and reducing cardiovascular risk. In patients who cannot tolerate CPAP, other treatment options are typically ENT surgery or oral (dental) devices. A variety of surgical techniques are available, but the low success rates make surgery a less appealing initial treatment in most cases.

Some adults will have significant tonsillar hypertrophy and be better surgical candidates. Tracheotomy has a very high success rate, but is a morbid procedure that has been much less frequently performed since CPAP has a high success rate. Oral appliances fitted and adjusted by an experienced dentist can maintain the tongue in a more forward position to improve airway patency in mild-to-moderate cases of OSA or for those who cannot tolerate CPAP (see Figure 31-1). Patients who have surgical or dental treatments should have a follow-up sleep study to document the efficacy of those treatments. The correct diagnosis and effective treatment of OSA can help improve quality of life, prevent serious accidents, and reduce cardiovascular risk.

Snoring is a common sleep symptom. Apart from being a nuisance to bed partners, snoring may herald the development of serious respiratory obstruction during sleep along a continuum of partial to complete airway closure. Men snore more than women, but the prevalence increases in women after menopause. Aside from male gender, other factors associated with snoring include anatomic narrowing of the airway, body habitus (obesity) and sleep position (supine), the use of alcohol and sedative–hypnotics, endocrinopathy (hypothyroidism, acromegaly), smoking, and, possibly, genetic factors. Since snoring is a common presenting symptom of OSA, it is important to ask questions regarding apnea and OSA symptoms in any patient who complains of snoring. Similarly to OSA, initial treatments to reduce snoring include weight loss, the avoidance of sedating medications and alcohol, and appliances to prevent back sleeping. If a sleep study confirms the absence of apnea, but snoring remains disruptive, then potential interventions include oral (dental) appliances, surgery, and nasal valve resistors. Oral appliances thrust the tongue or mandible forward during sleep, and are best fitted by an experienced dental provider. Ear, nose, and throat surgical techniques to reduce the uvula and soft palate are available, but the long-term effects are unknown. Because surgery can eliminate the noise of snoring without relieving airway obstruction, sleep study evaluation should be performed to rule out OSA prior to surgery.

Obstructive sleep apnea also occurs in 1–3% of younger children. Tonsil and adenoid hypertrophy are thought to contribute, since resection of these results in relief from OSA in the majority of children. However, the size of these tissues does not correlate with the presence or degree of OSA. Obstructive sleep apnea should also be considered in children with craniofacial abnormalities, macroglossia, neuromuscular disease, and obesity. As in adults, loud snoring, restless sleep, and witnessed pauses in breathing are symptomatic. Children with OSA may not complain of sleepiness; instead they may manifest daytime irritability, hyperactivity, decreased attention, or declining school performance.

Nasal Insert

A

Full Face Mask

C

Nasal Mask

B

Figure 31-1. Various positive airway pressure interfaces for patients who are CPAP-intolerant.
Source: McKean S, Ross JJ, Dressler DD, Brotman DJ, Ginsberg JS. *Principles and Practice of Hospital Medicine.* Accessed at www.accessmedicine.com.

Secondary nocturnal enuresis is another important symptom of OSA. Parents should be asked about snoring and breath-holding during sleep. Consultation with an ENT specialist is advised whenever OSA is suspected. Tonsillectomy is curative in up to 90% of cases and should be the first step in treatment. Other causes of OSA can be treated with CPAP, though careful monitoring for midface hypoplasia should be undertaken in children aged less than 12 years. Surgical approaches such as tracheostomy or craniofacial reconstruction may be necessary in rare cases.

CENTRAL SLEEP APNEA

Central sleep apnea (CSA) is defined as the cessation of airflow for at least 10 seconds with no ventilatory effort. In adults, central apnea accounts for approximately 5% of apnea cases, so CSA is much less common than OSA. Patients with predominantly central apnea tend to complain more of insomnia than of hypersomnolence, which may be a helpful distinguishing feature from OSA. The differential diagnosis of CSA includes congestive heart failure (CHF), hypoventilation (from chest wall, neuromuscular, or CNS disease), stroke, nasal obstruction, GERD, postnasal drip, and opiates. Congestive heart failure patients with reduced left ventricular function who show waxing and waning respiration during sleep are a particular type of CSA called Cheyne–Stokes respiration, which has been associated with reduced survival. Optimal treatment is unclear,

but options include servo-ventilation (a form of bilevel), CPAP, and nocturnal oxygen. In patients with hypoventilation due to neuromuscular disease, chest wall disease or neurodegenerative diseases that affect the CNS respiratory control, bilevel treatment can address both the central apnea and hypoventilation. Gastroesophageal reflux disease and postnasal drip are infrequent causes of CSA, but should be addressed if no other causes are present. Opiates can cause CSA in a minority of patients, and the risk appears to be dose related; these cases may be more frequently seen because more patients are being treated for chronic pain issues. Lastly, the term "complex" sleep apnea has been used to describe OSA patients who develop central apnea when they are treated with CPAP. Complex sleep apnea has been estimated to occur in 6% of OSA patients treated with CPAP, but usually resolves over time with continued CPAP treatment. If necessary, both opiate CSA and complex apnea can be treated with a bilevel machine that delivers a back-up rate. Complex sleep apnea remains difficult and challenging, but is much less common than OSA.

Central sleep apnea can also be seen in prematurity, neonates, and children, but the differential diagnosis is broad and complex. A detailed discussion is beyond the scope of this review. The differential diagnosis ranges from apnea of premature infants, to GERD, to neurologic syndromes, and to hypoventilation syndromes such as congenital central hypoventilation syndrome

(CCHS is caused by a *PHOX2b* mutation). Pediatric CSA may contribute to sudden infant death syndrome (SIDS). The cause of SIDS remains a mystery, but a wide variety of intrinsic and extrinsic factors are thought to play a role. A public information campaign to encourage mothers to avoid placing infants prone face down ("Back to Sleep") has been ongoing since 1995, and subsequent epidemiologic assessments have shown a dramatic decrease in the number of SIDS cases.

Narcolepsy

Narcolepsy is a disorder in which elements of sleep intrude into wakefulness and wakefulness intrudes into sleep. It consists of four primary symptoms: excessive daytime sleepiness, cataplexy, and less frequently, sleep paralysis and hypnagogic hallucinations. It occurs in approximately 1 in 2000 people. Narcolepsy usually begins in the teens or early twenties, but onset as old as the eighth decade has been reported. Prevalence is roughly equal in men and women, and a formal diagnosis is frequently not made until 5 or 10 years after the onset of symptoms.

The cardinal symptom is sleepiness that comes on suddenly and irresistibly in what are called "sleep attacks." Low-grade, persistent sleepiness affecting concentration, thinking, and memory may also occur. Sleep episodes may be brief (several minutes to an hour), but the person usually awakens feeling more alert, and the next sleep episode usually does not come on for at least an hour. Narcolepsy can impair nighttime sleep with frequent awakenings, vivid nightmares, and intense, realistic hallucinations prior to sleep onset (hypnagogic). The hallucinations are usually visual, but may involve any sensory modality. Cataplexy, the brief, sudden loss of muscle tone leading to neck muscle weakness, buckling of the knees, or rarely, complete collapse, is triggered by strong emotional reactions such as laughter or anger. Sleep paralysis is transient immobility on awakening, often accompanied by the vivid hallucinations of REM dreaming, all while the patient is lying in bed perfectly alert. The spells are brief, lasting several minutes at most. If the syndrome is not diagnosed and treated, people with the disorder may be perceived as lazy and unmotivated due to persistence of significant symptoms. Additional sequelae of a missed diagnosis include poor school and work performance, social stigma, and accidents.

Hypocretin-1 (Orexin), an alerting neuropeptide secreted by the hypothalamus, has been shown to play an important role in this disorder; a low CSF hypocretin-1 concentration below 110 pg/mL can be used as a diagnostic criteria. A combination of infectious, immune, and genetic factors appear to play a role in narcolepsy, and a human leucocyte antigen (HLA) linkage to DQB1*0602 has been demonstrated. Confirmation of the diagnosis should be undertaken with overnight PSG followed by a multiple sleep latency test (MSLT). The finding of mean sleep latency less than 5 minutes and REM periods during at least two naps confirms the diagnosis. Since diagnosis can be challenging in atypical cases, the testing should be supervised by a sleep disorders specialist who can integrate both clinical history and sleep testing data. Without the symptoms of cataplexy, the diagnosis is more difficult. An accurate diagnosis is advisable, since narcolepsy is a life-long condition that often requires a commitment to long-term treatment.

Excessive daytime somnolence (EDS) of narcolepsy may be treated with modafinil (200–400 mg) or armodafinil (150–250 mg) each morning, which can significantly improve daytime function. Sodium oxybate (Xyrem), a relative of gamma-hydroxybutyrate (GHB), is FDA-approved to treat cataplexy, and is used by some clinicians to treat EDS. The older CNS stimulants, dextroamphetamine (5–60 mg/day), methamphetamine (20–25 mg/day), and methylphenidate (10–60 mg/day), are commonly used as well. Scheduling brief naps into one's daily routine can be very helpful in improving function and reducing sleep attacks. Cataplexy and sleep paralysis can also be treated with REM-suppressant drugs such as TCAs and selective serotonin reuptake inhibitors (SSRIs). Joining a narcolepsy support group will help patients cope with the psychological sequelae, which result from the social and occupational stigma of having little control over sleep onset.

Kleine–Levin Syndrome

Kleine–Levin Syndrome is a condition characterized by periods of excessive hypersomnia and increased sleep time with frequent recurrences of the symptoms. The peculiar disorder is usually seen in people in their late adolescent years. These episodes can last from less than a week to 30 days. While the disease is active, some people experience other symptoms of excessive eating and hypersexuality. Social aspects of the patient's life will suffer during the active periods, such as not attending school or work. In between the flare-ups, the patient functions normally in all respects, but recurring symptomatic periods will begin to show sporadically. In most cases, the frequency and intensity of the spells decreases as the adolescent matures and eventually will resolve itself. It is thought to be caused by a virus or local encephalitis in the diencephalon region. Amphetamines, methlyphenidates, and modafinil have been used as treatment, but usually they are only effective for a few hours.

Patients With Abnormal Nighttime Behavior: The Parasomnias

An accurate diagnosis of the underlying cause of bizarre nighttime behavior can be challenging. Diagnostic considerations include seizure disorders, psychosis, delirium, and intoxication. Parasomnias, the least common class of sleep disorders, but perhaps the most dramatic in their presentation, need to be included in the differential.

Pavor Nocturnus

Sleep terrors (pavor nocturnus) are very disconcerting to parents but are usually quite benign. The child (usually aged 3–6 years) awakens with a scream and appears terrified, with signs of autonomic arousal: eyes bulging, heart racing, and sweating. Most episodes last only a few minutes. Attempts at comfort are to no avail and may exacerbate or prolong the episode. In the morning, the child is amnestic for the episode or may have a fragmentary memory of a bad dream. Sleep terrors involve partial arousals from stage 4 (deep) sleep. Reassurance of the parents is the usual treatment; in persistent night terrors, however, benzodiazepines may be justified.

Nightmares

True nightmares occur in REM sleep and occasionally occur in stage 1 or 2 sleep. The nightmares involve a narrative story people can often relate once awake. This story is not necessarily a recall of the day's actual events but a stressful episodic account that can be linked to the day's events. Nightmares are usually a transient problem, presumably triggered by a stressful personal incident. Persistent nightmares are a serious concern, however, and may require referral to a mental health specialist.

Post traumatic stress disorder has many accompanying symptoms, and one indication the patient is suffering from the disorder is persistent recurring nightmares (see Chapter 26). The nightmares of PTSD patients are distinguished from other nightmares because they are narratives of the actual traumatic event, usually set in a previous time, and mimic the memory of the experience. For example, many wartime veterans have persistent nightmares that they are on the battlefield, and they feel all the fear and terror they felt when they were actually taking part in the war. When a person is stressed from normal life expectancies, dreaming can be cathartic and help to sort out feelings. For people with PTSD, dreaming about what had caused them so much stress is detrimental and just reinforces the traumatic events they experienced. The other dreams they have that do not relate directly to the trauma also have negative emotional contents of threat, aggression, and are extremely vivid compared with control populations. There is no specific treatment for the nightmares that patients with PTSD experience, but by treating the disorder with medications and cognitive behavior therapy, the nightmare frequency will reduce. Controlled trial data and clinical experience supports the use of alpha-1 adrenergic receptor antagonists (e.g., prazocin) in reducing the intensity and frequency of nightmare in PTSD. Alpha-2 receptor agonists (e.g., clonidine and guanfacine) may help sleep and other autonomic arousal symptoms in PTSD. Antidepressant and mood-stabilizing atypical antipsychotic medications are generally used to help with daytime symptoms but can sometimes help sleep as well.

Somnambulism

Like sleep terrors, sleepwalking is a partial arousal from stage 4 sleep. Occasional sleepwalking is very common in childhood and may follow a period of stress or sleep deprivation. The main concern is accidental injury, and protective measures, such as placing gates in front of a stairwell, may be needed.

Rem Behavior Disorder

In this syndrome, loss of normal REM sleep muscle atonia leads to dream-enactment behavior. The diagnosis is made in patients with sudden bursts of excited, intense, sometimes violent activity during sleep. The syndrome may be subtle, in the form of leg movements and talking, or dramatic, with punching, kicking, grabbing, strangling, running, and moving about the bedroom. Dreams of an intense, violent nature are typical. REM behavior disorder is seen frequently in toxic or metabolic delirium, but the most persistent forms of the syndrome occur in old age, and are presumed to be idiopathic, ischemic, or neurodegenerative in etiology. The syndrome is especially common in patients with PD and dementia with Lewy Bodies and can start to develop even before other signs of the diseases. Once documented by PSG, the condition can be effectively treated with clonazepam, although there are reports of other agents, such as cholinesterase inhibitors, working as well.

Movement Disorders in Children

Other movement disorders such as rhythmic sleep disorders (head banging, body rocking, and head rolling) interestingly do not cause insomnia, but are usually brought to the examiner's attention by the caregiver for hazardous concerns. Rhythmic movements are observed in normal children at 9 months of age, and the occurrence decreases by 50% by the age of 18 months. By 4 years of age, the prevalence is only 8%. These movement disorders are usually seen on PSGs just before sleep onset and can persist into stage 1 non-REM sleep or after spontaneous arousal. Because these various movements can disrupt sleep, the child experiences excessive daytime sleepiness. Fortunately, between the ages of 2 and 4 years, the intensity decreases, and usually resolves spontaneously. Rarely is this disorder observed in healthy adolescents or adults.

Epilepsy

Epileptic discharges often occur during sleep and may be misinterpreted as other sleep arousal phenomena, such as somnambulism or pavor nocturnus. Onset of a seizure disorder can be at any age, but most commonly will begin in adolescence. Epileptic events generally occur in the non-REM stages of sleep and rarely in the REM stages. Nocturnal seizures may produce arousals that may or may not be remembered by the patient, and depending on the frequency and duration of arousals, can cause daytime sleepiness. Postictal sleepiness can also persist into daytime. In fact, daytime sleepiness in patients with epilepsy is not always attributable to antiepileptic medications.

There are particular types of seizures more prone to occur during sleep. Benign childhood epilepsy with centrotemporal spikes (BECT), or benign Rolandic epilepsy, is triggered by sleep and is recognized by unilateral facial paresthesias with tonic or tonic–clonic movement. If the pharyngeal muscles are involved, these symptoms will be coupled with drooling.

Seizures that involve the frontal lobe present themselves as peculiar behavior involving motor activity and unusual vocalizations. Autosomal dominant nocturnal frontal lobe epilepsy (ADNFLE) involves thrashing activity with spastic posture and speaking vociferously. These patients may also sleep walk and become violent. Nocturnal paroxysmal dystonia involves tonic spasms of the limbs and laughter as the vocalization. Pure tonic seizures also involve the frontal lobes and appear as insomnia or hypersomnia because of periodic arousals.

Diagnosis of seizure disorder involves routine EEGs or prolonged video EEGs combined with clinical symptoms to classify the seizure type. Anticonvulsant medications are given to those diagnosed to prevent further electrical discharges.

DIAGNOSTIC EVALUATION & REFERRAL

Most types of insomnia are diagnosed on the basis of history, and PSG evaluation of insomnia is rarely necessary or reimbursed. Clinicians should be able to accurately diagnose and treat transient insomnia without referral or consultation. Referral to a sleep specialist should be considered for patients with persistent symptoms who do not respond to initial treatment. Patients with severe RLS and chronobiological sleep disorders should usually be referred. Sleep-related breathing problems, periodic leg movements, narcolepsy, and the adult parasomnias all require PSG validation and expert management and will require a sleep specialist to validate the diagnosis and initial treatment plans.

SUGGESTED READINGS

Besteiro González JL, Suárez Fernández TV, Arboleya Rodríguez L, Muñiz J, Lemos Giráldez S, Alvarez Fernández A. Sleep architecture in patients with fibromyalgia. *Psicothema* 2011;23: 368–373.

Morin AK. Strategies for treating chronic insomnia. *Am J Manag Care* 2006;12:S2230–S2245.

Morin CM, Bellville G, Belanger L, Ivers H. The Insomnia Severity Index: psychometric indicators to detect insomnia cases and evaluate treatment response. *Sleep* 2011;34(5):601–608.

Pearson NJ, Johnson LL, Nahin RL. Insomnia, trouble sleeping, and complementary and alternative medicine. *Arch Intern Med* 2006;166:1775–1782.

Silber MH. Chronic insomnia. *N Engl J Med* 2005;353:803–810.

Vitiello MV, Rybarczyk B, Von Korff M, Stepanski EJ. Cognitive behavioral therapy for insomnia improves sleep and decreases pain in older adults with co-morbid insomnia and osteoarthritis. *J Clin Sleep Med* 2009;5:355–362.

Wickwire EM, Collop NA. Insomnia and sleep-related breathing disorders. *Chest* 2010;137:1449–1463.

WEB SITES

The National Sleep Foundation. www.sleepfoundation.org. Accessed February 2014.

The Society of Behavioral Sleep Medicine. www.behavioralsleep.org. Accessed February 2014.

American Academy of Sleep Medicine. www.aasmnet.org. Accessed February 2014.

Willis-Ekbom Disease Foundation. www.rls.org. Accessed February 2014

Sexual Problems

David G. Bullard, PhD; Harvey Caplan, MD; & Christine Derzko, MD

Sex is a problem for everyone. . . . Indeed, for a couple of weeks or a couple of months, or maybe even for a couple of years, if we are lucky, we may feel that we have solved the problem of sex. But then, of course, we change or our partners change, or the whole ballgame changes, and once again we are left trying to scramble over that obstacle with this built-in feeling that we can get over it, when actually we never can. However, in the process of trying to get over it, we learn a great deal about vulnerability and intimacy and love. . . . (Peck, 1993, Further Along the Road Less Traveled)

Rodin, "The Kiss" (545 x 800). Accessed at http://theroyalist10.wordpress.com/2010/10/

INTRODUCTION

Sexuality encompasses an enormous range of behaviors, beliefs, desires, experiences, and fantasies that patients may want to discuss with their health care providers. Sexuality also may have legal, medical, moral, political, and religious aspects. This chapter intends to give the practicing clinician basic practical knowledge of human sexuality and useful tools for managing common problems.

Patients with sexual concerns report feeling most comfortable discussing these issues with their primary care physician and expect to receive advice and treatment. In large studies of adult patients, more than 70% considered sexual matters to be an appropriate topic for the primary care provider to discuss. Yet, evidence of discussion about sexual problems has been found in as few as 2% of the notes of such providers.

Primary care practitioners are in an optimal position to evaluate sexual problems, as they often have the most comprehensive and long-lasting relationship with the patient. In contrast to most other medical diagnoses, however, it is the patient who usually defines when a sexual problem exists. That is to say, a "problem" exists only if and when the individual or the partner is troubled by his or her level of sexual desire, response, or function.

Levine (2010) posits that sexual issues can be usefully conceptualized within three broad categories: **sexual worries, problems, and disorders**. Although referral to medical or mental health specialists (or both) may be indicated in more severe situations of disorders and dysfunctions, many worries and problems can be successfully addressed by the primary care practitioner. When questions about sexuality are approached in an open, matter-of-fact manner, most people are relieved and respond positively. They appreciate the affirmation that these issues are valid and important, whether or not they have current sexual concerns or are sexually active (Table 32-1).

Table 32-1. Sexual concerns of patients.

- **Common sexual worries about normalcy**, such as: Am I OK? What is a "healthy" sex life? How do I compare? Is my sex life satisfactory?
- **Sexual identity questions** relevant to lifestyle, orientation, and preference.
- **Developmental issues of sexuality** for children, adolescents, parents, and the elderly, including the development of gender identity, masturbation, genital exploration, child sex play, sexuality, and the single life, marriage, divorce, and death of a partner.
- **Reproductive concerns** covering infertility, family planning, contraception, pregnancy, and abortion.
- **Sexual desire, satisfaction, and other problems**, such as a couple's differing levels of desire, and problems with vaginal lubrication, erections, orgasm, and pain.
- **Sexual changes** due to physical disability, medical illness, and treatment.
- **Sexual trauma** resulting from molestation, incest, and rape.
- **Safe sex practices:** AIDS and STDs.
- **Paraphilias and sexual compulsions**.

CHALLENGE FOR CLINICIANS

To provide patients with helpful responses to their sexual health concerns, health professionals need the following:

- Willingness and ability to discuss sexual topics comfortably.
- Awareness of the range and diversity of human sexual practices and concerns across and within cultures, as well as awareness of the importance of the circumstances or conditions under which individuals function best.
- Ability to separate their own personal beliefs and values from those of patients. Unless the practitioner encounters information indicating objective harm to someone involved, it is important to maintain a nonjudgmental demeanor.
- Skill at taking a history of sex problems in appropriate detail.
- Knowledge of simple interventions such as permission-giving, transmitting accurate information, providing specific suggestions (e.g., for making sex less pressured and more pleasurable), and making referrals to other resources, when appropriate.

As health professionals, we may have personally had limited sexual experience, as well as questions and problems of our own, and consequently may be uncomfortable in discussing particular sexual material. Time, thought, and experience, however, can build confidence and expertise in talking about sexual problems. Health care providers can increase their comfort level by examining their own attitudes, beliefs, assumptions, and experiences; reading the literature; discussing sexual issues with friends and colleagues; and routinely incorporating sexual health questions into the general health assessment of patients.

Of course, no one—patients *or* caregivers—should be forced to talk about sexuality. It is important for everyone to recognize the limits of their own interest, comfort, and competency. However, sexual health is an integral part of health care. All who deal with patients should be alert to the possibility of sexual concerns and, at a minimum, be able to respond with nonjudgmental listening and reassurance. When in the best interest of the patient, health care providers can refer to a colleague who is comfortable and competent in discussing sexual issues.

PERSPECTIVES ON HUMAN SEXUALITY

Knowledge of human sexuality has expanded remarkably since the modern pioneering efforts of Kinsey and Masters and Johnson—who published some of the earliest evidence-based treatment of sexual problems. While initially focusing on the range of sexual behaviors and the treatment of dysfunctional mechanical problems, the field has grown to include and better understand sexual motivations, the critical importance of sexual excitement and desire, and of the contexts required to produce sexual fulfillment.

Research in human sexuality has burgeoned, as has knowledge of the often-negative effects of long-accepted sex roles. And we are learning more about variations among individuals in terms of the role sexuality plays in life. A particular sexual problem may be perceived as central and significant to one patient, yet be seen by another to be peripheral or minor. Clinicians must be cautious to not make assumptions about the significance of various sexual problems, but rather assess and discover whatever meaning the issue has for that individual or within a particular couple.

Motivations for human sexual expression are complex and numerous. Different motivations exist throughout the life cycle, including variations in times of illness or periods of health. Motivations vary from culture to culture and from individual to individual. They may include the need to express love, the need for physical release, reproduction, recreation, the need to increase self-esteem—or combinations of all the above. Conversely, sexuality can also be used to coerce, control, or degrade others. Sexuality may be the focus of addictive or compulsive behavior.

Sexual worries or difficulties are likely experienced by most people at some period of life, and may result from developmental growth and changes in life circumstances rather than from pathology alone. Sexual problems are sometimes a blessing, such as when they compel a person to get help for symptoms that indicate underlying medical problems, problems with self-esteem, or problems with a relationship. Surprisingly, for some people, seeking help for problems involving erection or orgasm may be more acceptable than seeking help for issues involving self-esteem.

Because the language of sex is broad and varied, primary care practitioners will find it helpful to become familiar and comfortable with the vernacular and to be able to discuss calmly and in detail matters such as masturbation, sexual positions, oral sex, anal sex, penis size, and breast size. The following section discusses a few of the areas in which misconceptions about these subjects can be resolved.

COMMON SEXUAL ISSUES

From a medical viewpoint, **masturbation** is "normal," universal, and physically harmless at all ages. It is highly correlated with self-acceptance and sexual adjustment, and is often suggested as "homework" in sex therapy to further sexual self-awareness. Some people freely choose not to masturbate, perhaps following personal or religious tenets. Guilt about masturbation, however, continues to affect many patients. Some may use masturbation compulsively to avoid personal or relationship issues. Sex offenders may reinforce their antisocial fantasies via masturbation. Those who are truly addicted to some sexual behaviors may suffer from a variety of life difficulties common to other addictions.

There is no standard for what constitutes acceptable **sexual frequency**. Individuals who are celibate may still consider themselves sexual beings, whereas others may have sex rarely but find it satisfying and enjoyable when they do. Compulsive, frequent sex can become unrewarding for some, whereas others thrive on a frequent and active sex life. What is "right" for a particular individual or couple must be determined based on the various meanings and expectations they associate with sexuality.

Sexual fantasies are limited only by human imagination and may be enjoyed for their own sake. Fantasies may be exciting to a person who would never want to experience them in real life, or they may be yearned for. Obsessive and intrusive images that cause discomfort may need to be addressed with psychotherapy.

The majority of women enjoy and need direct **clitoral stimulation** manually or orally to reach orgasm. Unfortunately, many men assume that their female partners are fully satisfied with only intercourse. A result of this overemphasis on intercourse is that many women and men are uncomfortable with genital caressing alone. Couples can benefit from encouragement and permission to learn about and enjoy noncoital sex.

Most gay, lesbian, or bisexual patients do not wish to have their **sexual orientation** changed or challenged and often present the same concerns as heterosexuals about normalcy, dysfunction, and intimacy.

Life Changes: Menopause, Aging & Sexuality

Sexuality is an all-encompassing term that includes *sexual identity*, *sexual function*, and *sexual relationships*, *all of which* may be modified by a number of factors including both female *menopause* and *aging*.

Aging brings with it a number of recognized and normal changes in sexual response. These include the following:

1. In both men and women, more direct genital stimulation and more time are needed for arousal (lubrication or erection).
2. Women may experience irritation and pain with intercourse, especially after menopause or periods of abstinence.
3. Erections may become less rigid.
4. Orgasm may not occur with each sexual encounter and the urge to ejaculate may become less intense.
5. The refractory period (the time interval between a man's ejaculation and his next erection) increases.

Many adults in their 70s, 80s, and even later years are willing to experiment in response to changes in their interest, sexual physiology, and partner status. Some older men and women become less focused on intercourse, finding increased enjoyment in petting, oral sex, and masturbation. Others may be happy to have retired from an active sexual life.

Phosphodiesterase type-5 inhibitor (PDE5) oral medications such as tadalafil (Cialis), sildenafil (Viagra), and vardenafil (Levitra) enhance erectile functioning in many men. In women, results of studies looking for positive effects of these medications on sexuality, in general, have been inconsistent, in part because different end points have been used. However, some data show benefit with PDE5 therapy in those women with previously normal sexual function who developed low libido after starting antidepressant therapy. In the future, it may be found to benefit other select groups of women as well.

Testosterone or estrogen replacement may also be beneficial to correct decreases due to aging, and are discussed in greater detail below.

DISCUSSING SEXUALITY IN THE GENERAL MEDICAL EXAMINATION

Reasons given by health care providers who are reluctant to address sexual health issues include embarrassment, feeling ill-prepared, belief that the sexual history is not relevant to the chief complaint, and time constraints.

The prevalence of sexual concerns is consistently underestimated by physicians, which contributes to minimizing the importance of sexual health care. Patients report that physician discomfort and anticipated nonempathetic response to sexual problems are the primary barriers to discussing sexual health.

An assessment of problems related to sexual function requires a consideration of all relevant potential etiological factors in order that any appropriate therapeutic measures may be instituted, be they psychosocial, physical, and/or pharmacological.

Some patients may be more reluctant to discuss their diet or exercise patterns than the details of their sexual life, whereas others may feel they risk disapproval or judgment when talking with a medical authority about sexuality, and particularly about their sexual practices. When introducing the topic of sexuality, it is often helpful to acknowledge right away that the patient may feel some embarrassment. By routinely asking questions about sexual health in an initial history taking, a caregiver shows acceptance of sexual health as an integral part of a person's well-being.

Also, it may be helpful to explain that some diseases and conditions can be major factors in the etiology of sexual dysfunction, among them diabetes mellitus, cardiovascular disease hypertension, immunologic issues, arthritis, chronic back pain, and current and previously treated cancers.

The following is one way to initiate a discussion about sexuality:

Doctor: One area of health care that is often neglected is sexual health, yet it can be important to people. Do you have any questions about your sex life that you would like to discuss?

A "no" response can be accepted, without ruling out possible future discussion.

Doctor: If you have any questions later on, I'd be glad to talk with you or help you find someone with whom you would be comfortable talking.

When providers are uncomfortable about a sexual topic, they can make comments such as "I feel somewhat awkward bringing this up," or "I haven't had that experience, but let me find out," or "Can you educate me about that?" These phrases are acceptable to most patients and can extricate the clinician from some difficult situations, as well as foster patient rapport.

As part of the psychosocial component of the general medical examination, a brief sex history should cover the following:

- "Are you sexually active now?" "How many current partners do you have?" If none, "When was the last time you had sex?" "Is that O.K. for you at this point in your life?"

- "Are you sexually active with men, women, both, or neither?" To encourage the confidence of lesbian, gay, or bisexual patients, ask about the patient's "partner" rather than using the gender-specific terms "wife," "husband," "boyfriend," or "girlfriend." And ask about "sexual encounters" rather than "intercourse."

- "How satisfied are you with your sexual experiences and functioning?" (Frequency, variety, who initiates, etc.)

- "Do you experience any problems with lubrication, orgasm, erection, or ejaculation?"

- Rather than assuming contraception is necessary, ask, "Do you have a need for contraception?" Follow-up questions may include asking about the efficacy of or level of satisfaction with any current contraception method in use.

- "Have you ever been diagnosed and treated for sexually transmitted diseases (STDs)?" Discussion of human papillomavirus (HPV) vaccine and its relevance to cancer prevention of cervical and oral cancers can then be included.

- "Have you ever been tested for human immunodeficiency virus (HIV), and if so do you know if you are positive?" "Are you aware of safer sex precautions, such as the use of condoms and barrier protection, even when there is no risk of pregnancy or when other contraceptives (e.g., intrauterine device [IUD] or "the pill") are used?"

- "Have you ever been/or are you currently in a relationship in which you have been/or are being abused emotionally, physically, or sexually?"

Use questions that show openness to other than the modal heterosexual preferences. Making assumptions about a person's sexuality based on age, gender, race, ethnicity, marital status, or sexual orientation may be diagnostically misleading and send damaging messages to the individual. For instance, an elderly patient assumed to be sexually inactive may in fact have multiple sexual partners, and important risk factors for STDs and acquired immunodeficiency syndrome (AIDS) may be missed or a monogamous gay male may feel stereotyped or misunderstood if it is assumed that he has multiple partners.

Make sure that the terminology is mutually understood. Overly general or euphemistic terms such as "having sex," "getting it on," "making out," "making love," or "losing one's nature" may obscure important details. Terms that are too technical ("coitus," "copulation," and "cunnilingus") or too colloquial ("cunt," "cock," and "fucking") may be inappropriate for use in the professional relationship.

Avoid words that convey moral judgments or indicate little about what an individual is actually experiencing (e.g., *"adultery," "frigid," "impotent," "nymphomaniac," and "perversion"*). Clinicians can help patients discard demeaning labels by substituting behavioral descriptions such as "having sex outside of your primary relationship," "difficulty getting erections or getting aroused," or "trouble learning to have orgasms." Again, time and experience with a variety of patients provide a sense of what terms are most useful in conveying information to a given patient.

Patients may bring up vague or psychosomatic-like complaints (e.g., insomnia, fatigue, musculoskeletal aches, indigestion, headaches, or any specific symptoms of depression or anxiety) as a veiled request to talk about sexual concerns. Others mention a sexual concern at the end of a visit in an offhand manner, when there is little time for the problem to be adequately evaluated. *The provider may then choose to assess the problem briefly and validate the importance of investigating this as soon as a new appointment can be scheduled.*

Because sexual problems are often the result of a distressing gap between the patient's expectations and experiences, the effective sexual interview aims to elucidate both sides of the equation. *If expectations are unrealistic, the treatment is education; if the experience fails to meet realistic expectations, intervention or referral is indicated.* Often education and other clinical interventions are combined.

CASE ILLUSTRATION 1*
VALIDATION OF EXISTING SEXUAL PRACTICES

One couple sought help from a sex therapist because, after 30 years of enjoyable and satisfying sex (involving intercourse that would last less than 5 minutes), they had read an article extolling the virtues of extended intercourse and began to feel inadequate. When encouraged to value their own unique sexual patterns, versus what might be right for someone else, they were relieved and decided they did not have a problem after all. They then felt freer to build upon what was already satisfying to them in a spirit of exploration, rather than of attempting to be more "normal."

---

*Cases 1–10 described in this chapter were of actual patients seen in primary care settings as reported in consultation with the first author. Although some identifying characteristics of the patients have been changed to ensure confidentiality, the essential clinical issues presented are accurately portrayed. We thank all the patients and their health providers who helped us gather these examples.

SEX PROBLEM INTERVIEW

When getting a sex problem history and before proposing solutions, health care professionals need to ask questions about the relative importance of sex in the patient's life and what their expectations are for a fulfilling sex life.

The language of medicine is clinical, whereas issues of sexuality are associated with feelings and emotional vulnerabilities. Pay special attention to the case reports. They illustrate how cool clinical material can be translated to a warmer doctor–patient approach that allows for better trust and engagement with these vital human issues.

As with any other medical problem, five basic areas need to be addressed for the patient presenting with a sex problem (Table 32-2):

1. Explicit symptom or question
2. Onset and course of the symptom
3. Patient's perception of the cause and maintenance of the problem
4. Medical evaluation, including medical history, past treatment, and outcome—*(Specifically exclude such chronic health problems as diabetes mellitus, cardiovascular disease, hyperlipidemia, hypertension, the arthritides, past or current history of cancer)*
5. Current expectations and goals for treatment

Answers to the preceding inquiries can help guide the clinician to specific interventions.

PHYSICAL EXAMINATION

The detailed examination of the genitourinary system should include checking for signs of androgen or estrogen deficiency or excess, neurologic dysfunction, genital abnormalities, genital trauma, infections, condylomata (warts), and vascular disease.

For men, the examination should include the penis (to exclude conditions such as Peyronie disease, penile discharge, warts, other lesions, and hypospadias); testes and scrotum (for masses, atrophy, hernia, or varicoceles); and skin, prostate, and rectum. Testing should be conducted for evidence of gynecomastia, peripheral vascular disease, and neuropathy. Testicular self-examination can also be taught and information about prostate issues provided.

For women, look for evidence of atrophic changes, skin disorders (infectious or otherwise), developmental changes, urinary tract disorders, and general evidence of genital (internal and external) physical abnormalities, pelvic floor weaknesses, and postsurgical conditions. In case of genital pain, the woman should be encouraged to point out specific sites of pain, using a mirror to localize it.

Table 32-2. Sex problem interview.

Description of current symptom in detail

- Signal that you are glad the patient brought up the problem (to give approval, counteract shame, and encourage the patient).
- Help the patient specify exactly what the problem is, being careful to use understandable language—low desire, not getting wet or lubricating, difficulty getting or losing a "hard-on" or erection, difficulty "coming" or having orgasm, "coming too quickly" or rapid ejaculation, and so on.
- *I'd like to ask a few questions to help us sort it out.*
- *Tell me what happens.*
- *How is that a problem for you?*
- *Anything else that has changed?*

Onset and course

- *Does it happen alone with self-pleasuring or masturbation, with a specific partner, or with any partner?*
- *How does your partner respond when the problem occurs?*
- *Was there a time it was more enjoyable and then changed?*
- *Any situations when it's not a problem?*

Patient's perception of cause and maintenance of problem

- *Anything you think might be causing it or that you worry might be causing the problem or keeping it going?*

Medical evaluation, past treatment, and outcome

- *Do you smoke or use prescription or over-the-counter medications, drugs, or alcohol?*
- *Do you have any medical illnesses or treatments, depression, anxiety, or relationship problems?*
- *For women: Are your menses normal, regular? Have you had any children? Were any problems associated with pregnancy, delivery, breast-feeding?*
- *For men: Do you notice morning or nocturnal erections? Are they firm enough for penetration?*
- *Do you have a need for birth control; if so, what methods do you use?*
- *Are you concerned you might have gotten an STD?*
- *Any history of physical, emotional, or sexual abuse?*
- *What have you already tried to help to change the problem?*
- *Have you ever had psychotherapy, couple, or sex therapy? If yes, was this sexual problem addressed in the treatment?*
- *Have you discussed this problem openly with your partner?*

Current expectations and goals for treatment

- *How important is it to you to get help with this problem and are you interested in trying to change it now?*
- *What would be the minimum improvement you would need in order to feel it was worth your time and effort in dealing with this problem?*
- *Mostly, everyone has sexual concerns at one time or another. Talking about them is the most important first step. I'm glad you've felt comfortable talking with me and I suggest … (or will suggest some things after I've had a chance to review the best resources for you). Many people have been helped with these issues.*

The gynecologic examination provides an excellent opportunity for teaching patients about breast self-examination, discussing safe sex practices, protection against HPV and its consequences, and if appropriate, contraception.

Sexuality issues are rarely as clear-cut as a factual medical approach might yield. Generally, any condition or medication that is debilitating or energy depleting can be a contributory cause of sexual problems. Debilitation and/or anxiety are most frequently the final common denominators resulting in a sex problem. When going through the steps of Annon's (1976) P-LI-SS-IT model below, look for evidence of these final common pathways as a guide to making the best use of the model.

When pathology can be excluded, patients can be reassured that their genitals look "quite healthy" and are in the normal range. This can help counter the shame that many people feel about these vulnerable areas of the body. Naming specific genital parts, such as the foreskin and glans of the penis and the clitoris and labia as you examine them, may give increased permission for the patient to ask any questions or express any concerns they may have about them. Men concerned about the size of their penis or women with worries that their genitals are somehow abnormal are more likely to voice these concerns after the clinician has comfortably used these words.

LABORATORY TESTS

In general, few laboratory tests are necessary for patients presenting with the most common sexual problems. For complaints of low sexual desire, patients should be screened for depression and fatigue and also tested for anemia and endocrine, liver, and renal disease; or any other debilitating medical problems suggested by the history and physical examinations. Negative sexual side effects may be caused by gonadotropin-releasing hormone (GnRH) agonists, and narcotics (see "Medications"). Recognized underlying endocrine factors might include low thyroid, low estrogen, low androgen, or high prolactin levels. Whereas checking serum levels of thyroid-stimulating hormone (TSH) and prolactin is generally considered appropriate in women with sexual problems, routine measurement of serum estrogen and/or androgen concentrations generally is not recommended, as their measured serum levels do not correlate with sexual function.

Some authorities recommend evaluation of serum testosterone, TSH, and prolactin levels in all male patients with erectile failure or low libido. Elevated prolactin levels can be the result of many medical conditions, including pituitary tumors; renal dysfunction; sarcoidosis; thyroid disease; trauma; pelvic surgery; or use of medications such as cimetidine, haloperidol, and phenothiazine. If any of these tests is abnormal or other endocrine problems are suggested by the history or physical examination, specific, relevant additional tests should be performed as indicated.

In some men with erectile concerns, testing by a urologist may be indicated. These may include monitoring of nocturnal penile tumescence (NPT) in a sleep laboratory or, more commonly and less expensively, with a home monitoring unit or simple snap gauge. Increasingly, a trial with a PDE5, such as tadalafil (Cialis), sildenafil (Viagra), or vardenafil (Levitra), is recommended for both diagnosis and treatment.

ORGANIC & PSYCHOGENIC FACTORS

Rather than describing sexual problems with a simple differential diagnosis of either organic *or* psychogenic etiology, it is useful to identify *both* categories of causal factors. These can be assessed with the psychosocial history, sex problem interview, physical examination, and laboratory testing. A symptom that is generalized (occurring in all circumstances) may indicate major organic or psychogenic involvement, whereas situational symptoms tend to be psychogenic (Table 32-3).

ORGANIC FACTORS

Organic factors may be suspected when a man reports an absence of nocturnal or morning erections or is unable to get erect with masturbation. In women who find intercourse painful, important situational variables to identify include whether she has been adequately stimulated and aroused prior to penetration, whether precoital lubricants have been used if needed, whether

Table 32-3. Symptom patterns and etiology.

Symptom patterns suggestive of principally organic etiology
• Generalized (especially for absent desire, erectile problems, rapid ejaculation, and painful intercourse. Even when generalized, however, rapid ejaculation and primary female orgasmic problems in otherwise healthy individuals are rarely organic.)
• Gradual onset
• Rapid onset when associated with certain medications
Symptom patterns suggestive of principally psychological etiology
• Situational
• Rapid onset (unless medications are suspected)
• Sexual phobia and aversion

she feels pain with masturbation or when having sex with a partner, and whether she is able to direct the extent and timing of thrusting or is passive. Adequate vaginal estrogenization with local (estrogen) therapy, unless specifically contraindicated, should be ensured. Questioning should include possibilities that the problem is not physiological, but psychological, as is sometimes the case with vaginismus. Asking "under what circumstances have you felt pain?" might elicit "with one partner but not with another," "since I was raped," or "it has always been painful." Organic factors should also be considered when a patient has not responded to an adequate course of sex therapy.

MEDICAL CONDITIONS & TREATMENTS

Medical conditions and treatments affecting sexuality are listed in Table 32-4.

Table 32-4. Medical conditions commonly associated with sexual problems.

• Arthritis/joint disease
• Diabetes mellitus
• Endocrine problems
• Injury to autonomic nervous system by surgery or radiation
• Liver or renal failure
• Mood disorders, including depression, anxiety, and panic
• Multiple sclerosis
• Peripheral neuropathy
• Radical pelvic surgery
• Respiratory disorders (e.g., COPD)
• Spinal cord injury
• Vascular disease

Abbreviation: COPD, chronic obstructive pulmonary disease.

As we address the sexual needs of our patients, general health issues such as thyroid dysfunction, cardiovascular disease, and diabetes as well as hypertriglyceridemia, hypertension, neurological disease, genitourinary disease all need to be kept in mind, as do hormonal factors:

1. *Effects of low testosterone, primarily in men but occasionally in women with low sex drives*: Adequate testosterone is considered necessary for sexual drive and arousal in both genders. It also determines genital health and function in males. Although the traditional testosterone evaluation argues that testosterone levels falling within the "normal range" are **not** indicative of clinically insufficient testosterone levels, there have been recent suggestions that men who test within the normal range may indeed benefit from testosterone supplementation.

2. *Estrogen deficiency in women*: Severe estrogen deficiency can be associated with serious atrophic changes in the vagina and external genital tissues, and is a common cause of local dyspareunia, often correctable through adequate estrogen replacement. These changes commonly occur as a result of menopause, antiestrogen chemotherapy agents, wasting conditions such as anorexia nervosa, and even due to normal breast-feeding.

   Recent studies have been elucidating subtle **local** effects of estrogens at the cellular level, termed "intracrinology." DHEA (dehydroepiandrosterone), a precursor of androgens and estrogens, shows promise in ongoing studies when used as a vaginal cream by effectively treating hormone deficiencies at the local cellular level.

   While the effects of estrogen deficiency have focused on vaginal genital changes, it should be noted that these changes can also lead to serious pain with oral sex and clitoral masturbation.

3. *Centrally acting agents*: Although the intricacy of sexual functioning in women is not yet completely understood, hormones play an important role. Centrally, two major neurotransmitters, ***oxytocin*** and ***dopamine***, are known to be involved in sexual *desire* and *response* in women.

Oxytocin, which rises with sexual activity, results in relaxation and bonding, increasing a woman's interest in sexual activity and reducing her anxiety, as does dopamine, which acts centrally also to reduce anxiety about sexual activity. Both are said to act like an *"on/off switch."*

The sexual problems of women may be complicated by the physical and emotional changes of aging and menopause, especially surgical or premature menopause. Although hormone replacement, especially with surgical or premature menopause, may be useful (there is serious controversy about estrogen replacement post natural menopause), it is most often necessary to address the serious emotional and life crisis issues as well.

Medications

Medications of many kinds have been implicated in sexual dysfunction (Table 32-5). Older antidepressants such as amitriptyline (Elavil) and doxepin (Sinequan) have anticholinergic properties that undermine sexual arousal. The widely used SSRIs—antidepressants such as escitalopram (Lexapro), sertraline (Zoloft), and paroxetine (Paxil)—may inhibit orgasm for women and ejaculation and orgasm for men, while decreasing sexual desire for both. Certain cardiovascular and antihypertensive medications have been notorious for causing sexual dysfunction, as can any medication resulting in sedation or depressive effects.

In the case of antidepressants, strategies to alleviate such dysfunction include: (1) reducing the dosage; (2) taking a weekend "holiday" in which the last dose for the week is taken on Thursday morning and the medication is resumed at noon on Sunday; (3) switching to another medication; or (4) coadministering other medications, such as bupropion-SR (Wellbutrin-SR), neostigmine (Prostigmin), cyproheptadine (Periactin), bethanechol (Duvoid), and yohimbine (Yohimex) 1–2 hours prior to sexual activity. It is hoped that antidepressants currently in development will have fewer negative sexual side effects.

Table 32-5. Medication and drug categories commonly associated with sexual problems.

- Alcohol
- Anticancer drugs and hormones
- Anticonvulsants
- Antihypertensives, including beta-blockers (at high dosage), excluding ACE inhibitors
- Carbonic anhydrase inhibitors
- Cytotoxic drugs
- Digitalis family
- Diuretics
- H$_2$ receptor antagonists
- Nonsteroidal anti-inflammatory agents
- Opiates
- Pain medications
- Psychedelic and hallucinogenic drugs
- Psychiatric medications (benzodiazepines, tricyclic antidepressants, monoamine oxidase inhibitors, SSRIs, antipsychotics, lithium carbonate)
- Recreational drugs (tobacco, alcohol, and opiates)
- Sleep medications
- Tranquilizers

Abbreviation: ACE, angiotensin-converting enzyme inhibitors.

PSYCHOLOGICAL FACTORS

Psychological factors often play a causal role in maintaining sexual dysfunction. This possibility should be considered even in cases when a medical condition or use of a medication that is known to cause a problem has been identified as a cause (Table 32-6). For example, a female patient experiencing difficulty reaching orgasm since being treated with an SSRI antidepressant may continue to have this problem even after discontinuing the SSRI because she is now conditioned to performance anxiety.

Following hysterectomy, some women report increased sexual enjoyment because of the relief from uncomfortable physical symptoms and bleeding, whereas others find the surgery difficult and have a psychological response to the loss of these organs and to the loss of their reproductive capacity. These women may then experience a decrease in sexual desire, arousal, or orgasmic responsiveness. This is particularly so when concomitant oophorectomy is done, notably in premenopausal women.

CASE ILLUSTRATION 2 ERECTILE PROBLEM

Juan, a 38-year-old male patient, believing his erection problem was caused entirely by his type II diabetes,

Table 32-6. Psychological conditions commonly associated with sexual problems.

I. Immediate causes (of most concern for the general medical practitioner)
  A. Performance anxiety—fear of inadequate performance
  B. Spectatoring—critically monitoring one's own sexual performance
  C. Inadequate communication with partner regarding sex
  D. Fantasy—absence of fantasy, fantasy incompatible with sexual arousal, or distracting thoughts
II. Deeper causes (for referral)
  A. Intrapsychic issues—early conditioning, sexual trauma, depression, anxiety, guilt, fear of intimacy, or separation
  B. Relationship issues—lack of trust, power and control issues, anger at partner
  C. Sociocultural factors—attitudes and values, religious beliefs
  D. Educational and cognitive factors—Sexual myths or expectations (gender roles, age and appearance, proper sexual activity, performance expectations), sexual ignorance

---

Source: Adapted, with permission, from Plaut SM, Lehne GK. Sexual dysfunction, gender identity disorders, and paraphilias. In: Goldman HH, ed. *Review of General Psychiatry,* 5th ed. New York, NY: McGraw-Hill, 2000.

was helped to understand that he also had performance anxiety. Declining treatment with PDE5 inhibitors such as tadalafil (Cialis), he wanted to get help without more medication. By quitting smoking cigarettes and learning to engage in noncoital caressing (sensate focusing) with his partner to decrease his pressure to perform, he was able to experience satisfying erections firm enough for intercourse. In this case, the diabetes by itself was not the determining factor in maintaining the problem.

The research is mixed as to the effects of hysterectomy on orgasm in women. It has been proposed that women differ in the extent to which they perceive uterine and cervical contractions during orgasm, with differing sense of loss after the surgery. There is similar variability in men after prostatectomy. For many, orgasm may feel satisfactory even with a "dry" or retrograde ejaculation, with semen going into the bladder, but others may complain of a loss of orgasmic sensation.

Some medical illnesses and treatments are believed to decrease sexual desire or to cause sexual dysfunction *directly.* Psychosocial adaptations to virtually any medical condition, however, can *indirectly* affect sexual desire or functioning. For example, fears of rejection by a sexual partner because of a stoma or mastectomy or concerns about sexual functioning may lead to a suppression of sexual feelings and avoidance of sexual opportunities. Of course, many medically healthy men and women either choose to be sexually inactive or refrain out of a sense of inadequacy. The capacity to enjoy one's sexuality, therefore, cannot be predicted on the basis of medical diagnosis alone.

Psychological problems such as depression or anxiety can be either the *cause* or the *effect* of diminished sexual desire or functioning. Both may be true to some degree. In other instances, depression and sexual problems may both be the result of a third underlying factor, such as an endocrine disorder.

Sexual problems might have remote psychological causes, such as childhood trauma or prohibitions about sexual pleasure, but almost all such problems can be seen as having current maintaining variables of anxiety or depression. In general, psychological etiology is primarily suggested when the problem is situational; seems related to performance anxiety, depression, or guilt; is associated with significant relationship and communication problems; or there are indications of trauma from earlier sexual experiences.

PSYCHOLOGICAL MANAGEMENT & BRIEF SEX COUNSELING

A paradigm shift occurred in the treatment of sexual dysfunctions with the publication in 1970 of Masters and Johnson's signal work on sex therapy. The previous emphasis on the diagnosis and treatment of individual psychopathology, with somewhat poor treatment results for the sexual dysfunctions, gave way to an understanding of the importance of the **conditions** (internal variables such as attitudes, expectations, and lack of knowledge, as well as external factors related to the partner or the situation) under which people attempt to function sexually.

Education and suggestions for focusing on pleasure rather than on performance were found to lower anxiety and to promote improved sexual functioning and enjoyment.

Anxiety is considered one of the major psychological causes of the sexual dysfunctions, whether stemming from individual or relationship issues. Are patients comfortable, at ease, and feeling close to their partners? Or are they anxious due to lack of information, strained relationships, unrealistic attitudes about and focus on sexual performance goals, or other conditions? In these cases, modern sex therapy commonly provides anxiety-reduction interventions, many of which can be adapted for use by primary care providers. These include validating that most people at some time experience sexual problems and that such problems are often an understandable response to stress, worry, and concerns about performance; encouraging open communication between partners; dispelling maladaptive beliefs about sex; suggesting ways that patients can increase their level of comfort and safety and their ability to relax during sex; and encouraging the view that noncoital sex can be very satisfying and does not have to be considered "second best."

THE P-LI-SS-IT MODEL

Annon's P-LI-SS-IT model is a useful hierarchical guide to anxiety-reduction approaches to sexual problems and can be used by primary care practitioners. The letters in the acronym stand for different levels of intervention.

P = Permission

The fundamental intervention is to give patients permission to discuss their sexual concerns. Empathic listening, including verbal and nonverbal reassurance, helps give patients permission to talk openly about sexual issues and may encourage and enable them to discuss the problem more directly with a partner. Reassurance and permission can help validate that having a sexual problem is normal, rather than pathological. Inquire into positive exceptions: patients can describe those areas of sex about which they do feel good; for example, a woman can appreciate her ability to become aroused despite difficulty reaching orgasm, and a man can be a skillful lover despite his erectile problem. Permission to choose not to be sexually active may be very helpful for patients who feel pressured to have sex or

who feel inadequate if they do not care to be sexually active.

LI = Limited Information

Facts can add to the effectiveness of reassurance and can be at the disposal of any clinician who has done basic reading about sexuality and keeps up through the literature or review courses. Keeping responses focused and limited to the expressed concern saves time and does not overwhelm the patient with extraneous information (Table 32-7). Such information gives the patient the choice of maintaining or changing sexual practices or attitudes. A simple explanation of the psychophysiology of sexual arousal and the importance of conditions for relaxation helps "normalize" the symptoms and refocuses attention on conditions that can be changed to alleviate the problem, rather than on trying to determine what is wrong with the patient. One physician conveyed this information by the following "rhinoceros" story about sexuality:

Imagine you are lying on a blanket in a secluded meadow with a loving partner after a wonderful picnic lunch on a beautiful sunny day. You start kissing and feel arousal in your genitals, when, all of a sudden, a rhinoceros charges out of the jungle straight for you. What happens to your arousal (lubrication or erection)? The fight-or-flight response causes a rapid redirection of blood to the brain and large-muscle groups, with a corresponding loss of erection or genital arousal. The rhinoceros represents worrisome thoughts and anxieties about having erections, arousal, or orgasm, or fears that you won't please your partner or be seen as a good lover. Some simple suggestions can help you keep the rhinoceros out of your bedroom!

SS = Specific Suggestions

Where permission and limited information do not suffice, the patient may benefit from specific suggestions to help overcome a sexual problem. Most sex counseling interventions are designed to help the patient (and partner, if available) communicate better about sex and enjoy increased sexual pleasure by reducing performance anxiety about attaining the goals of arousal, lubrication, erection, and orgasm. Helpful interventions taken from sex therapy include: (1) temporary agreement not to have intercourse; (2) suggestions for focusing on pleasurable touch, genital caressing, Kegel exercises (tensing and relaxing the pubococcygeal [PC] muscles), and progressive muscle relaxation methods; (3) correction of cognitive distortions ("self-talk"); and (4) suggestions to improve emotional and sexual communication.

Table 32-7. Maladaptive ideas and therapeutic responses to them.

Maladaptive Idea	Therapeutic Response
My sexual problems are because I'm too old.	For those who are interested and willing to be creative, sex can be an enjoyable part of life in their 70s, 80s, and beyond!
I should be interested only in survival, not sex (for someone with terminal or chronic illness).	If sex was important to you before your illness it can remain so or become so again.
I am *asexual* because I don't have an active sex life.	We are *all* sexual beings. You can be aware of and enjoy your sexual feelings without being sexually active.
Sex equals love.	Many people have very loving relationships without being sexually active, and, of course, some people have sex without having loving feelings.
Sex equals intercourse.	There is no one *right* way to be sexual, and many people enjoy touching and caressing more than intercourse.
Having sex is the same as *enjoying sex.*	Many people have to learn to enjoy their sexuality.
It is not proper to talk about sex, either with your partner or a health care provider.	It is often a great relief when people can talk confidentially about their sexual feelings and concerns.
You shouldn't talk about sex because it will destroy the mystery.	Most people find that talking about their important feelings deepens intimacy, and trust develops when you know you can be vulnerable with another. You can create more mystery from deeper sharing.
You should be interested in having sex with any willing partner.	It is most important to be able to respect yourself. Your sexuality is a gift that you share only with those you truly want to share it with.
You should be able to enjoy sex with a partner even when you are tired, angry, or feel hurt.	We all have our own conditions for what makes a sexual encounter enjoyable, and feeling close to and loved by your partner is important to most of us.
I try not to masturbate and feel guilty when I give in because I have a partner and shouldn't need to do that.	Most married people continue to masturbate and find it does not interfere with the pleasure they have with their partner.
Sex is a performance, and it would be grim and catastrophic to "fail."	Sexual sharing can be playful, with the goals of giving and receiving feelings of pleasure and caring. If things don't go as planned, there is always next time!
A new partner will not like the size of my (breasts/penis).	Most men and women enjoy having sex with a person, not a body part. Most men compare themselves to other men when their penises are soft … size differences are usually not as great when erections are compared. Vaginas accommodate different penis sizes, with the outer third and the clitoris the most responsive areas for many women.
Sex should result in orgasm every time.	Does *not* having dessert ruin a fine meal? Orgasm is only one of the pleasurable aspects of a sexual encounter. Many people find it a relief to not have "shoulds" in their sex life.
Sex should never be a problem. Experiencing a problem is not normal.	Sex is perfectly natural, but not naturally perfect. Probably everyone has "problems" with sex at some time or another.

Even for couples who previously enjoyed certain patterns of lovemaking, predictable repetition over time can lead to sexual boredom. Suggesting that a couple agree, for example, to temporarily forego intercourse or otherwise change their usual sexual pattern often helps them focus on moment-to-moment pleasure. Rather than making assumptions about what the other wants, the couple can communicate their likes and dislikes. Many people remember how arousing and exciting it was when they were younger and were "making out" (sexual petting) without intercourse. If agreeable to both, they can take turns exploring other ways of caressing and pleasuring each other. The **sensate focus** exercise, from Masters and Johnson, is done for the interest of the person doing the touching, rather than for the pleasure of the receiver. To minimize performance anxiety, each is encouraged to take turns "savoring" the experience of touching and exploring the other's body, in contrast to worrying about "turning on" or performing for the partner. For many people, permission for **genital caressing** in this way increases sexual pleasure and satisfaction.

Arranging for follow-up after giving specific suggestions keeps the health care provider informed as to their effectiveness, helps the patient stay focused on problem solving, and informs the clinician about the necessity for further intervention.

IT = Intensive Therapy

This is the last step in the hierarchy and involves referral to an appropriate specialist when the previous three levels of intervention have not been effective (see "Indications for Referral").

ADDITIONAL PATIENT EDUCATION

Pamphlets detailing approaches for safe sex for the prevention of AIDS can supplement discussions and should be made readily available for patients. Many good self-help books dealing with common sexual problems enable patients to move at their own pace. Often people who are reluctant to enter counseling or who are hesitant about discussing their problems in depth are willing to read about the problems in the privacy of their home where they can be relaxed and comfortable. Several books are recommended at the end of this chapter. Educational videos are also available and useful for some patients.

INDICATIONS FOR REFERRAL

Refer patients to an appropriate medical specialist if the brief treatment suggestions in this chapter fail to help or if the history and physical examination suggest primarily an organic component. Refer patients to a mental health specialist trained in sex therapy if the problem is situational, occurring only with a certain partner; if functioning is adequate under certain conditions; or if significant emotional distress is present.

Primary care clinicians can develop a resource list of providers for sex-related problems. Colleagues, teachers, friends, and clinical societies can be asked for recommendations. Identify medical and mental health specialists with expertise in treating sexual issues. Practitioners can be licensed in psychiatry, psychology, social work, psychiatric nursing, or marriage and family counseling. Most states do not license "sex therapists" or "sex counselors."

COMMON SEXUAL PROBLEMS

Low or Absent Sexual Desire & Aversion

SYMPTOMS & SIGNS

The range of issues concerning sexual desire is wide (Table 32-8). As the etiology is multi-factorial, the approach to treatment will also need to be broad, ranging from counseling on basic sexual and possibly lifestyle issues, to consideration of pharmacotherapies including hormones.

It must be respected that some people normally put a low priority on sex or choose to not have any active sexual life. Others may be inhibited or find sex aversive, and some are clinically phobic. These problems can be of recent origin or reflect a long-standing pattern. Lack of desire may pertain situationally only to certain sexual partners or practices (such as oral sex). Couples with different levels of desire may disagree as to which partner's level is "abnormal." In this situation, each side has valid feelings, and it is important not to stigmatize the patient with the lower level of desire. Most couples occasionally deal with periods of discrepancy in desire or mutually low desire and feel they should have sex more often than they do. Demands of family, career, and friends often take precedence over sex.

Problems with desire or sexual aversion can derive from deeper relational power struggles or reflect childhood sexual, physical, or emotional abuse that requires couple counseling or individual psychotherapy for resolution. The following case example, however, demonstrates how permission and encouragement to talk about sex directly, together with specific suggestions, can have a powerful positive influence.

CASE ILLUSTRATION 3 LOSS OF SEXUAL DESIRE

Alice, a healthy 33-year-old primary school teacher, reported having lost her desire for sex. Her sex problem history established that although she had enjoyed sexual activity with her husband for the first 2 years of their marriage, in the past year it had become a chore that she never put on her extensive "to do" list. Because sex was seen as a bedtime activity, when she was usually tired, their sexual frequency dropped from weekly to once every several months. They did not address the problem directly, and Alice and her husband's feelings of estrangement from each other continued to grow.

*When asked what steps they had taken to address these problems, Alice disclosed that she and her husband had never had an open discussion about sex. Her primary care physician validated that this was common among couples and that most people have to learn to talk more comfortably about their sexual needs (**P**ermission and **L**imited **I**nformation). The physician also explained that everyone has certain conditions that need to be met to be interested in sexual activity (**P** and **LI**) and encouraged Alice to think about her conditions and then, with her husband, to "set some private time aside outside of the bedroom to let yourselves have a discussion about this, even if it is awkward" (**S**pecific **S**uggestions).*

Table 32-8. Common sexual problems and treatment approaches. (Distress levels can be more clearly delineated by a useful three-degree scale such as *no problem*—"never," *mild problem*—"hardly ever," or *significant problem* —"rather often," "often," "nearly always," and "always").

Problem	Diagnostic Criteria	Treatment Approach
Low sexual interest/desire	Diminished or absent sexual interest or desire in thoughts or fantasies and low or absent motivation to become sexually aroused.	After organic causes ruled out or if situational: **Permission and limited information:** Restate problem in behavioral terms Explore patient conditions for good sex (rhinoceros story), including whether patient receives adequate direct stimulation Validate patient's right to say "no" to sex
Sexual aversion	Extreme aversion and avoidance of genital sexual contact with a sexual partner.	May be secondary to depression, anxiety, panic, or phobic disorder (occasionally related to childhood sexual abuse), or May be symptomatic of hidden arousal or orgasmic problems (if so, treat appropriately) **Specific suggestions:** Listening exercises to *increase communication* with partner, *Suggested readings* (Barbach, 2000; Johnson, 2008,2013; Zilbergeld, 1999). **Intensive treatment:** Refer to mental health professional trained in sexual therapy.
Sexual arousal problems	Difficulty with adequate lubrication-swelling response of sexual arousal (female) or erection (male). Three subtypes include:	**Permission and limited information:** Give brief explanation of the physiology of arousal and the need for relaxation. Is sexual desire present? (if not, treat as desire problem).
Erectile or lubrication problems	*genital sexual arousal problems* characterized by minimal genital arousal and vaginal lubrication despite subjective excitement from nongenital sexual stimulation; *subjective sexual arousal problems* with absent or diminished sexual feelings despite vaginal lubrication and other signs of physiologic response; *combined genital and subjective arousal problems* with absent or diminished feelings of sexual excitement and pleasure as well as absent or diminished vulval swelling, lubrication, or erection.	**Specific suggestions:** Is there enough and the desired kind of direct stimulation by partner? Use of lubricants (Astroglide, K-Y, and so on) or vaginal moisturizers (Replens). For males: PDE5 inhibitors tadalafil (Cialis), sildenafil (Viagra), and vardenafil (Levitra). Suggest progressive muscle relaxation and Kegel exercises, explore ways other than intercourse of pleasuring the partner, temporary intercourse ban, genital caressing/sensate focus (nonde-mand pleasuring), hormonal therapy, low-dose beta-blocker (10 mg Inderal) if high-performance anxiety. **Intensive treatment:** Sexuality oriented psychotherapy, vacuum device (older male with organic etiology), intracorporeal penile injection or intraurethral application of PGE_1, penile implant.
Persistent genital arousal (female)	Spontaneous, intrusive, and unwanted genital arousal when not wanted by the individual. Can be secondary to neurologic pathology, onset or discontinuation of treatment with SSRIs and other mood stabilizers, beginning menopause, severe stress, and inactivity.	**Permission and limited information:** Psychoeducation and support that this is a physiologic and psychologically distressing experience, but one many women suffer and get help with. **Specific suggestions:** Anesthetizing agents or ice, pelvic massage and stretching, SNRIs. **Intensive treatment:** Mindfulness, body awareness, and cognitive behavioral exercises.

(Continued)

Table 32-8. Common sexual problems and treatment approaches. (Distress levels can be more clearly delineated by a useful three-degree scale such as *no problem*—"never," *mild problem*—"hardly ever," or *significant problem*—"rather often," "often," "nearly always," and "always"). (Continued)

Problem	Diagnostic Criteria	Treatment Approach
Persistent genital arousal (male) Priapism	Full or partial erection more than 4 hours after sexual stimulation and orgasm and unrelated to sexual stimulation.	**Intensive treatment:** May need penile blood aspiration.
Rapid ejaculation	Lifelong rapid ejaculation occurring prior to or within about 1 minute of vaginal or anal penetration after minimal sexual stimulation, with subjective distress, bother, frustration, or avoidance of sexual situation. (Occasional or temporary rapid ejaculation is not considered problematic when age, novelty, and frequency of sexual activity increase excitement to ejaculation).	**Permission and limited information:** As above, plus discuss masturbation patterns—he may have conditioned himself to ejaculate rapidly. Explain connection between rapid ejaculation and anxiety versus relaxation and longer-lasting erections. **Specific suggestions:** Above, plus increase frequency of ejaculation, stop–start exercises (Zilbergeld, 1999), clomipramine (Anafranil 25 mg as needed) or SSRI antidepressant medication, prilocaine–lidocaine cream with condom.
Orgasm problems	Difficulty or inability to reach orgasm, greatly diminished orgasmic sensations, or significant delay of orgasm despite significant sexual stimulation. Clinician should consider the age, sexual experience, and the adequacy of sexual stimulation received.	**Permission and limited information:** As above. **Specific suggestions:** For primary preorgasmic woman, recommend Barbach (2000); for male, Zilbergeld (1999). If orgasmic problem is secondary (at one time patient was orgasmic), then evaluate and treat for desire or arousal problem or relationship problems.
Delayed ejaculation	Unwanted delay in or difficulty reaching ejaculation (and usually orgasm) despite arousal and excitement.	**Permission and limited information:** As above, plus inquire about masturbation patterns—he may have conditioned himself to ejaculate to idiosyncratic fantasies, or with more vigorous stimulation than intercourse provides. Performance anxiety may exacerbate it. Rule out medications causing delayed ejaculation such as SSRIs. **Specific suggestions:** Encourage explicit communication with patient's partner about his need to have enough stimulation prior to ejaculation and orgasm. **Intensive treatment:** Sex therapy may be useful, focusing on sexual behaviors, fantasies, and relationship issues.
Genital pain Dyspareunia	Recurrent or persistent genital pain associated with sexual stimulation, such as intercourse in either a man or a woman.	**Permission and limited information:** As above. **Specific suggestions:** As above, plus encourage explicit communication with patient's partner about her need to have enough stimulation prior to penetration, with the partner experiencing pain having control to choose when penetration occurs and timing of thrusting.
Vaginismus	Persistent and recurring involuntary muscle spasm of the outer third of the vagina making penetration by a penis, finger, or other object difficult.	**Intensive treatment:** Sex therapy may be useful for long-standing dyspareunia and vaginismus, due to conditioned expectation of pain.

Doctor: It can be good for relationships when people risk being a little uneasy. You don't have to have the same perspective. You are each entitled to your own separate feelings about the situation, but together you can talk it out, try to understand each other, and see what other choices you have (**P**, **LI**, and **SS**).

At her 1-month follow-up appointment, Alice reported significant progress. When the couple set time aside to discuss their sex life, they had a very meaningful and tender talk. The husband was relieved to learn about the major sources of Alice's lack of desire and she acknowledged feeling resentful that he seemed unresponsive to her needs. He admitted that he had taken her lack of desire very personally, secretly and painfully interpreting the problem as her lack of desire for him. With these hidden resentments expressed, they could set aside their power struggles and cooperate in addressing these issues. Recognizing how they had both felt lonely and uncared for allowed them to take specific actions, such as planning a regular evening each week just for the two of them to talk and nurture their intimacy.

The physician also recommended a self-help book and offered to refer the couple to a therapist who treats couples, should their attempts to communicate falter.

Management

PERMISSION & LIMITED INFORMATION

For many individuals and couples, not being sexually active can be a choice and, if acceptable to the people involved, should not be judged by others to be dysfunctional.

Others may learn to accept that low desire may be understandable given their immediate circumstances (e.g., the months prior to and after childbirth, recovering from illness) and that their previous levels of desire can be expected to return over time. Validate the patient's right to say "no" to sex.

When a person presents diminished or lacking sex drive as a problem, questions can explore the conditions under which the person has previously felt the desire for sexual contact and release, and help her or him think about ways to reestablish some of those circumstances.

People raised within traditional sex roles can be helped to identify issues arising from sexual "suppression," wherein neither women nor men experience their sexual potentials. Questions about desire open the door to sexual fantasies and scripts, and can form reference points for reestablishing desire where it is low or absent. For example, if a woman has experienced desire and excitement during courtship, but none after marriage,

the doctor might help her understand why these changes have occurred and suggest potentially simple solutions.

SPECIFIC SUGGESTIONS

A "prescription" to go away on a weekend or to arrange a sleepover for children with relatives may help couples "break the ice" and reexperience intimacy. Suggest that the patient and their partner set time aside to talk about each other's feelings and discuss conditions for more enjoyable sex, with each taking an uninterrupted amount of time for self-expression. Self-help books may also be recommended.

INTENSIVE THERAPY

An assessment for couples or individual psychotherapy may be indicated when simpler discussions and behavioral changes have been unsuccessful.

OTHER MEDICAL INTERVENTIONS

Clearly, comorbid conditions should be excluded and, consideration given to readjusting current medications, if appropriate. Positive results in several domains have been obtained in some studies of postmenopausal women with sexual problems, treated with transdermal testosterone, usually in addition to menopausal hormone therapy (i.e., estrogen ± progestin).

Since none of the studied testosterone preparations has been approved by the Food and Drug Administration (FDA) for use in the United States (nor by Health Canada in that country), there are no approved testosterone products for women in North America. However, the transdermal preparations have been approved by regulatory agencies in Europe and South America where they are available and in use.

Testosterone products are sometimes used "off label" and may be helpful for select individuals, for example women postoophorectomy or those with premature menopause whose testosterone levels may be virtually undetectable. Vaginal or clitoral application of testosterone cream has been suggested for women who seek treatment for a troubling loss of desire following chemotherapy for breast cancer. However, this treatment is NOT universally accepted in the medical community.

DHEA vaginal preparations, currently still in clinical trials, have shown promising results and may prove useful in the future.

Sexual Arousal Problems

SYMPTOMS & SIGNS

Problems with female arousal are primarily manifested as vaginal dryness and may be reported separately from or together with lack of desire, difficulty reaching orgasm, or pain experienced during intercourse. The most common medical cause in older women is estrogen deficiency with resulting signs of vulvar irritation and atrophic vaginitis. Arousal may be inhibited by anxiety and depression, or shame resulting from early conditioning; it may also be a side effect of antidepressant medication. These possibilities should be explored (see Table 32-5).

Male arousal problems are manifested by erectile problems physically, but also include subjective inhibitions and performance anxiety as well.

CASE ILLUSTRATION 4

*Betty, a 78-year-old patient, had an appointment with her female physician. She brought along her 82-year-old husband because she wanted to discuss what she called her "sexual problems." Betty said she did not care about sex, that her husband was often angry with her lack of enthusiasm, and that this pattern had existed throughout the 50 years of their marriage. She believed she was not "a sexual person" because she had never been very excited by intercourse. She did enjoy kissing and caressing and mentioned that on several occasions she had been able to have orgasm when he stroked her labia and clitoris, but that she had never had orgasm from the "real sex" (intercourse) that he preferred. The physician responded that there really is no one way to be a "sexual person," that many people cherish the sensual and emotional aspects of sex, and that Betty did not need to consider herself asexual just because she preferred different aspects of sexual intimacy than her husband (**P** and **LI**). The physician further explained that the majority of women reach orgasm more often from manual caressing than from coitus, and that many couples enjoy bringing each other to orgasm without intercourse (**P** and **LI**). The couple was relieved and admitted to having curiosity about trying this petting more. They were given brief instructions to take turns at home touching and stroking each other without the goal of orgasm (sensate focus), to get reacquainted with each other's body, and to refrain from any attempts at intercourse for 2 weeks (**SS**).*

A follow-up telephone call confirmed that they were enjoying taking turns caressing each other, that orgasm often happened for each, and that they occasionally progressed to intercourse. A 1½-year follow-up was especially poignant—the husband reported that Betty had recently died from a stroke, and, although grieving her loss, he expressed profound appreciation for having gotten help for their sexual conflicts from the physician.

Husband: Settling those old battles over sex made our last year together more loving and caring than ever before in our marriage.

Management

PERMISSION & LIMITED INFORMATION

Is the patient getting stimulation in the way that works best for her? Feeling distant from or angry with a partner can inhibit sexual arousal, and such relationship concerns need to be addressed.

SPECIFIC SUGGESTIONS

Homework may be suggested for her to identify what stimulation works best. The goal is to experience the pleasure of arousal in that mode—not to reach orgasm. Inquiry should be made into the quality of the patient's relationship. Commercial lubricants (Astroglide, KY Jelly, and so on) and vaginal moisturizers (such as Replens) can be suggested and, if vaginal atrophy is present, a low-dose intravaginal estrogen preparation (cream, pill, or suppository) should be prescribed unless contraindicated.

As has been mentioned, an intravaginal DHEA preparation is undergoing further evaluation as a hormone replacement alternative without the usual contraindications. Labrie et al. (2009) have published extensively on DHEA use. The premise for safety of this cream for patients is that of "intracrinology," a term coined to describe the fact that DHEA, a relatively inert precursor substance ("a prehormone") inserted into the vagina, is absorbed and there transformed/converted "on site" in specific cells to active steroids (testosterone, estradiol) which act locally. The DHEA is then locally also deactivated, never entering the circulation, and thus not reaching other tissues. The endometrium which is close by remains unaffected, because it does not possess the necessary converting enzymes to act on the DHEA.

Self-help books also can be recommended, such as ones by Barbach (2000) and Johnson (2008, 2013).

INTENSIVE THERAPY

Recommend individual or couple therapy with a clinician skilled in human sexuality issues (where appropriate).

Other Medical Interventions

Referral to an ob–gyn or other women's health specialist.

Erectile Problems

SYMPTOMS & SIGNS

There have been more than a dozen studies in the past 12 years or so showing a growing link between erectile problems and cardiovascular disease in men, including younger populations. If a man presents in primary care setting with erectile complaints, the physician should always assess cardiovascular risk factors as potential contributing factors, and recommend aggressive risk factor reduction (e.g., weight loss, exercise) if relevant.

Generally, a man with a significant psychological component is aware of nocturnal or morning erections, is able to maintain his erection for a reasonable time and then ejaculate with masturbation, or has good erections in some situations but not in others. He may be able to get a firm erection but lose it after penetration or may not get an erection with a partner at any time. The original cause of the problem is often distinct from the maintaining variable, which is generally anxiety. Consider possibilities such as performance anxiety, lack of direct physical stimulation of the penis, conscious or unconscious guilt (e.g., "widower's syndrome"), anger at his partner or other relationship issues, or childhood issues such as sexual abuse.

 CASE ILLUSTRATION 5

Carl, a 58-year-old HIV-negative gay male, confided to his physician that he had been "impotent" since the death of his partner of 17 years, with whom he had had an active and monogamous sexual life. Attributing this problem to aging and worries about HIV infection, Carl nonetheless asked for any help the primary care physician could provide. A full session was scheduled for talking only. His partner had died suddenly from cardiac arrest a year before. In the past month, Carl had attempted sex on four occasions with two different men and was unable to get an erection. After a thorough socio-sexual history, Carl was seen to fit the "widowers' syndrome." Clearly, he was still grieving the loss of his partner but attempted to control his tears with statements such as "I should be over this by now" and "Life has to go on; he wanted me to go on." Carl then revealed that he was very afraid of feeling such loss, fearing that he would never be able to come out of the sadness. His grieving was acknowledged and validated (P), and it was explained to him that temporary sexual problems were common after such loss because of a number of factors: performance pressure of being with a new partner, continuing feelings of loyalty to a deceased partner, subsequent guilt at having sex with new people, and concerns about HIV infection with a new partner (LI). The physician encouraged Carl to join a grief support group or to contact a psychotherapist comfortable with gay sexuality (SS). In addition, the doctor referred Carl to a book on male sexuality, with suggestions on how to talk to a potential partner about both safer sex practices and ways they could reduce the pressure to have erections (LI and SS). At a follow-up visit 4 months later, Carl reported he had been able to cry more about his loss and was enjoying sex and intimacy with a new friend who had also lost a partner.

Management

PERMISSION & LIMITED INFORMATION

Many patients over 40 years old report previous successful sexual encounters when they were younger in which they became erect without direct physical stimulation of the penis. If their pattern for sexual interaction has rarely or never included direct touching by a partner, it might help them to learn that such touching becomes more necessary as men age, and that it can be an enjoyable part of sex.

SPECIFIC SUGGESTIONS

Institute a temporary ban on penetration and suggest sensate focus, progressive relaxation, and Kegel exercises. The couple should agree *not* to attempt penetration or intercourse even if the patient gets an improved erection.

> **Doctor:** For every minute you are relaxing with your partner and have an erection, your body is remembering just what it needs to do to get and maintain an erection. Your mind can be free to enjoy the pleasurable feelings and sensations of being caressed and kissing your partner. You might even allow your erection to go away. If you stay relaxed, it likely will return again with resumed stimulation.

INTENSIVE THERAPY

Recommend individual or couple therapy with a clinician skilled in human sexuality issues (where appropriate).

OTHER MEDICAL INTERVENTIONS

Referral to a urologist interested in male sexual functioning.
    PDE5 inhibitors. Tadalafil (Cialis), sildenafil (Viagra), and vardenafil (Levitra) are three oral medications popularly known to have revolutionized the medical treatment of male erectile problems. Although contraindicated in men taking organic nitrate medication for angina, these medications have been found to have broad-spectrum effectiveness across men of all ages and medical conditions, including diabetes, hypertension, neuropathy, postprostatectomy, and depression.

An important caveat is that, in spite of the evidence of PDE5 medications' demonstrated safety and efficacy, approximately 50% of men do not refill their prescriptions. Underlying psychological and interpersonal factors may need to be explored with these patients at follow-up visits.

Testosterone replacement therapy. For men with demonstrated low levels of serum testosterone, hormone replacement therapy may be helpful. This does not seem to benefit men whose serum testosterone is within normal limits, although recent work suggests there may be more subtleties to this. Side effects can be serious, including increase of any existing prostatic cancer, enlargement of the prostate, retention of fluids, and liver damage. Careful monitoring and follow-up prostate-specific antigen (PSA) screening and prostate examinations are necessary.

Antidepressant medication. Antidepressants, especially bupropion-SR (Wellbutrin-SR), can be effective treatment for some, but other patients may find that SSRI antidepressants hinder erection and ejaculation.

External penile vacuum device. With the aid of a vacuum cylinder, a tension ring is placed around the base of the penis after it has become erect. This device may work better for men who clearly have a major organic component to their erectile problem, such as severe diabetes, multiple sclerosis, or spinal cord injury. Although this device can create erections functional for intercourse, men with a more psychogenic etiology may be disappointed when the erections are not as firm as they had been expecting. Side effects may include bruising of the penis.

Intracorporeal penile injections or intraurethral delivery of prostaglandin E_1 (PGE$_1$). These methods were originally used diagnostically by urologists. However, patients can now be taught to inject themselves prior to sexual encounters, resulting in firmer erections that often do not disappear at orgasm or ejaculation and last about an hour. Side effects are priapism in less than 3% of patients and pain. In addition, scarring may be a concern with repeated injections over time.

Penile implant surgery. Since the advent of effective oral medications, implants with semirigid silicone rods or inflatable cylinders are less commonly utilized. Total costs are high, usually over $20,000. Complications include device failure (requiring additional surgery) and infection. However, for some men, this has been an effective and helpful treatment.

Rapid Ejaculation (Premature Ejaculation)

SYMPTOMS & SIGNS

Terms such as *rapid* or *early ejaculation* are clinically preferable to the established *premature ejaculation,* as they highlight the subjective nature of the problem and are less pejorative. No absolute measure—either in number of minutes or thrusts—is applicable to the diverse numbers of men presenting with this problem. Factors to be assessed include a patient's subjective evaluation, degree of sexual satisfaction, and sense of control.

CASE ILLUSTRATION 6

Donald, a 45-year-old divorced man, reported ejaculating after 1 minute or less of intercourse. This had been his pattern since becoming sexually active in his late teens. He reported proudly that he never masturbated but had a high sex drive, which led him to multiple sexual partners including prostitutes. His primary care physician gave Donald a supportive talk about how he could teach himself to last longer with certain physical exercises (P, LI, and SS). The patient was willing to do "self-stimulation" or "self-pleasuring" exercises for this "medical reason" and was comforted that as with the physical fitness regimen that he valued, he could tone up his PC muscles and learn to relax the pelvic muscles during sexual stimulation. Donald was advised to increase his frequency of ejaculation, was told about the importance of relaxation for maintaining erection, and was encouraged to read Zilbergeld's (1999) self-help section on "stop–start" exercises for lasting longer (P, LI, and SS). As his confidence grew through the solo exercises, and as he increased the frequency of ejaculation, Donald was able to try the stop–start exercises with a partner with increasing success. He said that it also helped him to read about the experiences of other men (getting validation from the universality of sexual concerns) and about how many women enjoy a variety of forms of sexual stimulation in addition to intercourse.

Management

PERMISSION & LIMITED INFORMATION

Point out that early ejaculation is a very common problem—one study found that 35% of married males reported that they ejaculated too quickly. Tell the patient that men with this problem have a high success rate when they try one or more specific suggestions for this problem. Give a *brief explanation of the psychophysiologic mechanism.*

> **Doctor:** Men aren't supposed to be able to have long-lasting erections if they are too nervous or distracted. The fight-or-flight response generally makes men more likely to ejaculate. Most men have trained themselves through rapid masturbation to get erect and ejaculate quickly; so it makes sense that they would continue to ejaculate quickly when they are with a partner.

Assure the patient that men often report more intense orgasms after they have learned to last longer and that it is highly likely that he will gain greater ejaculatory control by following these suggestions.

SPECIFIC SUGGESTIONS

The patient may need to *increase his frequency of ejaculations,* alone or with a partner, perhaps masturbating to orgasm earlier on a day that a sexual encounter with a partner is anticipated. Discuss *other ways he can please his partner,* so he does not feel pressure to do it all with an erect penis. Discuss the importance of muscle relaxation in achieving a prolonged erection. Suggest *breathing exercises and progressive muscle relaxation exercises*, targeting the PC muscles or those in the buttocks.

In contrast to common attempts by men to diminish sensations in hope of lasting longer, they actually need to *increase their tolerance for the good sensations and feelings* and can best do this by concentrating on their feelings and getting more "turned on." Focusing on these feelings in a relaxed "practice" atmosphere can increase the threshold of enjoyment before ejaculation and orgasm.

He and his partner can read about and practice the "*stop-start technique.*" Encourage the patient to change positions and to go from intercourse to oral or manual stimulation of his partner, and then back to intercourse (following the desires of his partner); changing positions and pleasuring a partner to orgasm without intercourse helps many men last longer.

INTENSIVE THERAPY

Recommend individual or couple therapy with a clinician skilled in human sexuality issues (where appropriate).

OTHER MEDICAL INTERVENTIONS

Clomipramine (Anafranil, 25 mg as needed) or SSRI antidepressants help men prolong their erections prior to ejaculation.

Prilocaine-lidocaine cream applied to the penis and then used with a condom has been recommended by some clinicians (although "numbing" of the genitals may detract from enjoyment for both partners).

Orgasm Problems

SYMPTOMS & SIGNS

Many women do not learn to have orgasms until they are in their 20s, 30s, or even later. A **primary anorgasmic** or **preorgasmic** woman is not yet able to reach orgasm reliably either with a partner or by herself. A woman with **secondary orgasmic problems** was previously able to reach orgasm but is no longer able to do so. **Situational orgasmic problem** refers to a condition in which a woman can have orgasm with masturbation but not with a partner, or with one partner but not with another. She may reach moderate-to-high levels of arousal without experiencing the pleasure and release of climax. If no arousal or interest is present, she should be evaluated for a desire or arousal problem.

Some males might report delayed or absent ejaculation despite prolonged intercourse or other stimulation. Some report ejaculation without the sensation of orgasm (see Table 32-8).

 CASE ILLUSTRATION 7

*Ethyl's complaint of low sexual desire and difficulty feeling aroused led the physician to do a brief sex problem interview. With this more open discussion, Ethyl revealed that she had never been able to climax, but had been highly aroused in the first year of her 5-year marriage. Their lovemaking style was focused on intercourse, and Ethyl's husband did not seem to understand why she did not enjoy it as much as he did. She had not faked orgasm but had never told him about her feelings of frustration about not reaching orgasm. Ethyl had never masturbated and remembered vague attitudes conveyed by her parents and her church that masturbation was not a correct thing to do. The physician then validated that many women first learn about self-pleasuring as adults and that the information she could get about how her own body worked would then be useful in her sexual relationship with her husband. It was suggested that Ethyl read a self-help book for women who want to learn to have orgasms (**P, LI,** and **SS**). At a visit 3 months later, Ethyl reported that she had proudly experienced her first orgasm by herself and felt so encouraged by this that she was able to talk more openly with her husband, who then agreed to go with her to see a marital/sex therapist to discuss ways they could bring more pleasure into their own lovemaking.*

 CASE ILLUSTRATION 8

*Frank, a 24-year-old man, confided that he had never reached orgasm with a partner. A sex problem history revealed that he had never ejaculated during intercourse and that his partners had never tried to bring him to orgasm manually or orally. Frank was able to ejaculate with masturbation, describing a vivid sexual fantasy (which he did not allow himself to have when with a partner) and a lifelong pattern of stimulation in which he rubbed his penis back and forth against a pillow without using his hands. He was congratulated for bringing this problem to his physician's attention (**P**) and was told that anxiety was often a cause of this problem, together with a masturbation pattern that did not simulate the type of sensations he would have during intercourse (**LI**). The physician encouraged Frank to take a stepwise approach to the problem by enlisting the help of a willing partner and starting with those elements that had been successful for him. He was also encouraged to expand on the kind of physical*

*stimulation he received during masturbation by gripping his penis with his hand and stroking it. With his partner, Frank was to focus on the goal of having high arousal while his partner stimulated his penis manually and he was imagining his "tried-and-true" fantasy. The next step was to reach higher levels of arousal in this manner and to stimulate an orgasmic response (**SS**). Frank was also referred to a self-help book (**P, LI, SS**). Follow-up indicated that Frank had successfully reached orgasm with manual stimulation with a partner in 3 weeks and was following suggestions in the book on his goal toward ejaculation during intercourse.*

Management

PERMISSION, LIMITED INFORMATION, & SPECIFIC SUGGESTIONS

Both men and women may present with difficulties in achieving orgasm because of a repeated pattern of masturbation that does not approximate the stimulation they receive from a partner. Although physical arousal may be apparent (erection or lubrication), these patients may not be feeling excited if they have to forego the fantasies or kinds of stimulation that had worked for them while masturbating. Encouraging them to incorporate the conditions under which they can reach orgasm when alone into their sexual play with a partner is the first step in their expanding their sexual enjoyment. In some instances, use of a vibrator may be recommended to provide the more intense stimulation needed for some people. Explicit communication with the patient's partner should be encouraged about the need to have enough stimulation prior to ejaculation and orgasm.

INTENSIVE THERAPY

Recommend individual or couple therapy with a clinician skilled in human sexuality issues (where appropriate).

OTHER MEDICAL INTERVENTIONS

The usual treatment of problems related to female orgasm is a combination of a good sex and psychosocial history, demythologizing, educating, behavioral treatments, and couples work where needed. There is no medication treatment available, since anorgasmia is rarely a physically caused problem.

As noted, Labrie et al. (2009) and the third author have had promising experience with intravaginal DHEA, whereas intranasal oxytocin (20–24 IU) is being studied as a potential stimulator of orgasm in women, and might hold promise for the treatment of delayed ejaculation.

Sexual Pain: Dyspareunia and Vaginismus

SYMPTOMS & SIGNS

Dyspareunia—pain for women or men associated with genital sex of all kinds may be one of the most common and perhaps most underreported of the sexual dysfunctions. **Vaginismus,** a specific cause of female dyspareunia, involves the involuntary spasm of muscles around the vagina. Vaginismus can usually be treated by teaching the patient exercises to establish personal vaginal control and remove sources of contributing associated anxieties, such as conditioning to previous genital trauma, fear of penetration, anatomical ignorance, and others.

A gentle, sensitive genital examination and demonstration should always be a part of the evaluation of vaginismus. The use of progressively sized vaginal dilators has been helpful in some cases, but treatment can often be successful without them.

 CASE ILLUSTRATION 9

*Nineteen-year-old Gina complained to her primary care provider that she had dyspareunia, was losing interest in sex, and was worried that her boyfriend was becoming impatient with her avoidance of sex. The physician then encouraged her to describe this problem behaviorally and in detail (**P**). Gina said that she had enjoyed intercourse since the age of 17 years and always used latex condoms, but on one occasion 6 months ago she suddenly felt as if her vagina "was being rubbed with sandpaper" when her partner penetrated her. Although the physical pain had not actually returned in subsequent lovemaking sessions, Gina's fear of the pain recurring diminished both her interest in and her enjoyment of sex. When asked what she would do if the pain happened again during intercourse, Gina replied that she "would have to ask him to hurry up, but sometimes he lasts longer then." The physician asked how she would feel about telling him to stop all movement immediately and to withdraw when she felt discomfort or pain. Gina expressed concern that an abrupt withdrawal from intercourse might result in her boyfriend having testicular pain. She was reassured that this would create no lasting discomfort for him, and that there were alternatives for reaching ejaculation and orgasm, either with her or alone (**P, LI, and SS**). She was also offered some suggestions for reading about how couples learn to increase their enjoyment of sex (**SS**). The physician also praised Gina for having shown the courage to discuss this personal issue and encouraged her to bring up any future concerns (**P, LI**).*

Management

SPECIFIC SUGGESTIONS

These issues can be approached gradually, by encouraging the woman to speak with her partner about her needs and to be a full participant in the sexual encounter. She and her partner should be educated about the need for sufficient stimulation and arousal prior to attempted penetration, and about the importance of her being in control of the sexual movement, so that she can stop it instantly if pain is felt. Instruction in Kegel's PC muscle exercises increases the woman's awareness and control of her vaginal muscles. Vaginal self-dilatation can be accomplished with graduated cylinders or with fingers, from the little finger to multiple fingers, while practicing muscle relaxation and calming mental imagery. The patient should be encouraged to be the one in control by bearing down on the finger(s) or penis as if pushing something out of the vagina, then relaxing. It helps for some women to imagine "capturing" the penis or other object in this manner, instead of being "penetrated."

OTHER MEDICAL INTERVENTIONS

Other medical suggestions include the use of artificial lubricants, such as Astroglide, Gyne-Moistrin, or KY Jelly (not good with latex); vaginal moisturizers, such as Replens; and vaginal and vulvar application of estrogen creams. Further evaluation of vaginismus includes assessment for developmental anatomical abnormalities; if deemed appropriate, surgical revision of the vulvovaginal region and/or excision of abnormal growths in the genital area may prove helpful. Diseases thought to cause the pain, such as vaginitis, condylomata, endometriosis, pelvic inflammatory disease, and other gynecologic or pelvic diseases, may all be treated directly. When painful intercourse has been a long-standing problem, however, medical intervention alone is seldom adequate and should be followed by sex therapy directed at the probable fear and expectation of pain that have been conditioned.

SEXUAL PROBLEMS DUE TO A GENERAL MEDICAL CONDITION

Many sexual issues of those with impactful medical conditions and physical disabilities may be treated like those persons who are nondisabled and healthy. In other cases, culturally competent health practitioners knowledgeable about the social and physical issues of disability may be most effective. Some studies, such as with women following gynecologic cancer surgery, suggest that Internet support groups can be as beneficial as actual group meetings. Other online resources that are appropriately monitored and proctored by health professionals may become available in the near future.

CASE ILLUSTRATION 10

When Hannah was 22 years old, she was diagnosed with clear cell adenocarcinoma of the vagina and had surgery that removed one ovary, her uterus, tubes, the upper two-thirds of her vagina, and her bilateral pelvic lymph nodes. None of her health care team was able to comfortably discuss sexuality with her. She was completely unprepared for the first attempts at intercourse several months following the surgery and was shocked and distraught to discover how little genital sensation she had left. She sought help from a male psychiatrist who listened as she expressed her grief and fears that she would never find a man because of her sense of diminished sexual self-worth. After rapport was established, he acknowledged her fears by saying that she might never have a "clitoral" orgasm again, but that there were other routes to orgasm and sexual pleasure. He discussed with her ideas that have been helpful to others who have sustained the loss of genital sensation: that her brain knew how to feel pleasure and have orgasms, that men and women can learn to focus on sensations from other, nongenital parts of the body, such as breasts, neck, ears, and lips, and that with or without accompanying fantasy, one can thus relearn to enjoy a sense of orgasmic release and pleasure. Twelve years after her surgery, Hannah wrote, "The growth in my ideas and experiments with sexuality have increased manyfold since my surgery. What was most helpful was being able to share my experiences with people who could understand and be accepting, and finding people who were trained and had accurate information on how I could help myself. Health professionals don't have to have all the answers, but they should know their own limitations and be able to refer when necessary."

For those patients who have undergone treatment for significant medical conditions such as cancer—with a potential altered body image and an understandable interruption or cessation of their sexual life—the following attitudes may be helpfully communicated to patients by their health care provider(s):

Whenever you are ready to become sexually active again, there are a few things you can keep in mind:

- *You are loved for who you are, not just for your appearance.* If you felt lovable or sexually desirable before you became ill, chances are that you will be afterward too.
- *We are all sexual beings.* Sexuality is part of who we *are*, whether we are sexually active or not. It is not defined just by what we do or how often we do it.

- *Survival overshadows sexuality.* It is normal and natural for stress, depression, worry, and fatigue to lower your interest in sex after major medical issues. Just coping with basic everyday decisions can seem like a burden. But take one day at a time and be patient. Sexual interest and feelings often come back when the immediate crisis has passed.

- *Share your feelings.* You may find yourself in the position of having to share your sexual feelings with someone, perhaps for the first time. This may be awkward at first, and learning how and when to talk about sexual issues may not come easily. You may feel shy or nervous about exploring new and different ways of finding sexual pleasure. You may each wait for the other to make the first move to resume sexual activities. This familiar waiting game is easily misunderstood and experienced as rejection by both people. It also may be frightening to think of breaking the silence yourself. Yet, a good move is to make the first move. Try sharing some of the myths or expectations you grew up with about sexuality. This can be humorous and may break the ice in starting a frank discussion about your sexual needs and concerns. Try not to make broad, generalized statements. Talk about what is important to *you* and about how *you* feel. The payoff is greater understanding of each other's needs and concerns, and that is worth the effort.

- *Expect the unexpected.* When you first have sex after a long time without it, physical limitations or fears about your performance, appearance, or rejection may keep you from focusing on the sheer pleasure of physical contact. On the other hand, you may be surprised by unfamiliar pleasurable sensations. If you expect some changes as part of the natural recovery process, they will be less likely to distract you from sexual pleasure if they do happen.

- *Give yourself time.* You and your partner may be frightened of, or even repulsed by, scars, unfamiliar appliances, or other physical changes. That's natural too. But such feelings are usually temporary. Talking about them is often the first step to mutual support and acceptance. Don't pressure yourself about having to "work on sex." A satisfactory and enjoyable sex life will happen one step at a time. You may want to spend some time by yourself exploring your body, becoming familiar with changes, and rediscovering your unique body texture and sensations. Once you feel relaxed doing this, move on to mutual body exploration with a partner.

- *Take the pressure off intercourse.* Almost all of us were brought up to believe that intercourse is the only real or appropriate way of expressing ourselves sexually. Yet sexual expression can encompass many forms of touching and pleasuring that are satisfying psychologically and physically.

Try spending some time in pleasurable activities—touching, fondling, kissing, and being close—without having intercourse. Reexperience the pleasure of playing, of holding and of being held without having to worry about erections and orgasms. When you feel comfortable, proceed at your own pace to other ways of being sexual, including intercourse if you like.

Experiment and explore to discover what feels best and what is acceptable. If radiation therapy, for example, has made intercourse painful, try oral or manual stimulation to orgasm, or intercourse between thighs or breasts. If you are exhausted by the disease or movement is painful, just cuddling or lying quietly next to your partner can be a wonderfully satisfying form of intimacy.

- *Your sexuality cannot be "diagnosed."* You will never know what pleasures you are capable of experiencing if you don't explore. Try new positions, new touches, and above all new attitudes."

OTHER SEXUAL PROBLEMS NOT OTHERWISE SPECIFIED

Serious sex-related problems may be best dealt with by a psychotherapist or health professional trained in sexual issues. A patient with **compulsive sexual behavior** or **sexual addiction** may be suffering from a form of obsessive–compulsive disorder and may require intensive psychotherapy, use of support groups, and medications such as SSRI antidepressants. Patients with **gender identity disorders**, patients who have experienced **spousal abuse, incest,** and **rape**, and patients troubled by **paraphilias** require referral for specialized treatment. Internet support groups for some people with some sexual problems can create new possibilities for support and provide hope and validation. **Infidelity** can be an extremely painful issue that affects many couples, yet many of them can be helped by couple therapy to address the pain, anger, and loss of trust.

CONCLUSIONS

For every human being, sexuality—like health—is a challenge at some point. Feelings of personal vulnerability are inherent in sexual interactions and help to make sexuality a powerful and unique part of life. Problems of sexual desire, arousal, or functioning can lead us to confront and overcome our fears of not being lovable and to seek better communication and increased intimacy with others. The deepest expressions of love often result from just sharing our vulnerabilities or problems.

ACKNOWLEDGMENTS

The authors thank Linda Perlin Alperstein, LCSW; Jean M. Bullard, RN, MS; Melissa A. Bullard, PhD;

Lisa Capaldini, MD; Deborah Grady, MD, MPH; Mary Rodocker, PhD, RN; & William B. Shore, MD for reviewing earlier drafts of this chapter. Finally, we benefitted from the comments on this chapter by Raymond C. Rosen, PhD; his career-long contributions to the study of human sexuality have been inspiring to us.

SUGGESTED READINGS

Readings for Patients

Barbach L. *For Yourself—Revised.* New York, NY: Signet, 2000.(A revised classic that empowers women to enjoy their own sexuality, with suggestions for women who want to learn to become orgasmic.)

Johnson, S. *Hold Me Tight: Seven Conversations for a Lifetime of Love.* New York, NY: Little, Brown, 2008.

Johnson S. Love Sense: *The Revolutionary New Science of Romantic Relationships.* New York, NY. Little, Brown. 2013

Levine SB. *Handbook of Clinical Sexuality for Mental Health Professionals,* 2nd ed. New York, NY:Routledge, 2010.

Perel E. *Mating in Captivity: Reconciling the Erotic and the Domestic.* New York, NY: Harper Collins, 2006.(Fresh, provocative, and intelligent exploration of the erotic imagination versus the sexless marriage.)

Schover LR. *Sexuality and Fertility after Cancer.* New York, NY: Wiley & Sons, 1997. (Compassionate and hopeful resource for women and men who have had cancer.)

Spring J (with Spring M). *After the Affair: Healing the Pain and Rebuilding Trust When a Partner Has Been Unfaithful.* New York, NY: HarperCollins, 1997. (A compassionate and hopeful resource for people grappling with the betrayal of infidelity.)

Zilbergeld B. *The New Male Sexuality—Revised.* New York, NY: Bantam, 1999. (A common sense, practical, and sane antidote to media pressures on males to be sexual superstars. Excellent discussion of the fantasy model of sex and myths of male sexuality, the importance of an individual's conditions for good sex, and specific self-help chapters dealing with common male sexual problems.)

Zilbergeld B, Zilbergeld G. *Sex and Love at Midlife.* Bethel, CT: Crown House, 2010. (Issues on aging and sexuality with a positive focus.)

General Reference Articles

Al-Azzawi F, Bitzer J, Brandenburg U, et al. Therapeutic options for postmenopausal female sexual dysfunction. *Climacteric* 2010; 13:103–120.

Caplan HW. An effective clinical approach to vaginismus—putting the patient in charge. *West J Med* 1988;149:769–770. PMID: 3250117.

Davis SR. Editorial: understanding female sexual function. *Menopause* 2009;16:425–426. PMID: 19225425.

Derzko C, Bullard D, Rosenbaum E. Changes in sexuality and sexual dysfunction.In:Spiegel D, Rosenbaum E, Fobair P, eds. *Cancer Survivorship.* New York, NY: Andrews McMeel, 2007.

Derzko C, Elliott S, Lam W. Management of sexual dysfunction in postmenopausal breast cancer patients taking adjuvant aromatase inhibitor therapy. *Curr Oncol* 2007;14:S20-S40. PMID: 18087605.

Labrie F, Archer D, Bouchard C, et al. Effect of intravaginal dehydroepiandrosterone (Prasterone) on libido and sexual dysfunction in postmenopausal women. *Menopause* 2009;16: 923–931.

Montorsi F, Basson R, Adaikan G, et al, eds. *Sexual Dysfunctions in Men and Women: 3rd International Consultation on Sexual Medicine – Paris.* Health Publication Ltd, 2010, 403–495.

Mulhall, JP, Incrocci L, Goldstein I, Rosen RC, eds. *Cancer and Sexual Health.* New York, NY: Humana Press, 2011.

SEXUAL MEDICINE WEB SITES

American Association of Sexuality Educator Counselors and Therapists Web site. www.aasect.org. Accessed February 2012.

Electronic Journal of Human Sexuality Web site. www.ejhs.org. Accessed February 2012.

International Journal of Transgenderism Web site. www.wpath.org/publications_ijt.cfm. Accessed February 2012.

Journal of Sexual Medicine Web site. http://onlinelibrary.wiley.com/journal/10.1111/%28ISSN%291743–6109. Accessed February 2012.

Kinsey Institute Web site. www.kinseyinstitute.org. Accessed February, 2012. Accessed February 2012.

North American Menopause Society(NAMS)Web site. www.menopause.org. Accessed February 2012.

Sexuality Information and Education Council of the United States Web site. www.siecus.org. Accessed February 2012.

Society for the Scientific Study of Sexuality Web site. www.sexscience.org. Accessed February 2012.

SECTION VI
Special Topics

Integrative Medicine

Kevin Barrows, MD & Tracy Ann Rydel, MD

INTRODUCTION

The term "Integrative Medicine" defines an approach to healing that utilizes conventional practices taught in traditional medical schools as well as practices taught outside of this conventional model. The term Complementary and Alternative Medicine (CAM) may be used to define the latter, whereas Integrative Medicine "refers to a practice that combines both conventional and CAM treatments for which there is evidence of safety and effectiveness." It is a patient-centered approach to care that not only seeks to eradicate disease or illness but also promotes optimal health and wellness.

A major focus of Integrative Medicine (IM) is on lifestyle, including nutrition and exercise, discussed in a level of detail not commonly explored in conventional medicine. Integrative Medicine also places a strong emphasis on the importance of sleep, stress, environment, social support, spirituality, and the effects that they may have on wellness. Many CAM disciplines also emphasize these holistic factors in their evaluation of the patient or client; it is this focus on holism that encourages many IM practitioners to frequently incorporate CAM modalities into their array of treatment options. Although many CAM modalities are utilized in the practice of IM, it is important to recognize that IM and CAM are not interchangeable terms. Integrative Medicine practitioners may call upon CAM modalities as part of their treatment plan, but they also utilize conventional medical practices and lifestyle modifications when deemed beneficial for the patient. The National Center for Complementary and Alternative Medicine (NCCAM), a center within the National Institutes of Health, has classified five domains of CAM listed in Table 33-1.

To practice IM, most clinicians seek formal training by way of university-based fellowship training and/or

board certification through the American Board of Integrative and Holistic Medicine. A new board certification, the American Board of Integrative Medicine, has been developed through the American Board of Physician Specialties. Some IM practitioners are trained in conventional practices and seek additional training and certification in one of the specific CAM modalities listed above. For example, some conventionally trained practitioners are also trained in acupuncture, naturopathy, or manual medicine, broadening their skill set. Self-guided study is also available via conferences or training seminars focused on particular areas of research or practice.

DISCUSSING INTEGRATIVE MEDICINE WITH PATIENTS

Epidemiology

A study performed by the American Association of Retired Persons (AARP) and the NCCAM revealed that more than half of all Americans over the age of 50 years use some form of CAM. The most commonly used CAM modalities in this survey were herbal medicines (37%), bodywork (e.g., massage, chiropractic; 22%), and mind–body techniques (e.g., meditation, guided imagery; 9%). It has been found that Americans spend approximately as much out-of-pocket expense on CAM treatments—over $25 billion per year—as they do on visits to all primary care physicians.

The reasons why patients use IM/CAM modalities have been evaluated in numerous studies. A holistic philosophy of health—one which values the mind, body, and spirit—is the most consistent predictor of who will pursue CAM therapies, and relief of symptoms is the most common benefit reported. Most patients say that they are looking to prevent illness and promote wellness,

Table 33-1. NCCAM classification of CAM.

Domain	Examples
Alternative medicine systems	Traditional Chinese medicine; acupuncture; ayurveda; naturopathy; homeopathy
Mind–body interventions	Meditation; hypnosis; guided imagery; dance, art, and music therapy; spiritual healing
Biological-based therapies	Herbal medicines and dietary supplements; special diets
Manipulative and body-based methods	Chiropractic; osteopathic manual medicine; massage; other "body-work" systems
Energy therapies	Reiki; therapeutic touch; magnets; methods that affect the body's "bioelectric" field

and over two-thirds are motivated to use CAM for the treatment or alleviation of pain. Interestingly, dissatisfaction with conventional treatment is not a significant predictor of the pursuit of IM/CAM modalities by patients.

Communication and Disclosure

While the percentage of Americans using CAM treatments continues to rise, a troubling yet consistent finding is the rate of nondisclosure from patients to their conventional physicians regarding CAM. The AARP/NCCAM study cited above found that less than one-third of the individuals using CAM modalities discussed it with their physicians. The reasons for nondisclosure are not completely understood; unfortunately the problem of poor communication on this topic continues to be quite pervasive despite the increasing utilization of IM and CAM practices.

Many patients report that they do not disclose their use of nonconventional therapies simply because their health professional did not ask them about it. Perceived clinician receptivity and nonjudgmental initiation of the discussion tend to be the most important factors in patients' willingness to talk about IM and CAM. Often patients do not realize that they can and should bring up the topic, instead expecting that their clinician should ask them about it. When surveyed, many practitioners report that their general lack of understanding of IM modalities prevents them from asking patients about their usage, fearing the lack of expertise to hold a proper discussion. However, most patients do not expect their physician or other conventionally trained practitioners to be well-versed in nonconventional modalities, understanding that this is out of the scope of traditional training. Also, perhaps because most

patients do not spontaneously offer this information, many clinicians have a falsely low perception of patient usage and, therefore, do not pursue discussing the topic.

The practitioner attitudes that seem to facilitate the most open discussions about IM with patients are ones of open-mindedness, holism, and a belief that it is possible to integrate different modalities of healing in the treatment of a given patient. Clinicians who embody these attitudes as well as the fundamental practices of IM—attention to nutrition, exercise, positive sleep habits, and the mind–body connection—may be more likely to achieve better outcomes with their patients. Leading by example may be a critical component in a clinician's ability to facilitate wellness in their patients. Medical students, who are astute observers of their mentors, overwhelmingly agree with the belief that doctors who lead balanced lives generate improved patient satisfaction.

An example of work–life balance and how personal physician behavior may affect patient outcomes is seen in the area of mind–body medicine. Such a concordance between clinician practices and patient/client outcomes has been observed in the use of mindfulness, a meditation practice devoted to awareness of the present moment. One study examined the effects on patients whose psychotherapists had received mindfulness training. Results showed that inpatients whose therapists practiced Zen meditation had improvement in understanding of their psychodynamics and treatment goals and showed significant reduction in a multitude of psychiatric symptoms. Cultivating attention to the present moment, practicing the fundamentals of a balanced, healthy lifestyle, and maintaining an attitude of open-mindedness and holism may be the best foundation for encouraging these very same behaviors and practices in one's patients (see Chapter 7).

TAKING AN INTEGRATIVE MEDICINE HISTORY

Integrative Medicine history-taking incorporates techniques from behavioral medicine and family medicine. Narrative Medicine, with its validation of the patient's experiential story, allows for a holistic, reflective, patient-centered approach to gathering information, concomitantly allowing for creativity and self-reflection on the part of the clinician (see Chapter 45). Motivational Interviewing uses empathy, discrepancy, and acceptance of client reluctance in order to motivate patients toward self-effective change (see Chapter 19). Rather than take an authoritative or paternalistic approach, this technique also allows for clinician creativity, avoiding a script and instead allowing the patient to highlight those influences in his or her life that are most relevant to their condition. The Biopsychosocial Model of medicine also emphasizes the varying influences on a patient's health and is inclusive of biomedical, psychological, social, and environmental factors and their effect on health and wellness.

A typical IM intake holds a broad definition of health and includes questions about diet, exercise, sleep, stress, biomedical illness, mental health, social connections, home and other environments, and spirituality. It is common practice to have the patient complete a standard form that includes such questions; this allows for better organization of this large amount of information and valuable background data, freeing clinicians to have a more narrative, conversational flow in their first meeting with the patient. A detailed visit to establish care, with a review of all of these barometers of health, is an optimal way in which to build rapport with a patient. If face-to-face time with the patient is severely limited, then such a detailed intake form can be even more useful since it can be reviewed by the clinician outside of the patient visit and still allow attention to these important aspects of the patient's health.

THE CLINICAL APPLICATION OF INTEGRATIVE MEDICINE: MAJOR DEPRESSION AS A CASE STUDY

Just as the IM intake described above is comprehensive and holistic, so too may be the treatment. The integrative treatment of major depression is an instructive example in which to explore the clinical application of IM to behavioral health, since it incorporates a broad spectrum of modalities that demonstrate well this holistic approach. The approach includes conventional therapies when indicated (e.g., pharmaceuticals, psychotherapy), though these are beyond the scope of this chapter (see Chapter 25). The key integrative therapies that are most frequently used are foundational health practices (nutrition, exercise, sleep, and stress management), light, mind–body therapies (e.g., meditation, guided imagery), and botanical medicines and supplements (e.g., St. John's wort). Some studies suggest that transcranial magnetic stimulation may be beneficial. Energy medicine therapies (e.g., Reiki), manual medicine techniques (e.g., osteopathy, massage), aromatherapy, and alternative systems (e.g., Traditional Chinese Medicine, homeopathy) may also be used, although there is less research evidence for these at present.

Foundational Health Practices: Nutrition, Exercise, Sleep, Stress Management

Nutrition: Food affects mood through a variety of mechanisms such as nutritional deficiencies, psychoactive foods (e.g., alcohol, caffeine), hunger (possibly including hypoglycemia), and food intolerances (e.g., celiac disease, fructose intolerance). Integrative treatment of depression, therefore, includes a comprehensive assessment of the patient's diet. General guidelines for nutrition in depression are:

- Eating mostly whole foods (e.g., grains, legumes) and few or no refined foods (e.g., processed cereal, sweetened beverages, and baked goods)
- Eating copious amounts of vegetables and fruits
- Reducing or eliminating alcohol, caffeine, and sugar
- Choosing healthy fats (e.g., fish and plant-derived) more often than unhealthy fats (polyunsaturated vegetable oils, animal-source saturated fats, trans fats)
- Using healthy snacks to avoid hunger between meals

Though results are mixed, some research has found a beneficial effect of supplementing with key nutrients, such as folate or omega-3 fatty acids from fish oil, either as monotherapy or as adjunctive therapy to pharmaceutical medicines for depression.

Exercise: Exercise has been shown to be beneficial for mild-to-moderate depression in some clinical trials. Many forms of aerobic exercise (e.g., running, walking, dancing), strength training, and mindful exercise (e.g., tai chi, qi gong) may be beneficial. Certainly, exercise should be a part of any wellness program for those who are able to participate.

Sleep: Sleep is another foundational health practice that affects mood (see Chapter 31). Chronic insomnia, for example, is a risk factor for depression. Integrative assessment of a patient with depression includes evaluation of sleep health. Recommendations for sleep health in a depressed patient, known as "sleep hygiene," are:

1. Awake-to-Sleep Transition
   - Light transition is helpful (gradually reducing amount of ambient light until ready for sleep). If this is too much trouble, then it is recommended to at least avoid bright light for the hour preceding bedtime. The sleep room should be thoroughly darkened. Illuminated clocks or any light-emitting devices should be off or facing away from the eyes.
   - It is recommended that the following be avoided in the period of time before sleep: vigorous physical exertion, mental stimulation, problem-solving or other task-oriented cognitive function, and loud or emotionally provocative stimuli. Meditation or prayer can be ideal. Relaxation exercises are useful. Listening to calming music or other calming sound can also be useful. Many people find aromatherapy helpful for falling asleep (e.g., lavender, chamomile).

2. Bed
   - The bed is for sleep or intimacy only. One should not read in bed, eat in bed, nor watch television in bed. This helps to condition the mind so that when one goes to bed the mind becomes calm rather than remaining active.

3. Caffeine
   • Anyone with sleep problems should consider eliminating caffeine from the diet entirely or at least avoid caffeine ingestion after 2 P.M.
4. Exercise
   • Studies show that vigorous aerobic exercise done in the morning or early afternoon improves sleep. Vigorous aerobic exercise done in the evening can worsen insomnia for some people, making it harder to fall asleep.

Stress Management: The last of the four foundational health practices, stress management, is very important in the integrative treatment of depression. Stress has a strong causal relationship with major depression, and mind–body therapies that reduce stress have proved to be beneficial (see Chapter 34).

Light

Light, or phototherapy, is an effective treatment for seasonal affective disorder (SAD), and may also be helpful as an adjunctive treatment of nonseasonal depression as well. Bright, full-spectrum light (10,000 lux) of 30–60 minutes in the morning from an appropriate bulb has been studied, but natural sunlight is likely to be effective also. This exposure to appropriate artificial or natural light is part of a comprehensive IM treatment plan for depression.

Mind–Body Therapies

Mind–body medicine is commonly defined as the field of medicine that uses processes of the mind to influence the health of the body. This is a useful definition with which to start, but it is important to note that it can perpetuate the mind versus body dualism, and it fails to acknowledge the bidirectional relationship of mind and body, that is, not only does the state of mind affect physical health (e.g., depression worsens coronary artery disease outcomes) but the state of the physical body can affect mental state (e.g., aerobic exercise improves mood). It may be more accurate to think of mind/body as a single entity, where the health of one part necessarily influences the health of the other. Examples of mind–body therapies are meditation, guided imagery, biofeedback, hypnosis, progressive muscle relaxation, breathing exercises, yoga, tai chi, and qi gong.

Mind–body therapies can be useful for treating depression. A Cochrane review and meta-analysis of 11 trials of relaxation therapies (e.g., progressive muscle relaxation, relaxation imagery, autogenic training) found significant reduction in *self-rated* depressive symptoms compared with no treatment. Mindfulness-based programs (mindfulness-based stress reduction [MBSR] and mindfulness-based cognitive therapy [MBCT]) have shown benefit in treating depression and preventing relapse.

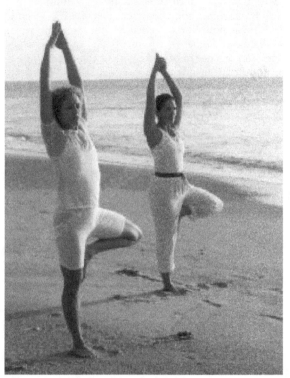

Beach Yoga

Botanical Medicines and Supplements

The botanical medicine St. John's wort and the supplement *S*-adenosylmethionine ("SAMe") are the two non-pharmaceutical medicines that have the most research evidence supporting their use in the integrative treatment of depression.

1. St. John's Wort (*Hypericum perforatum*)

St. John's wort is a perennial plant, with a yellow flower, native to Europe and naturalized to North America. It is one of the oldest medicinal botanicals of Europe. Over the past two decades, St. John's wort has been studied in thousands of patients for the treatment of depression. Several well-designed randomized, controlled clinical trials (RCTs) have found that St. John's wort is more effective than placebo for the treatment of mild-to-moderate depression and has fewer side effects than pharmaceutical antidepressants. Other recent RCTs have not replicated these findings, leading some experts to not endorse the use of St. Johns wort for this purpose. As with all treatment modalities, clinicians should discuss the potential risks and benefits of the treatment with their patients and come to a decision through a shared decision-making paradigm.

St. John's wort inhibits serotonin, norepinephrine, and dopamine reuptake in the central nervous system and may modulate autonomic system reactivity. As an oral medicine it is very well tolerated. Data from 35 double-blind randomized trials show that drop out and adverse event rates in patients receiving *Hypericum* extracts were less than that for tricyclic antidepressants or selective serotonin reuptake inhibitors (SSRI). Side effects include gastrointestinal upset, photodermatitis, mild headache, and restlessness. Cases of withdrawal symptoms similar to those that occur with SSRI antidepressants have been described, so gradual tapering of dose is recommended when therapy is terminated. Patients are advised to avoid taking St. John's wort in combination with prescription antidepressants because there have been case reports of serotonin syndrome. Importantly, St. John's wort also potently induces the cytochrome P450 system (isozyme CYP3A4), which may lower the blood levels of medications that are metabolized by this system (e.g., alprazolam, ethinyl estradiol, warfarin, cyclosporine, statins, and indinavir). St John's wort can also lower the serum level of medications by increasing activity of the P-glycoprotein transporter system, thereby increasing drug excretion through the gastrointestinal mucosa. St. John's wort has the potential for multiple herb–drug interactions through induction of the CYP3A4 and P-glycoprotein systems. Concurrent use of St. John's wort and medications metabolized by these systems should be avoided.

The usual dose of St. John's wort is 300 mg three times daily of a preparation standardized to hypericin (0.3%) or hyperforin (2–5%).

2. S-Adenosylmethionine

S-adenosylmethionine (SAMe) is a naturally occurring compound made in the human body that facilitates transmethylation reactions, such as those that occur in neurotransmitter metabolism. Levels of SAMe are dependent on B-vitamin concentrations. Although the exact mechanism of its antidepressant effect is not known, SAMe is associated with increased serotonin turnover and increased dopamine and norepinephrine levels in the brain.

There have been more than a dozen randomized controlled trials on SAMe for depression; although most of these studies show benefit, several examined parenterally administered SAMe, and there were methodological limitations to many.

S-adenosylmethionine appears to be safe. Side effects include gastrointestinal upset (nausea, vomiting, diarrhea) and psychomotor stimulation (insomnia, anxiety, restlessness). There have been cases of mania and hypomania in people with bipolar disorder who have taken SAMe, hence, it should be avoided in this population.

SAMe can lower blood glucose levels and, therefore, should be used cautiously in patients taking hypoglycemic agents. SAMe might interfere with the action of levodopa in those with Parkinson disease.

The dose of SAMe for depression is 800–1600 mg daily. The cost of this supplement is high, relative to other over-the-counter supplements.

CASE ILLUSTRATION

A 26 year-old male graduate student in the chemistry department of a university presents to an IM physician complaining of "feeling unhappy a lot", "stressed out", "just working all the time," and "out of touch with life." He confirms that his work and social life have suffered due to persistent low mood. He has no prior history of major depression, but does describe previous periods of "doldrums" in his adult life. He began weekly psychotherapy for the first time 1 year ago. He began taking an SSRI antidepressant for the first time 8 months ago, has never been hospitalized for mental illness, and has no history of suicidality. He does not drink alcohol nor use illegal substances. He prefers to work in the laboratory late in the evening, goes to bed between midnight and 1 A.M., has trouble falling asleep due to anxiety, awakens between 8 and 9 A.M., and does not feel alert until early afternoon. He either skips breakfast or eats a bagel with jam. In the mid-afternoon, he eats a burrito or sandwich, and he purchases take-out food from one of the local restaurants for dinner. He is anxious about a wide variety of things in his life (career, family, social life, health) and finds that his mind is mostly occupied with anxious thoughts when he is not focused on work. He was raised in the Catholic tradition and misses the participation that he recalls when he was younger. He exercises on the weekends occasionally, going to a local gym to run on the treadmill. He misses the team soccer he enjoyed regularly in his twenties. His weekly psychotherapy has been helpful, as has the SSRI, but he still feels lonely, anxious, and "not fully alive."

Because this patient may have major depression and possibly a generalized anxiety disorder, the IM approach to his case would include a discussion of pharmaceutical augmentation options. Nonpharmaceutical suggestions would address his foundational health practices, light, social and spiritual health, the use of mind–body medicine modalities, and supplements.

Regarding his nutrition, it would be recommended to never skip breakfast and to include all three macronutrients (protein, carbohydrate, fat) in that meal. To ensure adequate amount of B vitamins the patient could be asked to include more B vitamin rich foods in his diet or temporarily begin a B vitamin complex supplement. Increasing the quantity of whole foods, fruits, and vegetables would also be recommended for general nutritional benefit.

Regarding exercise, it would be strongly advisable to do more regular aerobic exercise. Due to his circadian rhythm phase shift, ideally this exercise would occur in the morning. His previous enjoyment of soccer and the social interaction that it offers as a team sport offer additional potentially therapeutic options. For example, he could do 30 minutes of vigorous aerobic exercise most weekday mornings and participate in soccer matches on weekends.

Regarding sleep, it would be important to address his behaviors around sleep (i.e., sleep hygiene) as well as the anxiety that interferes with falling asleep. Additionally, preliminary research suggests that shifting his circadian rhythm earlier would be helpful in improving mood.

At least 30 minutes of natural or appropriate artificial light in the morning would be another helpful adjunct in the treatment of this patient's mood. If an outdoor morning exercise routine could be established, then this may be accomplished naturally; however, a light box would be an effective alternative.

Exploring his nostalgia for the Church would be another important element in his integrative treatment plan. In addition to the benefit from spiritual practice, this could offer another social support and even a spiritually congruent way to introduce a mind–body practice. Centering Prayer, a method with ancient roots but developed in the 1970s, is a practice that shares much of the form and benefits of meditation.

Other mind–body practices that may be helpful for this patient are MBSR and the 4-7-8 breath. Mindfulness-based stress reduction is an 8-week program that is proven to help depression, anxiety, and sleep. It may also be particularly helpful with his complaint of "being out of touch with life," since mindfulness is an attentional training method that emphasizes present moment awareness (see Chapter 7). The 4-7-8 breath is derived from ancient breath practices known as pranayama, a branch of Ayurveda. The 4-7-8 method is easy, fast (2–3 minutes), and useful for acutely reducing anxiety and sympathetic tone.

Because the patient is on an SSRI, addition of St. John's wort would not be indicated. One could cautiously augment with SAMe; however, the anxiety component of this case argues against its use because SAMe can be stimulating and actually cause or exacerbate anxiety. Supplementation with fish oil may be useful for augmentation in this case and is very unlikely to be harmful.

Many other aspects of his case would of course also be explored, such as checking thyroid function if that has not already been done, checking testosterone and DHEA (dehydroepiandrosterone) levels if other symptoms of hypoandrogenism are present, addressing any other particular psychological tendencies of this patient (e.g., poor self-esteem), and discovering what most gives him a sense of meaning and purpose.

CONCLUSIONS

The field of IM is rapidly evolving and becoming more mainstream, as evidenced by the widespread use of integrative therapies by patients, the growth of research in this area, and by an ever-increasing number of practitioners seeking additional training in IM. The application of IM to behavioral health includes a common sense approach to physical, mental, and spiritual well-being, beginning with foundational health practices and potentially including conventional and multiple nonconventional therapies. Behavioral medicine, with its inherent awareness of the relationship between mind, body, and spirit is a field particularly amenable to incorporating the practices of IM.

SUGGESTED READINGS

AARP and National Center for Complementary and Alternative Medicine Survey Report. Complementary and alternative medicine: what people aged 50 and older discuss with their health care providers. April, 2011.

Chiesa A, Serretti A. Mindfulness based cognitive therapy for psychiatric disorders: a systematic review and meta-analysis. *Psychiatry Res* 2011;187:441–453. Epub September 16, 2010. Review. PMID: 20846726.

Jorm AF, Morgan AJ, Hetrick SE. Relaxation for depression. *Cochrane Database Syst Rev* 2008;(4):CD007142. Review. PMID: 18843744.

Linde K, Berner MM, Kriston L. St John's wort for major depression. *Cochrane Database Syst Rev* 2008;(4):CD000448. Review. PMID: 18843608.

Mead GE, Morley W, Campbell P, Greig CA, McMurdo M, Lawlor DA. Exercise for depression. *Cochrane Database Syst Rev* 2008;(4):CD004366. Review. Update in: *Cochrane Database Syst Rev* 2009;(3):CD004366. PMID: 18843656.

Shelley BM, Sussman AL, Williams RL, Segal AR, Crabtree BF. 'They don't ask me so I don't tell them': Patient-clinician communication about traditional, complementary, and alternative medicine. *Ann Fam Med* 2009;7:139–47. PMID: 19273869.

WEB SITES

National Institutes of Health. National Center for Complementary and Alternative Medicine Web site. http://nccam.nih.gov. Accessed February 2014.

The Bravewell Collaborative Web site. http://www.bravewell.org/integrative_medicine/what_is_IM. Accessed February 2014.

Stress & Disease

34

John F. Christensen, PhD

INTRODUCTION

Human history is replete with stories of the connection between stress and disease. A story about John Hunter (1728–1793), a surgeon and medical educator at St. George's Hospital in London, is that he stated publicly, "My life is at the mercy of any rogue who chooses to provoke me," and soon afterward died following a contentious meeting with hospital administrators.

A review of coroners' records in Los Angeles in 1994 revealed a marked increase in deaths, including sudden death, related to atherosclerotic cardiovascular disease on the day of the 1994 Northridge earthquake. In 1999 during a 7.3 magnitude earthquake in Taiwan, patients on Holter monitors showed heart rate variability derangement due to withdrawal of parasympathetic activity and increase in sympathetic arousal. In the quarterfinal of the 1996 European football championships between the French and Dutch teams, a draw at the end of overtime resulted in a sudden death penalty shoot out, which was won by the French. An analysis of mortality in the total population of Dutch men and women aged 45 years or more revealed a relative risk of death from acute myocardial infarction (MI) or stroke of 1.51 among the men on the day of the match, compared with the 5 days on either side. There was no such effect on French men. This gave new meaning to the term "sudden death penalty."

The *psychological* sequelae of exposure to life-threatening stressors are also problematic and disruptive to people's lives. The terrorist attacks on the World Trade Center and the Pentagon on September 11, 2001, were witnessed directly by an estimated 100,000 people and vicariously by millions of Americans and others worldwide. In the period of time between October 16 and November 15, 2001, it is estimated that 7.5% of Manhattan residents south of 110th street were suffering from posttraumatic stress disorder (PTSD) and 9.7% were suffering from depression. In a representative sample of the American population surveyed 3–5 days following the attacks, 44% reported one or more substantial symptoms consistent with acute stress disorder (ASD), and 90% had one or more symptoms to some degree. Refugees and prisoners of war who have been exposed to torture are also likely to develop symptoms of PTSD, anxiety, and depression.

Less dramatically, research since the late 1960s has demonstrated correlations between significant changes in individuals' lives and the subsequent onset of various types of physical and psychological illness. A consistent relationship has even been found between daily hassles and the onset of illness.

The interrelationship between mental stress and physical disease is complex and multifactorial. As a result, the study of stress and disease embraces a wide range of behavioral, emotional, cognitive, physiologic, hormonal, biochemical, cellular, environmental, and even spiritual interconnections, not easily understood or encapsulated in the controlled clinical trial.

It has been estimated that up to 70% of visits to primary care physicians are for problems related to stress and lifestyle. Most clinicians, however, have not been trained to extend their diagnostic workup and treatment interventions into the psychosocial context of these illnesses. Yet, adequate treatment and prevention require that providers regard their patients' illnesses and suffering in the context of their life struggles. This perspective allows the clinician to intervene at multiple points along the continuum from mind to molecule. The *biopsychosocial model* of medicine, originally proposed by Engel, regards illness as multidetermined—by biochemical alterations on the molecular level and by psychological and social events on the molar level. This model encourages clinicians to move conceptually up and down the hierarchy from patients' genetic susceptibilities and pathophysiologic processes to their unique life circumstances, stressors, and psychological meanings by which they construct their reality, to understand fully the origins of disease and the most appropriate therapies.

This chapter offers a framework for clinicians to think broadly and clinically about the stress–illness

379

connection and suggests some approaches to assessing and treating stress-related illness. It offers a brief background of the research base for this perspective; provides a conceptual framework to guide diagnosis and treatment; suggests methods for communicating with patients about stress; and offers some options for stress assessment, prevention, and intervention.

CASE ILLUSTRATION 1*

History: *A 54-year-old female with a history of chronic migraine headaches, hypertension, hyper-cholesterolemia, mild obesity, and smoking presented to a new primary care physician. She was treated by her previous physician with Tylenol #3, 1 tablet twice a day, for the migraines, and she routinely called in halfway through the month for extra refills. Other medications included atenolol 25 mg once a day for blood pressure elevation and migraine prophylaxis, as well as over-the-counter antacids for occasional heartburn.*

Patient Interview: The patient appeared angry and complained that the medication was not helping her pain. The new physician listened to her complaints and agreed at the end of the visit to refill her medications, but told her he would not prescribe more than the previous doctor. He asked her to return for her annual Pap smear, at which time he would take a history and do a physical examination.

This case is a common occurrence in primary care medicine, and the patient's chronic complaints pull for efforts by the new physician to ease her symptoms, especially with pain medication. Many physicians might regard this as a "difficult patient" (see Chapter 4). This physician astutely refrains from developing a treatment plan until after a complete history and physical, scheduled for the next visit. He provides a pain medication refill to meet the patient's immediate needs and elicits her agreement to return for the subsequent evaluation. That next visit will offer an opportunity, in addition to the physical examination, to explore the psychological and social stress pathways that contribute to the patient's symptom constellation. We will return to this case later, but first we will review the history and meaning of "stress," its research background, and the rich array of assessment and intervention tools available for the physician to help this patient steer a new course to health.

*I am grateful to Kerry Kuehl, MD, for sharing the case presented in Case Illustration 1.

DEFINITIONS

The concept of stress was borrowed by physiology and psychology from physics, where it generally refers to a force acting against some resistance. In materials science, stress is what is imposed on a material by the outer world; strain is the reaction of the material to the stress.

Hans Selye is generally credited with introducing the concept of stress into physiology. He defined stress loosely as "the rate of wear and tear in the body" and more rigorously as "the state manifested by a specific syndrome which consists of all the nonspecifically induced changes within a biologic system." In this specific syndrome, termed by Selye the **general adaptation syndrome** (GAS), glucocorticoids are secreted by the adrenal cortex in response to adaptational demands placed on the organism by such disparate stressors as heat, cold, starvation, and other environmental insults—hence the expression "nonspecifically induced changes."

A distinction is usually made between "stress" and "stressors." Although **stress** is sometimes loosely used to refer to the environmental sources of threat to the organism, the term **stressor** is more appropriate in reference to these agents, whereas "stress" refers to the organism's response.

More recent definitions of stress in humans emanate from a transactional model that takes into account the interactions between persons and their environment. In this view, stress occurs when a situational demand presents a call for action that the individual perceives as exceeding available resources. I have proposed the following working definition: "**Stress** is a process of interchange between an organism and its environment that involves self-generated or environmentally induced changes that, once they are perceived by the organism as exceeding available resources (internal or external), disrupt homeostatic processes in the organism–environment system." This definition includes the traditional notion of stress as originating with an external demand (environmentally induced change) that exceeds the coping resources of the organism. It also includes, however, those expectations of events that arise from within, that are seen as essential to one's life project, and that cannot be accommodated by the environment (exceeding external resources). The disruption of homeostasis in the organism–environment system can have its primary manifestation as a pathological end-state in the organism (illness or tissue damage) or as a destructive alteration of the environment (domestic violence as a stress response).

RESEARCH BACKGROUND

Psychoneuroimmunology

Psychoneuroimmunology (PNI) involves the study of the interactions of consciousness, the central nervous system (CNS), and the immune system (involving the

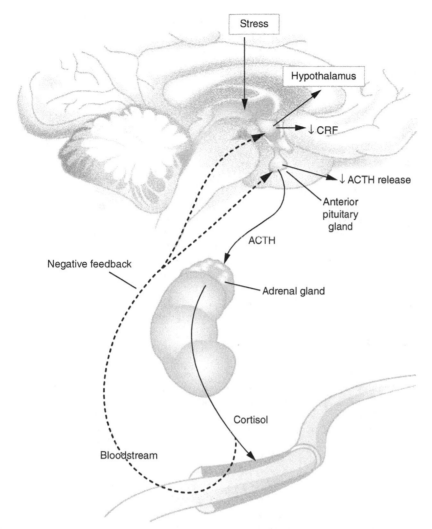

Stress

Hypothalamus

↓ CRF

↓ ACTH release

Anterior pituitary gland

ACTH

Negative feedback

Adrenal gland

Cortisol

Bloodstream

Figure 34-1. Hypothalamic–pituitary–adrenal (HPA) axis. Molina/Endocrine Physiology, 3e Chapter 6 (Adrenal Gland), Fig. 6-4, p.136. (Reproduced with permission from Molina, Patricia E. *Endocrine Physiology*, 3e New York, NY McGraw-Hill; 2009 Fig. 6-4.)

body's defense against infection and aberrant cell division). The compelling evidence of these studies is that the CNS influences immune function and that, conversely, the immune system can influence the CNS. The brain is normally part of the immunoregulatory network. Specifically, stimulation of the hypothalamic–pituitary–adrenal (HPA) axis leads to downregulation of immune system function in response to stress (see Figure 34-1). Stressful thoughts and emotions may reach the hypothalamus by axons projecting from the limbic system (primarily the amygdala) or from the forebrain. Corticotropin-releasing factor (CRF), produced in the hypothalamus under conditions of stress, acts on the anterior pituitary to release adrenocorticotropin hormone (ACTH), which in turn stimulates the production of corticosteroids in the adrenal cortex. Under conditions of acute stress, corticosteroids have immunosuppressive effects on the lymphoreticular system and marked antiallergic and anti-inflammatory effects.

In addition, CRF leads to release of catecholamines, which themselves may produce changes in lymphocyte, monocyte, and leukocyte functions. Opiates are also elevated with stress, and they are generally reported to be immunosuppressive. Finally, growth hormone and prolactin, which are immunoenhancing factors, are initially elevated at the onset of acute stress, but under conditions of prolonged stress their secretion is inhibited. Thus, the combined effect of elevated corticosteroids, catecholamines, and opiates, along with inhibition of growth hormone and prolactin, is to dysregulate the immune system.

Recent evidence indicates that chronic psychological stress can lead to increased production of proinflammatory cytokines, particularly interleukin-6 (IL-6), which is also triggered by infection and trauma. Proinflammatory cytokines have been implicated in a range of diseases in older adults that can be traced to inflammation, including cardiovascular disease, osteoporosis, arthritis, type 2 diabetes, certain lymphoproliferative diseases or cancers (including multiple myeloma, non-Hodgkin lymphoma, and chronic lymphocytic leukemia), depression, Alzheimer disease, and periodontal disease. IL-6 promotes the production of C-reactive protein, which is an important risk factor for MI. Depression and anxiety also enhance the production of proinflammatory cytokines, which is a possible mediator of the association of these disorders with increased morbidity and mortality (see Chapters 25 and 26). A recent study has shown that depressed subjects, compared with non-depressed controls, showed an impaired ability to regulate inflammation triggered by acute stress.

Another recent development in stress research involves the concept of "allostatic load," which is the wear and tear on organisms that results from chronic overactivity or underactivity of allostatic systems. Allostasis refers to the body's ability to produce hormones (e.g., cortisol) and other mediators (e.g., cytokines) that help it to adapt to novel situations or challenges. These systems, which include the autonomic nervous system (Figure 34-2), HPA axis (Figure 34-1), and the cardiovascular, metabolic, and immune systems, protect the body by responding to internal and external stress in an attempt to achieve stability through change.

Activation of allostatic systems in response to a stressor includes the release of catecholamines from nerves and the adrenal medulla, as well as the stimulation of cortisol release from the adrenal cortex via the HPA system described above. Four types of allostatic load can result from prolonged stress: (1) Repeated elevations of blood pressure over weeks or months accelerates atherosclerosis, increasing the risk of MI. (2) When adaptation to repeated stressors is lacking, there may be prolonged exposure to stress hormones. (3) There may be an inability to shut off allostatic responses after stress is terminated, leading to conditions such as hypertension or decreased bone mineral density. (4) Inadequate responses in some allostatic systems, such as cortisol secretion, may lead to compensatory increases in other systems, such as proinflammatory cytokines (which are downregulated by cortisol).

Stress, Food, & Inflammation

Inflammation is a common link for diseases high in mortality risk, including cardiovascular disease, cancer, and diabetes. Stress and depression, as well as dietary intake, can promote inflammation through proinflammatory cytokine production. Diet influences cytokine-induced inflammation by means of the balance between omega-3 (n-3) polyunsaturated fatty acids (PUFA) and omega-6 (n-6) PUFA, with n-6 (refined vegetable oils) promoting the production of proinflammatory cytokines and n-3 (fish, fish oil, walnuts, flax seed) mitigating their production. The link between depression and inflammation interacts with dietary balance, with higher n-6/n-3 ratios showing a relationship with depression. In epidemiologic studies, greater fish consumption has been associated with a lower prevalence of depression. A diet with higher n-6/n-3 ratio can also increase vulnerability to inflammatory responses to stress. Stress, in turn, promotes unhealthy food choices that promote inflammation, with higher stress associated with decreased fruit and vegetable consumption and increased consumption of sweets and fast food. Higher stress is also associated with higher peaks in postprandial lipidemia and delayed gastric clearing of these compounds, both associated with atherogenesis.

Effect of Psychological Interventions on the Immune System

In a series of studies on asymptomatic men following notification of human immunodeficiency virus (HIV) seropositivity, a 10-week program of cognitive behavioral stress management and aerobic exercise training programs buffered distress responses and immune alterations. The same intervention had positive effects on mood and immune function in gay men whose disease had become symptomatic. Meta-analyses of the placebo effect have shown positive effects in various inflammatory and immune-related diseases, including asthma, cancer symptoms (pain and appetite), Crohn disease, chronic fatigue, duodenal ulcer, irritable bowel syndrome, and multiple sclerosis (relapse frequency). A meta-analytic review showed that three classes of interventions could reliably alter immune function. *Hypnosis with immune suggestions* showed a positive influence on total salivary immunoglobulin A (IgA) concentration and neutrophil adherence, along with a modest suppression of intermediate-type hypersensitivity erythema. These effects were mediated through relaxation. Some studies have shown differential delayed skin sensitivity reactions on the right and left arm of subjects depending on which arm was suggested under hypnosis to show no changes. *Conditioning interventions,* in which a neutral stimulus is initially paired with an immune-modulating stimulus and later elicits the immune changes on its own, were able to enhance natural killer (NK) cell cytotoxicity. *Disclosure interventions,* which encourage patients to write essays about previously inhibited stressful experiences, have shown

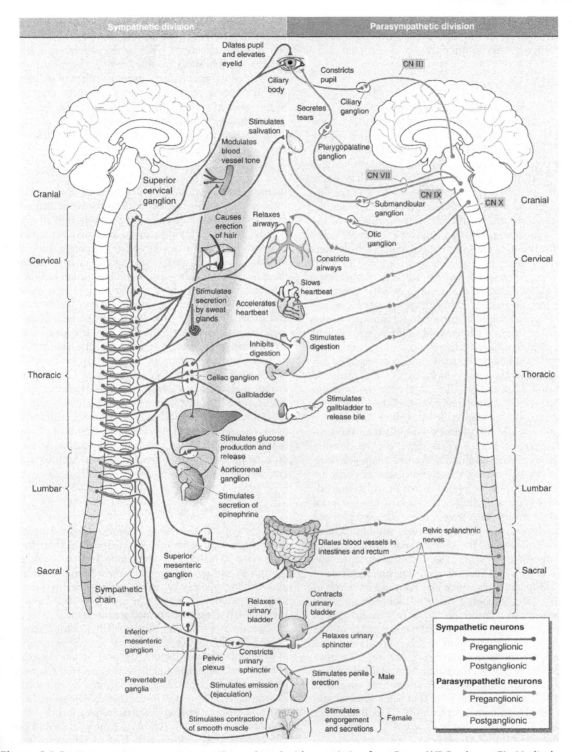

Figure 34-2. Autonomic nervous system. (Reproduced with permission from Boron WF, Boulpaep EL. *Medical Physiology.* Elsevier.)

some success in reducing antibody titers to Epstein–Barr virus and enhancing the body's control over latent herpes simplex virus production.

Stressful Life Events

In 1967, Holmes and Rahe published a scale of 43 life events, along with a method of quantifying life changes according to the amount of readjustment they require for the average person. This scale allowed greater quantitative precision in life change and illness studies and provided a pivotal methodological leap that broke through the circularity in which the stressful life changes had been measured in terms of illness outcome, rather than in terms of the inherent magnitude of the stressor. Questionnaires based on this and similar scales have gathered data on several populations globally. Retrospective studies have shown a relationship between recent life change and a host of pathological outcomes, such as sudden cardiac death, onset of MI, occurrence of fractures, pregnancy and birth complications, aggravation of chronic illness, tuberculosis, multiple sclerosis, diabetes, onset of leukemia in children, and onset of mental disorders such as depression and schizophrenia. Prospective studies, particularly those conducted on US Navy populations while deployed at sea, predicted future illness based on life change scores prior to deployment and subsequently verified the accuracy of those predictions by inspection of medical records.

Recent attention has focused on individual and situational variables that may mediate the relationship between life change and illness. Among the psychological variables that seem to mediate the stress response are locus of control (including the extent to which individuals prefer control in their lives and how much control they perceive they have over specific life events), need for stimulation, openness to change, stimulus screening, self-actualization, the use of denial, the presence of social supports, and emotional self-disclosure. In one study of Illinois Bell executives during the divestiture of AT&T, those executives who experienced high levels of stressors while remaining healthy differed from those with high stressors and high illness on a dimension of "hardiness." This personal characteristic consists of "the 3 Cs": a strong *commitment* to self, work, family, and other important values; a sense of *control* over one's life; and the ability to see change as a *challenge* rather than a threat. More recently researchers suggest a "fourth C": *coherence,* a belief that one's internal and external environments are predictable and that things will work out as well as can be expected.

More recent studies of *resilience* (a concept related to hardiness) have focused on the neurochemical and hormonal feedback systems that dampen or switch off the stress response (HPA axis and sympathetic nervous system response described above). Among these resilience chemicals are *DHEA* (dehydroepiandrosterone), which lessens the effects of cortisol, and *neuropeptide Y,* which counters the effects of CRF at the anterior pituitary. These stress inhibitory mechanisms may be more prevalent in people who show a greater resiliency or hardiness in response to stressful events. Yet to be examined is the question of whether levels of these feedback chemicals are modifiable in response to stress management training or other psychological interventions.

Technostress

Increased use of mobile phones, smartphones, and the Internet has established new norms for work and connectivity in industrialized countries. Although allowing broader and more rapid access to information than ever before in human history, as well as increasing flexibility for work location and hours among many workers, these technologies also exact a toll on human health. In a recent Swedish study of young adults, high mobile phone use was a predictor of stress, sleep disturbance, and depression at a 1-year follow-up. Increased use of social media to interact frequently with friends near and far presents a paradox. On the one hand these media facilitate engagement with social support networks, which are a well-established stress buffer. Chatting and instant messaging are among the high-frequency activities of those in Generation Y (born after 1980). On the other hand, these media also lead to communication overload, the taxing of working memory through multitasking, distractibility, and guilt induced by the social expectation of immediacy of response and constant availability.

Stress in America Survey

The Stress in America survey published by the American Psychological Association (APA) revealed that those who serve as caregivers—providing care to both the aging and chronically ill—for their family members report higher levels of stress, poorer health, and a greater tendency to engage in unhealthy behaviors to alleviate that stress than the population at large. According to estimates from the National Alliance for Caregiving, 65.7 million Americans served as caregivers for an ill or disabled relative in the past year. In the APA survey, 55% of caregivers (median age 49 years) felt overwhelmed by the amount of care required by chronically ill or aging family members. Caregivers were more likely than those in the general population to report that they are doing a poor or fair job of managing stress and getting enough sleep. Mean stress level of caregivers (on a scale of 1–10) was 6.5 compared to 5.2 for the general public. Caregivers reported being poorer in health than the rest of the nation, with greater rates of high cholesterol, high blood pressure, overweight/obesity, and depression. Other survey findings were that caregivers were more likely than the general population to have chronic illness, to lie awake at night, to have poor nutrition, to skip a meal, and to get sick five or more times a year.

Work-Related Stress and Burnout

The demands of the workplace in industrialized societies are a persistent and intense stressor. Job strain is defined as a combination of high job demands and low perceived control. In a prospective study of healthy young adults (Cardiovascular Risk in Young Finns study), job strain was associated with increased carotid atherosclerosis among the men, but not the women.

In another prospective study, the degree of job stress over time increased the risk of the metabolic syndrome in a linear fashion. Subjects with lower grades of employment suffered disproportionately from the effects of stress as a risk factor for the metabolic syndrome, with men showing more susceptibility than women. **Burnout** is a syndrome associated with unrelenting stress and has been studied extensively as a phenomenon in a variety of work settings and professions, including physicians. It includes symptoms of emotional exhaustion, depersonalization, and a decreased sense of personal accomplishment. In a prospective study, burnout was associated with an increased risk of type 2 diabetes in apparently healthy individuals.

In Japan, the concept of *karoshi*, or death from overwork, has received government attention in recent decades. Rapid growth in industrialization following World War II led to production efficiencies placing pressure on Japanese workers, who often worked overtime without additional compensation. A new phenomenon of sudden death among high-level businessmen who were previously healthy brought attention to these stressful work environments. In 2008 in a well-publicized case a company was ordered to pay 200 million yen to a man who overworked until he fell into a coma. Among statistics published by the Japanese Ministry of Health, Labor, and Welfare in 2007 for the previous year, 189 workers had died from overwork, many from heart attacks and strokes, and 208 more had become severely ill.

The Role of Acute and Chronic Stress in Cardiac Disease

Acute stress activates the sympathetic nervous system (Figure 34-2), which leads to increases in heart rate and blood pressure, coronary vasoconstriction, and decreased myocardial electrical stability. Several behavioral and emotional events have been implicated as probable triggers of acute coronary syndromes (MI and sudden cardiac death) in vulnerable individuals, especially events within a 1-to 2-hour period before the onset of symptoms.

Behavioral triggers include physical exertion (more common in men than women), sexual activity, sleep disturbance, and heavy consumption of alcohol. Well-studied emotional triggers include earthquakes, sporting events, war, high-pressure deadlines at work, and anger. In one study, the relative risk of acute MI in the 2 hours following an anger episode was 2.3, and in comparison with a control period 24 hours earlier it was 4.0. This effect was independent of age, sex, cardiovascular risk factors, and use of beta-blockers. The risk of anger triggering an MI was inversely related to socioeconomic status. In a large-scale study, the relative risk of anger triggering an MI was 9.0 compared to usual levels of anger, but when limiting the analysis to patients who had no premonitory symptoms the relative risk increased to 15.7.

Examination of the stored electrocardiograms of 200 New York area patients with implantable cardioverter-defibrillators showed differences in ventricular tachyarrhythmias triggering cardioverter-defibrillator therapy before and after the World Trade Center attack of September 11, 2001. There was a 2.3-fold increase in ventricular tachyarrhythmias during the month after 9/11, relative to other months between May 2001 and October 2002. Similar to the data from the 1996 European football championships mentioned above, in a study examining daily cardiovascular disease events in Munich during the 2006 World Cup, cardiovascular emergencies increased 2.7 times in men and 1.8 times in women on the days when Germany was participating in the quarterfinals and semifinals. On these days, MI and major arrhythmia admissions increased three times compared with the same day in previous years. The highest incidence of cardiac events occurred during the first 2 hours of the games.

In addition to promoting unhealthy behaviors, *chronic stress* activates and reactivates the sympathetic nervous system. Repeated sympathetic stimulation increases heart rate and blood pressure, and autonomic nervous system dysregulation leads to decreased heart rate variability and baroreflex dysfunction, which has been associated with cardiovascular disease events. Depression increases levels of inflammatory markers, including fibrinogen, C-reactive protein, IL-6, and tumor necrosis factor. Chronic stressors also activate the HPA axis producing hypercortisolemia, which in turn promotes central obesity and insulin resistance, risk factors for cardiovascular disease.

Chronic work stress, defined as high demands and low control, was associated with cardiovascular disease events in a study of 10,308 middle-aged London-based civil servants, with work stress contributing a relative risk of 1.68. Associations were found between work stress and negative behaviors, such as low physical activity and poor diet, and pathophysiologic consequences, such as decreased heart rate variability and an increase in morning cortisol.

In the Caregiver Health Effects study, 400 caregivers showed a 63% higher mortality rate than noncaregiving control subjects over a 4-year period. The increased mortality was particularly evident in caregivers who already had known cardiovascular disease. In a series of physiologically oriented studies, the San Diego Caregiver study examined possible pathways between caregiving and cardiovascular disease. Distressed caregivers had an increased risk for developing hypertension when followed over a 6-year period. Caregivers also had increased levels of D-dimer (a circulating procoagulant factor), more sleep disruption, and higher levels of circulating inflammatory cytokines.

Personality Influences on Cardiovascular Disease

Recent research has examined the relationship between coronary heart disease and a personality constellation that includes hostility, anger, cynicism, suspiciousness, and excessive self-involvement. Hostility is conceptualized as comprising three elements: the emotion of anger; its expression; and cognitions of cynical mistrust. Using well-validated measures of the cognitive aspect of hostility, studies have linked higher hostility scores with subsequent coronary events like hospitalizations for angina, nonfatal MI, stroke, and congestive heart failure. Higher hostility has also been associated with coronary risk factors, such as increased plasma homocysteine levels, triglycerides, body mass index, waist-to-hip ratio, glucose levels, alcohol consumption, and smoking. In a study of middle-aged women, each 1-point increase in hostility scores predicted a significantly higher intimal–medial thickening in the carotid arteries.

Gender Differences

Females have been noted to respond to stress with a "tend-and-befriend" way of coping, in contrast with the "fight-or-flight" model that may be more characteristic of males. When confronted with stress, females tend to engage in nurturing activities that protect themselves and their offspring and that enhance social support, which has been identified as a powerful stress buffer. In particular, there may be links between estrogen and a blunting of oxytocin, which is implicated in the fight-or-flight response. The "tend-and-befriend" response may also lower blood pressure.

Positive Cognitive Styles

Evidence is accumulating from a variety of studies that optimism, perceptions of personal control, and a sense of meaning are protective of physical health. These cognitive resources assume special significance in helping people cope with intensely stressful events. Even unrealistically optimistic expectations appear to slow down the progression of disease in men infected with HIV. In a study of healthy older adults, a sense of coherence (one indicator of resilience) moderated the association between anticipation of moving and reduced NK cell lysis, with a low sense of coherence associated with poorest levels of NK cell lysis. In a recent study of the cognitive and psychological sequelae of the 2011 Japanese earthquake and tsunami among survivors in the primary disaster area, posttraumatic stress had a major impact on self-perceived quality of life 3 months after the disaster. The study authors concluded that reducing negative cognitions would have a greater impact than positive re-appraisals on lowering depression and anxiety in this early stage of response. It was expected that positive re-appraisals leading to posttraumatic growth (PTG) would occur over longer time frames. Similar to the time course of recovery from other disasters, it was expected that PTG would include enhanced relationships with others, a sense of new possibilities, self-perceived personal strength, a sense of purpose in life, the concept of *ikigai* (meaningfulness), and a deepened spirituality.

Religion and Spirituality

Several studies have shown a relationship between religious or spiritual practice and health outcomes. "Religion" can be considered a collection of beliefs and practices that are external expressions of spiritual experience. These expressions can be organizationally based or private, but are usually grounded in a collective tradition. "Spirituality" can be considered an orientation toward or experiences with the transcendent, existential, or sacred dimensions of life. That which is transcendent or sacred is considered as something beyond oneself, whether it be conceptualized as a divine being, higher power, nature, spirit, or the ultimate ground of being. It is possible for people to engage in religious activities independent of having spiritual experiences, just as some people consider themselves intensely spiritual without being religious. Some consider their religious practice to be a pathway toward spirituality.

Types of studies on the religion–health connection have included cross-sectional as well as prospective and retrospective studies where participation in religious or spiritual practice is correlated with some health outcome measure, as well as intervention studies in which subjects were randomized into treatment and control groups. Correlational studies of religious or spiritual involvement and health outcomes have shown a positive association with longer life; less cardiovascular disease; less hypertension; more engagement in health-promoting behaviors; decreased risk of depression, anxiety, substance abuse, and suicide; better coping with illness; and better health-related quality of life. Among the intervention studies the best evidence for efficacy with health outcomes has been with religiously oriented cognitive therapy, meditation, 12-step fellowships, forgiveness therapy, and intercessory prayer. These studies need further replication with better designed controls.

Both religion and spirituality represent a heterogeneous group of belief systems, religious practices, and spiritual experiences. Most of the research linking religious or spiritual practice to health outcomes does not account for this heterogeneity, and thus the generalizability of results is limited. Nevertheless, the growing accumulation of evidence of positive health correlates of religion and spirituality warrants not only more sophisticated research but the attention of clinicians seeking to improve the health of patients.

 CASE ILLUSTRATION 1 (CONTD.)

Social History: *At the follow-up appointment, the physician took a social history, which revealed that the patient had been smoking a pack of cigarettes every day for the last 35 years but did not use alcohol or street drugs. Although never married, she had been involved in a 10-year relationship with her boyfriend, who suffered from severe emphysema and was dependent on oxygen. Three years previously this man had assumed responsibility for raising his two granddaughters (ages 8 and 11 years) because his daughter, the girls' mother, was a drug addict serving time in prison. The patient was not consulted about this custody decision. She accepted the stressor out of love for her partner, who was also dependent on her. The oldest granddaughter was now age 14 and had become unruly, rebellious, sexually active, and aggressive. She had asked the patient for help obtaining birth control. Although the patient wanted to leave this demanding social situation, she saw it as her responsibility to care for her partner and the two children. The history correlated these recent life events with increased frequency of migraines and initiation of daily use of Tylenol #3.*

Physician Facilitation of Emotional Self-Disclosure: *The physician actively listened to the patient's self-disclosure, which was accompanied by crying. At the end of the interview the patient thanked the physician, who noted that she had not complained of migraines during that visit.*

In allowing the patient to disclose her psychological and social stressors, the physician was able to gain relevant information within a biopsychosocial perspective of patient care. Relevant stressors potentially contributing to this patient's medical symptoms included caregiving for a disabled partner, having to assume a parenting role of grandchildren, and a self-expectation of a way of loving her partner that allowed no escape for her from an uncontrollable situation. In allowing the patient's emotional self-disclosure, there was an immediate effect on mitigating migraine symptoms. Going forward from this interview, it was important for the physician to have a pathway to navigate and orchestrate the various biological, psychological, and social interventions relevant to this patient's condition.

A STRESS MODEL FOR MEDICAL CARE

The etiology of illness and its waxing and waning course are multifactorial. Any given illness episode is determined by many circumstances. The complex pathway by which stress influences the outcome of illness is subject to the ongoing accumulation of data and elaboration of heuristic and clinical models. A model of stress that can aid diagnosis, prevention, and intervention is shown in Figure 34-3. Adapted from an optical model first proposed by Rahe and Arthur (1978), it depicts stressors as light rays filtered through successive lenses representing the individual's *perception* (threat appraisal), *coping, physiologic processes,* and *arousal reduction* activities, and then projected onto *illness outcome* screens. Each lens either augments or diminishes the intensity of light (heavy bold lines or dotted lines, respectively) on its pathway to illness outcome, and represents a potential focal point for the clinician's diagnosis of a stress influence or risk factor for patient illness. Each lens also represents a potential focus of preventive health care or intervention.

Perception refers to the person's appraisal of the threat involved in various stressors. Several personal variables that may affect the degree of perceived threat are shown in Figure 34-3. For example, the degree of a person's openness to change or the extent to which he or she values change influences whether a particular life change, such as a child leaving home, is perceived as a threat to the self or an opportunity for growth. The degree of control individuals prefer to have in their lives, as well as the amount of control they perceive they have over specific stressors, also influence their perception of threat. Thus, a parent with a high need to control an adolescent child's outside activities experiences more stress when the child struggles toward emancipation than does a parent who has less of a need for control and who trusts the child's judgment.

Coping refers to methods an individual uses to mitigate the influence of stressors perceived as threatening. One approach to coping is "exposure management," or attempts to increase or decrease the amount and intensity of stressors encountered. Thus, an overworked,

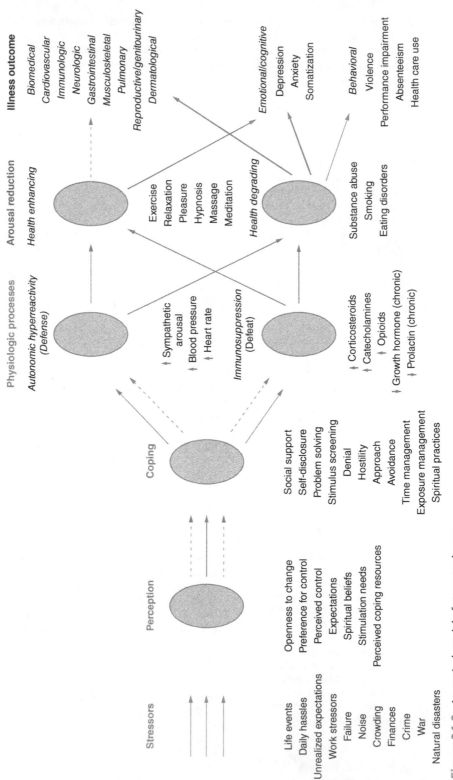

Figure 34-3. An optical model of stress pathways.

overcommitted manager might attempt to mitigate stress by withdrawing from some commitments, by reducing work hours, and by delegating more responsibility to subordinates. Social supports are an important stress buffer, and successful coping with stressors may involve both developing confiding relationships and increasing the amount of one's self-disclosure about the effect of stressors in one's life. There is some evidence that emotional self-disclosure about stressors enhances immune functioning. In the aftermath of the September 11, 2001 attacks, it is estimated that 98% of Americans coped by talking with others, 90% by turning to religious or spiritual practices, 60% by participating in group activities to memorialize the events, and 36% by making donations. "Stimulus screening" involves techniques to focus attention on relevant stimuli and to regulate the overall flow of stimulation to one's optimal level of functioning.

Two major classes of **physiologic response** to stressors that lead to target organ pathology are autonomic hyperreactivity and immunosuppression. Both are cortically mediated through the individual's perceptions and methods of coping. *Hyperreactivity* in the presence of stress, sometimes called the **defense reaction,** has been shown to be a factor in disease processes specific to vulnerable organ systems in persons with established disease. Thus, exaggerated pressor responses in hypertensives, increased electromyelogram responses in those suffering from tension headaches and chronic back pain, disturbances in glucose metabolism in insulin-dependent diabetics, and bronchoconstrictive responses in asthmatics are all examples of hyperreactivity in the presence of a definable stressor. In the case of hypertension, hyperreactivity is present in normotensives at risk for the disorder and in some studies has predicted future blood pressure levels. Other examples are increased levels of serum cholesterol seen in studies of tax accountants in the 2 weeks prior to April 15 and of fighter pilots landing on aircraft carriers compared with pilots on long commercial airline flights.

One of the adaptive functions of sympathetic activation (Figure 34-2) is to prepare the organism for large-muscle movement to either attack or flee a threat. In the twenty-first century human society, these somatomotor responses are often voluntarily suppressed or sublimated, leading to delayed elimination of released glucose and fatty acids and often bringing more powerful and prolonged increases in blood pressure. In addition, the relative absence of skeletal muscle exertion in affluent societies (without compensatory aerobic exercise) prevents the activation of endorphins that normally accompanies muscle exertion. Because these endorphins dampen mental arousal and sympathetic activity, in the absence of skeletal muscle exertion these arousal and activation states are prolonged.

Immunosuppression, as discussed previously, occurs through the mechanisms of increased levels of circulating corticosteroids, catecholamines, and opioids and decreased levels of growth hormone and prolactin under conditions of chronic or prolonged stress. Sometimes referred to as the **defeat reaction,** this response pattern occurs when patients are exposed to long-term stressful situations that tend to overwhelm ordinary coping mechanisms, thus leading to despair or deep sorrow in situations that appear to be beyond all hope and rescue. Rather than working directly on target organ systems as in the case of hyperreactivity, downregulation of the immune system in the defeat reaction increases vulnerability to external invasive organisms and endogenous neoplasms.

Several **arousal reduction** strategies are available to individuals to mitigate physiologic activation and disruption of homeostatic processes in conditions of stress. These include both **health-enhancing** and **health-degrading** activities. Among the health-enhancing arousal-reduction strategies are exercise, which expends accumulated corticosteroids and dampens sympathetic activation through the release of endorphins, and various approaches to stimulating the parasympathetic nervous system (Figure 34-2). This latter category includes relaxation exercises, abdominal breathing, self-hypnosis, meditation, soothing music, massage, and contact with nature (see Chapter 9).

Health-degrading activities, which may be attempts at physiologic arousal reduction but that actually magnify the stress response and lead to target organ disease, include substance abuse, tobacco use, and eating disorders. Intensification of all of these behaviors may coincide with stressful life episodes. An example is the mediating role of increased alcohol intake in the relationship between occupational stress and hypertension seen in studies of air traffic controllers.

Various **illness outcomes** of stress include **biomedical disease** manifested in specific organ systems, such as cardiovascular, immune, and neurologic disorders; **emotional and cognitive disorders,** such as depression, anxiety, and somatization; and **behavioral disorders,** such as violence, performance impairment, absenteeism, and overuse of health care resources. These stress outcomes are the usual focus of medical and mental health intervention, but the larger model of the stress pathway provides primary care clinicians with potent opportunities for comprehensive preventive health care.

HEALTH OUTCOMES OF STRESS

Each organ system has a unique susceptibility to stress. The following is a brief overview of some of the stress and treatment implications in specific diseases.

Cardiovascular

Cardiovascular disease is the leading cause of mortality in the United States. As reviewed above, stress contributes to all expressions of heart disease, including coronary artery disease, congestive heart failure, and sudden cardiac death. Because a third of sudden cardiac deaths and MIs cannot be fully explained by the severity of the standard cardiac risk factors—family history, hypertension, dyslipidemia, diabetes, or tobacco use—stress may explain some of this variance. As mentioned above, there is a connection between hostility and cardiac disease. It has been shown that hostility contributes independently of other risk factors to the pathogenesis of heart disease through lipid accumulation, increased blood pressure, and heart rate and platelet physiology.

Mind–body therapies show promise in the treatment of coronary artery disease. A meta-analysis of the use of psychoeducational interventions (health education and stress management) as a component of cardiac rehabilitation showed an overall 34% reduction in mortality, a 29% reduction in recurrent MI, and positive effects on dietary and exercise habits, weight, smoking, cholesterol, and blood pressure.

Immune

Clinical expressions of immune deficiencies are in part the result of stress. They range from the common cold to some forms of cancer. Although research on the relationship between stress and cancer is still inconclusive, there is some evidence that stress and surgical excision of the primary tumor can promote tumor metastasis by suppression of cell-mediated immunity. The perioperative period is a particularly important window during which psychological or pharmacological interventions to prevent or reduce stress may offer a reduced risk of metastasis. Other immune-mediated diseases, such as rheumatoid arthritis and systemic lupus erythematosus, may show a pattern of exacerbation brought on by stress.

HIV

More rapid disease progression in people infected with HIV has been associated with greater concealment of homosexual identity, more cumulative stressful life events, and less cumulative social support over a 5-year period. Alternatively, more deliberate cognitive processing about the death of a close friend or partner has been associated with greater likelihood of finding positive meaning in the loss, less rapid decline in CD4+ cell levels, and lower rates of AIDS-related mortality over a 9-year period in HIV-seropositive men.

Neurologic

All forms of stroke show a circadian expression in their presentation, with peaks during the early morning hours when catecholamines are highest. Dizziness, vertigo, and other balance disorders often have stress as a causative or contributing factor. One of the most common neurologic expressions of stress in clinical practice is headache. Both tension headache and migraine headache are substantially influenced by patient stressors. Meta-analysis has shown behavioral interventions (relaxation training and skin temperature biofeedback) to be as effective as medication in treatment of migraine headaches. Hypnosis with hand-warming imagery is an effective method to reverse the progression of migraine headache, especially early in the prodromal stage (see Chapter 5).

Gastrointestinal

Peptic ulcer disease may have an association with stress. Gastric hyperacidity and excess pepsin production are hallmarks of the sympathetic arousal that occurs during stress. Inflammatory bowel syndrome (IBS), which is characterized by abdominal pain with altered bowel habits (constipation or diarrhea) in the absence of a definable lesion or structural abnormality, frequently correlates with periods of emotional stress. The human "defense reaction" (fight-or-flight response) promotes activation of the cardiovascular system along with inhibition of gastric motility. The role of stress in promoting proinflammatory cytokines is a probable mechanism in the etiology of this disorder. Inflammation is also associated with depression, which is frequently a comorbidity with IBS.

Musculoskeletal

Some forms of arthritis show stress-related exacerbations. Complex syndromes such as fibromyalgia seem to have a psychosocial trigger. Temporomandibular joint (TMJ) dysfunction and its related pain syndrome are frequently associated with mental stress. Chronic pain tends to correlate with stress in a person's life. Persistent pain and psychological symptoms frequently seen after motor vehicle accidents (MVA) may involve the impact of acute stress interacting with past experience, post-MVA behavior, and cognitive/psychological consequences to alter activity in brain pathways that process pain.

Pulmonary

Asthma and chronic obstructive pulmonary disease appear to be worsened by stress. Conversely, one of the more powerful, self-regulatory, stress-control techniques is relaxed abdominal breathing. Asthmatics who participate in stress reduction programs have shown improved physical activity and decreased medical visits. Hypnosis has helped some asthmatics decrease their use of bronchodilators (see Chapter 5).

Reproductive & Genitourinary

The neurohormonal, vascular, and immunologic effects of stress significantly impact the reproductive and genitourinary systems. Changes in estrogen and testosterone levels can show marked association with environmental and psychological stressors. Amenorrhea frequently occurs during stressful times in the lives of women. Fertility also can be affected by stress. Dysmenorrhea, dyspareunia, endometriosis, and impotence all have substantial stress and strain connections.

Dermatological

A variety of skin lesions and rashes have been associated with the stress response. Stress-induced vasomotor changes may aggravate inflammatory dermatoses. Vasodilation is considered to be responsible for the thermal aggravation often expressed as pruritus. This lowering of the itch threshold by vasodilation may account for the pruritus seen with many dermatological syndromes. Emotional stress, fear, and pain are all accompanied by substantial drops in skin temperature of the fingers.

Wound Healing

Psychological stress has measurable negative consequences for production of proinflammatory cytokines, and stress-related delays in wound healing have ranged from 24% to 40% with effect sizes between 0.30 and 0.74. These effects on wound healing are consistent with other studies that have shown that greater fear or distress prior to surgery is associated with poorer outcomes, including longer hospital stays, more postoperative complications, and higher rates of rehospitalization.

Frailty in the Elderly

Elevated serum levels of the proinflammatory cytokine IL-6 have predicted future disability in older adults. These cytokines slow muscle repair after injury and accelerate muscle wasting. IL-6 and C-reactive protein play a pathogenic role in several diseases associated with disability among the elderly, including osteoporosis, arthritis, and congestive heart failure.

DIAGNOSIS

Given the multivariate, multiple-pathway nature of the stress response, clinical diagnosis of stress assumes a multifactorial approach. Traditional medical diagnosis and treatment occur at the point of illness manifestation in target organ systems. From the broader perspective of stress medicine, however, each of the lenses in the optical model (see Figure 34-3) is a potential focus of diagnosis.

The Medical Interview

The richest source of data concerning stressors, perception, coping, and arousal reduction strategies is the medical interview (see Chapter 1). Having the stress model in mind allows the clinician to inquire about current and recent life stressors and to make note of significant clusters of stressors that precede illness onset. A careful history should uncover whether life stressors are temporally related to the onset of chronic disease and to periods of disease exacerbation.

During the interview, the clinician can ask patients about their beliefs, expectations, self-perceptions, and needs that influence how stressors are perceived. For example, asking patients how much control they prefer in their lives and how much control they perceive that they have over specific life events can determine whether there is congruence or incongruence between preferred control and perceived control. Incongruence tends to amplify the effect of stressors. It is also helpful to ask patients how they view their own resources (internal and external) for coping with stressors, since the more the perceived threats exceed the perceived personal resources, the greater the stress involved.

Patients' approaches to coping with stressors should also be probed in the interview. The presence or absence of social supports as well as the ability of patients to access these supports through self-disclosure are critical data for facilitating stress management. The perceptual and coping styles uncovered in the interview have implications for management of the patient's health, both in prevention and intervention.

It is also important to assess patients' approaches to arousal reduction and to ascertain the balance of health-enhancing and health-degrading strategies. The following questions can be helpful in this regard: "What are the signs indicating that you are experiencing stress?" "What are your physical symptoms?" "What happens in your emotional life?" "How do you act differently when you are stressed?" Methods used to mitigate this arousal can then be ascertained: "When you notice these signs of stress, what do you do to reduce the intensity of the physical symptoms?" It is also important to elicit the short- and long-term outcomes of these strategies: "How does this strategy work for you?" "How does it affect the way you feel immediately? ... several hours later? ... the next day?" Sometimes it is helpful to ask about specific arousal reduction techniques: "Do you practice a form of meditation or relaxation exercise?" "Do you get regular physical exercise?" When questioning patients about substance use or tobacco use, it is helpful to ask whether their use is associated with periods of stress.

Self-Report Questionnaire

A multitude of self-report questionnaires and inventories have been developed for research purposes that measure stressors and many of the variables listed in Figure 34-3 related to perception and coping. Given the limitations of physician and support staff time, it is recommended that any questionnaire be simple, brief, and provide data that can be used by the clinician in counseling patients in the area of stress management. An example of such an instrument is the Life Stress Inventory shown in Appendix 34-A. Borrowing from the life event scaling studies and the critical role that perceived control plays in mediating stress, this inventory asks patients in an open-ended way to list the major events (and expected nonevents), changes, and stressors that have occurred during the previous year. They are asked to check those stressors that are current, ongoing problems. In addition, patients are asked to rate each stressor on a scale of 1–10, indicating the extent of perceived control they had over these events. The provider can take the mean of the control ratings and place that number (1–10) in the "control score" blank. This instrument provides both qualitative and quantitative data on the nature of patients' stressors, those that are a current source of struggle, and patients' perceived control over these events. The higher the external control score, the more at risk the patient is for adverse consequences of stress. Examining with patients those stressors that seem under their control can allow the clinician to suggest lifestyle changes in those areas. In some instances, patients can be counseled to adjust their perceptions of no control in the direction of greater control. For example, a patient who perceives that she/he has no control over her/his work hours can be helped to see areas in which limits can actually be set. In other cases, patients can be led to consider changing their expectations and accepting areas that are truly beyond their control.

CASE ILLUSTRATION 1 (CONTD.)

*Having reviewed the optical model of stress prior to the patient's second appointment, the physician had a number of options to recommend after eliciting her psychosocial history. In the **coping** category, an obvious first step was to intervene in the dysfunctional family relationships that were a major stressor for the patient. Increasing support from her boyfriend and enlisting professional support in managing the hormonal challenges of the adolescent grandchild seemed an obvious starting point, so referral to family therapy was high on the agenda for that visit.*

Brief Counseling and Referral for Family Therapy: *The physician counseled the patient to realize that she was not isolated. He validated her efforts to work with the situation, even though she had the real option of leaving. He recommended family therapy, to which the patient agreed. Further medical treatment was deferred until after the family had engaged in therapy. The patient made no mention of pain medication during this visit.*

Change of Medication and of Lifestyle: *Prior to the next visit there were no further calls for pain medication refills. At that visit the patient stated that the migraines, although still present, were not as disabling. The focus of the visit was on improving management of hypertension, high cholesterol, and migraines. They discussed starting an exercise program, initiating a low-fat diet and weight loss, and quitting smoking. The physician remarked that the patient appeared to be gaining control over the life events involving her family.*

Disposition: *After several months of family therapy the patient had established a primary care relationship with a pediatrician to help her with the medical and hormonal issues of the grandchildren. Her boyfriend had increased his level of help. She had lost 8 lbs over 4 months, started walking 4 days a week for 30 minutes, and began a low-fat diet, all without pain medication. She agreed to start a smoking cessation program. The patient demonstrated a marked change in attitude and treatment of office staff, and the primary care provider developed a changed perception of her and an appreciation of the healing potential in "drug-seeking patients."*

MANAGEMENT: PREVENTION & INTERVENTION

Stress Management in the Intensive Care Unit

The immune system of many patients in the intensive care unit (ICU) is suppressed due to trauma, sepsis, or profound physiologic and psychological stress. Increases in cortisol levels have been found to correlate with severity of injury in minor and moderate trauma immediately after injury and hours later. Sepsis often begins as a local process of inflammation involving cytokine upregulation. These cytokines eventually, however, may move into circulation, leading to inflammatory processes systemically. Psychological stressors reported by ICU patients include pain, sleep deprivation (due to noise, disturbances by health care staff, and pain), and fear or anxiety (which may manifest in the extreme as delirium, confusion, and other unreal experiences), each of which is associated with decreased immune functioning. The implications for the ICU team are that intervening to reduce these psychosocial stressors may help prevent nosocomial infection. Feelings of anxiety and isolation can be buffered by a nurse providing a nurturing presence. Anxiety can be decreased through the use of benzodiazepines, which may also aid sleep. Nurses can attempt to minimize noise levels as much as possible and decrease the number of times patients are disturbed. Although many analgesic drugs used in the ICU can suppress immune function, alternative approaches to reducing pain should be attempted, since pain itself is immunosuppressive.

 CASE ILLUSTRATION 2

Deborah Jones, an ICU nurse with 10 years' experience in critical care, joined a process improvement team (PIT) to examine an increased trend in nosocomial infections among ICU patients over the previous 12 months. Having recently completed a continuing education course in PNI, she was sensitized to the effect of stressors in the ICU environment on patients' immune functioning. Deborah shared this information with the team, and the group (including a physician critical care specialist, a pharmacist, the ICU nurse manager, a pulmonologist, and the chief medical resident) came up with some suggested modifications in the environment and administration of care. Staff entering the ICU were reminded verbally and with a posted sign to speak softly near patient beds. A review of all mechanical noise sources was conducted, and it was determined that a few changes could reduce ambient noise by 30%. Rounding on patients was coordinated to cluster around certain times of the day, and an attempt was made to have greater predictability to staff disturbance of patients when resting. Different staff members, regardless of discipline, were assigned to specific patients for brief visits of a nonmedical nature to provide support and nurturance, either verbally or through appropriate touch. A palliative care specialist was consulted to develop a menu of pain medications and doses to minimize the risk of immunosuppression, and alternative procedures such as acupuncture were sometimes ordered in collaboration with the patient. Within 3 months it was noted that the rate of infection in the ICU had dropped by 40%. In the face of that data, Deborah was delegated by the PIT to make a formal presentation to hospital administration, and the changes became hospital policy.

Stress Management in Primary Care

The model of stress, shown in Figure 34-3, offers the clinician various foci for illness prevention and intervention, just as it does for diagnosis. The clinician familiar with this model should be able to tailor specific psychological, social, behavioral, and pharmacological strategies to the unique needs of individual patients. This is preferable to referring the patient for "stress management," since this generic term does not address the multiplicity of stress-related variables and pathways discussed earlier.

Communicating with Patients about Stress

A primary component of stress prevention and treatment involves the way stress is discussed with patients. Avoiding the implication that "it's all in your head" is of great importance. Equally important is avoiding the message that "you are responsible for your illness," which implies greater personal control over somatic processes than is realistic. Here the risk is inducing guilt in patients who become ill and who feel they have failed at being a "better person." Avoiding negative emphases, for example, "Your hectic pace is going to kill you," in favor of a positive framing of the health benefits of stress management is more likely to have a positive influence (see Chapter 5). For example, the clinician can express optimism about the patient's ability to influence health as follows: "Fortunately there are many avenues available for examining and changing your habits of thought and ways of responding to life challenges. I'd like to give you an overview of some strategies that we can discuss now and in future appointments." Showing the patient a model such as that in Figure 34-3 can be helpful as part of this discussion.

It is also important to frame beneficial lifestyle changes as the patient's choice. Rather than using the stress model to assume more responsibility for patients' lives, the primary care provider can act as a consultant and coach, clearly giving feedback to patients about the patterns of stress revealed by the diagnostic workup and offering concrete strategies for health promotion along with likely consequences for adherence and nonadherence (see Chapters 19 and 20).

Counseling about Perception & Coping

The perception and coping variables listed in Figure 34-3 represent potential topics for primary care counseling with patients. Depending on the clinician's expertise, inclination, and time, this could be done during a portion of several primary care visits. For example, a parent who is feeling stressed because of a teenager's oppositional behavior could be invited to reflect on how much parental control is needed and coached on ways of setting realistic limits. With an accountant feeling overwhelmed about a recent promotion to senior management, the clinician could elicit the patient's recollections of previous adaptations to challenging life

Table 34-1. Nonpharmacological interventions related to perception and coping.

1. Improve time management.
2. Improve sense of humor.
3. Pursue personal and vocational activities consistent with life values.
4. Explore the meaning and purpose of life.
5. Cultivate spiritual and transcendent activities:
   a. Prayer
   b. Communal religious observances
   c. Spiritual retreat
   d. Seasonal ritual celebrations.
6. Increase emotional self-disclosure.
7. Pursue short-term psychotherapy.
8. Clarify values.
9. Cultivate social support network.
10. Increase assertiveness.
11. Reduce exposure to unnecessary stressors.
12. Monitor sensory input.
13. Help others.

Table 34-2. Health-enhancing arousal reduction techniques.

1. Meditation
2. Self-hypnosis
3. Relaxation exercises
4. Time in nature
5. Massage
6. Abdominal breathing
7. Singing
8. Tai-chi
9. Listening to soothing music
10. Yoga

changes to help him become cognizant of his own resources.

Referring a parent of a child with recently diagnosed leukemia to a support group of other parents is an example of a coping strategy. Encouraging a widower to confide feelings of sadness to close friends is an example of helping a patient improve his use of social supports. Referring a teacher with a chronically explosive temper for short-term anger management therapy would potentially reduce a cardiac risk factor.

Counseling patients about time management offers a rich opportunity for clinicians to raise questions concerning the patients' values and missed opportunities for personal renewal. For example, the clinician can ask the patient to reflect on those important but nonurgent activities that can contribute to personal well-being (e.g., time spent playing with a child), but which are consistently postponed in favor of more urgent but less important tasks (e.g., keeping track of the performance of stocks). A list of potential nonpharmacological strategies related to perception and coping that can be suggested to patients is shown in Table 34-1.

Arousal Reduction Strategies

For patients showing a high degree of autonomic hyperreactivity, the clinician can provide or suggest several arousal reduction strategies that can work synergistically with perception and coping skills, as well as with pharmacological interventions. These strategies are listed in Table 34-2. Mindfulness meditation in particular is an effective method of stress reduction that not only activates the parasympathetic response, but builds a mental habit of staying present to the task at hand while assuming a nonjudgmental stance toward the progression of one's thoughts and emotions (see Chapter 7). Referring patients to introductory books on mindfulness meditation, such as those listed at the end of this chapter, or encouraging them to take a meditation class, can provide them with a powerful stress management resource. One study showed that 16 weeks of transcendental meditation improved components of the metabolic syndrome (blood pressure, insulin resistance, and heart rate variability) among patients with stable coronary heart disease.

Referral for Psychotherapy

The clinician may choose to refer patients for psychotherapy or to educational groups to achieve some of the desired outcomes in the areas of perception, coping, and arousal reduction techniques. These referrals are more effectively targeted to the unique needs of patients if the clinician uses the multifactorial model in Figure 34-3. This model can also aid the primary care clinician in communicating with the psychotherapist about possible foci for treatment. Psychotherapy may be more effective than primary care counseling for altering dysfunctional belief systems (e.g., a perception of no control in one's life) or coping habits (e.g., excessive need for achievement) that amplify stress. In addition, it may offer focused training in the acquisition of arousal reduction skills such as meditation and self-hypnosis.

CONCLUSIONS

The relationship between stress and disease is well established, although the specific pathways are complex and multifactorial. Clinicians increasingly are asked to examine the cost-effectiveness of the time spent with their patients with a view to improving outcomes within the constraints of available financial and human resources. Attention to the function of stress in patients' illnesses creates the potential for improving treatment outcomes and preventing or delaying the onset of costly target organ disease or the exacerbation of chronic illness. Applying a multidimensional stress model that includes patients' perceptions, coping strategies, physiologic arousal mechanisms, and arousal reduction strategies offers the health care professional multiple opportunities for influencing the ecology of disease.

SUGGESTED READINGS

Anderson NB, Johnson SB, Belar CD, et al. *Stress in America: Our Health at Risk*. Washington, DC: American Psychological Association, 2012. (www.stressinamerica.org)

Christensen JF. The assessment of stress: environmental, intrapersonal, and outcome issues. In: McReynolds P, ed. *Advances in Psychological Assessment*, Vol. 5. San Francisco:Jossey-Bass,1981.

Cohen S, Janicki-Deverts D, Doyle WJ, et al. Chronic stress, glucocorticoid receptor resistance, inflammation, and disease risk. *PNAS* 2012;109:5995–5999. www.pnas.org/cgi/doi/10.1073/pnas.1118355109

Engel GL. The need for a new medical model. *Science* 1977;196:129–136.

Figueredo VM. The time has come for physicians to take notice: the impact of psychosocial stressors on the heart. *Am J Med* 2009;122:704–712.

Kiecolt-Glaser JK. Stress, food, and inflammation: psychoneuroimmunology and nutrition at the cutting edge. *Psychosom Med* 2010;72:365–369.

Kyutoku Y, Tada R, Umeyama T, et al. Cognitive and psychological reactions of the general population three months after the 2011 Tohoku earthquake and tsunami. *PLoS ONE* 2012;7:e31014.

McEwen BS. Protective and damaging effects of stress mediators. *N Engl J Med* 1998;338:171–179.

Nishiyama K, Johnson JV. Karoshi—death from overwork. *Int J Health Services* 1997;27:625–641.

Rahe RH, Arthur RJ. Life change and illness studies: past history and future directions. *J Hum Stress* 1978;4:3–15.

Schuster MA, et al. A national survey of stress reactions after the September 11, 2001, terrorist attacks. *N Engl J Med* 2001;345:1507.

Spickard A, Gabbe SG, Christensen JF. Mid-career burnout in generalist and specialist physicians. *JAMA* 2002;288:1447–1450.

Steptoe A, Kivimaki M. Stress and cardiovascular disease. *Nature Reviews Cardiology* 2012;9:360–370.

Thomee S, Harenstam A, Hagberg M. Mobile phone use and stress, sleep disturbances, and symptoms of depression among young adults—a prospective cohort study. *BMC Public Health* 2011;11:1–11. (http://www.biomedcentral.com/1471-2458/11/66)

SUGGESTED READINGS FOR PATIENTS

De Mello A. *The Way to Love: The Last Meditations of Anthony de Mello*. New York: Doubleday, 1991.

Kabat-Zinn J. *Full Catastrophe Living: How to Cope with Stress, Pain and Illness Using Mindfulness Meditation*.15th anniversary ed. London: Piatkus Books, 2004.

Kabat-Zinn J. *Wherever You Go There You Are: Mindfulness Meditation In Everyday Life*. New York: Hyperion, 1994.

Thich Nhat Hanh. *The Miracle of Mindfulness: A Manual on Meditation*. Boston: Beacon Press, 1987.

Thich Nhat Hanh. *Peace is Every Step: The Path of Mindfulness in Everyday Life*. New York: Bantam, 1991.

WEB SITES

PsychoNeuroImmunology Research Society. http://www.pnirs.org/. Accessed January 2014.

Center for Mindfulness in Medicine, Health Care, and Society. http://www.umassmed.edu/cfm/. Accessed January 2014.

Appendix 34-A Life stress inventory.

In the blanks below list the major events, changes, or stressors that have happened to you within the last year. Also list those events that you expected but that failed to occur. In the next column, place a check next to those stressors that are current, ongoing problems. In the last column opposite each stressor, indicate the degree to which this event has been under your control by writing a number corresponding to the scale at the top.

Life Event or Stressor	Current Problem	Within Your Control	Outside Your Control
		1 2 3 4 5 6 7 8 9 10	
1._____	_____		_____
2._____	_____		_____
3._____	_____		_____
4._____	_____		_____
5._____	_____		_____
6._____	_____		_____
7._____	_____		_____
8._____	_____		_____
9._____	_____		_____
10._____	_____		_____
		Control Score_____ (mean of ratings)	

John F. Christensen, PhD

Pain

Matthew J. Gonzales, MD; Gregory T. Smith, PhD; Michael W. Rabow, MD; & Steven Z. Pantilat, MD

INTRODUCTION

Most pain is acute and short lived. Acute pain is primarily a symptom of a pathological process or injury. Typically treating the illness or injury will reduce or eliminate acute pain symptoms. Analgesic medications are often used in this setting for comfort during the healing process. For the most part, treatment of the underlying pathology or injury and medication management are effective in the treatment of acute pain. Many resources exist for assisting clinicians with acute pain management strategies.

Despite even the best efforts, *acute pain* evolves into *chronic pain* in approximately one out of five patients. The management of chronic pain is complex and often involves both pharmacological and nonpharmacological interventions. Because chronic pain is also modulated by psychological status (e.g., depression and anxiety), environmental consequences (e.g., stressors or reinforcers), and prior conditioning history, a comprehensive, multidisciplinary approach to management of this condition is of critical importance.

Management of patients with chronic pain is often challenging and can lead to complex patient–physician relationships. Often these relationships engender strong reactions from primary care providers. This chapter focuses on helpful strategies for the management of chronic pain and approaches for facing the particular challenges of caring for patients with chronic pain.

CHRONIC PAIN PREVALENCE/ BACKGROUND DATA

The International Association for the Study of Pain (IASP) defines pain as an "unpleasant sensory and emotional experience associated with actual or potential tissue damage." The transition from acute to chronic pain is defined by duration. Acute pain may last up to 3 months at most, whereas chronic pain is any pain that lasts more than 3 months. Although pain from untreatable malignancies often lasts many months and is progressive, the terminal nature of the underlying condition leads most to consider cancer-related pain separately from chronic noncancer pain. Roughly 20% of the patients with acute pain will eventually seek treatment each year for chronic noncancer pain. Of these, 62% will report having pain for longer than 1 year; 57% report that their pain is episodic (e.g., migraine, neuropathy), whereas 43% will report having constant pain.

Chronic noncancer pain accounts for more than 70 million office visits per year in the United States, with annual direct medical costs of $125 billion. The cost of treating low back pain alone averages almost $86 billion annually. Although the diagnosis of low back pain represents only 5–10% of all disability claims, these claims account for 80–85% of the costs of disability.

CLINICIAN–PATIENT RELATIONSHIP/ GOALS OF THERAPY

Taking care of patients with chronic noncancer pain can be problematic for the primary care provider. Even the most experienced practitioners occasionally find the clinical relationship with a patient with chronic pain to be challenging and frustrating. Some patients with chronic pain are engaged in living active lives with modest and stable doses of medication. Others are inactive and passive, seeking to rely only on escalating doses of medication, and often put their lives on hold as a result of pain. Primary care providers can find themselves in an oppositional relationship with the latter group of patients, which can lead to feelings of inadequacy, frustration, and anger for both the clinician and the patient.

Chronic pain typically has no cure and is poorly managed by medications alone. Although the etiology of chronic pain varies with each patient, there are

Figure 35-1 Harvested Poppy Capsules, Afghanistan.

usually comorbid psychological, social, and functional variables that contribute to the difficulty of managing patients with chronic pain. These comorbid conditions often need clinical attention as well. Treatment strategies limited to pharmacological interventions usually fail.

The effectiveness of the physician–patient relationship is defined largely by the physician's ability to acknowledge the patient's problem, address the patient's goals, and establish a collaborative management strategy on which both the physician and the patient can agree. Because the primary concerns of the physician and the patient can be different, there is marked potential for miscommunication. An important first step for clinicians is to seek patients' expectations of treatment before sharing their own approach and philosophy of chronic pain treatment. Establishing a clear clinician–

patient relationship is central to successful management of chronic noncancer pain.

Patients dealing with chronic pain present for medical attention with a number of possible feelings and goals:

1. They may simply want to discover the cause of the pain to allay fears about an underlying serious disease.

2. They may be interested only in relief from the pain.

3. They may want to regain impaired function to return to normal work, social, or recreational activities.

4. They may want medical and social acknowledgment that the pain is preventing normal activities.

The "three-function model of the medical interview" (Table 35-1) can be utilized as a format for the ongoing

Table 35-1. The three-function model of the medical interview.

1. *Data gathering*: Elucidate the physical and psychological etiology of pain. Arrive at a tentative working diagnosis even while considering alternative hypotheses.
2. *Relationship building*: Using empathy skills and active listening, determine the meaning the pain has in the patient's life, including the role of "pain behaviors" and pain dysfunction, both physical and social.
3. *Management*: Explain the role of pain medications, including the duration of their use, the importance of time contingency, and an expectation of the degree of relief.
   a. Plan the use of physical and other therapies designed to improve function.
   b. Acknowledge the roles and limitations of rest periods.
   c. Establish the value of return to normal work and recreational activity to overcome pain behavior and dysfunction.

Table 35-2. Key elements in a typical pain contract.

Establish goals of treatment, particularly that (1) pharmacotherapy is only one part of therapy, and that (2) medication is not expected to completely eliminate pain.

Only one provider will write prescriptions for pain medication.

Patient agrees to use a single pharmacy for all opioid and nonopioid analgesics.

Refills for pain medication are not provided for lost or stolen medications and are only provided during regular business hours with appropriate lead time.

Random urine drug screening is to be performed without prior notice.

Patient agrees not to give or sell medications to others.

Warnings regarding sedating effects and long-term side effects of medications.

Warnings to avoid any and all illicit substances.

Breaking one or more of the elements in the contract will result in discontinuation of opioid prescriptions after an appropriate taper; however, all other elements of care will continue.

Adapted from publicly available contracts, including from www.dora.state.co.us/medical/policies/10-14SampleContract.Doc. Accessed November 20, 2011.

evaluation and reevaluation of patients with chronic pain (see Chapter 1).

Pain management is based on a number of basic guidelines.

1. Obtain a description of the pain and the meaning or impact the pain has on the patient's life and the life of others around the patient.
2. Assess for comorbid psychiatric conditions such as depression and anxiety.
3. Perform a focused physical examination based on pain history.
4. Review or obtain diagnostic studies that might rule in treatable physical pathology.
5. Use communication and empathy skills to discuss pain treatment.
   a. Explain rationale for nonuse of opioid analgesics for chronic noncancer pain.
   b. Provide nonpharmacological alternatives in context of "stages of change" model.
   c. Negotiate goals of treatment as restoring function and quality of life versus only eliminating nociception.
6. Provide relief and comfort through medication and reassurance.
7. Use multiple management modalities.
8. Assess for change in pain behavior and overall function.
9. Reinforce improvement in function and reduced pain (the goals of treatment) and discontinue ineffective treatments that do not achieve these goals.

The use of a "pain contract," which defines conditions for prescription of opioid medications, is also helpful in the management of patients with chronic noncancer pain. The contract aims to thoughtfully establish the goals of management prior to the initiation of any therapy. Key elements of a chronic pain management contract are included in Table 35-2. Both the physician and patient should sign the contract prior to therapy initiation and both individuals should retain a copy. Violation of the contract by the patient can be met initially with a single written warning, but any subsequent violation should be met with the cessation of opioid therapy, after a brief taper to avoid opioid withdrawal. It is critical to make clear to the patient that care with other management strategies and interventions can continue even if opioids will no longer be prescribed.

PHARMACOTHERAPY

Pharmacotherapy is often the first technique employed by the primary care provider for the management of chronic noncancer pain. It is an important technique in the treatment of pain, but should not be the mainstay of treatment. For mild-to-moderate pain, acetaminophen, aspirin, and nonsteroidal anti-inflammatory drugs (NSAIDs) may be sufficient. For moderate-to-severe pain, these agents combined with opioids may be helpful. Severe pain may require full opioid agonists.

Acetaminophen & NSAIDs

Acetaminophen and NSAIDs are in many cases the first-line pharmacotherapy for chronic noncancer pain. Appropriate doses of acetaminophen may be just as effective an analgesic and antipyretic as NSAIDs, but without the risk of gastrointestinal bleeding or ulceration. Hepatotoxicity is of particular concern because of how commonly acetaminophen is also an ingredient in various over-the-counter medications. Total acetaminophen doses should not exceed 3–4 g/day long term or 2 g/day for older patients and for those with liver disease.

Aspirin is an effective analgesic, antipyretic, and anti-inflammatory medication. Gastrointestinal irritation and bleeding are side effects, which are lessened with enteric-coated formulations of aspirin and concomitant use of proton pump inhibitor medication. Bleeding from other sources, allergy, and an association with Reye syndrome in children and teenagers further limit its use.

Commonly used NSAIDs and their dosages are listed in Table 35-3. Like aspirin, the NSAIDs are antipyretic, analgesic, and anti-inflammatory. NSAIDs increase the risk of gastrointestinal bleeding by 1.5 times normal. The risks of bleeding and nephrotoxicity from NSAIDs are both increased in elders. Topical formulations of diclofenac (patch or gel) result in lower blood levels of the NSAID and may be associated with decreased systemic side effects. NSAID gastrointestinal bleeding and ulceration may be prevented with the concurrent use of proton pump inhibitors or with the class of NSAIDs that inhibit only cyclooxygenase (COX)-2. Celecoxib is the only COX-2 inhibitor available and should be used with caution in patients with cardiac disease. The NSAIDs, including COX-2 inhibitors, can lead to fluid retention and exacerbations of congestive heart failure and should be used with caution in patients with that condition.

Opioid Medications

Opioid therapy has its place in the management of chronic noncancer pain, yet it is important to note that opioids alone will rarely be sufficient to adequately manage the pain and in this clinical setting should be used in conjunction with the other management strategies outlined in this chapter. Certainly, however, this class of agents is effective for pain management and should be used in select patients with chronic persistent or debilitating pain that is not well controlled with nonopioid treatment strategies. In certain populations, particularly chronic low back pain, consideration should be given to limiting or reducing opioids over time as other modalities are likely to be more effective.

Opioid medications are listed in Table 35-4. Full opioid agonists such as morphine, hydromorphone, oxycodone, methadone, fentanyl, hydrocodone, and codeine are used most commonly. Hydrocodone and codeine are typically combined with acetaminophen or an NSAID. Short-acting formulations of oral morphine sulfate, hydromorphone, or oxycodone are useful for acute pain not controlled with other analgesics. For chronic stable pain, long-acting medications are preferred, such as oral sustained-release morphine, oxycodone, or methadone. Methadone is inexpensive, available in a liquid formulation, and may have added efficacy for neuropathic pain. However, equianalgesic dosing is complex because it varies with the patient's opioid dose, and caution must be used at higher methadone doses because of the risk of QT prolongation. Consultation with a pain or palliative care specialist may be appropriate.

A useful technique for opioid management of chronic pain is equianalgesic dosing (see Table 35-4). The dosages of any full opioid agonists used to control pain can be converted into an equivalent dose of any other opioid. In this way, 24-hour opioid requirements and dosing regimens established using shorter-acting opioid medications can be converted into equivalent dosages of long-acting medications or formulations. Cross-tolerance is often incomplete, however, so less than the full calculated equianalgesic dosage is generally administered initially when switching between opioid formulations. Equianalgesic dosing for methadone is more complex and varies by dose and duration of use.

Although some clinicians and patients inexperienced with the management of severe chronic pain may feel more comfortable with combined nonopioid–opioid agents, full agonist opioids are typically a better choice in patients with severe pain because the dose of opioid is not limited by the toxicities of the acetaminophen, aspirin, or NSAID component of combination preparations. There is no maximal allowable or effective dose for full opioid agonists.

As opioids are titrated upward, increasing difficulty with the side effects can be expected. Constipation is common at any dose of opioid, and tolerance to this side effect does not develop over time. Opioid-induced constipation should be anticipated and prevented in all patients.

Neuropathic Pain

It is essential when taking a patient's history to listen for descriptions such as burning, shooting, pins and needles, or electricity, and for pain associated with numbness. Such a history suggests neuropathic (as opposed to nociceptive) pain, which is treated with some medications not typically used for other types of pain. Whereas opioids are effective for neuropathic pain, a number of nonopioid medications have been found to be effective in randomized trials (Table 35-5). The tricyclic antidepressants (TCAs) are good first-line therapy. They usually have an effect at lower doses than are needed for an antidepressant effect.

Table 35-3. Acetaminophen, COX-2 inhibitors, and useful NSAIDs.

Drug	Usual Dose for Adults weighing >50 kg	Comments
Acetaminophen (Tylenol, Datril, others)	650 mg q4h or 975 mg q6h	Not an NSAID because it lacks peripheral anti-inflammatory effects. Equivalent to aspirin as analgesic and antipyretic agent. Limit dose to 3–4 g/day and to 2 g/day in older patients and those with liver disease. Be mindful of multiple sources of acetaminophen as in combination analgesics, cold remedies, and sleep aids.
Aspirin	650 mg q4h or 975 mg q6h	Available also in enteric-coated form that is more slowly absorbed but better tolerated.
Celecoxib (Celebrex)	200 mg once daily (osteoarthritis); 100–200 mg twice daily (rheumatoid arthritis)	COX-2 inhibitor. No antiplatelet effects. Lower doses for elderly who weigh less than 50 kg. Lower incidence of endoscopic gastrointestinal ulceration. Not known if true lower incidence of gastrointestinal bleeding. Possible link to cardiovascular toxicity. Celecoxib is contraindicated in sulfonamide allergy.
Choline magnesium salicylate (Trilasate, others)	1000–1500 mg three times daily	Salicylates cause less gastrointestinal distress and kidney impairment than NSAIDs but are probably less effective in pain management than NSAIDs.
Diclofenac (Voltaren, Cataflam, others)	50–75 mg orally two or three times daily; 1% gel 2–4 g four times daily; 1.3% patch two times daily	May impose higher risk of hepatotoxicity. Enteric-coated product; slow onset. Topical formulations may result in fewer side effects than oral formulations.
Diclofenac sustained release (Voltaren-XR, others)	100–200 mg once daily	
Diflunisal (Dolobid, others)	500 mg q12h	Fluorinated acetylsalicylic acid derivative.
Etodolac (Lodine, others)	200–400 mg q6–8h	
Fenoprofen calcium (Nalfon, others)	300–600 mg q6h	Perhaps more side effects than others, including tubulointerstitial nephritis.
Flurbiprofen (Ansaid)	50–100 mg three or four times daily	Adverse gastrointestinal effects may be more common among elderly.
Ibuprofen (Motrin, Advil, Rufen, others)	400–800 mg q6h	Relatively well tolerated and inexpensive.
Indomethacin (Indocin, Indometh, others)	25–50 mg two to four times daily	Higher incidence of dose-related toxic effects, especially gastrointestinal and bone marrow effects.
Ketoprofen (Orudis, Oruvail, others)	25–75 mg q6–8h (max 300 mg/day)	Lower doses for elderly.
Ketorolac tromethamine (Toradol)	10 mg q4–6h to a maximum of 40 mg/day orally	Short-term use (less than 5 days) only; otherwise, increased risk of gastrointestinal side effects.
Ketorolac tromethamine (Toradol)	60 mg IM or 30 mg IV initially, then 30 mg q6h IM or IV	Intramuscular (IM) or intravenous (IV) NSAID as alternative to opioid. Lower doses for elderly. Short-term use (less than 5 days) only.
Magnesium salicylate (various)	467–934 mg q6h	
Meclofenamate sodium (Meclomen)	50–100 mg q6h	Diarrhea more common.
Mefenamic acid (Ponstel)	250 mg q6h	
Nabumetone (Relafen)	500–1000 mg once daily (max dose 2000 mg/day)	May be less ulcerogenic than ibuprofen, but overall side effects may not be less.
Naproxen (Naprosyn, Anaprox, Aleve [OTC], others)	250–500 mg q6–8h	Generally well tolerated. Lower doses for elderly.
Oxaprozin (Daypro, others)	600–1200 mg once daily	Similar to ibuprofen. May cause rash, pruritus, photosensitivity.

(Continued)

Table 35-3. Acetaminophen, COX-2 inhibitors, and useful NSAIDs. (Continued)

Drug	Usual Dose for Adults weighing >50 kg	Comments
Piroxicam (Feldene, others)	20 mg daily	Not recommended in the elderly due to high adverse drug reaction rate. Single daily dose convenient. Long half-life. May cause higher rate of gastrointestinal bleeding and dermatological side effects.
Sulindac (Clinoril, others)	150 200 mg twice daily	May cause higher rate of gastrointestinal bleeding. May have less nephrotoxic potential.
Tolmetin (Tolectin)	200–600 mg four times daily	Perhaps more side effects than others, including anaphylactic reactions.

Source: Adapted from Jacob AK et al. *Management of Cancer Pain: Quick reference Guide for Clinicians No. 9.* AHCPR Publication No. 94-0593. Rockville, MD. Agency for Health Care Policy and Research, Public Health Service, U.S. Department of Health and Human Services, March 1994.

Desipramine and nortriptyline are good first choices because they cause less orthostatic hypotension and have fewer anticholinergic effects than amitriptyline. Start with a low dosage and titrate upward every 4 or 5 days.

The calcium channel a2-d ligands gabapentin and pregabalin are also considered first-line therapy for neuropathic pain. Both medications can cause sedation, dizziness, ataxia, and gastrointestinal side effects but have no significant drug interactions. Both drugs require dose adjustments in patients with kidney dysfunction. Both drugs are relatively safe in accidental overdose and may be preferred over TCAs for a patient with a history of congestive heart failure or arrhythmia or if there is a risk of suicide. Gabapentin plus morphine in combination is more effective at lower doses of each drug than when each is used as a single agent.

The selective serotonin norepinephrine reuptake inhibitors (SSNRIs), duloxetine and venlafaxine, are also considered first-line treatments for neuropathic pain. These should not be combined with other serotonin or norepinephrine uptake inhibitors, but it can be combined with gabapentin or pregabalin. Because venlafaxine can cause hypertension and induce ECG changes, patients with cardiovascular risk factors should be carefully monitored when starting this drug.

The 5% lidocaine patch is effective in postherpetic neuralgia (PHN) and may be effective in other types of localized neuropathic pain. A new patch is applied to the painful region daily for up to 12 hours.

Successful management of neuropathic pain often requires the use of more than one effective medication.

Interventional Pharmacotherapy

Injection Therapies: Injections include trigger point injections, epidural injections, and nerve blocks. Trigger points are localized areas of muscle tenderness and pain, often injected in the treatment of myofascial complaints for temporary short-term relief. Epidural injections utilize local anesthetics or steroids into the epidural space and can be used for both diagnostic purposes as well as to provide short-term relief. Trigger point and epidural injections should not be used in the treatment of chronic pain. Nerve blocks are typically used for peripheral neuropathy for short-term relief of pain. Nerve blocks are often provided in a series of three injections over a period of 3–18 weeks.

Implantable Pumps: Intraspinal infusion of opioid into the intrathecal area through an implanted pump is available. Small levels of opioid are introduced into the intrathecal area, lowering the dose required to provide relief. The efficacy for the use of an implantable pump has not been shown in rigorous trials.

Spinal Cord Stimulator: Neurostimulation is provided by an implanted pulse generator through electrodes that are targeted to the spinal cord with the intent of blocking the pain signal. There is some evidence for the use of spinal cord stimulators for complex regional pain syndrome; however, the efficacy for the use of this procedure is yet to be shown for other pain conditions.

Behavioral Medicine Approaches

Cognitive behavioral therapy (CBT) has been proven as a primary evidence-based approach in the treatment of chronic pain in multiple randomized controlled studies. Cognitive behavior therapy is a form of psychological treatment that focuses on thinking as having an important role in determining how we feel and what we do. CBT and other therapies that have been demonstrated to be effective in the treatment of chronic pain include: Biofeedback Therapy, Hypnosis, Mindfulness Therapy, and Acceptance and Commitment Therapy (ACT). Table 35-6 summarizes behavioral therapy approaches used in treatment of chronic pain.

Table 35-4. Useful opioid agonist analgesics.

Drug	Approximate Equianalgesic Dose (compared to morphine 30 mg orally or 10 mg IV/SC)[a]		Usual Starting Dose Adults ≥50 kg Body Weight		Potential Advantages	Potential Disadvantages
	Oral	Parenteral	Oral	Parenteral		
Opioid agonists[b]						
Fentanyl	Not available	100 mcg q1h	Not available	50–100 mcg IV/IM q1h or 0.5–1.5 mcg/kg/h IV infusion	Possibly less neuroexcitatory effects, including in kidney failure.	
Fentanyl transdermal	Conversion to fentanyl patch is based on total daily dose of oral morphine[b]: morphine 60–134 mg/day orally = fentanyl 25 mcg/hour patch; morphine 135–224 mg/day orally = fentanyl 50 mcg/hour patch; morphine 225–314 mg/day orally = fentanyl 75 mcg/h patch; and morphine 315–404 mg/day orally = fentanyl 100 mcg/hour patch	Not available	Not available orally 12.5–25 mcg/h patch q72h;	Not available	Stable medication blood levels.	Not for use in opioid-naïve patients.
Hydromorphone[c] (Dilaudid)	7.5 mg q3–4h	1.5 mg q3–4h	1–2 mg q3–4h	1.5 mg q3–4h	Similar to morphine. Available in injectable high-potency preparation, rectal suppository.	Short duration.
Levorphanol (Levo-Dromoran)	4 mg q6–8h	2 mg q6–8h	4 mg q6–8h	2 mg q6–8h	Longer-acting than morphine sulfate.	
Meperidine[d] (Demerol)	300 mg q2–3h; normal dose 50–150 mg q3–4h	100 mg q3h	Not recommended	100 mg q3h	Use only when single dose, short-duration analgesia is needed as for outpatient procedures like colonoscopy. Not recommended for chronic pain or for repeated dosing.	Short duration. Normeperidine metabolite accumulates in kidney failure and other situations, and in high concentrations may cause irritability and seizures.

Drug					Comments	
Methadone (Dolophine, others)	10–20 mg q6–8h (when converting from <100 mg long-term daily oral morphine[e])	5–10 mg q6–8h	5–20 mg q6–8h	2.5–10 mg q6–8h	Somewhat longer-acting than morphine. Useful in cases of intolerance to morphine. May be particularly useful for neuropathic pain. Available in liquid formulation.	Analgesic duration shorter than plasma duration. May accumulate, requiring close monitoring during first weeks of treatment. Equianalgesic ratios vary with opioid dose.
Morphine[c] immediate release (Morphine sulfate tablets, Roxanol liquid)	30 mg q3–4h (repeat around-the-clock dosing); 60 mg q3–4h (single or intermittent dosing)	10 mg q3–4h	4–8 mg q3–4h	10 mg q3–4h	Standard of comparison; multiple dosage forms available.	No unique problems when compared with other opioids.
Morphine controlled-release[c] (MS Contin, Oramorph)	90–120 mg q12h	Not available	15–60 mg q12h	Not available		
Morphine extended release (Kadian, Avinza)	180–240 mg q24h	Not available	20–30 mg q24h	Not available	Once-daily dosing possible.	
Oxycodone (Roxicodone, OxyIR)	20–30 mg q3–4h	Not available	5–10 mg q3–4h	Not available	Similar to morphine.	
Oxycodone controlled release (Oxycontin)	40 mg q12h	Not available	20–40 mg q12h	Not available		
Oxymorphone[f] oral, immediate release (Opana)	10 mg q3–4h	Not available	5–10 mg q3–4h	Not available		New formulation with less known about equianalgesic dosing.
Oxymorphone[f] extended release (Opana ER)	30–40 mg q12h	Not available	15–30 mg q12h	Not available		New formulation with less known about equianalgesic dosing.

(Continued)

Table 35-4. Useful opioid agonist analgesics. (Continued)

Drug	Approximate Equianalgesic Dose (compared to morphine 30 mg orally or 10 mg IV/SC)[a]		Usual Starting Dose Adults ≥50 kg Body Weight		Potential Advantages	Potential Disadvantages
	Parenteral	Oral	Oral	Parenteral		
Combination Opioid–NSAID Preparations						
Codeine[g,h] (with aspirin or acetaminophen)[i]	130 mg q3–4h	180–200 mg q3–4h	60 mg q4–6h	60 mg q2h	Similar to morphine.	Closely monitor for efficacy as patients vary in their ability to convert the prodrug codeine to morphine.
Hydrocodone[f] (in Lorcet, Lortab, Vicodin, others)[i]	Not available	30 mg q3–4h	10 mg q3–4h	Not available		Combination with acetaminophen limits dosage titration.
Oxycodone[g] (in Percocet, Percodan, Tylox, others)[i]	Not available	30 mg q3–4h	10 mg q3–4h	Not available	Similar to morphine.	Combination with acetaminophen and aspirin limits dosage titration.

[a]Published tables vary in the suggested doses that are equianalgesic to morphine. Clinical response is the criterion that must be applied for each patient; titration to clinical efficacy is necessary. Because there is no complete cross-tolerance among these drugs, it is usually necessary to use a lower than equianalgesic dose initially when changing drugs and to retitrate to response.

[b]Conversion is conservative; therefore, do not use these equianalgesic doses for converting back from fentanyl patch to other opioids because they may lead to inadvertent overdose. Patients may require breakthrough doses of short-acting opioids during conversion to transdermal fentanyl.

[c]*Caution:* For morphine, hydromorphone, and oxymorphone, rectal administration is an alternative route for patients unable to take oral medications. Equianalgesic doses may differ from oral and parenteral doses. A short-acting opioid should normally be used for initial therapy.

[d]Not recommended for chronic pain. Doses listed are for brief therapy of acute pain only. Switch to another opioid for long-term therapy.

[e]Methadone conversion varies depending on the equivalent total daily dose of morphine. Consult with a pain management or palliative care expert for conversion.

[f]*Caution:* Recommended doses do not apply for adult patients with kidney or hepatic insufficiency or other conditions affecting drug metabolism.

[g]*Caution:* Doses of aspirin and acetaminophen in combination products must also be adjusted to the patient's body weight.

[h]*Caution:* Doses of codeine >60 mg often are not appropriate because of diminishing incremental analgesia with increasing doses but continually increasing nausea, constipation, and other side effects.

[i]*Caution:* Monitor total acetaminophen dose carefully, including any OTC use. Total acetaminophen dose maximum 4 g/day. If liver impairment or heavy alcohol use, maximum is 2 g/day. Data from Jacox AK, et al. *Management of Cancer Pain: Quick Reference Guide for Clinicians No. 9.* AHCPR Publication No. 94–0593. Rockville, MD. Agency for Health Care Policy and Research, Public Health Service, US Department of Health and Human Services. March 1994, and from Erstad BL. A rational approach to the management of acute pain states. *Hosp Formul* 1994;29(8 Part 2):586.

Source: Adapted from Jacox AK et al. *Management of Cancer Pain: Quick reference Guide for Clinicians No. 9.* AHCPR Publication No. 94–0593. Rockville, MD. Agency for Health Care Policy and Research, Public Health Service, U.S. Department of Health and Human Services, March 1994.

Table 35-5. Pharmacological management of neuropathic pain.

Drug[a]	Starting Dose	Typical Dose
Antidepressants[b]		
Nortriptyline	10 mg orally at bedtime	10–150 mg orally at bedtime
Desipramine	10 mg orally at bedtime	10–200 mg orally at bedtime
Calcium channel a2-d ligands		
Gabapentin[c]	100–300 mg orally once to three times daily	300–1200 mg orally three times daily
Pregabalin[d]	50 mg orally three times daily	100 mg orally three times daily
Selective serotonin norepinephrine reuptake inhibitors		
Duloxetine	60 mg orally daily or 20 mg orally twice daily in elders	60 mg orally daily
Venlafaxine[e]	75 mg orally daily divided into two or three doses	150–225 mg orally daily divided into two or three doses
Opioids	(see Table 35-4)	(see Table 35-4)
Other medications		
Lidocaine transdermal	5% patch applied daily, for a maximum of 12 hours	1–3 patches applied daily for a maximum of 12 hours
Tramadol hydrochloride	50 mg orally four times daily	100 mg orally two to four times daily

[a]Begin at the starting dose and titrate up every 4 or 5 days.
[b]Begin with a low dose. Pain relief may be achieved at doses below antidepressant doses, thereby minimizing adverse side effects.
[c]Common side effects include nausea, somnolence, and dizziness. Take medication on a full stomach. Do not combine with serotonin or norepinephrine uptake inhibitors, or with TCAs.
[d]Common side effects include dizziness, somnolence, peripheral edema, and weight gain. Must adjust dose for kidney impairment.
[e]*Caution*: Can cause hypertension and ECG changes. Obtain baseline ECG and monitor.
Source: Adapted with permission from Rabow MW, Pantilat SZ. Palliative Care & Pain Management, 50th ed. Editors: McPhee SJ, Papadakis MA. Current Medical Diagnosis and Treatment: Lange Medical Books/McGraw-Hill, New York, NY 2011.

Table 35-6. Behavioral treatment methods for pain.

1. Cognitive behavioral therapy	This approach often involves the monitoring of automatic thoughts that are negative; recognizing the connections between thoughts, affect, and behavior; and alternatively replacing dysfunctional thoughts with more reality-oriented interpretations. Recent advances in CBT for the treatment of chronic pain have resulted in behavioral and cognitive methods to challenge dysfunctional beliefs about pain and the impact that pain has on normal functioning and replace them with more accurate reality-based beliefs.
2. Biofeedback	Computer-assisted measurement of physiologic changes previously thought to be involuntary, for the purposes of training the patient to bring them into voluntary control. Measurements often include surface electromyelography, skin temperature, galvanic skin response, respiration, heart rate, pulse time, distal polysomnography, and electroencephalogram.
3. Autogenic and relaxation training	A series of mental exercises designed to produce relaxation imagery that may be guided by a practitioner through suggestion or can be coupled with relaxation and exercise.
4. Progressive muscle relaxation	A systematic approach to relaxation with exercises involving the tensing and relaxing of muscle groups from head to foot.
5. Mindfulness	In this context, a type of CBT that emphasizes bringing nonjudgmental attention to the patient's present experience at each moment, with a focused awareness of thoughts, emotions, and sensations, including pain. In this way, the patient can develop an observing mind, to be aware of thoughts or judgments and emotional reactions to the changes in physical pain and to notice that one can respond in different ways that allows for a more complete or satisfying physical and emotional life together with acceptance of pain.
6. Hypnosis	A state of enhanced focus or awareness that can lead to increased levels of suggestibility. This can be helpful in the blocking of painful sensations (hypnoanalgesia).

Table 35-7. Patient self-help resources.

1. Caudill M. *Managing Pain Before it Manages You*, revd ed. New York, NY: Gillford Press, 2002.
2. Catalano E, Hardin KN, eds. *The Chronic Pain Control Workbook: A Step-by-Step Guide for Coping with and Overcoming Pain*, 2nd ed. Oakland, CA: New Harbinger Publ., 1999.
3. Butler DS, Moseley GL. *Explain Pain*. Adelaide, Australia: Noigroup Publications, 2010. http://www.noigroup.com/en/Store. Accessed June 2013.
4. American Pain Foundation. www.painfoundation.org. Accessed June 2013.
5. Internet support group. www.chronicpainsupport.org. Accessed June 2013.

There are also patient self-help resources to which the clinician can refer patients who are literate and motivated to take an active role in managing their pain (Table 35-7).

Mindfulness training is a primary modality for the treatment of chronic pain. Mindfulness is the practice of

CASE ILLUSTRATION

Michael is a 50-year-old concrete construction crew leader who experienced an injury on the job resulting in lumbar disc herniation with a multiple-level nerve root compromise and was treated with fusion including instrumentation with a quick recovery and return to work within 6 weeks. Six months later Michael experienced a reoccurrence of low back pain. Imaging studies revealed a solid fusion with no other abnormalities, and he was referred for injection therapies.

Michael has a strong work ethic and is in need of continued full-time employment to support himself and his family. He has few easily transferable skills; concrete is all he knows. He benefited from steroid injections every 3 months and remained on the job. In between injections he used oral opioids, gradually requiring increasing amounts to provide a measure of pain relief. After 5 years he was found to be totally disabled by his doctors and referred for CBT to assist with his adjustment to disability.

After an initial period of anger toward his doctors, he began to take steps to manage his pain. He realized in treatment that his initial goal of total pain relief was unrealistic. He learned to observe his pain, his reactions of anger and fear to his pain, and how he made himself anxious and depressed by concluding that he was severely and permanently functionally impaired. He decided what level of pain was acceptable to him and learned what functional activities he

wanted to pursue regardless of the pain. He learned self-management skills to reduce the pain without using medications or procedures when it was elevated. He then returned to work full time, less than a year after being declared disabled, in a less physically demanding job, armed with skills to live with his pain.

bringing complete attention to one's present experience. It recognizes the primacy of the present moment, whereas memories of the past and anticipated future events are mere mental constructs. As such, living only in the present moment is critical. Mindfulness also teaches that although thoughts are useful tools, they alone do not define an individual. Often pain as a private sensory experience is *reified* (made into a static thing), analyzed, and reacted to by our thinking. Our analysis and reaction to the sensory experience of pain is called suffering and is entirely in our control. The practice of mindfulness allows us to relax into the pain and to observe or even alter our reactions to the sensory experience of pain. In this way, patients learn to accept the pain as a natural part of their experience and limit or reduce reactions to it. This technique also emphasizes the need to make decisions about present and future activities or life plans despite the pain.

Acceptance and commitment therapy is an approach to treating chronic pain that uses mindfulness training as well. It combines mindfulness with *cognitive defusion* (the process of separating or defusing thoughts and images from emotions and memories). It teaches acceptance, which in this context is allowing painful thoughts, images, and memories to come and go without struggling with them. In this therapy, a values exploration is pivotal in helping each person discover what is most important. This approach promotes the individual's ability to accept pain, as well as thoughts and reactions to the pain.

Biofeedback is a computerized audio and visual feedback system that uses physiologic measures to amplify the individual's awareness including muscle contraction (through electromyography (EMG); sympathetic arousal; skin temperature change; heart rate (HRV); and brain activity (through electroencephalogram [EEG]). With this increased awareness individuals are taught to increase and decrease the physiologic feedback to gain greater control over their levels of arousal. Biofeedback has been shown to be quite useful in the treatment of headache and has also been shown to be useful in conjunction with active physical therapy for musculoskeletal back pain, as well as assisting with stress management training.

Relaxation and stress management have been shown to be useful in reducing comorbid anxiety and report of pain (see Chapter 34). Hypnosis can also be utilized through imagery and relaxation to focus attention and assist with reduced pain and improved sense of well-being (see Chapter 5).

When patients present with comorbid psychiatric conditions, such as depression or anxiety, a referral to a clinical psychologist or psychiatrist who works with chronic pain patients should be considered. In addition, CBT has been shown to assist patients in reducing pain and suffering, as well as improving function and coping skills. CBT can be provided in collaboration with other rehabilitative and medical techniques.

Pain Rehabilitation

Physical therapy treatment for acute pain is typically passive at first (hot packs, ultrasound, myofascial techniques, etc.) but then becomes more active (stretching, strengthening and endurance techniques, etc.) over a 6- to 12-week period. Physical therapy is useful for musculoskeletal pain complaints. Active physical therapy has been shown in combination with other behavioral approaches and education to be most effective in the treatment of chronic low back and upper back pain.

Occupational therapists often evaluate and treat dysfunction in the activities of daily living and daily functioning, both at home and in the work setting. Work site and home modifications and use of adaptive equipment can be established by an occupational therapist to improve independent functioning.

Transcutaneous electrical nerve stimulation (TENS) unit provides an electrical current topically and is commonly used for pain relief. The TENS unit can be beneficial in the treatment of neuropathic pain and when provided within an interdisciplinary pain treatment program.

Interdisciplinary Pain Programs

Interdisciplinary pain rehabilitation programs (IPRPs) utilize the services of a pain physician, pain psychologist, physical and occupational therapist, nurse, biofeedback therapist, and often employ several healing modalities, including hypnosis, mindfulness, ACT, or TENS units. These professionals work together on interdisciplinary teams to provide coordinated and collaborative care. These programs often involve primary behavior change and rehabilitative strategies while adjusting medications and improving function. The efficacy for the use of these programs with chronic pain conditions is evidenced based and well documented. In fact, the combination of CBT with rehabilitation in IPRPs has shown the best outcomes in the treatment of chronic pain.

Multidisciplinary pain procedure programs utilizing primarily injection therapies, medications, implantable pumps and stimulators, together with physical therapy and psychological treatment, work collaboratively to provide pain relief and to assist with improved mobility and coping skills.

Alternative medicine techniques, including acupuncture, chiropractic manipulation, and homeopathy have been shown in specific cases to be useful in reducing pain on a long-term basis when provided in conjunction with other treatment modalities or as part of an interdisciplinary program. Clinicians should rule out underlying medical causes for chronic pain, such as malignancy or rheumatologic disease, prior to referral.

CHRONIC PAIN CASE EXAMPLES

The following case illustrations highlight major issues related to chronic pain management.

In this way, the primary care physician helped Lisa redefine the headache treatment regimen: it does not

CASE ILLUSTRATION 1
CHRONIC HEADACHE PAIN

Lisa is a 39-year-old woman who sought care for her long-standing headaches. These headaches first appeared at the age of 18 years, at which time they were characterized by severe left orbital and temporal pain associated with nausea, nasal stuffiness, and photophobia. They were often preceded by a scintillating scotoma in the right temporal/visual field. Her workup included a normal lumbar puncture, several normal EEGs, computerized tomography (CT) scans, and blood chemistries. She was virtually headache-free for 1 year following a pregnancy in her early 20s. Headaches gradually recurred but remitted again for a year after a hysterectomy for endometriosis in her early 30s. She now reports that the headaches have increased in frequency, duration, and severity over the past 2 years with more photophobia, nausea, and vomiting.

Treatment modalities have included analgesia (aspirin, acetaminophen, NSAIDs, opioids), abortive agents (sumatriptan and topiramate), prophylactic medications (amitriptyline, cyproheptadine, phenytoin, valproic acid, propranolol), and vitamins, all of which have had only transient benefit. Dietary and activity prescriptions have also been of minimal success. Her main source or relief over the past year has been repeated emergency room visits for intravenous opioids. She has seen multiple internists, neurologists, anesthesiologists for trigger point injections and nerve blocks, allergists and emergency room physicians.

Long-standing, recurrent, incapacitating, nonmalignant pain creates a number of challenges in management:

1. Seeking assistance from a series of caregivers without resolution.
2. A clear fluctuation in the frequency and intensity of the headache seemingly due to physiologic changes, but without an exploration of the possible behavioral or social changes associated with these fluctuations.
3. Failure to explore the impact the headache has had in the patient's life.

A pain history revealed that Lisa's headaches in early adulthood were infrequent (several per year) and were managed conservatively. Her single severe attack resulted in a hospitalization that was a source of embarrassment to her and her husband. During the early years of her marriage she continued to have infrequent but more severe headaches. During a period of 6 months of treatment with oral contraceptives her headaches became more frequent and severe. As her daughter grew older and her job responsibilities increased, the frequency and severity of the headaches grew. She further reported that she was best able to control her pain by being alone in a quiet room, reading, or listening to quiet music.

The patient is now identifying what may be a clear relationship between marital or social stress and her headache complaint. The headache can provide "timeout" from the conflicts at hand, and she can ease the pain by listening to music or reading. She further indicates that the headaches did not have a significant impact in her early life.

The headache pattern remained unchanged until 1½ years ago. At that time Lisa and her husband relocated as a result of her husband's work and they moved into a home that required major remodeling, the responsibility of which was largely the patient's. She had difficulty replacing her former employment and considered a new career. Although she reported enthusiasm for the remodeling and the relocation, Lisa also reported a marked increase in the frequency of the headaches. She was unable to work around the house remodeling or participate in family discussions when she had the headache, but was otherwise able to prepare meals, do housework, and drive as far as 30 miles one way for social and medical visits. She reported that when she retreats to her room with a headache her husband and children attend to her until she starts to improve. She also indicated that her husband returned home early from work during times of a severe headache. She has seen a cascade of physicians in various specialties with a variety of unremarkable diagnostic tests and specialty workups. Her average length of treatment with any one physician was five visits. She reported with embarrassment that she had been unable to keep up with her diet and exercise program and was increasingly overweight. Otherwise, she was in good health with no other medical problems.

Although the headache event is likely to have muscle contraction, endocrine, and vascular components, there appear to be a number of clear situations or conditions that accompany its onset and severity. Moreover, it is clear that as life stress has increased, Lisa's headaches have also increased in severity and frequency. There seem to be behavioral factors that reinforce the headache complaint: (1) avoidance of stress and (2) increased attention from others.

The following treatment course of action was undertaken:

1. *The physician explained to the patient that she wanted to work with her to ease her headaches. She reassured Lisa that she thought that by working together and taking a broad view they could ease the frequency and severity of headaches and improve her quality of life overall.*
2. *It was agreed that the best course of treatment was to use as little opioid medication as possible. Even though opioids were found to be useful by the patient, she recognized that ultimately they were not changing the overall pattern of her headaches and decided to use them only for severe headaches that did not resolve with other measures. Patient and physician medication management responsibilities were outlined in the medication agreement, which specified the number and frequency of opioid medications.*
3. *It was agreed that the patient would not seek additional medical evaluation or treatment without discussing it with her primary care physician first.*
4. *The primary care physician agreed that she or her designee would be available within a 12-hour period of being contacted about a headache to discuss the headache and the possible situation surrounding it. It was agreed that these conversations would generally be brief and not longer than 5–10 minutes.*
5. *The physician discussed a comprehensive approach to the headaches, including a course of biofeedback training and instruction for neck exercises in physical therapy. Lisa agreed to participate actively in these treatments.*
6. *The physician also referred Lisa for CBT.*
7. *If this plan did not show significant reduction in headaches within 3 months, referral to a multidisciplinary pain rehabilitation program would be considered.*

8. Finally, the physician would attend to all of Lisa's medical needs, including preventive care, which had been somewhat neglected due to a singular focus on the headache and the frequent changing of doctors.

need immediate or intensive medical care; it does not need further diagnostic evaluation (because a detailed medical evaluation had already been done); and it does not need further multiple/different medication trials (these have also been tried). By creating an effective relationship with the patient, acknowledging the severity of her complaint, setting expectations for how to respond to symptoms, explicitly stating a desire and intent to help, and securing the patient's commitment to work within this setting, a productive patient–physician partnership was established to address Lisa's pain complaint.

CASE ILLUSTRATION 2
CHRONIC INTRACTIBLE PAIN:
CHRONIC LOW BACK PAIN

Michael is a 45-year-old man with controlled hypertension who presented with low back pain. He reported that while working on a farm 2 years ago he experienced a motor vehicle accident that resulted in a herniated disc in his lumbar spine. A lumbar laminectomy and discectomy followed with some relief of pain for approximately 3 months. Since that time he had 6 weeks of passive physical therapy (hot packs, ultrasound, massage, gentle stretching) and was receiving oral opioids and NSAIDs from his surgeon. He had low back pain and no other complaints. He had not returned to work since the day of the injury and was currently involved in a vocational rehabilitation plan.

On physical examination, the patient was tender to palpation across his low back bilaterally. Passive straight leg raising was normal. Sharp, dull, and light touch sensations were intact throughout, with symmetric reflexes in both the lower extremities. The CT scan of the lumbar and sacral spine revealed old surgical repair of a herniated disc without other abnormalities. Recent nerve conduction studies were unremarkable for nerve slowing. The patient's surgeon, who had "nothing more to offer," referred him back to his primary care physician for continued treatment. The primary care physician referred him

for a series of three epidural injections. The first injection resulted in partial pain relief for 2 weeks. The last two injections produced no relief of pain.

Chronic low back pain often has the following characteristics:

1. Subjective complaint of pain with minimal objective findings.
2. Use of "passive" rather than "active" physical therapy.
3. Continuous use of opioid medication in escalating dose to manage the pain.

The patient reported that he spends much of the day sitting in his reclining chair, either watching television or reading except for when he attends the vocational training. He moves from the chair two or three times each day, primarily for meals. He frequently naps during the day and reports disrupted sleep at night, averaging 5–6 hours. He feels depressed and hopeless about his recovery and believes that unless his pain is relieved he will be unable to return to work. He acknowledges that his spouse and children are angry with him and his inability to return to work.

On further questioning it was discovered that the social "cost" of the pain is high. Michael's daily activities are greatly impaired. His self-esteem and affect have plummeted, and he is further emotionally isolated from his family. In a circumstance in which a patient's chronic pain is associated with the patient belief that pain relief is necessary to return to a degree of normal living, the doctor must accurately establish expectations for recovery and the probable outcomes of treatment. Because the patient is usually still focused on the pain as a continuation of the original precipitating injury, it becomes necessary to identify and deal with the patient's pain beliefs while focusing on improving function.

Although Michael reported feelings of depression, it is inaccurate to say that the pain is caused by the depression or vice versa, but rather it is comorbid to the pain. It has been shown, however, that the intensity of pain often diminishes with a trial of antidepressant medication, which can improve sleep as well.

The goals of treatment for chronic low back pain are primarily focused on improving the patient's activity level; diminishing their reliance on medications because, as in this case, they have not improved functioning despite escalating doses; and reducing pain behaviors (e.g., changing the focus of treatment from decreasing pain to increasing activity level for meaningful tasks). In this way, the doctor assists in "managing" the pain behavior.

At the same time the doctor should challenge the commonly held belief that increased opioid medication is necessary for increased activity. Whereas this is often the case for acute pain conditions, the same is not necessarily true for chronic noncancer pain conditions, and in some cases increasing opioid dose is associated with worse overall functioning. The doctor also should help the patient recognize that increases in pain with activity do not mean that an underlying condition is getting worse. The doctor should also reinforce the use of nonpharmacological methods of pain control while the patient is increasing his functional activity levels.

After a careful explanation by the doctor of the anatomy, physiology, and possible/probable causes of Michael's low back pain, a collaborative discussion followed, leading to an agreement on the following treatment plan:

1. *A course of physical therapy using primarily active exercises (e.g., aerobic exercise, walking, strengthening, and stretching). In addition, the patient agreed to take progressively longer walks each day. It was expected that with increased activity there would be an initial increase in pain. For that reason it was agreed that the patient could continue to use his opioid medication at the same dose during this period.*

2. *Although there was no evidence of addiction or abuse of opioids, it was also clear that increasing opioid doses and prn use had not improved the patient's pain or function. The physician realized that the sole reliance on opioids for management was not working. On the other hand, given prolonged use of opioids, discontinuation was also not a realistic option. Oral opioid medication was managed with a long-acting preparation with no short-acting or "breakthrough" dosing. This approach avoided linking the patient's pain with the timing and amount of dosing. The physician wrote monthly prescriptions. It was agreed that any request for change in his medication regimen would be directed only to the primary care physician and not to emergency rooms or other physicians. This was outlined and signed in a patient medication agreement.*

3. *The patient would be seen once a month by the doctor. A primary focus of future visits would be discussion about daily activities or return-to-work goals, if appropriate, rather than pain interferences with life.*

4. *Progress toward increased functional activities and reduced reliance on medications was monitored monthly through a brief activity-oriented questionnaire filled out at each doctor's visit.*

5. *The patient and the physician agreed that reducing opioid use was a goal and would be done gradually over time as tolerated. The physician reassured the patient that he would continue opioids if necessary but expected that a more comprehensive approach would lead to improvement that would obviate the need for opioids.*

The doctor has now, in collaboration with the patient, established the parameters of treatment, clarified the expected outcomes in terms of function, developed a more rational plan for the use of opioids, and progressed toward meaningful employment goals if appropriate, all in the context of reassuring the patient that the physician was invested in helping him and would work with him. This approach is a far cry from the previous message of "there is nothing more to do" and provides hope to the patient. These steps define the treatment effort to reducing pain perception and pain behaviors and changing beliefs about pain impact. Patients who respond favorably to this treatment of chronic pain usually report either that the pain is significantly reduced or that it does not bother them as much as it used to. When pain behavior is more entrenched (the patient is unresponsive to treatment due in part to beliefs about pain impact or secondary gain or both), referral to a multidisciplinary pain rehabilitation facility is recommended.

Cognitive-behavioral therapy and other behavioral approaches (Table 35-6) are often useful therapies independent of the multidisciplinary pain rehabilitation programs and would be reasonable adjuncts for this patient.

CASE ILLUSTRATION 3
FIBROMYALGIA

Kim is a 46-year-old woman with a known history of gastroesophageal reflux disease (GERD), who presented with total body pain. She reported that while lifting some baked goods in her kitchen 20 years ago she felt an acute snap coming from her right shoulder. She was later diagnosed with thoracic outlet syndrome and underwent removal of her first rib. She experienced pain relief for approximately 8 months with a recurrence of symptoms followed by an additional supraclavicular surgery. She continued to report having neck and shoulder pain. She was then diagnosed with cervical spondylosis and underwent a cervical laminectomy 5 years later with good benefit. Thereafter, she was tapered from her pain medications and returned to normal life, including work as a baker. For approximately 10 years following her surgery she reported essentially no recurring symptoms. She then had an onset of "achiness" in her shoulders and upper extremities bilaterally.

Kim now presents with pain in all four quadrants of her body and was positive for increased sensitivity for 16 of 18 tender points when applying 9 lbs of pressure. Kim also reports having an increased sensitivity to pain especially in her neck and shoulder.

Fibromyalgia is a clinical syndrome or cluster of symptoms for which there is little agreement as to cause or etiology. Complaints of total body achiness in all four quadrants of the body plus tenderness in 11–18 tender points when applying 9 lbs of pressure are sufficient to make a diagnosis. Report of symptoms of fibromyalgia can occur with no known traumatic event or illness.

On physical examination, sensation was intact throughout with symmetric reflexes without evidence of clubbing, cyanosis, or edema. She had full range of motion in the bilateral upper and lower extremities with no motor deficits identified. An MRI of the cervical spine showed old cervical repair with no abnormalities. Kim was then referred to a pain relief specialist (anesthesiologist) at a multidisciplinary pain procedure program.

A detailed history taken at the multidisciplinary pain procedure program documented pain symptoms, together with chronic fatigue, sleep disturbance, intermittent headaches, loss of weight, subjective feelings of weakness, intermittent report of irritable bowel, and anxiety. The multidisciplinary evaluation included a psychological evaluation, which diagnosed comorbid depression and anxiety with an above-normal arousal response to stress.

The multidisciplinary evaluation identified a number of other symptoms that are commonly seen with fibromyalgia, including fatigue, sleep disturbance, intermittent headaches, weight loss or weight gain, complaints of weakness, irritable bowel, and anxiety and depression. Not uncommon with fibromyalgia is an abnormal startle response as well as decreased coping in the presence of increased stress or stimulation.

Kim reports that she is a single mother of three teenage daughters, two of whom are living at home. She reports her ex-husband to be estranged from her and her children. He has not provided child support, requiring that Kim work full time as the sole support of the family. As her daughters grew to their mid-teen years, an increasing number of conflicts occurred between them. Kim reports that she is most worried about her eldest, 17-year-old daughter, who has recently dropped out of school and is living with a boy. Kim fears that she is using recreational drug. Kim reports having missed several days of work due to her pain and has been warned by her employer on two occasions that further absences might lead to disciplinary action. Finally, she reports that she is involved romantically with a man who seems to like her daughters and has been responsive to her needs for support as her pain problems seem to worsen.

While it is unknown if stress is one of the triggers of fibromyalgia, it is not uncommon to find comorbid environmental or personal situations that promote symptoms of anxiety and depression.

Treatment initiated at the multidisciplinary pain procedure clinic included SSRI antidepressant medication, gabapentin, a trial of muscle relaxant medication, and a series of myofascial trigger point injections. She was also seen for a course of CBT designed to improve problem-solving capabilities and teach stress management techniques. She also engaged in passive physical therapy modalities (such as ultrasound, massage, and gentle stretching). Kim reported improved mood and greater relaxation in response to the passive physical therapy techniques and muscle relaxant medications. There was no benefit from the trigger point injections. Finally, it was reported by the psychologist that her decision making about her 17-year-old daughter was improving, with evidence of better coping skills. She also had scheduled relaxation into her daily routine. She has begun a course of oral, short-acting opioid medications; and Kim decided to take a leave of absence from her employer on short-term disability.

In the absence of a true etiology, the tendency is to treat the symptoms of pain. The symptoms are often vague and transient and do not respond well to an acute pain treatment approach. Though Kim does benefit from treatments that are designed to reduce arousal and improve coping skills, she continues to report the symptoms of pain leading to increased disability.

Kim discharged from the multidisciplinary pain procedure program and returned to the care of her primary care physician. In collaboration with her doctor, Kim agreed to continue with her use of the antidepressant medication and to gradually reduce and discontinue her use of muscle relaxant and opioid medications. Consideration was given to use of low-dose NSAIDs. She continued physical therapy that now included walking in the swimming pool three times a week for 1 month, followed by light aerobic exercises three times a week, and, finally, active physical therapy for muscle fitness. It was agreed that she would use hot packs and massage for temporary relief in lieu of the opioid or muscle relaxant medication. She was to continue her relaxation practice throughout the day and agreed to continue CBT to assist with coping.

The doctor agreed to meet with Kim once a month to review progress. Kim agreed to keep records of her daily exercises and her medication use. Kim also agreed in her medication contract that any flare-ups or changes in her medication would be managed by her primary care physician, who agreed to be responsive to her within 24 hours of initial contact between monthly visits.

After 6 months of treatment Kim was able to improve her function and daily activity sufficiently to return to work on a full-time basis. She was able to plan for her future wedding with her now fiancé and reported that her total body pain had reduced substantially, but "waxed and waned" intermittently.

CASE ILLUSTRATION 4
POSTHERPETIC NEURALGIA

Lynn is a 63-year-old woman with well-controlled hypertension and elevated cholesterol. Lynn works as a social worker and also volunteers with social service agencies. Twelve years ago, she developed a vesicular rash on her left frontal scalp and forehead. The area was severely painful. She presented to her general medicine physician 4 days after the rash appeared, having thought it was a reaction to a new shampoo.

She was diagnosed with varicella zoster virus infection (shingles). A careful evaluation was conducted to make sure she did not have any ocular involvement. Despite the delay in her presentation, she was treated with acyclovir and a 10-day course of prednisone.

For her acute pain, she was treated with hydrocodone/acetaminophen and ibuprofen. She received moderate control of her pain but felt somewhat dizzy with the hydrocodone/acetaminophen medication and experienced gastrointestinal upset with the NSAID.

Five weeks after onset and after complete resolution of the lesions, Lynn returned to her primary care physician with the complaint of continued pain on her scalp and forehead. The pain was described as "burning" and "searing." The patient was most aware of the pain at night, in bed before sleep and it sometimes kept her awake. When she was more active, she reported that she had less pain. However, sometimes the pain was so severe it was difficult for her to go about her usual activities. Lynn was diagnosed with PHN.

Post herpetic neuralgia is an unfortunate complication of varicella zoster infection that is more likely to develop in patients older than 60 years. It can last for months or years or be permanent. The actual cause of the PHN is not known and, therefore, treatment is directed at managing the pain symptoms. People with PHN benefit from an honest explanation of the disorder, the typical course of the condition, and a multidisciplinary approach to management.

Lynn tried gabapentin but experienced little benefit. Moreover, she was burdened by severe sedation at a dose of 900 mg three times daily. Pregabalin was ineffective. She refused a trial of the lidocaine transdermal patch due to cosmetic concerns. Capsaicin cream was difficult to use on her scalp. Nortriptyline up to 150 mg nightly had only a modest effect. Other TCAs, SSRI, and SNRI medications were tried. Duloxetine proved most helpful among these. She continued to use hydrocodone/ acetaminophen when the pain was incapacitating; however, she did not like the idea of using an opioid medication regularly and also reported some dizziness even at low doses. Pain relief was only partial at best. The mainstay of her pharmacological treatment was ibuprofen 400 mg two to three times daily. She added a proton pump inhibitor to help with stomach upset.

The side effects of analgesic medications often require management with other medications. Even patients who wish to limit their use of medications may soon find that their pharmacological regimen has become complex and burdensome. Moreover, as in this case, medications alone may not adequately treat the pain and behavioral medicine approaches should be considered.

Lynn tried acupuncture without success as well as a mindfulness-based stress reduction practice, with some benefit. She noted that her Mindfulness exercises were especially useful to her at night when she was going to sleep. She was referred to physical therapy, where modalities including contrast heat/cold treatments were used, followed by a trial of the transcutaneous nerve stimulator (TENS), all with only temporary benefit. She was referred for CBT where she learned to accept her pain, be mindful of her life with pain, and to live a normal life despite the pain.

In cases such as these, where pain is refractory to multiple medications, the focus is on chronic pain management. Chronic pain typically has no cure and is poorly managed by medications alone. Combining CBT techniques with physical rehabilitation and medications has shown the best outcomes in the treatment of neuropathic chronic pain.

After 6 months of managing her symptoms, Lynn settled into a regular medication regimen of ibuprofen, omeprazole, and duloxetine, and needed hydrocodone/acetaminophen only rarely. She recognized that being as active as possible at work and at home greatly improved her quality of life, including the management of her pain. After 12 weeks of CBT and 6 weeks of physical therapy, she now a has an active life despite the pain, a number of self-management approaches that she employs as needed, and an acceptable pharmaceutical regime with few side effects—all of which enhance her well-being and resilience.

SUMMARY

In this chapter, we presented several approaches to the treatment of persons suffering various types of noncancer chronic pain, which emphasize the evaluation and treatment of not only the biological but also the psychological and social implications of the problem. The primary care provider is encouraged to make good use of the three-function model for interviewing and ongoing communications with his or her patient (see Chapter 1). The following key factors should be attended to in the treatment of chronic pain:

- **Identifying pain as an issue:** Deal with it in a comprehensive medical, social, and psychological way at onset, instead of when it becomes a problem.

- **Pain behaviors:** Whereas the patient may be quick to understand the pain largely as derived from the precipitating event or factors, the treating physician must always attend to the social causes and consequences of the pain and its implications in the life of the patient at work, at home, and during play.

- **Meaning and impact of the pain:** Cultural influences may dictate differing attitudes and roles in the expression of pain. Changes in lifestyle or work can have a profound effect on the quality of life.

- **Doctor as "change agent":** In addition to providing direct treatment and advice, the doctor, through the patient/doctor relationship, can improve adherence to treatment.

- **Function not dysfunction oriented:** The interests and attention of the doctor influences greatly the thoughts and behaviors of the patient. By commenting on improving function as an indicator of healing, the doctor can redirect the patient's attention away from the pain and toward increased functioning.

SUGGESTED READINGS

Pain Control in the Primary Care Setting. American Pain Society. Glenview, Illinois, 2006.

Chou R. Clinical guidelines for the use of chronic opioid therapy in chronic noncancer pain. *J Pain* 2009;10:113–130.

Chou R. Diagnosis and treatment of low back pain. A joint clinical practices guideline from the American College of Surgeons and the American Pain Society. *Ann Intern Med* 2007;147:478–492.

Catalano E, Hardin KN, eds. *The Chronic Pain Control Workbook: A Step-by-Step Guide for Coping with and Overcoming Pain,* 2nd ed. New Harbinger Publications, Oakland, CA. 1999.

Gatchel RJ, Okifuji A. Evidenced-based scientific data documenting the treatment and cost effectiveness of comprehensive pain programs for chronic nonmalignant pain. *J Pain* 2006;7:779–793.

Rabow MW, Pantilat SZ. *Palliative Care & Pain Management,* 50th ed. *Current Medical Diagnosis and Treatment.* New York, NY: Lange Medical Books/McGraw-Hill, 2011.

Turk DC. Clinical effectiveness and cost effectiveness of treatment for patients with chronic pain. *Clin J Pain* 2002;18:355.

Turk, D, Meichenbaum, D, Genest, M, eds. *Pain and Behavioral Medicine: A Cognitive-Behavioral Perspective.* Guilford Press, New York, NY. 1983.

Winterow C, Beck A, Gruener D. *Cognitive Therapy with Chronic Pain Patients.* Springer Publishing, New York, NY. 2003.

HIV/AIDS

36

Lisa Capaldini, MD, MPH & Mitchell D. Feldman, MD, MPhil

INTRODUCTION

Infection with the human immunodeficiency virus (HIV) is associated with a range of psychosocial and neuropsychiatric complications. While HIV/AIDS has become a manageable chronic disease for many patients, living with HIV/AIDS continues to be a practical and psychospiritual challenge. Persons at highest risk for HIV/AIDS (we use the term HIV/acquired immunodeficiency syndrome [AIDS] to designate the entire spectrum of clinical manifestations of HIV disease, from asymptomatic infection through advanced AIDS) are disproportionately likely to suffer behavioral and mood disorders and to be socially disenfranchised and economically disadvantaged. Once infected, they must contend with a still stigmatized, and if untreated, a progressive medical condition. In addition, many people with HIV have other significant comorbidities, such as chronic hepatitis, psychiatric problems, and/or substance use, which may make adhering to HIV treatment more difficult. Although patients with HIV/AIDS can present with life-threatening neuropsychiatric sequalae of HIV (central nervous system [CNS], opportunistic infections, HIV dementia), most patients' behavioral concerns are focused on maintaining medication adherence, maximizing quality of life, and managing lifestyle issues.

EPIDEMIOLOGY & PREVENTION

Human immunodeficiency virus is primarily transmitted through sexual exposure or shared injection drug paraphernalia (sharing needles). Initially, the epidemic was concentrated among gay men in cities; now new cases of HIV infection are disproportionately seen in socioeconomically disadvantaged populations, especially women and men of color. Some patients do not fit "classic" risk factor profiles. For example, a monogamous woman may be infected through her husband who is bisexually active. Although past HIV prevention programs successfully reduced rates of new HIV infections in gay men, incidence of new HIV infection in multiple patient populations is significant. These patient groups include men who have sex with men but who do not self-identify as "gay," speed users who share straws for intranasal use, teenagers, elders, and women. In the United States, about one-quarter of the over 1 million HIV-positive persons have never been tested and are not aware of their seropositive status. In spite of the great advances in treatment, HIV/AIDS remains underdiagnosed and undertreated in the United States and worldwide.

In 2006, the Centers for Disease Control (CDC) formally modified its HIV screening recommendations from that of focused testing in high-risk groups and in high-prevalence settings to universal screening. In this paradigm, *all* patients between the ages of 18–64 years are encouraged to be tested as part of routine preventative care, and detailed consent procedures have been modified to an opt in or out of HIV testing as part of routine care. Newer rapid testing procedures allow for patients to receive their results at the time of testing, improving the number of patients who receive their results and facilitating triage for medical follow-up. Evolving HIV treatment paradigms stress early and even universal treatment of HIV-infected patients. Theoretically, "test and treat" strategies will benefit patients by optimizing immune function, and benefit communities by reducing HIV transmission. At the same time, getting HIV-infected patients tested and engaged in long-term treatment is a persistent challenge. "Engagement in care" is emerging as a model in which patients feel connected with their care providers and their medical care institutions, and correlates not only with retention in treatment but also with treatment success.

Integrating HIV screening and HIV prevention counseling into routine health care activities can facilitate this discussion in primary care settings. For example, following discussion of other lifestyle/health-related issues like cigarette smoking and exercise, sexual practice and substance use questions have a practical context. As in all patient interviews, open-ended questions with the use of specific and understandable language are most likely to put the patient at ease and generate accurate information. For example: Are you sexually active with men, women, both, or neither? How about in the past? What, if any, street drugs do you currently use, for example, speed, pot, etc? How about in the past?

The purpose of these screening questions is not only to identify which patients to test but to identify high-risk behaviors that may be modified, for example, through condom use or needle exchange. Thus, HIV testing is paired with HIV prevention counseling, pairing screening with harm reduction education. Harm reduction programs like needle exchange reduce the spread of HIV infection. Substance use, including alcohol, is highly correlated with unsafe sex behaviors, and patients need to be educated about the risk of combining recreational substances and sexual activity. Preexposure prophylaxis is a harm reduction strategy in which persons at high risk for HIV acquisition receive antivirals to prevent HIV infection. While studies document the biological effectiveness of this strategy, many operational challenges limit its widespread implementation.

Because HIV/AIDS is a significant underrecognized and undertreated public health problem in the United States, generalist practitioners in both outpatient and inpatient settings should be competent in screening and prevention. In addition, in an era in which HIV treatment has become simplified, more durable and better tolerated, another important role for the primary care provider is to help evaluate and address barriers to patient's adherence to treatment. Mental health conditions from preexisting psychiatric disorders like bipolar disorder or from incident conditions like adjustment disorders are common in HIV-infected patients and require active diagnosis and treatment. In addition, cohort studies document a bidirectional relationship between HIV infection and mental health disorders: patients with psychiatric disorders are more likely to engage in high-risk behavior, whereas HIV acquisition can exacerbate mental health disorders.

THE PSYCHOSOCIAL IMPACT OF HIV/AIDS

Overview

Although the course of HIV/AIDS is different for every patient, some common clinical and life events are associated with psychological distress, ranging from mild anxiety and discouragement to feelings of despair and suicide. Although untreated HIV infection is generally fatal, it is now rare for treated HIV patients to die from their infection. However, many "successfully" treated patients may have disabling neurocognitive disorders (mild dementia, neuropathy) profound fatigue, chronic pain, and other disorders. Although the mechanism of some of these symptoms is unclear, it is evident that they are increasingly common. Whether these disorders are due to long-term HIV infection itself, HIV-induced autoimmune sequelae or HIV treatments remains unresolved. However, some HIV-infected patients are asymptomatic and able to lead normal lives: working full time, completing school, and having children.

Women and men with HIV benefit from empathic relationships with their medical providers and from connections with other HIV-positive people. For example, in adherence studies of adult women with HIV, a robust predictor of medication compliance was the patient's perception of her relationship with the clinician. In addition, women who meet other women with HIV (through retreats, support groups, newsletters) are more likely to be medication adherent and to keep medical appointments.

In many urban areas, support groups exist for HIV patients from diverse risk groups (e.g., patients in recovery, gay men with HIV, and so on). In more rural and underserved areas, public health departments may offer case management services for people with HIV. In some cases, these case managers may be the only local source of information, clinician referral, and psychosocial support for patients.

COUNSELING PATIENTS WHO TEST POSITIVE FOR HIV

For most patients, being told that they are infected with HIV is traumatic. Practitioners should anticipate this distress and counsel patients with up-to-date information, and arrange referrals to appropriate HIV care sources, including medical providers and support groups. Web sites can be excellent resources and are best complemented by local support services. Patients who test HIV positive may experience and express a variety of emotional responses. In general, practitioners should allow the patient to express his or her feelings, and should actively listen to the expressed emotions in a nonjudgmental manner. Effective use of empathic statements such as: "I can understand how difficult this must be for you" and "We can work on this together" can help the patient to feel a little less overwhelmed and helpless.

Clinicians should be alert to the potentially wide range of emotional responses expressed by patients and then check their understanding with a reflective statement such as "You seem quite saddened by this news." Often, the emotion that unexpectedly wells up in the physician (e.g., sadness, anger, panic) may be indicative of what the patient is feeling. Physicians can use their own emotions as diagnostic information to gain insight into the patient's feelings (see Chapter 2, "Empathy" and Chapter 3, "Giving Bad News").

Paradoxically, although many persons seek testing to relieve the uncertainty of not knowing their status, testing positive for HIV can create additional uncertainty. Suddenly, they are confronted with not knowing how long they will remain well, who will care for them if they become ill or debilitated, how they will support themselves, and many other unknowns. The physician can help the patient cope with this sudden uncertainty by providing both information and emotional support. It may be helpful to say: "Many people who test positive are concerned because they do not know what to expect—is this true for you?" Some patients are comforted by the physician's acknowledgment that they are the same person they were before the test, but now they possess new information about their health that can be addressed. For example, the clinician can say: "You are the same person today as you were yesterday, only now you *know* that you are HIV-positive. It is important that you have this information so that we can now work together to keep you healthy." Patients should be given up-to-date information about treatment, prognosis, and other medical data, especially if they request it. It has been shown that distress can be decreased if patients are informed about their disease and the treatment options.

Other emotions that the seropositive patient may express include anger, fear, denial, and depression. Patients may feel angry for many reasons: about having an incurable illness, about perceived loss of control, about current or future discrimination. Some patients are angry at themselves for having become infected or at the partner who may have transmitted the virus to them. Allow patients to express their anger and frustration; often the anger dissipates with empathic listening.

Fear is often a less evident emotion and may need to be elicited with questions such as: "What are your major fears about HIV?" and "From your experience with other people with HIV, what kinds of things are most frightening for you?" These fears should be acknowledged as legitimate, and when possible, the physician can help the patient to deal concretely with those problems that can be anticipated and ameliorated. It may be helpful to have the patient make two lists dividing the current or anticipated problems into those that are to some extent controllable and those that are basically uncontrollable. The controllable problems can be addressed through specific **problem-solving** strategies, and the clinician should focus on **emotion-handling skills** for the uncontrollable problems and emotions that may arise (see Chapters 1 and 2).

Denial is a common response to the news of a positive HIV test. For some patients this initially may be a healthy way of not allowing themselves to feel overwhelmed. In fact, some people may need several months to a year to come to terms with the diagnosis. If, however, denial leads patients to harm themselves (e.g., by refusing potentially life-enhancing or life-extending treatment) or to harm others by exposing them to HIV, the physician should challenge the denial. This can be done gently, for example, by saying: "I can understand why you would wish that you were not HIV infected, but you are, and we need to deal with it." Such statements may need to be repeated at subsequent visits until the patient is ready to accept the fact and consequences of their seropositive status.

Depression and anxiety are also common responses in persons who test positive for HIV. The clinician should assess the severity and duration of these symptoms to determine the appropriate treatment. Some studies have found that the risk of suicide is increased in the 3–6 months following a serologic diagnosis, so all patients should be screened for *reactive depression and suicidal ideation*. It is best to use direct, open-ended questions such as: "How are you handling your HIV diagnosis?" and "What fears or concerns do you have?"

In the weeks and months following a positive test, the clinician can assist patients in coping more effectively by assessing their social support system. This can be done by asking: "Who are you talking to about your concerns and issues?" If patients are isolated, provide them with phone numbers of local AIDS service organizations. Family members can also provide valuable support, but often HIV-infected people avoid seeking their help, or the family has previously rejected them because of their lifestyle. Clinicians can help patients by offering to have family or significant others attend medical appointments, and by integrating supportive others into the treatment team.

Managing Substance Use

Active substance use is a risk factor for HIV acquisition, for medical nonadherence, and for reexposure to HIV through unsafe sex and needle sharing. Many cases of new HIV infection are correlated with unsafe sex during alcohol or drug binges. Patients in drug and alcohol recovery have been shown to be able to achieve good adherence. All patients with current or past drug or alcohol problems should be screened for comorbid psychiatric disorders.

Methadone has significant interactions with nonnucleoside reverse transcriptase inhibitors (NNRTIs) and protease inhibitors (PIs). These interactions are not always predictable (e.g., one agent, nevirapine, can both raise and lower methadone levels). When antiviral drugs are changed, patients should be monitored for both methadone intoxication and withdrawal, and their methadone treatment center informed of the need to adjust the methadone dosage.

Many street drugs, for example, heroin and ecstasy, are metabolized by cytochrome P450 3A4 and 2D6 enzymes, enzymes that may be downregulated by a PI booster, ritonavir and cobicistat, an integrase booster. Inadvertent drug overdoses have occurred due to these interactions. Patients who continue to use street drugs and who are on antiretroviral therapy should be counseled in a harm reduction model about these potentially fatal interactions.

WORKING WITH ASYMPTOMATIC & SYMPTOMATIC PATIENTS

 CASE ILLUSTRATION 1

Juan, a 27-year-old Hispanic man with HIV infection is admitted with shortness of breath and fever and diagnosed with PCP (Pneumocystis carinii pneumonia). He was started on HAART but reported that his antivirals made him "dizzy" and "sleepy" and that he stopped them because he was unable to work while taking them. He was unaware that he needed to take the regimen at bedtime to avoid these symptoms. An HIV genotype test showed no resistance and a plan was made to reinitiate the antivirals once his PCP treatment was completed. While hospitalized, he was visited by an adherence counselor and a case manager who helped review his regimen and identify adherence barriers, as well as help with scheduling his clinic follow-up.

Involving patients in the timing and choice of antiviral medications may reduce their anxiety and improve long-term adherence. When patients know what side effects are possible and what the demands may be of different treatment regimens, they can assist the clinician in selecting the most workable antiviral combination. Adherence to a medication regimen is often a challenge for patients with chronic illness (see Chapter 20) and adherence to HIV medications is especially crucial for HIV-positive patients. Newer HIV treatment paradigms may be more or less "forgiving" of patient nonadherence, so skilled clinicians take these differences into account when selecting and reformulating an appropriate treatment regimen.

Ironically, although HAART adherence is critical to success, it is difficult to predict or measure. Multiple studies have revealed that even skilled HIV/AIDS practitioners are often inaccurate at assessing or predicting any individual patient's medication compliance. Across studies, active substance use, untreated psychiatric and behavioral disorders, isolation, transportation problems, health system barriers (to visits or to pick up medications), and changes in routine are all risk factors for nonadherence. On the positive side, patients who experience their clinicians as knowledgeable, trustworthy, and approachable are more likely to comply with their medications, reinforcing the importance of the clinician–patient relationship. In institutions where medical turnover is high (e.g., residency programs, fellowships) engagement in care can be enhanced through continuity with another provider such as a case manager or social worker.

Clinicians should assess and address adherence initially and on an ongoing basis. Open-ended and supportive questions are useful: "How are you doing with remembering your meds?" "How many doses did you miss yesterday? Last week?" "Are you having any side effects that cause you to skip doses?" This assessment provides important clinical information and reinforces the critical importance of medication adherence for the patient.

For most patients, linking doses to routine activities (walking the dog, brushing teeth, waking the children) is helpful. Medisets, beepers, and periodic adherence checks by case managers may also be helpful. Clinicians can regularly reassess each patient's regimen, considering off-label but studied dosing schedules that may be more user-friendly than on-label dosing. During periods when the patient is at high risk of nonadherance, temporarily suspending antivirals (a structured treatment interruption) may be preferable to poor adherence.

SPECIAL ISSUES & POPULATIONS

Hepatitis B & C Coinfection

All patients with HIV should be screened for chronic hepatitis B and C. For some patients learning they have chronic viral hepatitis, in addition to HIV, can be overwhelming. In addition, evaluation for treatment of hepatitis B and C may involve liver biopsy, and currently available treatments for hepatitis C (interferon, ribavirin) can cause severe flu-like symptoms and exacerbate major depression.

The clinician should assess each patient's ability to cope with another diagnosis and plan diagnostic studies accordingly. Patients on an interferon-containing regimen should be closely monitored for depression. Although interferon treatment can exacerbate mental health conditions, many patients can tolerate these exacerbations and a mental health diagnosis alone should not preclude a patient from treatment. A recent study of patients with hepatitis C showed that those with mental health diagnoses had comparable adherence and virologic outcomes compared with patients without psychiatric diagnoses. In fact, with the advent of interferon-sparing hepatitis C (HCV) treatment regimens, most HIV/HCV co-infected patients will be candidates for HCV treatment.

Women

Isolation and stigma are especially common in women with HIV. Women may be especially fearful about disclosing their HIV status for fear of domestic abuse, loss of child custody, or loss of employment. Referral to local and national organizations is often helpful. Pregnant women with HIV benefit from multidisciplinary care teams that can both optimize their HIV care and provide appropriate perinatal care to mother and baby. They should be advised about the risks and appropriate management of perinatal transmission of HIV.

Chronic Pain

Chronic pain is a common complication of HIV disease. Specific causes of chronic pain include postherpetic neuralgia, peripheral neuropathy, avascular necrosis (AVN), and HIV myelopathy (spinal cord dysfunction). In 10% of HIV patients with chronic pain, a specific etiology is not found. Untreated pain can contribute to insomnia, depression, substance use, and medication nonadherence. Patients at highest risk of undertreatment are women, minority patients, and patients with prior or active substance use. Depression is a risk factor for chronic pain and should be screened for in all patients with pain disorders.

General pain management principles (see Chapter 35) can be applied in treating HIV-associated pain. Treatments for chronic pain include agents that elevate neurotransmitters both in the spine and brain; these include older treatments like low-dose tricyclic antidepressants (TCAs), and newer agents like serotonin norephinephrine reuptake inhibitors (SNRIs). Many analgesic and adjunctive medications (e.g., TCAs, carbamazepine, methadone) are metabolized through cytochrome P450 and may interact with NNRTIs and PIs. Gabapentin (Neurontin), Lamictal (lamotrigine), Lyrica (pregabalin), nonsteroidal anti-inflammatory drugs (NSAIDs), acetaminophen, and aspirin have no significant interactions, but their use may be complicated by rash, sedation, renal dysfunction, and other side effects. In patients requiring narcotic therapy, longer-acting agents supplemented by fast-acting narcotics as needed for breakthrough are generally most effective.

Fatigue

Many patients with HIV, even those successfully treated with antivirals, suffer from disabling fatigue. Typically, patients wake with a good deal of energy only to develop severe fatigue with minor activities. Many patients will need to nap and sleep longer than was usual for them. Researchers have speculated that this fatigue may be due to cytokine effects in the brain, neuroendocrine dysregulation, and/or autonomic/circadian rhythm dysregulation.

Before ascribing fatigue to idiopathic HIV-associated fatigue, an extensive differential diagnosis should be considered including depression, anemia, testosterone, deficiency, sleep apnea, chronic hepatitis, hypothyroidism, chronic pain, and medication side effects. Idiopathic HIV-related fatigue may respond to bupropion (Wellbutrin), modafinil (Provigil, Nuvigil), or stimulants. Patients who are otherwise well and wish to resume a full life need validation that their fatigue is real and need to be informed that even with aggressive treatment their stamina may remain limited.

NEUROPSYCHIATRIC COMPLICATIONS

Management of Neuropsychiatric Complications of HIV/AIDS

Clinicians caring for HIV-infected patients must be able to identify specific syndromes (e.g., depression, psychosis), formulate preliminary differential diagnoses, and make appropriate psychotherapy and psychopharmacological referrals. HIV-related neuropsychiatric syndromes are evaluated and treated with the following guidelines:

1. HIV-associated opportunistic infections, which may present as behavioral disorders, are very uncommon in patients with more than 200 CD4 cells or in patients with less than 200 CD4 cells and low or undetectable viral loads.

2. Side effects of prescription or over-the-counter medication commonly cause neuropsychiatric symptoms.

3. Drug interactions (both with prescription and recreational drugs) are of special concern in patients receiving potent suppressors of cytochrome P450 3A4 and 2D6, particularly ritonavir.

4. Recreational drug use and withdrawal can cause symptoms directly or exacerbate preexisting disorders (e.g., bipolar affective disorder).

5. With a few exceptions, HIV-associated neuropsychiatric symptoms are guided by the same treatment principles as for the general population; most psychiatric medications are used at the same dosages and for the same indications.

DRUG EFFECTS

Some of the medications used to treat HIV/AIDS and its complications have common neuropsychiatric side effects. Side effects may be related to cumulative dose or to peak levels or may be unpredictable and idiosyncratic. Furthermore, in patients with advanced HIV disease, the homeostatic mechanisms responsible for maintaining therapeutic drug levels may be disrupted by end-organ involvement, such as decreased renal excretion, hepatic metabolism, or cardiac output; diminished body fat; immunologic dysregulation; and a predisposition toward dehydration. These patients with HIV are, therefore, also more susceptible to side effects from more commonly used medications. The rule of thumb for prescribing to persons with advanced HIV is "say no, start low, and go slow," that is, avoid unnecessary medications, use reduced dosages of those that are necessary, and increase doses slowly and cautiously. Most patients, however, *will* require conventional doses of medications used to treat psychiatric disorders, so the edict "go slow" includes reaching therapeutic doses eventually.

Drug effects and toxicities must always be considered in the initial differential diagnosis of any neuropsychiatric abnormality. A few general principles should be kept in mind. First, use agents with favorable side effect profiles. Second, use caution in the coadministration of medications with similar side effect profiles or those that significantly affect one another's pharmacodynamics. An example of the first situation is the simultaneous use of any combination of antidepressants, antihistamines, neuroleptics, or antimotility agents, all of which have substantial anticholinergic effects. The second concern arises in the use of agents, such as rifampin or rifabutin, which induces the hepatic cytochrome P450 enzyme system and thereby accelerates metabolism of many other drugs or conversely, agents such as ritonavir or delavirdine which inhibit the P450 enzyme.

A third concern is that adherence to complex medication regimens is often unreliable. Incorrect dosing may result in undertreatment for some conditions, but confusion may also result in inadvertent overdosing. Always simplify the regimen and use the lowest dose of the fewest drugs likely to be effective. The assistance of a pharmacist is invaluable in addressing these concerns. If possible, the regimens of patients with advanced HIV/AIDS or on multiple medications should be periodically reviewed by a pharmacist.

Persons with HIV/AIDS on average have higher levels of substance use, in part because of the association between preexisting drug use and the risk of acquiring HIV/AIDS, and perhaps because of self-medication for depression or anxiety. Stimulant drugs such as cocaine or amphetamines can cause agitation, psychosis, or delirium, as can withdrawal from sedating drugs such as benzodiazepines and alcohol. Sedatives and narcotics can not only cause somnolence, confusion, and psychomotor slowing but can also cause paradoxical reactions, including agitation, paranoia, and rage. This may be especially true of the short-acting benzodiazepines.

With regards to specific antiviral agents, two specific points need emphasizing. First, cobicistat or ritonavir-containing regimens, through inhibition of cytochrome P450 enzymes, *may* dramatically raise the level of many prescribed and recreational drugs. These substrates include many anticonvulsants (carbamazepine, valproic acid, phenytoin), narcotics (meperidine, methadone), recreational drugs (3,4-methylenedioxymethamphetamine [MDMA] or Ecstasy), and other agents (warfarin, digoxin, estrogen). Patients receiving these antivirals should be monitored for potential interactions (see Table 36-1).

Second, 2 weeks after starting efavirenz, patients may experience disrupted sleep, depression, agitation, and exacerbation of previously stable psychiatric disease. Whereas case and cohort studies report delayed or persisting neuropsychiatric symptoms due to efavirenz, a prospective double-blinded study failed to show any lingering or delayed CNS side effects attributable to the medication. Conversely, a recent cohort study showed an increased risk of suicidal ideation in patients taking efavirenz long term. Patients with stable psychiatric disorders may be prescribed efavirenz, but should be monitored for drug-associated agitation or depression. All patients who are starting efavirenz should be provided with sleeping medication for the first 2 weeks, either a standard benzodiazepine, or if substance misuse is a concern, a low-dose atypical antipsychotic.

Depression

 CASE ILLUSTRATION 2

Marjorie, a 36-year-old ex-intravenous drug user with a 5-year history of stable HIV disease (undetectable

Table 36-1. Clinically important cytochrome P-450 psychotropic interactions in the treatment of patients with HIV/AIDS.

Psychotropic Medication	Key Enzyme	Clinical HIV Implications
Fluoxetine, paroxetine	2D6, 3A4	May raise PI levels, but not to a clinically significant extent; increased TCA levels
Steraline	2D6, 3A4	Milder effects, not significant
Citalopram	3A4, 2C19	Not clinically significant
Venlafaxine	3A4, 2D6	Few drug–drug interactions
Mirtazapine	3A4, 2D6, 1A2	Not clinically significant
Bupropion	2B6, 3A4	Levels raised with PIs; seizure risk
Lithium	None	Renally excreted ion
Valproate	2D6	Ritonavir interactions
Alprazolam, triazolam, zolpidem, zaleplon	3A4	Increased sedation with PIs
Risperidone	2D6	Avoid with ritonavir
Olanzapine	1A2, 2D6	Cigarettes will decrease levels
Seroquel	3A4	No reported PI or NNRTI interactions
Ziprasidone	Not significant	Check QTc duration
St. John's wort	3A4	May lower levels of PIs

viral load, T cells 500 on HAART), is noted to have a viral load of 14,000. On interview, she reports missing "a few" doses due to "spacing out," "just forgot." She has maintained her sobriety but is not attending Narcotics Anonymous (NA) meetings—"too tired." On further questioning, she reports morning fatigue, insomnia, anhedonia, and hopelessness. A diagnosis of depression is made and she is offered initial treatment with therapy or medication. After attending a support group she recognizes that she has been "depressed a long time" and agrees to both counseling and psychopharmacologic treatment. Because she also has chronic pain from peripheral neuropathy, a dual-active/serotonin norepinephrine reuptake inhibitor (SNRI) medication is initiated with the hope of decreasing pain, improving sleep, and treating her depression.

Major depression is the most common psychiatric disorder in persons with HIV/AIDS. The lifetime incidence is unknown but rises dramatically as the disease progresses. As with non-HIV-infected depressed patients, the cardinal symptoms include depressed mood, anhedonia, feelings of worthlessness and hopelessness, disturbances in sleep and appetite, weight loss or gain, fatigue, psychomotor slowing, agitation, and preoccupation with morbid thoughts (see Chapter 25). A family history of an affective disorder or alcoholism may be present. Depression may be more difficult to diagnose in the presence of HIV/AIDS, however, for several reasons. First, its manifestations, and particularly the vegetative symptoms (fatigue, weakness, weight loss, and loss of libido) commonly overlap with the constitutional symptoms attributable to HIV infection or its complications. Second, organic impairment due to the HIV-associated dementia complex may have affective manifestations. Third, HIV-associated hypogonadism (low testosterone) may cause fatigue, impaired libido, and other depressive symptoms. For some patients, testosterone supplementation has been shown to reverse depressive symptoms. Finally, some medications and the use of or withdrawal from other psychoactive substances, can have mood-altering effects as described previously. Nevertheless, depressive disorders including major depression and dysthymia are diagnosed by the same criteria for HIV-infected as for non-HIV-infected persons and should never be treated as a normal finding. Indeed, recent surveys have documented that untreated depression is a major correlate of poor quality of life in people with HIV disease, and is an important risk factor for noncompliance with treatment.

Certain clues may help to distinguish depressive from constitutional symptomatology. For example, progressive fatigue that worsens with exertion and over the course of the day is characteristic of somatic disease (e.g., anemia), whereas an inability to get going in the morning, which improves with activity, may suggest depression. Similarly, nondepressed patients may report that nausea or dysgeusia (an abnormal sense of taste) interferes with their appetite, whereas depressed patients often report simply no interest in eating. Nondepressed patients often report their symptoms and limitations with frustration and concern, whereas apathy and resignation are more characteristic of major depression. Anhedonia and a sense of worthlessness are rarely symptoms of a somatic condition, and should therefore be directly investigated as specific indicators of depression. Depressed patients may appear more anxious or preoccupied than sad. Patients with depression and anxiety may self-medicate with recreational drugs or alcohol; patients with substance use should be screened carefully for depression and anxiety disorders.

The treatment of depression in HIV/AIDS does not differ from the non-HIV-infected population. Regular, empathic listening and short-term psychotherapeutic techniques may be effective. Explicit recognition and validation of the patient's losses and fears help to establish a trusting therapeutic relationship and may permit developing joint strategies to cope with them. Emphasizing that depression is a common ailment in the setting of HIV/AIDS and is amenable to treatment is important. As with other patients, choosing among the many available agents should be largely a matter of selecting the most desirable or tolerable side effect profile.

The clinician must be alert to how the activity and toxicity profile of particular agents may help in simultaneously addressing other concerns of the patient. For example, appetite and sleep-stimulating medications such as mirtazapine may be effective in patients who suffer from insomnia. A TCA such as nortriptyline or an SNRI may be an ideal choice in a patient with neuropathic pain, who may also benefit from the drug's pain-modulating effects. The risk of cardiac arrhythmias associated with tricyclic drugs may be increased in persons taking ritonavir. Bupropion is especially useful in patients with fatigue, and along with mirtazapine is unlikely to cause sexual dysfunction. Selective serotonin reuptake inhibitors (SSRIs) are especially useful in patients with anxious depression or comorbid anxiety disorders.

Stimulants may be used with other antidepressants in patients with severe refractory fatigue, and can also be used to palliate narcotic-associated fatigue and sedation. Because of their abuse potential, these agents must be used selectively, and their efficacy varies considerably from patient-to-patient.

Isolation from family, religious or spiritual community, or friends can result in demoralization. Because of the stigma of HIV within certain communities, HIV-infected patients may feel cut off from the usual sources of fellowship and support. Support groups, pets, engaged case management, and counseling can help prevent isolation.

Anxiety

As with some depressive symptoms, anxiety may be a normal response to many of the stressors associated with living with HIV. Symptoms of anxiety may include poor concentration, restlessness, preoccupation or intrusive thoughts, insomnia (particularly trouble falling asleep), and fatigue. Persons with poor coping skills may be particularly prone to periods of uncontrollable anxiety. Withdrawal from nicotine, alcohol, or illicit drugs, or overuse of caffeine may cause symptoms of anxiety.

Treatment is indicated if anxiety impairs social or occupational functioning, or is persistently uncomfortable. Pharmacotherapy generally involves the use of SSRIs and other serotonergic antidepressants, or benzodiazepines. For episodic and unpredictable bouts of anxiety, short-to medium-acting benzodiazepines, such as lorazepam (Ativan) or alprazolam (Xanax) are generally more effective, due to their more rapid onset of action. The physician should carefully monitor the frequency of refilling of anxiolytic prescriptions; a pattern of escalating use may suggest that a longer-acting agent or antidepressant therapy is preferable. For chronic disabling anxiety, longer-acting benzodiazepines such as clonazepam (Klonopin), which maintain more stable blood levels, may be more effective and better tolerated. Selective serotonin reuptake inhibitors are useful maintenance agents in the treatment of anxiety syndromes like panic disorder, obsessive-compulsive disorder (OCD), and posttraumatic stress disorder (PTSD).

Patients with anxiety symptoms should be screened for PTSD. A recent study found that PTSD was the most robust predictor of medication and appointment non-adherence. Posttraumatic stress disorder symptoms include easy startling, flashbacks or nightmares, and dissociative symptoms. For some patients, the trauma of living with HIV rekindles memories of prior traumas (abuse, rape, accidents). Studies of incarcerated women with HIV have demonstrated a high rate of PTSD. Posttraumatic stress disorder is best treated with focused counseling, although SSRIs have been shown to help alleviate some of its symptoms.

PRIMARY CNS DISEASE: THE HIV-ASSOCIATED DEMENTIA COMPLEX

Human immunodeficiency virus-associated dementia is a subcortical dementia initially characterized by cognitive and behavioral dysfunction, and in its most advanced stages by motor dysfunction. Advanced HIV dementia is rarely seen in patients with more than 200 CD4 cells or who are on effective antiviral therapy. Although antivirals differ in their penetration of cerebrospinal fluid (CSF), all combinations of antivirals that suppress serum viral load are likely to prevent HIV dementia. Rarely, genotypic analysis of CSF and blood reveals the presence of different HIV strains. In these cases, some experts recommend that antiviral medication may need to be adjusted to treat the CSF strains.

All patients with HIV dementia should be evaluated for comorbid depression, as depressive symptoms can easily be misattributed to dementia. A trial of antidepressants may result in gratifying functional improvement in these patients. As in all patients with organic brain disease, sedating agents like antihistamines and benzodiazepines should be used with great caution and in general avoided.

HIV-Associated Minor Cognitive Disorders

Although HIV dementia is rare in HIV patients undergoing treatment and in patients with more than 200 CD4 cells, minor cognitive problems can persist and even progress in patients with good surrogate markers (e.g., adequate CD4 cells and/or suppressed viral load). HIV-associated minor cognitive disorders are characterized by word-finding problems, difficulty sequencing complex tasks, and immediate memory dysfunction. Patients may note pauses in conversations while searching for words, difficulty performing clerical tasks, and difficulty multitasking.

Minor cognitive disorders may persist or progress in patients who are otherwise responding well to antiviral therapy. Although minor cognitive disorders tend not to progress, they are often disabling, despite patients appearing "normal." These cognitive symptoms need to be carefully recorded in patients' charts should disability status need to be assessed. Formal neuropsychiatric testing can document subtle cognitive dysfunction. Neuroimaging studies performed in research settings have correlated loss of both frontal lobe volume and frontal metabolic activity in patients with these symptoms. Standard mini-mental status tests are not appropriate diagnostic tools to diagnose minor cognitive disorder; the cognitive domains addressed in this tool are different from the executive task domains impaired in minor HIV cognitive disorder.

Mania

Mania can be a terrifying and dangerous complication of HIV/AIDS. As in non-HIV-infected persons, mania is characterized by hyperactivity and psychomotor restlessness, euphoric or irritable mood, insomnia and perceived decreased need for sleep, pressured or rapid speech, grandiosity or paranoia, racing thoughts, distractibility, hypersexuality, and reckless or disinhibited hedonistic behavior. Mania in HIV/AIDS can be due to a preexisting bipolar diathesis precipitated by substance use, stress, or intercurrent illness. Less frequently, mania may be an initial manifestation of HIV-associated organic brain disease like opportunistic infections or dementia. Medications reported to cause mania include high-dose corticosteroids, antidepressants, zidovudine, efavirenz, and stimulant drugs such as cocaine and amphetamine derivatives.

Treatment involves first discontinuing any potential pharmacological precipitant and ensuring a safe social environment. No specific antimania drug is best for HIV-associated mania—pragmatically, agents should be selected with the goal of calming the patient without undue sedation. Lithium, a mainstay of treatment for bipolar affective disorder in non-HIV-infected patients, may be more risky for patients with advanced AIDS in whom levels appear to fluctuate unpredictably. Dehydration, due to diarrhea, fever, or poor intake can quickly result in toxic lithium levels, further complicating management. However, lithium can be used safely in medically healthy HIV patients.

Psychosis

As with mania, psychotic symptoms are generally due to underlying psychiatric disease (schizophrenia) or drug (prescription, recreational) side effects. Psychotic symptoms include hallucinations, typically auditory rather than visual; delusions, which tend to be paranoid in content; looseness of association; and flight of ideas. Personal care and hygiene may be neglected, and medication adherence is poor. Use of or withdrawal from many illicit drugs, including amphetamines, phencyclidine, cocaine, alcohol, marijuana, and opiates, may cause a transient psychosis, and psychosis caused by methamphetamine in particular may last for days or weeks. Psychosis may complicate administration of the anticytomegalovirus drugs ganciclovir and foscarnet, anabolic or corticosteroids, zidovudine, efavirenz, opiates, other psychoactive pharmaceuticals including sedatives and antidepressants, and, very rarely, many ordinary antimicrobial agents. Psychosis is a rare manifestation of underlying secondary CNS infection or neoplasm.

Treatment of HIV/AIDS-associated psychosis involves identification and removal of precipitating drugs and treatment as appropriate. Psychiatric consultation is essential to confirm the diagnosis, identify possible secondary causes, and optimize management. Atypical antipsychotic agents are effective in acute and maintenance treatment of psychosis. These atypical agents are less likely to cause tardive dyskinesia and are less sedating than older agents.

Many patients with schizophrenia and HIV are "triply diagnosed," that is, they also use recreational substances. These patients often benefit from day treatment programs where medical treatment is integrated with their mental health care, and where medication adherence can be facilitated through directly observed therapy.

CONCLUSIONS

Similar to all chronic medical disorders, HIV disease can be complicated by a myriad of psychiatric and spiritual challenges. Some patients acquire HIV as a consequence of their psychiatric disorders; others face psychospiritual challenges as they live with HIV. Although all patients benefit from accurate psychiatric assessment, patients also benefit from an ongoing relationship with a clinician they perceive as knowledgeable, caring, and trustworthy. In the authors' experience, no other area of medicine requires such a skillful integration of the science and the art of medicine, nor offers such rewards for doing so.

SUGGESTED READINGS

Letendre S. Central nervous system complications in HIV Disease: HIV associated neurocognitive disorder. *Topics Antiviral Med* 2011;19:137–142.

Valcour V. Evaluating cognitive impairment in the clinical setting: practical screening and assessment tools. *Topics Antiviral Med* 2011;19:175–180.

Altice FL, Kamarulzaman A, Soriano VV, Schechter M, Friedland GH. Treatment of medical, psychiatric, and substance-use comorbidities in people infected with HIV who use drugs. *Lancet* 2010 Jul;376(9738):367–387.

WEB SITES

HIV Insite Web site. http://hivinsite.ucsf.edu/InSite. Provides comprehensive up-to-date information on HIV/AIDS treatment, prevention, and policy with links for clinicians and patients. Accessed June 2013.

Project Inform Web site. http://www.projinf.org. An HIV advocacy organization that issues up-to-date information about HIV research. Accessed June 2013.

WORLD Web site. http://www.womenhiv.org/. A national support group for women with HIV. Accessed June 2013.

Errors in Medical Practice

Albert W. Wu, MD, MPH; John F. Christensen, PhD; & Stephen J. McPhee, MD

INTRODUCTION

Errors are inevitable in the practice of medicine. The most obvious causes are failures in individual performance related to attention, memory, knowledge, judgment, skill, and motivation. However, they also result in part from the nature of medical work, such as the complexity of medical knowledge, the uncertainty of clinical predictions, and the need to make timely treatment decisions in spite of limited or uncertain knowledge. And importantly, mistakes are caused by system factors that influence working conditions. Although much attention has been focused on the harmful effects of errors on patients, it must be understood that these incidents can be correspondingly distressing for physicians, evoking shock and feelings of remorse, guilt, anger, and fear.

If dealt with effectively, errors can provide powerful learning experiences for physicians; however, difficulty in dealing with mistakes may impede both learning and efforts to prevent future errors. Professional norms that assume physician infallibility and treat mistakes as anomalies pose significant barriers to learning. Judgmental institutional responses and fear of litigation are further disincentives to the open discussion of mistakes and reduce the potential for wider learning.

Definitions

It is useful to define several terms related to what are commonly referred to as errors or mistakes. The Institute of Medicine (IOM) defines an **error** as "the failure of a planned action to be completed as intended (i.e., error of execution), or the use of a wrong plan to achieve an aim (i.e., error of planning). An error may be an act of commission or an act of omission." An **adverse event** is an injury due to health care. Errors differ from adverse events because they do not necessarily cause harm. They differ from **negligence** or **malpractice**, which require both preventable harm and violation of the standard of practice.

Prevalence

Most studies of medical errors have focused on the hospital setting and on adverse events. Although the overall prevalence of errors is difficult to ascertain, it appears that they are common. Studies conducted in multiple states and countries suggest that the rate of adverse events may be as high as 10%. The Canadian Adverse Events Study reported on the incidence of adverse events among hospital patients in Canada. The authors randomly selected four hospitals (one teaching, one large community, and two small community hospitals) in each of five Canadian provinces and reviewed a random sample of charts for nonpsychiatric, nonobstetric adult patients hospitalized in each hospital during 2000. Trained reviewers screened all eligible charts, and physicians reviewed the positively screened charts to identify adverse events and to determine whether they were preventable. After adjustment for sampling, the adverse event rate was 7.5 per 100 hospital admissions (7.5%). Among the adverse events experienced by patients, 36.9% were judged to have been preventable; 20.8% of these preventable events resulted in death. According to the physician reviewers, the adverse events were associated with an estimated 1521 additional hospital days.

In a study of 254 medical residents (conducted by the authors), 45% reported a significant mistake made during the prior year. In a survey of 2637 US and Canadian physicians, 55% reported involvement in a serious error.

The prevalence of errors in outpatient practice is less well studied, but one investigator has documented a prescription error rate of 7.6%, and another suggests errors in at least one-quarter of the encounters, with a rate of adverse drug events of 27 per 100 patients. A literature synthesis found that the median preventable adverse drug events prevalence rate was 16.5% in ambulatory care-based studies. A study of ambulatory oncology care found that medication reconciliation resulted in 31 changes per 100 prescriptions. A survey of patients attending primary care clinics found that nearly one in three reported experiencing a mistake or diagnostic error by a physician in the previous 10 years, with 14% of patients having changed physicians as a result.

Types

Mistakes occur in every aspect of medical practice—diagnosis, decision making (often because of ignorance of facts), the pace of evaluation or its timing, prescribing medications, and performing tests and procedures (Table 37-1). In the Harvard Medical Practice Study, the most common adverse events involved performance of or follow-up of a procedure or operation (35%). Failure to take preventive measures (e.g., failure to guard against accidental injury) was the next most common error (22%), followed by diagnostic errors (e.g., failure to use indicated tests, act on test results, or avoid delays in response; 14%), errors involving drug treatment (9%), and system errors (2%).

Cognitive Errors. Cognitive errors may result from failures in perception, faulty pattern recognition, and common biases in thinking. Two broad areas of cognitive functioning are relevant in these errors: the schematic and attentional control modes. In the *schematic control* mode of functioning, which is typical of the expert, sequences of thinking and acting are embedded in unconscious subroutines that allow more mental energy to be available for other activities. Examples would be speaking one's native language or driving a vehicle. In medicine, some procedural skills as well as pattern recognition skills (such as an intuitive appreciation of a patient's condition or hunch about a diagnosis) are under schematic control. When an anomaly occurs, or when the physician is fatigued or stressed, a shift occurs to the *attentional control* mode, which is more energy intensive and requires more deliberate thinking and action. This model is more prevalent in the novice learning any new skill (a foreign language, a new procedural skill). The attentional control mode can more quickly degrade over time. Errors can occur in each of these cognitive modes. A momentary break in a skilled routine in surgery, or a lapse in attention that leads to missing data are common examples.

Other cognitive errors result from biases inherent in human thinking. Among these are thinking tendencies such as the "availability" bias, in which the first diagnosis that comes to mind is deemed most likely; the "confirmatory" bias, in which only data supportive of the first hypothesis is entertained; the "recency" bias, in which the last serious diagnosis managed looms large in probability estimates; and the "gambler's fallacy," in which a series of similar diagnoses leads the clinician to expect that the next presentation will be of a different disease.

Procedural Errors. Procedural errors occur in both surgical and nonsurgical procedures. One study suggested that major complications occurred in 3.4% of surgical operations. Wrong site surgeries and retained foreign bodies are rare, but can have devastating consequences for patients. Causes include individual errors—such as surgical technique (including slips and fumbles), judgment errors, inattention to detail—and incomplete understanding of the case. Other causes occur at other levels of the system, including poor communication among members of the perioperative team, poor planning (e.g., surgical implant not available on the day of surgery), lack of teamwork, and surgical site infection. Surgical site infections are common, with overall incidence rates in the United States of about 3%, and there is great variability associated with procedure and site. Contributions to error in nonsurgical procedures (e.g., endoscopy, lumbar puncture, line placement) include fatigue and disruptions. Many might have been prevented by use of the Joint Commission Universal Protocol or by simulation training.

System Errors. Errors occur throughout the health care system, many arising from the inherent fallibility of human beings working within systems not primarily designed for safety. Errors occur at the level of patient, task, individual practitioner, team, unit, organization, and beyond. They also occur in multiple locations, such as in the clinical diagnostic laboratories, the pharmacy, and the preparation and maintenance of medical devices. Identification errors, which involve confusing one patient, test, or treatment for another, are a common element in many adverse events. Another common occasion for errors is in the handoffs between different health care providers and locations of care. Communication problems are at the root of many adverse events as are problems with team functioning.

Table 37-1. Types of medical mistakes.

Error	Example
Diagnosis or evaluation	Missed diagnosis
Medical decision making	Inappropriate or premature discharge
Treatment	Waiting when treatment is indicated
Medication	Incorrect dosage
Procedural complications	Faulty technique
Faulty communication	Failure to convey information during sign-out
Inadequate supervision	Failure to review treatment plan

Source: Adapted, with permission, from Wu AW, Folkman S, McPhee SJ, LoB. Do house officers learn from their mistakes? *JAMA* 1991;265:2089–2094.

Medication Errors. Medication errors are very common, in part because of the ubiquity of the use of medications. In the United States, more than four out of five adults take at least one medication in a given week, and almost a third of adults take at least five different medications. The goal of safe and effective medication use is referred to as "the five rights": the right drug, right dose, right route, right time, and right patient. However, errors can occur with any drug product at any point in the medication use process. It is estimated that over 1.5 million people are injured by medication errors each year and that, on average, hospitalized patients are subjected to an average of one medication error per day.

Causes

A combination of individual human and system-related factors can lead to adverse events. Human error, which occurs at what is sometimes referred to as the "sharp end" of adverse events, happens close to the patient and includes deficits in skill (attention, memory, and execution), knowledge, decision making, and following of rules. System errors, the "blunt end" of adverse events, occur at multiple levels, including at the levels of patient, task, individual provider, team, unit environment, department, and institution. Examples of system errors include use of handwritten prescriptions, team members who are unfamiliar with one another, inadequate communication at change of shifts, understaffed units, inadequate equipment, long work hours, and production pressures. It should be kept in mind that individuals are part of and function within the system of health care delivery.

Individual physicians report a variety of reasons for their mistakes and frequently attribute the mistakes to more than one cause. In one study, house officers most often reported that mistakes were caused in part because they did not possess specific essential knowledge (e.g., being unaware of the significance of a prolonged episode of ventricular tachycardia). Almost as often, they cited "too many tasks" (one resident neglected to continue a required medication because he was "too busy with other sick patients, and supervising interns and students"). Fatigue was a significant factor (after inadvertently ordering potassium replacement as a bolus, one resident commented, "It was 3:00 A.M., and I'm not sure I was completely awake."). Fatigue can interfere with the clinician's ability to rely upon the "schematic control" mode of cognitive functioning, leading to more reliance on the less efficient "attentional control" mode, which is more vulnerable to decay. The common cognitive biases mentioned above also contribute to diagnostic and decision making errors by the individual clinician.

Many errors are caused by conditions in the workplace and organizational processes largely independent of clinician attributes. Studies of system factors demonstrate the predictive power of these characteristics independent of physician identity. One study of an inpatient medical service found cross-coverage to be a significant predictor of preventable adverse events. Recent studies suggest that staffing ratios tend to be related to patient outcomes. The pressures of practicing medicine in a managed care setting, especially in prospective payment systems with higher demands for productivity, may increase the risk that a hurried physician will overlook important diagnostic information or make an error in prescription. Similarly, the incentives offered by third-party payers to order fewer diagnostic tests and to limit the number of referrals to subspecialists can lead to errors of omission.

An overlooked contributor to the prevalence of medical errors is the culture of medicine itself. Historically the "hidden curriculum" in medical training has held up an ideal of perfectionism that is heroic in fantasy but unattainable in practice. This perspective views mistakes as a failure of character, often leading to a "blame and shame" response to individual physician error. This habit of over-focusing on individual perfection has led to an unrealistic reliance on error-free performance. It underplays the "blunt end" of system errors and overemphasizes the "sharp end" of clinician error. These cultural biases tend to drive discussion of mistakes underground, thus avoiding the reporting and discussion of error that can lead to meaningful change.

A systems-oriented view acknowledges that errors are expected even in the best of organizations. Lucian Leape, a leading scholar of medical error, has suggested, "*Any system that relies on error-free performance is doomed to fail. We need to build systems that assume errors will occur, but that can identify and absorb them before they become catastrophes.*"

Circumstances

Mistakes seem to occur particularly frequently during residency training, possibly because interns and residents are learning new skills, honing their clinical judgment, and accepting new responsibilities. Additionally, they are caring for patients who are acutely ill. However, although first-year residents made the highest proportion of prescription errors (4.25 per 1000 orders) according to one study, even more experienced physicians have reported making serious medical mistakes.

Many mistakes happen in the inpatient or emergency department setting. The surgical specialties and intensive care units have also been identified as areas of high risk for patient safety. Severely ill patients require rapid assessment of a complex clinical picture as well as multiple procedures, evaluations, and decisions, thus affording many opportunities for mistakes to occur. One study found that patients in intensive care units had on average 178 activities performed on them, with 1.7 errors observed per day.

Patient characteristics can also increase the risk of mistakes. The risk of adverse events increases with increased age, severity of illness, length of hospital stay, and number of drugs prescribed. Older patients, for example, are likely to have advanced disease and comorbid conditions and are more likely to be taking numerous medications. These factors increase both the risk of errors and the likelihood that these errors will cause harm.

Serious medical mistakes also occur in office practice. In the United States, the main source of medical care for patients is in ambulatory settings. Due to the decentralized structure and diverse nature of events, medical errors can be common. Three top patient safety concerns are medication adverse events, diagnostic errors, and surgical errors. A study of malpractice claims showed that the former two errors are of concern for outpatient treatment and diagnosis of cancer. Some patients may be at increased risk. For example, patients older than 64 years of age are more vulnerable to medication errors. Some practicing physicians contend that the probability of making a serious error increases with more years in practice and particularly with greater pressures to increase productivity.

THE OUTCOMES OF MEDICAL MISTAKES

Consequences for Patient & Family

Some errors may have no major consequences for patients. In such cases, clinicians may not even be aware that an error has occurred. Often, however, errors have significant consequences for the patients involved, such as physical discomfort, emotional distress, need for additional therapy or procedures, increased and prolonged hospital stay, worsening of disease, permanent disability, or death. Mistakes can also cause distress for family members, including worry, anger, and guilt, particularly if they were involved in making treatment decisions.

Consequences for Physicians

Physicians may also experience emotional distress in reaction to a medical mistake, often reporting a variety of emotional responses from remorse, anger, guilt, and feelings of inadequacy to shame and fear—particularly the fear of negative repercussions, such as malpractice suits. After a fatal mistake involving a young patient, one house officer wrote, "This event has been the greatest challenge to me in my training."

Self-perceived errors have been associated with decreased quality of life, depression, and burnout among physicians. Some physicians report persistent negative psychological effects and impact on their career from mistakes that they have made. After a mistake caused the death of a patient, one house officer commented, "This case has made me very nervous about clinical medicine. I worry now about all febrile patients, since they may be on the verge of sepsis." For another house officer, a missed diagnosis made him reject a career in subspecialties that would involve "a lot of data collection and uncertainty."

Consequences for the Physician–Patient Relationship

In some cases, depending on the severity of the outcome for the patient and the quality of communication between physician and patient, the physician–patient relationship may be harmed by a mistake. For the physician, feelings of guilt and shame or shaken confidence may lead to avoidance of the patient or to a diminution of open and frank discussion. One physician, for example, reported that his guilt from the death of a patient led him to act like an indentured servant to the patient's family, attempting to expiate his "crime" over a prolonged period of time by spending more time with the family and reducing his fees.

For the patient, learning about a mistake may cause alarm and anxiety, destroying the patient's faith and confidence in the physician's ability to help. There may be anger, erosion of trust, decreased respect, or feelings of betrayal that diminish openness. Patients may become disillusioned with the medical profession in general, causing them to reduce their adherence to beneficial treatments or habits.

If the doctor and patient can discuss their emotions directly and with mutual understanding and acceptance, the relationship is likely to endure; it may even deepen with time. The negative effect of a mistake on the doctor–patient relationship may also be mitigated if there is a history of shared decision making, which diffuses the responsibility of the physician, especially when there has been uncertainty about treatment.

Mistakes that are nationally—or even locally—reported in the press can damage public trust in the medical profession. Any loss of credibility can be harmful to public health by creating cynicism about medical care and research, as well as discouraging individuals from seeking care or adopting healthful behaviors. Vilification by media coverage can also have adverse effects on individual professionals.

RESPONDING TO MEDICAL MISTAKES

The way in which physicians respond to mistakes can turn these experiences into powerful opportunities for learning and for personal growth. Figure 37-1 outlines a strategy for handling a mistake, whether made by oneself or by a colleague.

Figure 37-1. Strategy for Handling Mistakes

Individual Responses

After recognizing that a mistake has occurred, the first step is to take any corrective action possible. Other important steps include beginning one's own coping process, disclosure to the patient and family, disclosure to colleagues and the health organization's risk management department (sooner if there is a serious adverse outcome), and attempting to learn from the incident.

Individual Coping With Mistakes

Two major modes of coping are *problem focused*, in which coping is directed at the problem causing the distress, and *emotion focused*, in which coping is directed at managing the emotional distress caused by the problem. Effective coping can prevent unhealthy responses such as denial, cynicism, and excessive concern. The use of effective coping strategies can also play a role in modulating physician stress and increasing physician work satisfaction.

Table 37-2 briefly summarizes some of the many possible strategies for coping with medical mistakes. Among these, accepting responsibility and problem-solving techniques may be those most often used. As an example, "accepting responsibility" would include statements such as "I made a promise to myself that things would be different next time"; "I criticized or lectured

Table 37-2. Potential strategies for coping with medical mistakes.

Approach	Strategy
Problem focused	Acceptance of responsibility
	Consultation to understand nature of mistake
	Consultation to correct mistake
	Planned problem solving (e.g., obtaining extra training)
Emotion focused	Pursuance of social support
	Reframing of mistake (e.g., recognizing it as inherent in practicing medicine)
	Disclosure to colleague, friend, or spouse
	Disclosure to patient
	Emotional self-control (e.g., repressing one's emotional response)
	Escape/avoidance
	Distancing

Source: Adapted, with permission, from Wu AW, Folkman S, McPhee SJ, et al. How house officers cope with their mistakes: doing better but feeling worse? *West J Med* 1993;159:565–569; Christensen JF, Levinson W, Dunn PM. The heart of darkness: the impact of perceived mistakes on physicians. *J Gen Intern Med* 1992;7:424.

myself"; and "I apologized or did something to make it up." Seeking social support and controlling emotions may be somewhat less frequently employed, and escape/avoidance and distancing are used even more rarely.

Accepting responsibility is a prerequisite to an individual learning from a mistake, and physicians who cope by accepting responsibility for their mistakes seem to be more likely to make constructive changes in practice. They may also be more likely to experience emotional distress, however, as in the case of the resident who described persistent feelings of guilt and shame after realizing that inappropriate management of a diabetic patient's foot ulcer led to an amputation.

Disclosure to Patients & Families

It is difficult to disclose mistakes to patients or their families, and several reports suggest that physicians are reluctant to tell patients about mistakes. Studies suggest that physicians and trainees have conflicting feelings of responsibility to the patient, colleagues, institution, and themselves. These feelings are complicated by fears, anxieties, and an uncertain self-efficacy and outcome expectancy. There are many barriers to disclosure, including fear of damaging one's reputation as well as fear of disciplinary action and litigation. Even the National Practitioner Databank, designed to improve quality of care, provokes fear and resentment among physicians. In one study, disclosure of mistakes to patients or families was reported by less than 25% of house officers.

Professional societies, including the American Medical Association and American College of Physicians, as well as legal and ethical experts suggest that in general physicians should disclose errors to those involved. In 2001, the US Joint Commission on Accreditation of Healthcare Organizations (JCAHO) announced an "unanticipated outcome" policy that demands disclosure of a critical event by the provider or the institution. The Canadian Disclosure Guidelines (Canadian Patient Safety Institute, 2011) state that "when a harmful incident occurs, the patient should be told what happened. Disclosure acknowledges and informs the patient, which is critical in maintaining the patient's trust and confidence in the healthcare system." Disclosure of a mistake also fosters learning by compelling the physician to acknowledge the error truthfully. In addition, when there are serious adverse consequences, disclosing a mistake to the patient may be the only way for the physician to achieve a sense of absolution. Lazare has suggested a framework for the use of apologies that includes four parts: (1) acknowledgement of the offense; (2) explanation for committing the offense; (3) expression of remorse, shame, and humility; and (4) reparation.

In the past, physicians have been unaware of the guidelines that exist on disclosing adverse events to patients, leaving them to develop their own approach to each case. Disclosure and discussion of an error with the patient or family can be made easier by several techniques. Physicians should first try to acknowledge their own emotions. Before approaching the patient or family, it may be helpful for physicians to perform a simple relaxation exercise and to remind themselves that the event and present feelings do not define them as either a healer or a person. Rehearsing a few simple, direct statements ahead of time can provide a road map in this awkward moment. When meeting the patient or family, the physician should make a brief, direct statement, accompanied by a genuine apology. Such directness may help avoid the kind of long and rambling discussion that often increases anxiety for both physician and patient.

The physician who has mistakenly prescribed a medication without checking the patient's allergies, for example, might tell the patient: "Mr. Jones, I've discovered what made you sick last week. I regret to say that I failed to check whether you were allergic to the antibiotic before I prescribed it. You are allergic to it, and that information is clearly in your medical record. I feel awful that my not checking has caused you so much distress. I am truly sorry." It would then be appropriate to pause and allow the patient to respond. Reflecting and accepting the patient's feelings can help to heal the relationship more effectively than overwhelming the patient with information. The doctor–patient relationship can be enhanced by honesty and empathy in this difficult and sensitive moment (see Chapter 3).

It is possible that disclosure of an error of which the patient had been unaware may lead to a lawsuit, particularly if there was serious harm. It is certain, however, that the risk of a lawsuit is multiplied when a cover-up comes to light. Limited evidence suggests that risk may be reduced if disclosure is made promptly, if the patient appreciates the physician's honesty, if it is part of an ongoing dialogue about the patient's care, and if there is a sincere apology. In the event of serious injury, a prompt and fair settlement may be essential.

Several organizations have reduced costs and litigation as a result of a policy of full disclosure. One study that modeled the potential litigation consequences of disclosure found that an increase in litigation volume and costs was highly likely. However, the favorable experience of the Lexington Kentucky VA Medical Center, which instituted a proactive policy of full disclosure and assistance for the patient in filing claims, as well as a reduction in claims experienced at the University of Michigan, suggests that this strategy may decrease the institution's losses. Based in part on both of these models, the University of Illinois Medical Center (UIMC) in Chicago has adopted institutional guidelines toward initiating a full disclosure policy. The UIMC emphasized five principles, including effective and honest communication to patients and families, a sincere apology and rapid compensation for inappropriate care, learning from mistakes, quick disciplinary action for recklessness, and proper support for physicians and staff. There were seven pillars of their guidelines. First, they emphasized patient safety incident reporting. Second, in the case of an incident there was immediate, standardized investigation. Third, a risk manager or patient safety officer would aid physicians in communication and full disclosure. Fourth, if harm came from unreasonable care, there was early compensation, apology, and remediation. Fifth, there was prompt system improvement following a root cause analysis. Sixth, there was data tracking and performance evaluation of the system improvement. Seventh, there was education and training for all personnel on the system improvement. The results of these guidelines revealed no increase in litigation or compensation. There was also direct extrapolation from transparency to the pursuit of safety in risk management. Another result was increased recognition of provider stress leading to peer support. Finally, these guidelines emphasized the crucial importance of timeliness in responding to any patient safety incident.

Empirical research on the disclosure of medical errors to patients and their families has been limited. Published studies have focused primarily on the decision stage of disclosure. Fewer have considered the disclosure process, consequences of disclosure, or relationship between the two. More research is needed to understand how disclosure decisions are made, to give physicians guidance on the process of disclosure, and to help all involved anticipate the consequences of disclosure.

Many publications have examined why patients sue their doctors. Although they suggest that some lawsuits may be averted by disclosure of medical errors, these publications do not allow us to estimate the additional lawsuits that could be created by disclosure. More studies are needed to determine the effect of disclosure on physicians' malpractice liability. One recent study using video vignettes suggests that full disclosure is likely to have a positive or no effect on how patients respond to medical errors. Some survey data suggest that patients confident in a doctor's commitment to disclosure are less likely to pursue litigation and will be more likely to recommend the doctor to other patients.

Disclosure to Colleagues & the Institution

It may be very important for colleagues to know about a mistake, particularly if they are also participating in the care of the patient as a supervisor or other member of the team. Knowing about a mistake can also benefit the institution, enabling it to provide assistance in handling the mistake, to help individuals appreciate the causes or significance of the incident and learn from it, and to prevent future occurrences. Physicians, however, seem reluctant to tell their colleagues about mistakes. Some physicians report that they find this kind of discussion both threatening, because of the fear of judgment by colleagues, and unhelpful, because of the tendency of colleagues to minimize the event. Discussing mistakes with colleagues, however, serves the purpose of problem-focused coping: correcting the situation that led to the mistake. Sharing mistakes with colleagues can also prevent isolation and start the necessary healing process of remorse and learning.

Changes in Practice

Table 37-3 summarizes changes in practice that often follow medical mistakes. These changes can either be constructive or they can be defensive—and maladaptive—in nature. Constructive changes cited by physicians include paying more attention to detail, confirming clinical data personally, changing protocols for diagnosis and treatment, increasing self-care, changing methods of communication with staff, and being willing to seek advice. Additional constructive action includes attempting to effect institutional change to prevent future incidents.

Physicians also report making defensive changes. These include an unwillingness to discuss the mistake, avoidance of similar patients, and—in some circumstances—ordering additional tests. Defensive changes in practice

Table 37-3. Common changes in practice following mistakes.

Constructive Change	Defensive Change
Increasing information seeking • Asking advice • Reading Increasing vigilance • Paying more attention to detail • Confirming data personally • Changing data organization • Ordering additional tests as appropriate • Improving screening for disease Improving communication with patients Improving self-pacing Improving communication with staff Supervising others more closely	Being unwilling to discuss the error Avoiding patients with similar problems Ordering additional but unnecessary tests

are more likely to occur if the institutional response to a mistake is punitive or judgmental.

Learning from Errors

Several factors may determine the extent to which physicians learn from mistakes. When negative emotions such as shame, guilt, or humiliation follow from the mistake, the physician's energy may focus on the emotional aspects of coping. Addressing these negative emotions directly can enhance the physician's ability to learn new information or new approaches to the problem. Failure to appreciate these emotions can lead to denial. The cause to which the physician attributes the mistake can also affect learning. Physicians in one study were more likely to report constructive changes if the mistake was caused by inexperience or faulty judgment in a complex case; they were less likely to do so if they believed that the mistake was caused by job overload. Physicians who responded to the mistake with greater acceptance of responsibility and more discussion were also more likely to report constructive changes.

Responding to Colleagues Who Make Mistakes

When responding to a colleague who discloses an error, it is important to elicit or accept the colleague's self-assessment and not to minimize the importance of the incident. At this point, a selective and discreet disclosure of one's own mistakes can reduce the colleague's sense of isolation and legitimize the discussion. It is then appropriate to inquire about the emotional effect of the mistake and how the colleague is coping with it. An important consideration here is that negative emotions are not necessarily problems to be solved, and they can often be mitigated by acknowledging them. The clinician should return to the content of the mistake and help the colleague to correct it with problem-solving techniques, making the necessary changes in practice and incorporating the new lessons that have been learned.

Providing a safe setting in which clinicians can share mistakes and their emotional impact can correct the culture of perfectionism and provide a mutually supportive approach to learning from these experiences. One of the authors (JFC) has developed a workshop format in which physicians from various specialties have reflected in small groups on their mistakes. After writing a brief narrative of the event, they discuss in a confidential format the emotional impact the mistake had on them, how they coped with these emotions, whether they disclosed the error to anyone, the personal beliefs underlying their emotional responses, and the changes in clinical practice that ensued.

One institutional approach to supporting clinicians suffering emotionally in the wake of errors is the development of a "second victim" support team. In this approach, a team of clinicians is trained to provide emergency peer support to clinicians involved in a traumatic patient-related event. Additional levels of support are then offered in the days and weeks following the event, depending on the clinician's needs.

Witnessing Mistakes by Others

A physician who sees an error made by another physician has several options: passively waiting for the physician to disclose to the patient, advising the physician to disclose the mistake, actively telling the patient oneself, or arranging a joint meeting to discuss the mistake. Although some physicians may feel an obligation to report mistakes they have seen, most are reluctant to say anything. There are many barriers to such a discussion, including fear of eliciting anger and threatening relationships with colleagues or referral sources.

The simplest option, of course, is to wait for the physician who made the mistake to report it. There is no assurance, however, that the patient will actually be informed. Telling the patient directly may be awkward, particularly if the observing physician does not know the patient, and may interfere with the existing doctor–patient relationship. Advising the physician who made the error to tell the patient may fulfill the observing physician's responsibility for disclosure, but the patient may still not be informed. Simultaneously advising the physician and the hospital or clinic quality-assurance or risk-management personnel increases the likelihood that the patient will be told. Arranging a joint conference can satisfy the observer that appropriate disclosure is made while preserving the primacy of the relationship between the patient and the treating physician (see Figure 37-1).

INSTITUTIONAL RESPONSES

Hospitals

A goal for institutions is to develop a "safety culture" that allows learning from adverse events. A safety culture encourages clinicians to be aware of the potential for error and to include system thinking in their everyday practices, and it provides adequate data regarding errors to managers. Physicians sometimes feel that the hospital's atmosphere inhibits them from talking about their mistakes and that its administration is judgmental about mistakes. To avoid a vicious circle of blame, denial, and repeated problems, it is crucial for senior leadership in hospitals to assume a blame-free attitude that encourages the reporting and handling of errors. Some institutions have formal settings for discussing mistakes, such as morbidity and mortality conferences. However, important issues such as a discussion of the

physician's feelings about the mistake and disclosure by colleagues of how they coped with their own mistakes are commonly avoided in these conferences. The risk management departments of hospitals could take a leading role in this area—promoting comprehensive, supportive forums for discussing mistakes and using emotion-focused coping to maximize problem-focused learning and to minimize future errors.

Graduate Medical Education

In spite of fears of public disclosure of mistakes, there is growing consensus that patient safety, physician fallibility, and methods of handling medical errors are appropriate topics for medical school, residency, and fellowship training. Although they may experience initial reluctance, physicians sometimes find that discussing a mistake is a positive experience: "Presenting this case at interns' report was difficult—I felt under a lot of scrutiny from my peers. In the end, I felt as though I had gotten more respect from presenting this kind of case rather than one in which I had made a great diagnosis."

Mistakes can be discussed in attending rounds, at morning report, or at morbidity and mortality conferences. When mistakes are discussed in these conferences, it is important to address issues such as overwork, shared responsibility with other physicians (e.g., consultants, attending physicians), and appropriate protocols for communicating with staff. These discussions also present a good opportunity to expose cognitive biases and explain strategies to reduce them. In addition, although ensuring that everyone involved learns from the mistake, care should be taken that errors are seen as an unfortunate inevitability in the practice of medicine and that there are appropriate ways of coping with them and of responding to colleagues who make them. A few institutions have begun to organize regular "patient safety rounds"—interdisciplinary conferences focused on promoting patient safety that recognize the many factors that contribute to errors. To address variability in faculty response and local culture, institutions can disseminate clear, accessible algorithms to guide behavior when medical errors occur.

Greater attention should also be given to practicing physicians who may be unaware of patient safety issues that occur in the outpatient setting. Although there has been a federal mandate on increasing patient safety, studies have shown that textbooks still do not adequately address patient safety education at the graduate level. Evidence shows that a short formal curriculum could improve attitudes and comfort toward full disclosure of medical errors, allowing cultural change in patient safety. There are now resources available to help educators develop educational materials, such as the World Health Organization (WHO) Patient Safety Curriculum and *Doc.com*, an interactive web-based curriculum developed by the American Academy for Communication in Healthcare. Future work could focus on identified themes such as learning from errors and near misses, learning and teaching in emotionally charged situations, and balance between individual and systems responsibility.

Primary Care Practice Groups

As primary care patient-centered medical homes become the norm, it is important that such groups implement procedures for responding to mistakes. Collegial support should be an explicit rule, providing a safe and confidential setting for discussion of the mistake (see the guidelines discussed earlier for responding to a colleague's mistake). It would also be wise for the practice group to formalize—and thus legitimize—periodic discussions about mistakes; these could broaden the scope of the emotion-focused support, allow members to learn from colleagues' mistakes, and address system flaws that contribute to the mistakes. A bonus of this approach is the gain in personal well-being of the group members—a nonspecific yet significant contribution to the practice climate.

PREVENTING MISTAKES

Reducing the frequency and severity of mistakes is the highest priority. There are several ways to help physicians learn from their mistakes and to make constructive changes in practice. The majority of improvements, however, need to occur at the system level.

Individual Physician Performance

As noted earlier, physicians should be encouraged to accept responsibility for their mistakes. Although those who do so seem more likely than those who do not to make constructive changes in practice, accepting responsibility for mistakes can engender emotional distress. It is therefore important for colleagues and supervising physicians to respond with sensitivity to the distress of practitioners acknowledging their mistakes. The probability of future mistakes can be reduced if the current error can be reviewed in a way that decreases emotional distress, invites disclosure of uncertainty in diagnosis and management, and leads to a discussion of appropriate changes in practice.

Many medication errors are caused by poor communication or misunderstandings about the use of medication. Physicians should place greater emphasis on reconciling their own lists with the patients, and informing patients about appropriate medication use. They can also encourage patients to become more active members of the health care team. For example, the IOM recommends that patients maintain lists of their own medications and allergies, and that they take every opportunity to share these with their clinicians.

Developing self-awareness can be a vital corrective to the cognitive biases mentioned above. Both in medical training and continuing medical education, learning the skills of mindfulness (see Chapter 7) can help clinicians be aware of the emotional and contextual conditions in which they are more likely to engage in cognitive shortcuts (low-level decision rules) that lead to diagnostic errors. They can learn to default to high-level decision rules, for example, looking beyond early hypotheses, when they perceive themselves as impatient, fatigued, or anxious for a quick resolution.

Simple, easily implemented safety strategies to prevent errors should not be overlooked. These include consistent use of a reliable method to verify patient identity, use of metric measurements, and adequate workplace illumination and organization. An interim step is for all drug orders to be in plain English, rather than in arcane Latin, apothecary script, with the old shorthand abbreviations that are subject to misinterpretation. Other strategies include elimination of abbreviations and acronyms, provision of up-to-date information at the point of care, and partnering with patients regarding their own safety. At the level of individual tasks, thoughtful standardization can enhance patient safety.

Reading back laboratory results during telephone calls is a cost-effective way of reducing miscommunication. Using auto racing and Formula 1 pit stops as a model, standardizing handoffs of patients can reduce technical errors, improve information handoffs, and reduce the duration of handoffs in an easy to teach protocol.

Administration & Supervision

Efforts to forestall errors must begin at the highest administrative levels. Leadership acknowledgment of the inevitability of errors and making patient safety an explicit priority are crucial in helping institutions learn from mistakes. Clinically, more active supervision may prevent some mistakes or mitigate their adverse effects. Senior physicians should be more available to their less experienced colleagues for help in making critical decisions about patient care, especially in complex cases that require more mature clinical judgment. Group practice administrators and training program directors should address problems in staffing, scheduling, and nature of work—which may all contribute to mistakes. Optimizing handoffs between different providers and care locations is an important goal.

Serious attention must be paid to the workload. Sleep deprivation has been shown to be a source of errors; job overload and fatigue can also lead to mistakes. Working under these conditions may induce house officers to tolerate and rationalize errors; in addition, it may make them less likely to seek the corrective information that could help prevent future mistakes. Not only residents, but senior clinicians are also vulnerable to the effects of sleep deprivation, which erodes the executive functions of the brain and leads to more failures of attention.

Using protocols, standardizing procedures, and employing checklists can help physicians do the right thing. Examples of such protocols include a "Sign Your Site" protocol for surgeons to eliminate the risk of wrong-site surgery, the WHO Safer Surgery Checklist to reduce other problems in surgical care, a "central line cart" providing needed supplies to reduce catheter-related bloodstream infections, and a simple checklist to improve medication reconciliation as patients move from surgical recovery room to the ward.

Changes in staffing can also improve safety. Having a dedicated nurse for discharge facilitations in close cooperation with residents and primary care physicians can increase hospital discharges, increase patient satisfaction and medication reconciliation, and reduce work hours for residents. The addition of specialist nurses and specialist support roles such as dietary assistants also have an important impact on positive patient outcomes. Decreasing the patient-to-nurse (PTN) ratio can decrease mortality rate, although it increases hospital costs. Hospital administrators need to carefully balance costs with workloads and allow nurse supervisors more control in setting staffing levels to ensure patient safety. A 10% rise in occupancy has been shown to increase the risk of adverse events by up to 15% in hospitals that are continually overcapacity.

Identifying & Reporting Errors

Investigation and root cause analysis to elucidate the causes of adverse events often suggest specific strategies for preventing future harm. This is aided by routine mechanisms to identify adverse events, such as anonymous reporting by physicians and nurses or computerized feedback about adverse drug reactions, which are beginning to prove useful in providing information about the frequency and nature of mistakes. Developing routine methods of conveying information, such as computerized cross-coverage templates that standardize the type and amount of information exchanged between covering physicians, can also reduce errors.

It is important to take special care with newer medications, "look-alike/sound-alike" medications, and "high alert" medications that should be handled with deliberation, particularly in the high acuity settings of emergency department, operating room, and intensive care unit.

Workplace Design

Interventions can be applied at the level of specific tasks and clinical microsystems. A "human factors" approach seeks to "optimize the relationship between humans and systems by studying human behavior, abilities, and limitations and using this knowledge to design systems for safe and effective human use. Assuming that the human component of any system will inevitably produce errors, human factors engineers design human/machine interfaces and systems that are tough enough to reduce both the rate of errors and the effects of the inevitable error within the system.

Changes can be made to the physical design and layout of work areas to improve safety. Some of these changes are intended to overcome barriers to following good practice. For example, compliance with hand hygiene guidelines can be improved by optimizing design features of alcohol hand gel dispensers. Improving air quality using laminar floor ventilation and automatic doors and using single bedrooms can reduce airborne pathogens and infections. Lighting that follows night/day cues can increase patient comfort, whereas noise reduction using sound absorbing tiles can reduce distraction and subsequent degradations in performance and burnout.

Computerized Systems

Computerized systems can detect and avert medication errors, including overdoses, incorrect routes of administration, drug interactions, and allergies. Computerized order entry systems, automated medication-dispensing machines, and bar coding of medications, blood products, and patients have been shown to reduce the incidence of adverse events.

As part of a comprehensive set of recommendations, a 2006 report from the IOM suggested the elimination of handwritten prescriptions by 2010, with the adoption of computerized prescription writing that would also utilize clinical decision support systems.

It is essential, however, that new technology be introduced in a way that acknowledges the risks as well as benefits of such change. Health care workers must receive sufficient preparation and training so that technologies are not disruptive or that they themselves do not become inadvertent sources of error. There are risks entailed in an overreliance on automation in which vigilance becomes dulled, as was the case in the Chernobyl nuclear disaster.

System-wide adoption of IT interventions, such as computerized prescriber order entry (CPOE), bar coding of medications and patients, and the use of Electronic Health Records—with drug interaction alerts and clinical support system—can reduce cognitive errors in diagnosis as well as pharmaceutical errors. Bar codes used to identify medication, blood transfusions, and patient identification have reduced the rate of errors in medication administration and order transcription. They have also improved documentation and improved the confidence of health care providers in complex and laborious procedures like blood transfusions. Bar codes force nurses manually and electronically to verify patient identities and provide a procedure that can reduce memory lapses and associated errors. Bar codes have a complementary role with decision support systems in computerized order entry, which prevent errors associated with bad judgment and lack of knowledge. A study showed that implementation of a commercial order entry system was associated with reduction in hospital-wide mortality. However, it is important to note that workflow redesign is an important factor in the successful implementation of CPOE. Although it is expensive, it allows for standardization of communication with hospital staff and can lead to improved turnaround times for patients.

SUMMARY

Individual physicians, managers, and institutions should make whatever changes in practice are warranted to prevent new mistakes and to prevent the recurrence of similar events. Providing emotional support to clinicians in the wake of a mistake can reduce distress and increase the likelihood of meaningful learning that leads to constructive changes in practice. The training of health care clinicians should include confidential, nonpunitive opportunities for discussing mistakes and their emotional impact on both clinician and patient. Recognizing and dealing with mistakes honestly and directly can improve the quality of patient care and lead to more rewarding practice.

SUGGESTED READINGS

Borrel-Carrio F, Epstein RM. Preventing errors in clinical practice: a call for self-awareness. *Ann Fam Med* 2004;2:310–316.

Butler M, Collins R, Drennan J, et al. Hospital nurse staffing models and patient and staff-related outcomes. *Cochrane Database Syst Rev* 2011 Jul;(7):CD007019.

Christensen JF, Levinson W, Dunn PM. The heart of darkness: the impact of perceived mistakes on physicians. *J Gen Intern Med* 1992;7:424–431.

Gillies R, Speers S, Young S, et al. Teaching medical error apologies: development of a multi-component intervention. *Fam Med* 2011;43:400–406.

Helmchen L, Richards M, McDonald T. How does routine disclosure of medical error affect patients' propensity to sue and their assessment of provider quality? *Med Care* 2010;48:995–961.

Institute of Medicine. *Preventing Medication Errors.* Washington, DC: National Academies Press, 2006.

Joseph A, Rashid M. The architecture of safety: hospital design. *Curr Opin Crit Care* 2007;13:714–719.

Kachalia A, Kaufman SR, Boothman R, et al. Liability claims and costs before and after implementation of a medical error disclosure program. *Ann Intern Med* 2010;153:213–221. PMID: 20713789.

Kohn LT, Corrigan JM, Donaldson MS, et al, eds. Committee on Quality of Health Care in America, Institute of Medicine. *To Err is Human. Building a Safer Health Care System.* Washington, DC: National Academy Press, 2000.

Lazare A. Apology in medical practice: an emerging clinical skill. *JAMA* 2006;296:1401–1404.

McDonald T, Helmchen L, Smith K, et al. Responding to patient safety incidents: the "seven pillars." *Qual Saf Health Care* 2010;19:e11.

Patient Safety Advisory Group. Health care worker fatigue and patient safety. The Joint Commission Sentinel Event Alert2011;(48):1–4. (www.jointcommission.org)

Poon E, Keohane C, Yoon C, et al. Effect of bar-code technology on the safety of medication administration. *N Engl J Med* 2010;362:1698–1707.

Sibinga EM, Wu AW. Clinician mindfulness and patient safety. *JAMA* 2010;304:2532–2533. PMID: 21139116.

Taché SV, Sönnichsen A, Ashcroft DM. Prevalence of adverse drug events in ambulatory care: a systematic review. *Ann Pharmacother* 2011;45:977–989. Epub June 21, 2011. Review. PMID: 21693697.

West CP, Huschka MM, Novotny PJ, et al. Association of perceived medical errors with resident distress and empathy: a prospective longitudinal study. *JAMA* 2006;296:1071–1078.

Woodward H, Mytton O, Lemer C, et al. What have we learned about interventions to reduce medical errors? *Annu Rev Public Health* 2010;31:479–497.

Wu AW, ed. *The Value of Close Calls in Improving Patient Safety: Learning How To Avoid and Mitigate Patient Harm.* Oak Brook, IL: Joint Commission Resources, 2010.

Wu AW, Cavanaugh TA, McPhee SJ, et al. To tell the truth: ethical and practical issues in disclosing medical mistakes to patients. *J Gen Intern Med* 1997;12:770–775.

Wu AW, Folkman S, McPhee SJ, LoB. Do house officers learn from their mistakes? *JAMA* 1991;265:2089–2094.

OTHER RESOURCES

Barnett P. Dialogue about unwanted and tragic outcomes. *Web-Based Learning Module in Doc.com: An Interactive Learning Resource for Healthcare Communication.* American Academy on Communication in Healthcare. www.aachonline.org. Accessed February 2014.

Canadian Disclosure Guidelines. Canadian Patient Safety Institute, 2011. http://www.patientsafetyinstitute.ca/English/toolsResources/disclosure/Documents/CPSI%20Canadian%20Disclosure%20Guidelines.pdf. Accessed February 2014.

WHO Patient Safety Curriculum Guide. http://www.who.int/patientsafety/education/curriculum/tools-download/en/index.html. Accessed February 2014.

Intimate Partner Violence

Mitchell D. Feldman, MD, MPhil & Gina Moreno-John, MD

INTRODUCTION

Intimate partner violence (IPV), is defined as any intentional, controlling behavior consisting of physical, sexual, or psychological assaults in the context of an intimate relationship. The data on IPV underscore the magnitude of the problem. In a landmark study, 28% of a random nationwide sample of couples reported violence at some point in their history; almost 4% of the women reported severe violence. If these figures are extrapolated to the general population, it is estimated that about 4 million women are subjected to violence each year in the United States (a woman is beaten or assaulted every 9 seconds in the United States), with about 500,000 women requiring medical treatment. Women visiting outpatient medical and obstetric/gynecologic clinics as well as the emergency department (ED) are often there for complaints directly attributable to IPV. Because they are frequently misdiagnosed, they may return time and time again, often with increasingly severe trauma.

Despite its magnitude in society and in medical settings, until recently IPV could be described as a "silent epidemic." Considered a private, family problem by the government, and a social problem by the medical establishment, victims often had nowhere to turn. This predicament has gradually improved. Intimate partner violence is now acknowledged to be an important public health problem, and medical practitioners have a variety of diagnostic and treatment guidelines available to them. All practitioners must be knowledgeable about and comfortable with the evaluation and care of patients who are subjected to IPV.

EPIDEMIOLOGY

Research conducted in a variety of medical settings has reported on the prevalence of IPV. Cross-sectional studies from outpatient primary care clinics and ED settings have found the prevalence of IPV among women to be from 6% to 28%; lifetime prevalence rates up to 50% have been reported and IPV accounts for more than half the murders of women in the United States every year.

A recent systematic review reported lifetime estimates of 22–39% in the United States, with similar rates having been reported by studies conducted in obstetric/gynecologic outpatient clinics. In fact, pregnancy may double the risk of IPV. Differences in prevalence of IPV among various studies can be explained, in part, by their use of different definitions of IPV.

Most studies ask about violence exclusively in the context of heterosexual relationships. However, a similar prevalence of IPV appears to exist in LGBT (Lesbian, Gay, Bisexual, Transgender) relationships, with the same physical and emotional consequences. Primary care providers should be aware that it may be more difficult for LGBT patients to disclose that they are in an abusive relationship for social and legal reasons, and they are less likely to actively seek help compared with heterosexual victims. In addition, the commonly held bias that violence does not occur in these relationships ("women can't hurt women") further lowers detection rates.

Men report being physically abused by their female partners at rates just below those reported by women. The injuries inflicted by women on men, however, are generally less significant when compared with same-sex or male-on-female violence.

DIAGNOSIS

Many women seek medical care both for the direct and indirect consequences of IPV, but only a small percentage of them are diagnosed and treated appropriately. The following case is illustrative of the type of patient commonly seen in medical settings.

 CASE ILLUSTRATION 1

A 40-year-old nurse presents to the ED with a chief complaint of a headache. She reports having been in a motor vehicle accident 3 days earlier and striking her head on the dashboard. She says that her friends

encouraged her to come in, and she is accompanied to the ED (but not the office) by her partner. On physical examination, she appears tense and sad, with bilateral, periorbital ecchymoses.

History

A thorough history is the cornerstone of the diagnosis of IPV. Because the presentation is often subtle, with few dramatic injuries, detection requires a high index of suspicion. There are many clues in the medical history, as shown by the case illustration that should prompt the physician to evaluate the patient for IPV (Table 38-1). Patients who have been assaulted often delay seeking medical attention, in contrast to accident victims who generally seek out medical attention immediately. Injuries that are attributed to a mechanism that seems illogical should always raise concern. For example, periorbital ecchymoses ("black eyes") generally are not caused by a motor vehicle accident, a "doorknob," or anything other than a fist.

MULTIPLE SOMATIC COMPLAINTS

Some women may present with vague somatic complaints as their only symptom of IPV. Fatigue, sleep disturbance, headache, gastrointestinal complaints, abdominal and pelvic pain, genitourinary problems such as frequent urinary tract and genital infections, chest pain, palpitations, and dizziness are just some of the complaints with which women present. IPV should be considered as a sole or contributing cause of these problems.

DEPRESSION, ANXIETY, AND OTHER MENTAL DISORDERS

Depression, eating disorders, and anxiety disorders such as posttraumatic stress disorder (PTSD) and panic disorder are more common among victims of IPV than among the general population. If present, the medical practitioner should always screen for IPV. These mental and behavioral disturbances should be thought of as a consequence, not a cause, of the IPV. Some patients may feel hopeless and turn toward suicide as a way out. One of every 10 battered women attempts suicide. Of those, 50% try more than once.

PREGNANCY

Many studies have demonstrated that women are at increased risk of physical and sexual abuse during pregnancy. Clues to be alert for include delay in seeking prenatal care, depressed or anxious mood, injuries to breasts or abdomen, frequent spontaneous abortions, and preterm labor. In addition to the physical and emotional trauma to the pregnant woman, these assaults can result in placental separation, fetal fractures, and fetal demise.

SUBSTANCE ABUSE

Although violence and substance abuse may coexist, it is inaccurate and generally not helpful to frame IPV as secondary to the substance abuse. Although the perpetrator, and at times the woman herself, often assert that the violence was a consequence of altered behavior from drugs or alcohol, in fact, the violent behavior must be addressed as a separate issue and is unlikely to end even if the substance abuse does.

Conversely, some studies have found an increased rate of substance use in victims of IPV. At times, this may take the form of increased use of pain medications or anxiolytics in an effort to cope with the assaults. It is even more imperative in this instance that physicians do not attribute the IPV to the substance use; it is precisely this mentality of "blaming the victim" that has often prevented the appropriate evaluation and treatment of IPV in all medical settings.

RECENT DIAGNOSIS OF HIV

Some women report an initiation or escalation of IPV after informing their partner of their human immunodeficiency virus (HIV) seropositive status. Although every attempt should be made to notify sexual partners of HIV-positive results, practitioners should assess their patient's risk of violence while discussing the issues surrounding notification. Discussion of IPV and review of a safety plan should always be part of posttest counseling.

FAMILY HISTORY OF IPV

Patients who report a family history of IPV, particularly those who witnessed parental violence as a child or adolescent, are at increased risk themselves even if they are not presently in an abusive relationship. Such women should, therefore, be educated and screened more carefully.

OVERBEARING PARTNER

An overbearing partner who, for example, insists on accompanying the patient into the examining room, acts overly solicitous or concerned (sometimes to the

Table 38-1. When to screen for IPV.

- Delay in seeking care
- Illogical explanation of injury
- Multiple somatic complaints
- Depression, anxiety, and other mental disorders
- Pregnancy
- Substance use
- Recent diagnosis of HIV
- Family history of IPV
- Overbearing partner

point of knocking on the examining room door to inquire about her well-being), or is hostile to the health care team may be a clue to the presence of IPV. Never probe about IPV if the perpetrator is in the examining room as this may unintentionally escalate the violence and put the patient in extreme danger.

SOCIOECONOMIC OR ETHNIC STATUS

Many health care providers mistakenly believe that IPV disproportionately affects persons from particular ethnic or socioeconomic groups; in fact, it cuts across all ethnic groups and all economic strata. Although some studies have found that women who are uninsured or on medical assistance are at increased risk of IPV, this is most likely due to selection bias in the studies. Women from lower socioeconomic status (SES) groups may be overrepresented in some statistics because those from higher SES groups have more resources available to them and the abuse is, therefore, more likely to remain hidden. Women with fewer resources are forced to take refuge in shelters or county hospital EDs, for example, whereas their middle-class counterparts may flee to a hotel or their offices and are, therefore, underrepresented by some of the surveys.

CASE ILLUSTRATION 2

A 28-year-old postdoctoral fellow presents to her primary care practitioner (PCP) complaining of new-onset insomnia and headache. On physical examination, the PCP discovers bruising on her chest and back and inquires about IPV. The patient breaks down and reports that her partner, a professor at the university, has been emotionally and physically abusing her for years and that only one friend was aware of this history. When the abuse escalated, the patient would seek refuge in her laboratory, sometimes conducting experiments all night.

Physical Examination

The physical examination may provide the first clues of the presence of IPV. These include what appears to be inappropriate behavior, multiple injuries, central pattern of injury, and injuries at different stages of healing (Table 38-2).

INAPPROPRIATE BEHAVIOR

Behavior that appears to be inappropriate at the time of the physical examination may be a sign of IPV. Fright, inappropriate embarrassment or laughter, anxiety, passivity, shyness, and avoidance of eye contact may all be clues that the patient has been battered.

Table 38-2. Physical examination clues to the presence of IPV.

- Inappropriate behavior
- Multiple injuries
- Central pattern of injury
- Injuries at different stages of healing

MULTIPLE INJURIES

Intimate partner violence victims are more likely to have multiple injuries than are ordinary accident victims. Women who have been subjected to IPV, for example, typically have injuries to the head, neck, abdomen, and chest, whereas accident victims often present with less widespread trauma. The common emotional reaction to an IPV assault of denial, confusion, and withdrawal may also lead to more extensive injuries.

CENTRAL PATTERN OF INJURY

Victims of IPV often experience injuries such as bruises, lacerations, burns, bites, and more severe injuries secondary to assaults with a deadly weapon or repeated beatings that cause massive internal injuries and fractures. Injuries are most commonly seen in the central areas of the body—the head, neck, chest, abdomen, breasts—and occasionally upper arms from fending off blows.

INJURIES AT DIFFERENT STAGES OF HEALING

As with child abuse, multiple injuries at different stages of healing should always prompt an inquiry about IPV.

In summary, medical providers must be alert to the signs and symptoms of IPV. It is important to remember that most IPV victims do not present with injuries that require emergency treatment or lead to hospitalization. In fact, for many patients, even in EDs, the presenting complaint is often medical or psychological, rather than an actual physical injury. For this reason, detection of IPV will increase only if practitioners include it on the differential diagnosis and actively screen for it during the medical encounter.

Screening for IPV

Many experts and national groups such as the US Preventive Services Task Force and the Joint Commission on Accreditation of Healthcare Organizations advocate screening for IPV in health care settings, along with improved provider education. Since the potential benefits of screening appear to outweigh the potential harms, and since research has demonstrated that most abused and nonabused patients favor routine screening by their health care practitioners, questions about IPV should be incorporated into the routine history and physical examination for all female patients. Some practitioners also screen men, particularly men in intimate relationships with other men. The optimal method of screening, whether by including questions about abuse on the electronic medical record (EMR) or intake medical history questionnaire, or verbally as a part of the social or past medical history, or both, is a subject of ongoing research. The HITS screening instrument is widely used and consists of four questions ("Have you been **h**it, **i**nsulted, **t**hreatened, or **s**creamed at?) on a 5-point Likert scale from "never" to "frequently"; it is available in several languages and has been validated for use with men and women. Some patients may feel more comfortable revealing IPV by screening with the following questions that seek to normalize the problem:

> **Doctor**: "We all fight at home. What happens when you or your partner fight or disagree?"

> **Doctor**: "Because abuse and violence are so common in women's lives, I've begun to ask about it routinely. At any time, has a partner hit or otherwise hurt or threatened you?" (See Table 38–3 for suggested screening questions.)

If the answers are vague or evasive, more direct questions must be asked to determine if abuse is taking place. If this is done in a supportive, nonjudgmental manner, most patients will feel comfortable and respond honestly.

TREATMENT

When IPV is detected, five basic tasks must be accomplished (Table 38–4). First, **validate the problem** by making a clear statement to the patient that violent behavior is unacceptable and illegal, and that nobody has the right to abuse her. The physician's acknowledgment of the IPV as a real issue may be the first step in helping to free her from the abuse. Under all circumstances, avoid language that could be interpreted as blaming the victim for the violence.

Table 38-3. Screening questions.

- We all fight at home sometimes. What happens when you or your partner fight or disagree?
- Do you feel safe in your home and in your relationship?
- Do you ever feel afraid of your partner?
- Because abuse and violence are so common in women's lives, I've begun to ask about it routinely. At any time, has a partner hit or otherwise hurt or threatened you?
- Does your partner ever force you to engage in sex that makes you feel uncomfortable?
- Does your partner threaten, hit, or abuse your children?

Table 38-4. After detection: five tasks to accomplish.

1. Validate the problem.
2. Assess the patient's safety, and review an emergency escape plan.
3. Document clearly and completely.
4. Provide information and appropriate referral.
5. Be aware of reporting and other legal requirements.

Because the majority of women are not ready to leave the relationship when the IPV is detected, a main task for the primary care provider is to build the relationship with the patient. Statements that express empathy can be an effective way to accomplish this task, for example: "I really respect the way you have been dealing with this" and "we can work on this problem together." Research has shown that even brief discussions with physicians are therapeutic and health outcomes are improved when the conversation is conducted in a concerned way. It is important to help the patient set short-term goals (e.g., to obtain the skills required for a particular job) so that she is not distressed when it takes time to realize her long-term goal of ending the abuse and/or the relationship. Above all, avoid recapitulating the power and control dynamics that so often characterize the patient's abusive relationship. Never insist that she leave the relationship and always allow her the autonomy to make her own decisions.

Second, it is essential to **assess the patient's safety**. Is it safe for her to go home? Other options (such as friends, shelters, and so on) should be explored and an emergency escape plan reviewed if she chooses to return home. For women not returning home, advise them to inform one or two coworkers about the situation as the perpetrator may attempt to find her at work. It is important to ask if there are children who are potentially at risk. Risk factors for escalating violence such as an increase in the frequency and severity of assaults, an escalation in threats, and the availability of a firearm should be carefully assessed.

Third, it is imperative that practitioners **document clearly and completely** when they uncover IPV. The medical record should include a complete description of the assault with quotes, if possible, from the patient's own account. Include relevant details in the past medical history and social history. Be sure to document clearly; successful prosecution should never be compromised by sloppy recordkeeping. Injuries should be described and visually documented, either with a body chart or with photographs, if the patient consents (include the patient's face in at least one photograph). If the police are called, always include the name of and any actions taken by the investigating police officer.

Fourth, the patient must be provided with **information and appropriate referral**. Health care providers should be familiar with the social and legal services available for battered women in their area. Information about shelters should be offered even if the woman intends to return home (though it is important to understand that discovery of such information by the perpetrator may lead to an escalation of the abuse). All patients should be assessed for the presence of psychiatric or substance abuse problems that would benefit from treatment or referral. Practitioners should have a basic understanding of legal options, such as restraining orders, so that they can help advise women who wish to take immediate action to ensure their safety.

Finally, understand the IPV **reporting requirements**, if any, in your state. For example, in California, health practitioners are required to report to the police all incidents of IPV that result in an injury. The usual doctor–patient privileged communication is explicitly preempted by this law. Providers should work with their ED, hospital, or clinics to be sure that information about reporting requirements as well as other patient education literature is freely available and in multiple languages.

CASE ILLUSTRATION 3

A 32-year-old man was admitted to the hospital for treatment of injuries and bleeding after reporting that he "fell through a glass door." He required an emergency operation to repair lacerations to internal organs and 2 units of packed red blood cells. Five days postoperatively, he was visited in the hospital by his male partner who became belligerent when the surgical residents attempted to obtain additional history. Later that day, the patient revealed that he had been in a long-term abusive relationship, and that the abuse had been escalating over the past 6 months, and in fact he had been pushed through the door by his partner. The hospital social worker was called to speak with the patient and told him that she would report his case to the domestic violence hotline. The patient said that he had finally made the decision to leave the relationship and was intending to press charges and was grateful for the support of the hospital doctors and staff.

What to Avoid

There are four pitfalls to avoid when caring for victims of IPV:

1. Do not insist that the patient terminate the relationship, even if you believe that this is the most appropriate action. Only she can make that decision. Trying to

control her behavior, albeit subtly, recapitulates the same negative dynamic that is taking place in the abusive relationship.

2. Recommend couple counseling *only* when the perpetrator acknowledges the problem, wants to change his or her behavior, and both partners want to preserve the relationship.

3. Do not use the word *alleged* in the medical record. It implies that you do not believe the patient's story, and you may inadvertently impede her ability to bring her case to court.

4. Do not ask what the victim did to bring on the violence.

BARRIERS

Physician Barriers to Detection

Many studies have revealed that physicians and other health care practitioners do a poor job of detecting IPV, with detection rates rarely exceeding 10%. Several factors are responsible for this dismal record. First, many practitioners lack the appropriate knowledge and training to effectively detect and treat victims of IPV. The first step in improving their ability to do so is to disseminate information more widely about its prevalence and consequences and to include IPV in medical school, residency, and continuing medical education curricula.

Lack of institutional support is another important barrier. Despite the enormity of the problem and the increasing requirements that all health care institutions have IPV protocols in place, most hospitals and clinics have few, if any, adequately trained support staff, accessible guidelines for practitioners, or information for patients. In addition, with growing pressure to see more patients and use fewer resources, issues such as IPV may be overlooked. Many of the physicians interviewed in one study identified time constraints as the major deterrent to opening the "Pandora's box" of IPV.

It should be noted, however, that the total annual costs related to IPV are estimated to be between $2 and $7 billion. In addition, the diagnostic and treatment strategies outlined here are not particularly time intensive. Inquiry about IPV adds less than 1 minute to the typical new patient evaluation; if widely employed, it could yield potentially enormous savings through prevention of injury and decreased health care usage.

The third barrier to detection of IPV arises from practitioner discomfort. Many practitioners feel uncomfortable addressing issues that do not fit neatly into the traditional medical model. Numerous studies have shown that many do a poor job discussing issues with their patients having to do with sex, violence, mental disorders, and substance use. Delving into the cause of a suspicious injury may make them uneasy: it is often not amenable to a straightforward solution and may raise embarrassing or uncomfortable feelings. All practitioners must reflect on the feelings that IPV raises in them to be effective in caring for these vulnerable patients.

Patient Barriers to Terminating an Abusive Relationship

Providers often have difficulty understanding why more patients do not terminate their abusive relationship. Why they remain in these relationships is complex. Some of the reasons include the following:

1. *Fear.* Fear for their own safety or for their children. One-third of the women are not at home when the assault takes place, so it is clear that leaving is no guarantee of safety.
2. *Economic.* Many battered women lack employment skills or experience and would find it very difficult to support themselves and/or their children outside of the relationship.
3. *Psychological.* Some may find it difficult to leave because of the "psychological dependence" the years of repetitive abuse have created. Battered women are told overtly and covertly that they are "worthless"; some eventually internalize this and come to believe that they are incapable of surviving on their own.
4. *Social support—or the lack thereof.* Women are often encouraged by well-meaning friends and family members to "try to work things out," or they are advised to stay "for the children's sake."
5. *Lack of other options.* Shelters are often full, friends and family unavailable, and legal counsel not accessible.
6. Not all women want the relationship to end, just the violence.

PERPETRATOR PROGRAMS

In some cases, a patient may self-disclose violence perpetration in a health care setting. These patients may be more amenable to behavior change. However, very few studies have looked at interventions for perpetrators of violence. Few evaluation studies have been done on outcomes and recent reviews show only a small effect size for prevention of future abuse. Most interventions are ordered by the criminal justice system and, unless mandatory, have very high dropout rates. Nonetheless, women find these programs to be useful and primary care providers can contact local IPV or legal resources to find programs for perpetrators.

NEW TECHNOLOGIES

Most patients believe that computer-based health technologies, such as electronic health records, are effective

means to improve the quality and safety of health care. In particular, patients find computer-based IPV screening methods acceptable and IPV screening done on a computer leads to substantially higher rates of IPV detection compared with a usual care. Computer-based screening methods may help to detect IPV in emergency and primary care settings. One research group was able to build a model based on symptoms that can predict the risk of future diagnoses of abuse. Next steps might be a warning system for clinicians through the EHR for such high-risk patients.

Videoconferencing-based health interventions (also called telemedicine) has been shown to help trauma and abuse victims by providing psychological services via telemedicine. Rates of symptom improvement (reductions in depressive and PTSD symptoms) are comparable to effect sizes documented for traditional cognitive behavioral therapy and appear to be a viable future option for underserved populations.

CONCLUSIONS

Along with the criminal justice system, physicians and other health care providers are most likely to come into contact with victims of IPV. They have a professional and ethical obligation to recognize IPV and intervene appropriately as well as to exert their influence on a broader level. This may be to lobby for more funding for shelters or to advocate for teaching about IPV at all levels of medical education. Screening for and treating IPV should be a routine part of the practice and training of medicine. We all have the obligation to confront the epidemic of IPV and strive to lessen its impact as one of the most important public health issues of our time.

SUGGESTED READINGS

Hegarty K, O'Doherty L, Taft A, et al. Screening and counseling in the primary care setting for women who have experienced intimate partner violence (WEAVE): a cluster randomized controlled trial. *Lancet* 2013.doi:pii: S0140–6736(13)60052–5. 10.1016/S0140–6736(13)60052–5. [Epub ahead of print]

Moyer VA. Screening for intimate partner violence and abuse of elderly and vulnerable adults: A U.S. Preventive Services Task Force recommendation. *Ann Intern Med* 2013;158:478–486.

Taft A, O'Doherty L, Hegarty K Ramsay J, Davidson L, Feder G. Screening women for intimate partner violence in health care settings. *Cochrane Database Syst Rev* 2013;(4):CD007007.doi: 10.1002/14651858.CD007007.pub2.

WEB SITES

http://www.futureswithoutviolence.org. Accessed July 2013.

http://www.thehotline.org. Accessed July 2013.

http://www.ncadv.org. Accessed July 2013.

Chronic Illness & Patient Self-Management

39

Susan L. Janson, PhD, RN, NP, FAAN; Roberta K. Oka, PhD, RN, NP;
& Thomas Bodenheimer, MD, MPH

INTRODUCTION

CASE ILLUSTRATION 1

Alicia Romero is a 45-year-old woman from El Salvador who works as a nursing assistant at a nursing home. If she has an acute complaint such as back or knee pain, she will make an appointment to see her primary care nurse practitioner, but even then there is little time in the 15-minute visit to address her chronic medical issues such as diabetes, hypertension, and hyperlipidemia. The nurse practitioner has done her best to explain the importance of healthy eating, physical activity, and taking the five prescribed medications, but Senora Romero is busy with her job and caring for her sick mother and 8-year-old son and has not been able to take good care of herself. Her hemoglobin A1c (HbA1c) is 9.5, her blood pressure (BP) is usually 150 over 95 mm Hg, and her low-density lipoprotein (LDL) cholesterol is 140 mg/dL.

About 130 million people in the United States live with at least one chronic illness, a number expected to top 150 million by 2020. Over half of that population have multiple chronic conditions. People with chronic illnesses account for 80% of total health care expenditures. By 2023, 48 million people are expected to have diabetes and 47 million will have a chronic mental health problem. About one-half of the people with hypertension and two-thirds of those with diabetes are in poor control of their disease, demonstrating that even with proven treatments for most chronic conditions, the health care system is poorly organized to care for these conditions.

Chronic disease is a primary care problem. Of the visits for chronic illness, 83% for hyperlipidemia, 79% for hypertension, 72% for diabetes, 76% for asthma, and 71% for depression are visits to primary care practitioners rather than specialists. The rushed 15-minute visit, which on average needs to address three or more medical issues, is entirely inadequate to care for chronic conditions. Primary care practitioners are constrained by the "tyranny of the urgent," the need to prioritize acute problems over chronic care management. As the case of Senora Romero reveals, the 15-minute visit constrains the nurse practitioner from helping her patient gain control of her three chronic conditions. To improve the care of chronic disease, primary care needs to be transformed, moving beyond the 15-minute visit and creating new ways to manage chronic illness. A vibrant movement within primary care has taken on this task, hoping to transform primary care practices into "patient-centered medical homes."

Much of this chapter is devoted to a discussion of the Chronic Care Model (CCM), the guide to improving chronic care management. The end of the chapter describes the innovations taking place in primary care practices to implement the CCM.

THE CHRONIC CARE MODEL

The CCM (Figure 39-1) incorporates the community, health care system, health care team, and patients in a unified model designed to improve patient outcomes for those with chronic illness. Developed by Ed Wagner in the 1990s, the model describes six components or dimensions of care that are necessary to maximize effective use of resources and coordinate care. The six components are: (1) community resources and policies; (2) the health care organization; (3) self-management support; (4) delivery system design; (5) decision support; and (6) clinical information systems. The last four components exist within the health care organization, generally within a primary care practice. Implementation of this system of care, with linkages to community resources, provides a network of

The Chronic Care Model

Figure 39-1. *The Chronic Care Model.* (Reproduced, with permission, from Edward H. Wagner Chronic Disease Management: What Will It Take to Improve Care for Chronic Illness? *Effective Clinical Practice,* Aug/Sept 1998, Vol. 1.)

support for a knowledgeable, prepared health care team to work in partnership with patients to manage and control chronic diseases. Since many chronic diseases are directly linked to behaviors (e.g., tobacco use, sedentary lifestyle, and unsafe sexual behaviors), a key component of the CCM is self-management support—assisting patients to gain the knowledge, skills, and confidence to self-manage their disease and/or risk behaviors. Yet, to offer self-management support requires realignment of health care providers into a system of care delivery that uses an integrated team approach.

The Community: Resources & Policies

The health care organization exists within a local community where individuals with chronic illnesses live. An integral component of the CCM is the cultivation and maintenance of relationships with community resources and agencies. Many community organizations provide additional resources and support for individuals with chronic illnesses and their families, such as patient education classes, exercise classes, smoking cessation programs, and home health services. These programs can bridge the service gap between health care organizations and patients and their families. Community agencies also can be partners in setting priorities and achieving goals that enhance the health of the community by

advocacy. On a macro level, public policies that promote health care for chronic conditions or encourage primary prevention are also essential in reducing the burden of long-term illness. Examples of these policies include: raising tobacco taxes, the creation of smoke-free environments, banning trans fats in restaurants, and creating bike paths to encourage physical activity.

Health Care Organization

The foundation of the CCM rests on the values and policies that govern health care provider organizations and set the tone for attitudes toward patients with chronic illnesses. If the leadership within the organization supports the importance of chronic care management, innovations are likely to be instituted. Such buy-in and support require commitment to the goal of controlling chronic illness and willingness to fund practice innovations. In addition, reimbursement policies can either facilitate or hinder quality chronic illness care. For example, fee-for-service payment creates the incentive for many 15-minute visits performed by clinicians and fails to pay for longer planned visits with nurses, health educators, or health coaches. Moreover, strong links between primary and specialty care are needed for patients with a high degree of complexity. The CCM cannot be implemented without concrete buy-in and support from the senior leaders of health care organizations that encourage redesign of the outpatient care delivery system.

Delivery System Design

To provide more efficient and proactive health care, the delivery system must change from care delivered by one clinician to an expanded primary care team in which roles and responsibilities are clearly delineated. For patients with chronic illness, planned visits are a key component of practice redesign because they provide opportunities for patients to work with the health care team to address self-management goals and disease control proactively rather than only during acute exacerbations of illness. These planned visits—generally led by nurses, pharmacists, educators, nutritionists, or social workers, as well as physicians and nurse practitioners—enable adequate time for teaching and reinforcing patient self-management skills. When acute exacerbations occur, they are handled within the context of an ongoing chronic care plan, individualized for each patient. The success of this component depends on patients' understanding and acceptance of the partnership in proactive chronic care management, which requires patients' active participation.

The primary care practice should be designed to ensure patient access to regular follow-up care that fits with the patient's cultural background, and which could be group visits, individual face-to-face visits, phone, e-mail, or web-based encounters. These creative strategies have been demonstrated to be effective in improving clinical outcomes including diabetes, hypertension, and hypercholesterolemia. For patients with one or two chronic conditions, health coaches—who may be nurses, health educators, trained medical assistants, or motivated peer patients—can assist patients in behavior change and medication adherence. For more complex patients with multiple concurrent illnesses, nurses trained in complex care management are needed. Care management has been demonstrated to be an effective strategy to improve patient outcomes and reduce costs for elderly patients with multiple chronic conditions. Care managers can monitor patients more closely, provide patient education, and intervene directly if the patient's condition does not improve or worsens. Another important function of care managers or health coaches is systems navigation, assisting the patient in successful negotiation of the health care system and access to system resources.

Decision Support

Decision support for the health care team is critical to ensure best practices in chronic illness management. It includes the provision of current clinical education and national guidelines. Ready access to individual patient clinical data and aggregated registry data must be provided so that adherence of the health care team to national practice guidelines is made available and tracked. Guidelines from national organizations can be implemented more easily if they are embedded in electronic medical records so that key decisions are supported in daily practice. Access to specialist expertise should be integrated with primary care and facilitated. Evidence-based guidelines and goals of treatment should be shared with patients to encourage their agreement and their participation in care.

Clinical Information Systems

Clinical information systems provide timely and pertinent data about both individual patients and the entire population of patients cared for by a medical practice. This information is most easily provided through electronic registries. These information systems are capable of tracking clinical data by patient or panels of patients and by disease or preventive maintenance needs and results of care processes over time. They can be programmed to alert clinicians and the care team to values outside normal ranges, allowing the health care team to identify subpopulations that need proactive care and monitoring to improve clinical outcomes. Several studies have demonstrated that the use of registries for both chronic and preventive services improves clinical outcomes. A well-designed clinical information system also allows monitoring of the performance of the practice team and the health care system in meeting national guidelines for processes of care and clinical outcomes by creating a feedback system for selected quality performance measures. Electronic feedback in the form of graphs allows the care team to work on continuous performance improvement. Sharing clinical information with patients as well as the care team is essential to enlist patient participation in their own care and helps to support the patient–clinician relationship.

Self-Management Support

The final CCM component is self-management support for patients with chronic illnesses; assisting patients and their families in developing the knowledge, skills, and confidence to effectively manage problems, set goals, and actively participate in a partnership with their clinicians and health care team is the goal. People with chronic conditions spend 99.9% of their lives with their families, at work, or in the community, and 0.1% in the health care system. People with chronic conditions decide whether to eat healthy or unhealthy foods, whether to be sedentary or physically active, and whether or not to take their medications. For chronic disease, the patient, not the clinician, makes most of the decisions. If people are not informed, active participants in the management of their chronic condition, the efforts of the health care team will be of no avail. The health care team must assist patients to be informed and activated, but patients have the ultimate say.

The outcome of successful implementation of the CCM is a prepared, proactive health care team interacting with informed, activated patients. Because all CCM components are designed to encourage patients to be informed and activated, the next section of this chapter provides more details on patient self-management and the importance of patient-centered care.

SELF-MANAGEMENT & PATIENT-CENTERED CARE

 CASE ILLUSTRATION 1 (CONTD.)

Alicia Romero's nurse practitioner asked her to attend a six-session Spanish language diabetes self-management group at her clinic one evening per week, and provided childcare at the clinic to allow parents to attend. At the first session, the 12 participants in the group talked about their challenges in controlling their diabetes, hypertension, and cholesterol. Senora Romero was inspired that everyone faced the same challenges, and toward the end of the meeting, everyone made an action plan to do something realistic to improve their health. Senora Romero's action plan was to commit to taking all her medications every day. The group divided into buddies, who call each other twice a week to check on the action plans. Senora Romero's next HbA1c had gone down from 9.5 to 8.2 and her BP was now controlled. She felt good.

Overall, the success of chronic disease management lies in fostering a patient-centered partnership between the patient and health care team. This is particularly important when caring for patients with behavioral health problems and difficult lives. The ultimate goal of this approach is to empower patients to develop the skills and behaviors that will help them self-manage their diseases to achieve better health outcomes. Several clinical trials and systematic reviews have concluded that collaborative care models in which decisions are made jointly between clinicians and patients are significantly more effective in improving clinical outcomes than care in which clinicians tell patients what to do.

Patient-Centered Care for the Clinician

Patient-centered care is a critical concept for effective management of chronic illnesses. The concept includes

Table 39-1. Self-management support.

Self-management support is what providers do to assist and encourage patients to be empowered and able to manage their illness. This paradigm shift requires building a partnership—with shared responsibility for making and implementing health-related decisions—between the provider(s) or care management team and the patient.

engaging patients in care planning as well as giving patients tools, skills, and knowledge. It means the health care team and primary clinician elicit and accept the patient's beliefs and concerns about illness and teach key information and self-management skills in the context of the patient's family, community, and culture, taking into consideration individual needs. The patient's concerns are identified and addressed first (Table 39-1). The team and primary care clinician involve the patient directly in negotiating and implementing the treatment plan, making adjustments and providing options that will meet the patient's goals. Ask: "What do you want to do this week to improve your health?" Working in collaboration with the patient, the primary care clinician and health care team design a treatment program that fits within the context of the patient's life (Table 39-2). Potential solutions and feasible options are offered and patients are invited to choose those they are willing to accept and pursue or modify. For example, to reduce high cholesterol levels, patients are asked if they would be willing to eat more healthy foods, do more exercise, or regularly take medications. When patients can choose their treatment program, it is more likely they will implement it. The keyword in this context is "collaboration" to work toward goals that are acceptable to both the care team and the patient. Additionally, primary care practitioners should be aware of patients' culturally based understanding of the disease and its treatment. Every effort should be made to deliver critical information and self-management instruction in the patient's native language. A patient-centered partnership means that health care providers collaborate with patients to design a treatment program that takes into consideration the patient's

Table 39-2. Lessons learned from dialogue.

- The provider allows the patient to set the agenda.
- The provider assesses the patient's levels of importance and confidence and explores what it would take to improve confidence in behavior change. This information also allows the provider to explore the activities patients are interested in pursuing.

Table 39-3. Key elements to goal setting/action plans.

- Collaborative between patient and provider, using tools of motivational interviewing.
- Actions are highly specific.

---

attitudes, beliefs, lifestyle, and culture to promote positive treatment outcomes (Table 39-3).

Clinician behaviors may contribute to better patient self-management, particularly in subpopulations with specific needs. A survey of an ethnically diverse, low-income sample of 956 adult patients with diabetes or asthma in 17 academic outpatient practices revealed a strong relationship between higher patient assessments of provider support and patient self-efficacy for self-care. Within the diabetes subgroup, patients who gave high ratings of provider support were significantly more likely to perform self-management tasks than those with low ratings. The findings provide support for the belief that health care providers can successfully promote patient self-management of chronic illnesses.

Problems of Living with a Chronic Illness

Living with a chronic illness presents the patient with a number of medical, social, emotional, and physical challenges that include adjusting to the natural course or progression of the disease, preventing social isolation, normalizing activities and communication within the boundaries of the illness, preventing exacerbations, controlling chronic symptoms, following complex treatment regimens, and finding the necessary financial and tangible resources to pay for treatments and potential loss of employment. To manage these problems, patients must develop a set of strategies for self-managing the disease and for coping with the problems. Teaching, facilitating, and supporting the patient's attempts at self-management of the chronic condition is at the core of the patient–clinician–health care team relationship.

The partnership paradigm is based on acknowledging the expertise of both the clinician and team in understanding the disease, its psychological and physical impact on patients, and therapeutic interventions; and patients' expertise about their own lives. The new paradigm of clinician/team–patient partnership supports interactions that are primarily based on the patient's agenda, not the clinicians.' It purports a belief that increased self-efficacy for self-care tasks facilitates behavior change that education alone cannot accomplish. In the patient-centered approach, enhanced self-efficacy is the goal rather than adherence to clinician advice. Finally, mutually agreed upon decisions are made together by the patient and clinician.

Self-management support encourages patients to become more actively engaged to adopt health behaviors and develop necessary skills.

Self-Management Support Strategies

Research has demonstrated that activated patients are more likely to adopt healthy behaviors and thus have improved clinical outcomes. Several strategies to activate patients are discussed here.

COLLABORATIVE AGENDA SETTING

In traditional clinical encounters, the visit is guided by the chief complaint provided by the patient and the agenda is established by the clinician. In the collaborative paradigm, the agenda is negotiated between the clinician and the patient.

INFORMATION GIVING USING ASK-TELL-ASK

One technique that has been used in providing patients with information is based upon the "elicit-respond-elicit" motivational interviewing technique first described by Miller and Rollnick (see Chapter 19). This method is more popularly called "ask-tell-ask," a strategy based on adult learning theory in which individuals learn best when provided with information that they are interested in learning. Rather than giving patients a didactic lecture on diabetes, the nurse or health educator asks "What do you know about diabetes?" and "What would you like to know about diabetes?" and gives patients the information they want to know, after which they ask again whether the patient understands or has other questions. In addition, rather than telling patients that they must exercise and change their diet, the health care team member asks patients what they are willing to do to improve their health. For many health professionals who are used to telling patients what to do, this shift to collaborative interactions and shared decision making is a challenge.

INFORMATION GIVING: CLOSING THE LOOP (TEACH BACK METHOD)

A simple but much overlooked strategy is asking the patient to restate instructions provided by the practitioner. It is known that 50% of patients leave a medical visit without understanding or remembering what the clinician said. "Closing the loop" or "teach back" assesses a patient's understanding of the information provided by the practitioner. Rather than asking, "Did you understand how to take your medication?" which does not assess understanding, closing the loop involves asking, "Just to make sure I was clear, how will you be taking that new medicine?" Teach-back or check-back is a relatively simple strategy that has been associated with improved outcomes in patients with diabetes; yet few clinicians actually close the loop in practice.

0	1	2	3	4	5	6	7	8	9	10
Not sure									Very sure	

Figure 39-2. **Self-Efficacy** Scale indicating confidence in ability to make a change in behavior (diet, exercise, etc.).

BEHAVIOR CHANGE ACTION PLANS

Traditionally, clinicians tell patients that they must eat healthier foods, exercise, and take all their medications without their input to the treatment recommendations. Motivational interviewing studies suggest that telling patients what they are supposed to do generates resistance on the part of the patients and is thereby ineffective in encouraging behavior change. Keys to motivational interviewing technique include: (1) assessing readiness to change by determining the relationship between level of importance and level of confidence for change and (2) encouraging patients themselves to talk about a behavior change they are willing to entertain. To assess level of confidence and importance, a 0–10 scale or a picture graph can be used (Figure 39-2). Once individuals are motivated to change a behavior, they can set goals for themselves, and then agree to a specific action plan that begins the process of meeting the patient-generated goals.

Action plans are developed through collaboration between the clinician or health care team member and the patient. The action plan is very specific with identified behaviors, a start date, and frequency. For example, a patient may wish to walk 3 days per week (Monday, Wednesday, and Friday) at lunchtime, for 20 minutes, beginning next Monday. Another example may include reducing candy bar consumption to 1 per day from 3 per day and eating one piece of fruit daily.

The primary purpose of action plans is to achieve behavior change through a series of successes. Self-efficacy is defined as an individual's level of confidence in performing a specific behavior or activity. If self-efficacy is high, the behavior is likely to be performed. Thus, enhancing self-efficacy is of primary importance in achieving long-term behavior change. Therefore, the action plan should be simple and achievable. If the patient has a low level of confidence in achieving the action plan, the team member can suggest a more achievable goal to insure success. Additionally, if self-efficacy is low, this provides an opportunity for the clinician to explore barriers to change and to develop specific strategies to promote success. In a randomized controlled trial, patients with diabetes who made action plans had significant lowering of HbA1c compared with patients who were given patient education without action plans. The key to success in implementing action plans is to engage the patients by eliciting their input and to increase their self-confidence to act.

THE CYCLE OF CHRONIC ILLNESS EXPERIENCE FOR PATIENTS

Even with well-planned patient self-management support and the best intentions of the care team, chronic illnesses go out of control, exacerbations occur, and life events happen that compromise patients' ability to cope. Psychosocial stress, new symptoms, progressive disease, and increased disability place additional burdens on patients with chronic illness. Increasing stress in an individual's life, such as greater work demands, might lead to an increase in activity level, greater fatigue, muscle tension, increased or new symptoms, and the psychological experience of feeling overwhelmed. These developments may contribute to high levels of pain, dyspnea, or depression, which in turn can lead to a decline in daily functioning, immobility, and the perception of heightened disease activity. These symptoms, perceptions, and loss of control may make the individual aware of the debilitating aspects of the chronic illness and negatively affect self-esteem, contributing to a cycle of further depression, poor coping responses, worsening adherence, and an inability to adapt.

Clinicians can empower patients to be alert to the interplay of these factors in their lives. Once aware, patients can make short-term goals and action plans that interrupt the cycle, reducing stress and symptoms and increasing psychological well-being and control of the illness.

The natural history of chronic disease can be discouraging for patients and their families and for clinicians, which is why development of an effective health care team approach directed at supporting patients and their families is essential. In the end, chronic care management requires concentric circles of surveillance and care management supported by the health care system and endorsed by the community.

PSYCHOLOGICAL IMPACT OF CHRONIC DISEASE

CASE ILLUSTRATION 2: SELF-MANAGEMENT

Maria is a 68-year-old Spanish-speaking woman with adult-onset diabetes and depression. She also has been told that she has high BP and high cholesterol.

She takes several oral medications for these conditions but does not know what they are and has not brought them with her to her appointments. She has a glucometer at home but has not checked her blood glucose for several months. She is out of glucometer strips and has not been able to figure out how to obtain them through her new Medicare Part D plan. She is currently living with her husband and daughter. Her meals consist of beans, rice, chicken, and tortillas. Her BP is 150/100 mm Hg.

Patients with chronic illness encounter a number of challenges that impact every aspect of their lives. Care teams must be able to understand their patients' internal experiences and outward expressions of their emotions and intervene in ways that promote adaptive coping, that is, having available a repertoire of responses that can be used to modulate the ebb and flow of the disease.

The goal of coping is to respond cognitively or behaviorally to manage, tolerate, or reduce the effect of a stressful acute or chronic event (see Chapter 34). The two major methods of coping are problem focused and emotion focused. Problem-focused coping consists of active efforts to change something about oneself or the environment. Emotion-focused coping involves efforts to regulate emotional distress. Most often, people tend to take action to solve problems, but when a stressful experience is uncontrollable, problem-focused coping can be counterproductive. In these situations, efforts at emotional regulation or minimizing emotional distress may be more successful at providing relief.

The problem-focused/emotion-focused distinction in coping is useful not only in understanding people's coping efforts, but in providing guidelines to primary care practitioners about how to facilitate patients' active involvement in their care and adaptation to chronic disease. Asking questions about patients' concerns and helping them to develop coping solutions are integral to developing a patient-centered partnership that will maximize the potential for positive treatment outcomes.

Key aspects to consider for Maria include:

- Facilitating effective communication between the primary clinician, health care team, and the patient by scheduling her with a team member such as a health coach who is bilingual.
- Assessing and monitoring her depression with regular checks of the Patient Health Questionnaire (PHQ-9) by a member of the health care team.
- Monitoring Maria's progress on her action plan through regular follow-up phone calls by the health coach.
- Checking and sharing the results of her HbA1c testing at regular intervals to provide her with feedback about her progress.

COLLABORATIVE DECISION MAKING: GOAL SETTING/ACTION PLANS

 CASE ILLUSTRATION 2 (CONTD.): SETTING AN AGENDA

Provider: I just checked your HbA1c and it is 8.5.

Maria: It seems high, I remember that it should it be lower, like about 7?

Provider: Yes, that is correct. What would you like to do about this?

Maria: I have been taking my medicines. I don't have time for anything else. I don't know what else to do.

Provider: We could talk about a number of different things, for example, medications, diet, exercise, or something else that you would prefer?

Maria: I would be interested to hear about exercise.

Provider: OK, now using a scale "0" to "10," how confident are you that you can make a change in your activity level or exercise? A "0" means you aren't sure you can make a change in your activity level and a "10" means you are 100% sure you can change your activity level (see Figure 39-2).

Maria: It is a "4," I don't have a lot of time and I am not sure what to do.

Provider: Why did you say a 4 and not a "1"?

Maria: It might be nice to take a walk with my husband or daughter, they walk together sometimes.

Provider: What would it take to improve your confidence to around a 7 that you can exercise more?

Maria: Maybe if I could walk with my husband, I would enjoy that and it would encourage me to do it.

Provider: Great! Do you want to set a short-term goal about your exercise? We could come up with an action plan together.

Patients who rate their confidence level at less than 7 on a 10-point scale are unlikely to maintain a change in that behavior. Here the health coach is working with Maria to identify a patient-centered and achievable behavior change that will contribute to her goal of improving her diabetes management. Goal setting is performed on behaviors that patients feel they are ready to attempt and action plans that are realistic, concrete, and short term to achieve the goals. In Maria's case, the action plan may include walking with her husband or daughter beginning the next day for 20 minutes four times a week.

Other key elements to consider for this case as it relates to the CCM are:

- Matching of language in verbal and written communication.
- Goal setting and action planning can be performed by other key members of the care team. This can take place after the visit with the primary care clinician.

- Closing the loop is key in this case and can be performed by other team members as well as the primary clinician. Closing the loop assesses the patient's understanding of the visit and what, how, and when to take medications.

- System navigation is an important health coaching function. It is important to find out if patients know where to go to get their labs drawn and whether the tests need to be performed after 12 hours of fasting. Patients need to know where they go to fill the prescriptions for medications and what assistance they can request from the pharmacist.

- Follow-up (planned) visits should be scheduled to assess progress with action plans, revise and update goals, and to address management of other chronic conditions. These visits do not need to be with the primary care clinician when it may be more appropriate for other team members with special skills to be involved. Follow-up should also be conducted by phone calls.

- Community resources may provide support outside the health care system. Maria may have access to other resources such as a park, community center, or church that organizes walking groups or other health-related activities. Referrals can be made to these organizations and may be more convenient for her than returning to the clinic at regular intervals.

- Assessment and treatment of comorbid behavioral health problems is critical for enhancing self-management. Like many patients with diabetes mellitus, Maria is also being treated for depression. The clinician knows that inadequately treated depression can contribute to worsening glycemic control and that conversely, assessing and managing depression is a key component of the overall management of Maria's diabetes.

Final key points to remember are as follows:

- After Maria's visit is complete, her information should be entered into a computerized system that will then allow the care team to follow her BP, HbA1c, PHQ-9, weight, and so on. This information can be pulled and collated prior to her next visit as a cue to optimal management.

- Additionally, her health maintenance activities will be recorded, and the clinician or other team member will be prompted to review her health maintenance needs at the next visit.

IMPLEMENTING THE CHRONIC CARE MODEL IN PRIMARY CARE

For a primary care practice to implement the CCM requires a major transformation that has been labeled the patient-centered medical home. Fundamental to this transformation is a two-part paradigm shift: (1) From concern only with individual patients to concern with the entire panel of patients, whether or not they come for care and (2) from I (the individual practitioner) to We (the team). Practices increasingly have clinical registries with lists of patients including clinical data. Practices can train personnel to be panel managers, who regularly search the registries for people overdue for preventive and chronic care services that are recommended by practice guidelines, and who contact those patients to receive recommended services. To overcome the tyranny of the urgent and the 15-minute visit syndrome, practices must create well-trained teams so that patients with chronic conditions can receive planned visits led by nurses, health educators, pharmacists, psychologists, or other team members who provide self-management support, which can also be called health coaching. A health coach is any team member who interacts with patients to provide information using the ask-tell-ask model; to collaboratively set goals and action plans; to close the loop to ensure patient understanding of the care plan; to assist patients with medication understanding and adherence; and to provide support to ease the emotional burden of chronic disease. Transition to patient-centered, team-based primary care provides a health care home for patients who require ongoing collaborative care to survive and manage their chronic illness problems. This transition requires system-wide delivery design change and the support of system-based administrative leaders.

IMPLEMENTING THE CHRONIC CARE MODEL GLOBALLY

The challenge of managing chronic conditions is one that is faced by health care leaders around the world. In many countries, noncommunicable diseases and mental health disorders account for approximately 47% of the global burden of disease, with a projected increase to 60% by 2020. Historically, public health concerns for developing countries were limited to infant mortality, population control, and malnutrition. However, concerns are growing over the additional burden of chronic noncommunicable diseases, such as tobacco-related illnesses. Although there is a surge in need for treatment of chronic conditions, delivery of care to these individuals is lacking. Developing countries often struggle with the complexity of insufficient resources and poor access necessitating creative solutions to address the increased shifting demand in health care. To address these issues, the World Health Organization (WHO) considered a variety of programs. WHO convened a group of experts from around the world to review and adapt the CCM from their countries' perspectives. The result was the Innovative Care for Chronic Conditions (ICCC) framework. The framework includes components at a micro (patient and family), meso (health care organization and community), and macro (policy) level. The focus of the framework is to highlight the need for a comprehensive design for change to deliver effective care. The ICCC has been adapted and has been shown to be effective in improving outcomes in a number of countries. Thus, although the burden of chronic health conditions is increasing globally, changes to the health care system as demonstrated with the ICCC have great potential for improving global health.

SUGGESTED READINGS

Bodenheimer T, Chen E, Bennett HD. Confronting the growing burden of chronic disease: can the U.S. health care workforce do the job? *Health Affairs* 2009;28:64–74. PMID:19124856.

Bodenheimer T, Wagner EH, Grumbach K. Improving primary care for patients with chronic illness: the chronic care model. *JAMA* 2002;288:1775–1779. PMID:12365965.

Glasgow RE, Kurz D, King D, et al. Outcomes of minimal and moderate support versions of an internet-based diabetes self-management support program. *J Gen Intern Med* 2010; 25:1315–1322. PMID:20714820.

Stange KC, Nutting PA, Miller WL, et al. Defining and measuring the patient-centered medical home. *J Gen Intern Med* 2010; 25:601–612. PMID: 20467909.

Wagner EH, Glasgow RE, Davis C, et al. Quality improvement in chronic illness care: a collaborative approach. *Jt Comm J Qual Improv* 2001;27:63–80. PMID: 11221012.

WEB SITES

Institute for Patient- and Family-Centered Care. www.ipfcc.org. Accessed February 2014.

Patient-Centered Primary Care Collaborative site. www.pcpcc.net. Accessed February 2014.

MacColl Institute. Improving Chronic Illness Care. www. improvingchroniccare.org. Published 1996-2010. Accessed February 2014.

Palliative Care, Hospice, & Care of the Dying

Bethany C. Calkins, MD; Michael Eisman, MD; & Timothy E. Quill, MD

INTRODUCTION

The goals of medical practice based exclusively on cure and restoration of function are frequently called into question when patients are irreversibly ill and potentially dying. New goals, such as pain and symptom management, enhancing quality of life, and finding meaning in the face of death may take precedence, becoming an increasingly important part of the treatment plan. Some clinicians may wonder if death is something to be fought at all costs, or if relieving suffering is a central part of our responsibility as clinicians.

Enhancing the quality of life for those afflicted with serious chronic illness is the cornerstone of the rapidly developing specialty of palliative care. As illustrated in Figure 40-1, palliative care can be provided alongside aggressive treatment of a patient's underlying disease, but as the patient becomes sicker and closer to death, palliation often becomes the primary objective.

CASE ILLUSTRATION 1

Ella, a 71-year-old woman, develops pains in her lower chest for a month before visiting her personal physician. When a chest film shows several nodular masses suggestive of widespread lung cancer, the physician phones Ella and tells her there is a problem, making an office appointment for the next day. At this visit, the doctor discusses the results of the chest film with the patient and her son. Ella, having long suspected she might get lung cancer from smoking heavily, weeps openly upon hearing the results. Bronchoscopy is recommended, and she is referred to a pulmonologist. Bronchoscopic biopsies show a small-cell lung cancer. The pulmonologist refers Ella to an oncologist who recommends chemotherapy.

The patient and her son return to her primary care doctor to discuss her options. Ella says she would like to proceed with chemotherapy but wants to stop it if she becomes too ill from the treatments. A Roman Catholic, she has discussed with her priest the morality of refusing extraordinary care, including feeding tubes, if she were to have a terminal condition. She has appointed her son as her health care proxy, and discusses her desire not to undergo cardiopulmonary resuscitation (CPR). The physician gives Ella a living will and a do-not-resuscitate (DNR) document; she and her son complete them together. She wants to try all other potentially effective disease-directed treatments, and she also agrees to have her pain and shortness of breath treated aggressively as well. She also knows that cure is very unlikely with this treatment, so she begins to work with a financial planner to get her affairs in order.

Ella undergoes chemotherapy for several months, but gradually grows thinner and weaker. She and her son visit her doctor, and they are told that treatment is not controlling the disease and that the only options left for cancer treatment are experimental. She is referred to a home hospice program and agrees to a plan that is now directed exclusively at relieving her suffering. Ella lives alone and does not want to die in her apartment. Neither does she want her son to have to provide home care for her when she becomes too dependent to live alone. She also wants to know whether she could move to a hospice house or a nursing home for the very last phase of her illness when she is unable to care for herself at home. Her doctor and her son agree to find other placement when the need arises.

When she becomes confused 1 month later and is unable to stay at home, she is admitted to a comfort care floor at a local nursing home. An intensive palliative treatment regimen is initiated, and she dies 2 weeks later with her son at her bedside, 6 months after the initial diagnosis.

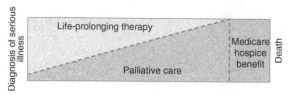

Figure 40-1. The place of palliative care in the course of illness. (Adapted from Clinical Practice Guidelines for Quality Palliative Care. Available at: www.nationalconsensusproject.org.)

Early after this patient's initial diagnosis, she received palliative care alongside aggressive treatment of her disease. Withholding aggressive pain and symptom management until referral to hospice is misguided and unfair, depriving patients of optimal treatment of their suffering from the beginning of their illness. This "both/and" approach has been one of the most important conceptual breakthroughs for palliative care, for it allows quality-of-life issues to be addressed for all seriously ill patients, not just those who are referred to hospice. It also allows patients simultaneously to "hope for the best" (that even improbable or experimental treatment might affect their disease and prolong their life) and "prepare for the worst" (make sure that financial affairs are settled and consider religious or existential issues should they wish to do so). It may be easier for some patients to make the transition to hospice if they have had this "both/and" conversation with their physician from the start of their illness.

Nonabandonment

When a patient is given the diagnosis of a life-threatening illness, a wide spectrum of feelings may emerge, including denial, anxiety, fear, sadness, and anger. If practitioners are surprised by the diagnosis, feel as though they missed a clue to the diagnosis earlier on, or are discomfited by death, they may feel inclined to withdraw from the patient's care or to minimize the meaning and impact of the diagnosis. The commitment not to abandon the patient requires that clinicians learn to work through their own feelings, become knowledgeable about palliative care, and recognize that the process of dying can be a unique spiritual and personal experience for both doctor and patient. The goal should be to form a partnership that will help the patient face the future with courage and dignity.

The goals of partnership and shared decision making are sometimes limited by strong emotional reactions as well as long-standing personality traits that can isolate the patient from the clinician, friends, and family. In addition, physicians may be unable to commit the time and energy needed to develop close personal contact with the seriously ill and dying patient. Clinicians need

to realize that extraordinary effort is sometimes required to be a partner with patients and their families through what initially may be a vigorous fight against disease, but eventually may end in the patient's death.

The goal of palliative care is to provide the best possible quality of life for patients and their family. Palliative care addresses the biological, psychosocial, and spiritual dimensions of suffering, emphasizing state-of-the-art pain and symptom management, as well as a fresh look at goals and prognosis. Unlike Medicare-sponsored hospice programs, palliative care does not require patients to give up on aggressive treatment of their underlying disease, to accept a prognosis of lesser than 6 months, or to accept palliation as the central goal of therapy. Thus, it allows "hospice-like" treatments to be made available to those seriously ill patients who want to continue some or all disease-directed treatments. For example, patients who are highly likely to die, but want to try improbable experimental therapy in hopes that it might prolong their lives, could receive palliative care, but would not qualify for a Medicare-sponsored hospice program. Hospice programs enroll patients with a terminal disease who are more likely than not to die within the next 6 months' time once they agree to forgo curative treatments for their disease and focus only on improving quality of life. Palliative care allows better pain and symptom management, careful attention to quality of life, an examination of the goals of treatment, and an opportunity to provide a much broader range of patients' reflection on issues of life closure. Unfortunately, the medical infrastructure that supports the patient and family receiving palliative care at home is much less comprehensive than the medical infrastructure supporting hospice.

Patients confronting a severe illness may opt for an all-out, disease-oriented medical treatment, or a trial of aggressive medical care with set limits (such as a DNR order). Optimally, both of these patient pathways would also receive palliative care consultation from the time of diagnosis. When undergoing time-limited trials of aggressive care, patients have the opportunity to gauge and discuss with their provider whether the suffering involved with the treatment, given the odds of success, is worth it. When treatments begin to fail, or if supposedly curative treatments become too burdensome, patients can stop at any time and consider a transition to an approach that emphasizes pure palliation with their palliative care provider. This would be the time to consider referral to hospice, where relieving symptoms and alleviating suffering take precedence over attempts to treat the underlying disease.

Hospice

Hospice programs provide comprehensive care to dying patients, with a multidisciplinary team of nurses, physicians, social workers, volunteers, and clergy. These programs, which accept only patients who are more likely than not to die in the next 6 months and are willing to forgo disease-directed therapies and hospitalizations, help patients and their families live as fully as possible by providing quality palliative care. In the United States, only about 30% of deaths occur in hospice programs, and many of these patients are referred to a hospice too late in the course of their illness to take full advantage of the resources and supports available to them. The palliative care philosophy underlying hospice can be applied in a range of settings including acute-care hospitals, skilled nursing facilities, and within the homes of patients. The advantage of hospice programs is the expertise brought to techniques of palliative care by the multidisciplinary staff, as well as the added support for patient and family at home, including payment for palliative medications and medical equipment. In most outpatient hospice programs, the primary care physician and the hospice team form a partnership to care for the patient. The primary care provider, with whom the patient may have a long-term relationship, should be intimately involved in both the decision for hospice referral and the patient's ongoing care. Once distressing symptoms are controlled, the hospice team may then help the patient find avenues for hope, meaning, and ways of saying good-bye.

Dealing with Grief

At times it may be difficult to distinguish normal grief reactions to the dying process from pathologic states that may require consultation and special treatment. There is a natural sadness that human beings experience with regard to death. This sadness, which may be a way of preparing for death, has been called **preparatory** or **anticipatory grief**. Grieving over the loss of physical abilities, social position, and contact with pleasurable routines—whether one's own or those of a loved one—is a natural reaction. The absence of grief over these losses may indicate denial and emotional numbing. Sharing and exploring the grief can help both the patient and the clinician enter into a relationship that acknowledges each other's humanity. Having the courage to explore these feelings assists the patient in coming to terms with death and may prevent the isolation and subsequent clinical depression to which some patients are prone.

Depression

Distinguishing clinical depression from the natural grieving process that accompanies a terminal illness may be difficult, as they share many common symptoms. The vegetative symptoms of depression—fatigue, changes in appetite, sleep disorders, decreased sexual drive—are all common in serious illness. As much as 80% of the psychological symptoms that occur in cancer patients go untreated simply because it is difficult to diagnose depression in this population. Providers should have a high index of suspicion for depression in patients with serious disease. The affective and cognitive signs of depression, such as loss of interest, withdrawal, sadness, inability to concentrate, and hopelessness may be realistic assessments in the face of severe suffering, fear of a loss of dignity, and the expectation of death. Major depression should be considered when the cognitive symptoms of dysphoria, shame, guilt, isolation, or suicidal ideation seem out of proportion to the patient's situation (see Chapter 25). Depression in the terminally ill can be very responsive to pharmacotherapy as well as counseling even when it is part of a normal reaction. Depending on the expertise of the physician and other members of the multidisciplinary team, more challenging cases of depression and anxiety should be referred to a mental health professional. Psychotherapists who are familiar with the dying process and are experienced with medically ill patients can provide an invaluable resource, both diagnostically and therapeutically, in the care of the terminally ill.

Transitions

In terminal illness, patients frequently decline in health in a stepwise fashion. These transitions near the end of life result in feelings of loss for patients and their families, and provide the potential for personal growth and the acceptance of death. Progressive declines initially may be treated as another form of bad news, but they provide the opportunity for enhanced meaning and control in the dying process. Physicians caring for terminally ill patients must explore and work through these transitions with their patients. Questions that clinicians can ask their patients in exploring their views on end-of-life issues are listed in Table 40-1. These can be asked as hypothetical questions to explore the patient's beliefs about life and death. In patients with more advanced illness, the questions and their answers may be highly relevant to immediate treatment decisions.

 CASE ILLUSTRATION 2

Carlos, a 70-year-old man, has been diagnosed with advanced hepatocellular carcinoma. In exploring the treatment options with his physician, he is clear about wanting only palliative measures, and referral to a home hospice program is initiated. Carlos is not a verbal man, and discussions about death and dying meet with little response.

Table 40-1. End-of-life issues to be discussed with patients.

Life support
- Do you have an advance directive (a living will or health care proxy)?
- Do you know what CPR is? It may not work very well for people in your condition, and it is very painful. Should you choose to forego CPR, we can focus our treatments on anything that has a good chance of helping you without harming you.
- In the event an illness led to your being unable to eat or drink on a permanent basis, would you want to be fed with feeding tubes?
- Do you want your medical care primarily geared to prolonging your life, or is improving or maintaining your quality of life more important?

Personal beliefs
- What life experiences have you had around death and dying?
- How have these experiences affected your own attitudes about death?
- What are your worst fears about dying? What are your biggest hopes?
- What would be a "good death" for you?
- What do you believe happens to you when you die?
- If you were to die sooner rather than later, what would be left undone?

Long-term care and support systems
- If you become too ill to take care of yourself, who will take care of you?
- Who would you want to make health care decisions for you if you became unable to do so?
- If you were dying, would you prefer to be at home or in an institution such as a hospital or nursing home?
- Do you know what hospice care is? Would you want that kind of care if you were terminally ill?
- Who would you want to be present at the time of your dying and death?
- Is there anything you need to get done before you die?

At first, periodic nursing visits are all that is needed. He has an antique tool collection and spends countless hours labeling and ordering the tools. His nurse talks to him about this process, which has come to symbolize his anticipatory grief. As he deteriorates, nursing visits become more frequent, and home health aides come to help with his personal care. Carlos gradually becomes bed bound. Although his family initially feels uncomfortable with his dying at home, a family meeting with the physician and hospice nurse sets up a rotation of visits to provide for both company and supervision. Children who had been estranged are in the rotation, and it becomes a time of family healing. Although little is explicitly said about his approaching death, the presence of family and talk about the tools provide a vehicle for saying good-bye. Carlos dies quietly at home with his family present.

Patients' willingness and ability to enter into deep discussions about death and dying vary considerably; clinicians need to be flexible in their expectations about how much exploration is desirable or even possible. It is unusual for a life-long pattern of behavior to be altered by the dying process; therefore, those who lived very private lives may not be able to open up significantly at the end of life. For some, dying may be a time for personal growth, reflection, and meaning; but for others, personal factors and emotional reactions block an acceptance of death. The most frequently encountered

of these reactions are denial, anger, depression, fear, and anxiety. These reactions may be present in different degrees and at different times in the dying process. Clinicians need to acknowledge, explore, and eventually understand what function the reaction is serving for the patient. Empathy, rather than withdrawal, is the way to deepen the patient–clinician relationship and create an atmosphere in which personal growth is more likely to occur (see Chapter 2).

 CASE ILLUSTRATION 3

At 68 years old, Albert has severe end-stage emphysema, complicated by mitral regurgitation, congestive heart failure, cardiac arrhythmias, alcoholism, and years of smoking. He lives with his wife, whom he has bullied and dominated throughout their 40-year marriage. He has been on home oxygen and has had multiple hospital admissions for shortness of breath.

Admitted to the emergency room with severe shortness of breath, Albert is found to have pneumonia and heart failure. He had previously decided not to have CPR and wanted "no part of any of those damned machines." He is admitted to the hospital and treated with aggressive medical means but is not put on a respirator. Albert regularly yells and curses at the respiratory therapists, nursing staff, physicians, and his family for not taking care of him, for making him suffer, and for not being prompt enough with meals, medicines, and treatments. He insists that the only thing wrong with him is that the medicines are making him sick.

Efforts to engage Albert in a dialogue that explores his feelings meet first with an unwillingness to talk and then a life history of feeling abandoned, powerless, betrayed by employers, and subject to bad luck. He describes himself as an "ornery son of a bitch." He fears lingering and suffering in the hospital, and although he hopes he will die quickly, he is also afraid to die. One of Albert's fears is of being buried alive, a phobia fed by a television program he had seen about the difficulty of determining when someone was dead and the possibility of being sent to the undertaker while still alive. The anxiety of being trapped in a "tight" place is overwhelming to him.

Albert's physicians had initially resisted placing him on anxiolytic drugs or narcotics out of fear they would compromise his breathing. The palliative care consultant recommended that both be started, and reassured both the treating physicians as well as the patient and family of the safety and effectiveness of these treatments as long as they are started at low doses. Low-dose opioids and anxiolytic medications are eventually started around the clock, and his dyspnea and anxiety are dramatically improved. Placed in a room with a large picture window to the outside, he spends long periods of time staring out the window. His complaints diminish and he seems much more relaxed. He allows the hospital chaplain to visit and to pray with him, though he does not otherwise want to talk about the nearness of death or any regrets he has about his life. He eventually tells his wife he has suffered enough, and does not want to live any longer. He gradually becomes more confused as a result of the rising carbon dioxide levels and dies several nights later.

Patients with difficult personality traits who are experiencing the dying process can be especially challenging to caregivers. As represented on palliative care teams, the use of multidisciplinary specialties to brainstorm potential approaches and to share expertise may facilitate providers' commitment not to abandon these particularly challenging patients and families.

Information, Prognosis, Alternatives

Clinicians need to provide the patient with information about the disease, the prognosis, the treatment options, and the anticipated course of the illness. Most patients and their families want to know how much time is left when a terminal diagnosis is made. Providing ranges of survival times and allowing for outliers on either end is better than predicting an exact amount of time. Refusing to give time estimates or withholding other grim information to protect the patient is usually not productive and may not allow the patient and family to prepare for death. The possibility of a miracle or an exception to the usual course of the illness allows a glimmer of hope for some patients. However, clinicians giving prognostic information must discipline themselves to discuss the possibility that death may also come sooner than expected, so that patients are not unprepared for this possibility as well. In general, the physician should be guided by patients and their families in determining how detailed the information about the course of the illness should be.

Alternative healing methods may offer hope to some patients when traditional methods are not working, have proven too burdensome, or are not consistent with the patient's preferences. Patients who are interested in pursuing alternative methods of treatment should be supported in doing so, particularly if those treatments are noninvasive, and are therefore unlikely to harm. There is nothing to preclude combining nontraditional treatments with traditional treatments as part of an individually tailored plan. Aggressive therapeutic alternatives offer some patients a degree of hope. However, clinicians and patients should explore the tradeoffs of this type of hope together. Examining the risks and benefits of both traditional and nontraditional therapies is frequently enough to begin the dialogue, which can then continue by exploring the possibilities and probabilities of improvement and by distinguishing false hope from a meaningful alternative (see Chapter 33).

  CASE ILLUSTRATION 4

Max, a 63-year-old, recently retired, and previously healthy man, develops abdominal pains and is found to have widely metastasized colon cancer. He goes to a physician and is advised that no treatment would be beneficial and that he has approximately 6–12 months to live. He is given acetaminophen and codeine for pain and told to come back when the combination no longer relieves the discomfort. Max and his wife cannot bear the thought of just waiting for him to die and decide to cast a wider net in seeking a cure—or at least some kind of treatment. They hear of a cancer treatment clinic out of the country and go there for a 6-week program of intensive vitamin and herbal treatments, coffee enemas, a variety of teas, and dietary supplements. Max is also given a long list of treatments to follow when he returns home; this keeps him busy trying to "beat" the cancer. The clinic is supposed to provide follow-up by mail or telephone; however, several *months go by and there is no contact from the clinic.*

Discouraged, Max and his wife go to another physician in their hometown when the abdominal pain intensifies and ascites and jaundice set in. The physician and the couple discuss the available options and agree on purely palliative care measures. Max is referred to a home hospice program and dies 4 weeks later, approximately 9 months from the time of diagnosis. His family feels he received superb care for his last 4 weeks; however, they feel abandoned and betrayed with regard to his prior treatment. His wife never receives any follow-up information from the overseas clinic, nor does anyone from the original physician's office call to offer condolences on her husband's death.

The patient in case illustration 4 has been abandoned twice. The first treating physician failed to explore all treatment alternatives (such as a second opinion, experimental therapy, and guidance in exploring nontraditional treatments) and then offered inadequate follow-up (asking him only to come back when his pain is uncontrollable at home). The alternative clinic offered the patient an active treatment approach which he and his wife desperately sought, but then deserted him by failing to follow through after the treatment was completed. The third physician finally helped the patient and family come to grips with the reality of his condition, and arranged for a program that provided caring and follow-up for his final weeks. Nonabandonment is always a key element in the care of the dying patient.

Hope & Meaning

Throughout the dying process, the search for hope and meaning is always present, even if it is not dominant. Hope aids patients and their loved ones in enduring suffering when faced with a terminal illness. It comes in many forms, not simply through cure or recovery: to hope for a peaceful death, to hope for more time to finish business, to find new meaning and the possibility of personal growth, and to hope for more emotional closeness with loved ones or with God. None of these hopes are dependent on cure of the body.

CASE ILLUSTRATION 5

Rhea, a 64-year-old woman with metastatic breast cancer, is on high-dose long-acting morphine because of bone pain. She has fractures of the clavicle and both femurs and has requested no

resuscitation in the event of cardiac or pulmonary arrest. She hopes to be able to die at home, where she has very close family support, without more painful episodes or fractures. She is enrolled in a home hospice program, and her sister moves in with her to serve the role as primary care provider.

Rhea eventually shows signs of increasing confusion and dehydration. She expresses the strong wish not to die yet, because her children and their families are arriving in 2 weeks. She wants not only to see them, but also to be as alert and pain free as possible while they visit. Blood work is done to see if she has anything that might be easily reversed, and hypercalcemia is found. Because she wishes to die at home with only palliative measures taken, she remains at home for another day. She knows that she will likely die from the effects of the untreated hypercalcemia, but that she then would likely not get to see her children. Despite attempts at oral treatment, she becomes progressively less alert, and is brought to an acute hospice unit when her oral intake stops.

In hope of having her alert for her family's upcoming visit, treatment is initiated with intravenous fluids, diuretics, and bisphosphonates. The hypercalcemia is corrected, her confusion clears, and she is able to go home after a week. By the time her children arrive, Rhea is alert and able to communicate coherently. She is quite elated that she can have last words with them and her grandchildren. Despite the need for increased doses of morphine and multiple other medications to control her symptoms, she is not readmitted to the acute hospice unit when her hypercalcemia and the associated confusion recur. She dies quietly at home several days later.

Fortunately, the hope for more time in case illustration 5 could be achieved, because the patient was willing to endure relatively aggressive treatment, and the hospice program allowed flexibility to meet her short-term goals. Invasive interventions that exceed the usual boundaries of hospice care but that extend meaningful life and improve quality of life are sometimes appropriate even within a hospice approach, as long as the patient consents. Remaining flexible in the face of changing, difficult situations and allowing the patient's goals to guide the treatment permit the clinician to hope along with the patient for a death with as little meaningless suffering as possible.

Trying to find and maintain hope when the patient's goal of recovery is futile calls for personal and spiritual exploration. It may be necessary to probe in depth the patient's feeling of hopelessness before possible new avenues for hope and meaning can be examined. It is important not to provide false hope through simple or formulaic solutions to complex problems; hopeful solutions are often uniquely personal and may be discovered through the patient's continuing exploration with family, friends, health care providers, and clergy.

PLANNING FOR THE FUTURE

Advance Directives

Advance directives are formal documents that direct health care decisions should patients lose the capacity to speak for themselves in the future. There are two types of advance directives: living wills and health care proxies (also called durable powers of attorney).

A living will allows a patient to direct the kinds of treatments wanted if the capacity to make decisions is lost. Some living wills focus on general goals, whereas others specify exact treatments (CPR, artificial ventilation, artificial hydration, and nutrition) and explicit circumstances (terminal illness, persistent vegetative state, unable to make decisions for oneself). Living wills become operative only when patients are unable to communicate for themselves, and when the circumstances specified in the document are realized.

A **health care proxy** or **durable power of attorney** allows patients to designate a person to make decisions on their behalf should they become unable to do so. These directives allow much more flexibility than do living wills, as it is difficult to anticipate all possible medical conditions and treatment options that might be in question for a particular patient.

Many people complete both documents: a living will to represent an overarching philosophy to guide care, and a health care proxy to designate a person to help interpret that philosophy when the patient can no longer do so. For healthy persons, discussing a living will or a health care proxy may be the first time they have had to face their own mortality. For those with terminal illness, completing an advance directive may be seen as another indication of their inevitable deterioration.

Involving family members in the discussions of advance directives is useful. A proxy who is uninformed about the values and wishes of the patient has an arduous job when difficult care decisions must be made. Although they cannot cover every situation, living wills with clear statements about goals, values, and directions help the clinician and the designated proxy formulate a care plan. In addition, having a form to fill out helps many patients and their families discuss death-and disability-related issues. For severely ill patients, the advance directive decisions can provide a starting point for discussions about limitations on care and the burdens of suffering as well as orders not to resuscitate.

Do Not Resuscitate

The "do-not-resuscitate" (DNR order refers to the withholding of CPR, specifically closed-chest cardiac massage, defibrillation, and artificially supplied respiratory support. For most patients with a terminal disease, CPR is ineffective, and its harshness makes it a cruel, expensive, technological death ritual. Many studies have shown that CPR provides no increase in out-of-hospital survival for patients with multisystem disease, particularly patients with advanced cancers and renal failure.

Unfortunately, many patients and their families equate DNR with abandonment or "giving up," and agonize over its issuance. This is in part due to the way medical personnel emphasize what will be withheld rather than what will be done. When alternative treatment strategies are not explained, patients and families think that a DNR order means nothing will be done to treat potentially reversible conditions or to relieve uncomfortable symptoms. They sense that second-class treatment will be given—which may indeed happen if clinicians and the institutions they work in are not knowledgeable about the narrow focus on a DNR directive. It should be understood that agreement to a DNR order in no way limits other treatment options. A way of articulating this is to say: *"We want to do everything possible to help you, but we also do not want to harm you. CPR would not work given your condition, and it is very harsh. I would recommend that you set that limit while we continue to provide any and all treatments that will help you."*

DNR orders do, however, signal that things are different. The notion that being resuscitated from cardiopulmonary arrest will not add appreciably to the quality and or quantity of life is an open acknowledgment that death might be near—and that reversing the dying process is not within the power of medicine. Although some patients are initially frightened by this discussion, many feel relieved and appreciate the opportunity to avoid treatment that would not help them.

Emergency rescue crews are obligated to attempt resuscitation unless they have specific instructions not to proceed. DNR orders that are valid in the inpatient setting may not be valid in the outpatient setting unless special forms, which vary by locality, are completed. These issues should be addressed with terminally ill patients who want to remain at home, as resuscitation may be carried out in times of crisis if the proper documentation is not on hand. In New York and other states, the Medical Orders for Life Sustaining Treatment (MOLST) has been accepted as a legal document that must be honored by emergency medical technicians and first responders. This ensures portability to other settings of the patient's explicit wishes recorded in physicians' orders.

Restricted Interventions

Patients at the end of life, or patients with a high degree of suffering, may elect through their advance directives not to undergo treatments that may be considered routine under other circumstances. Patients have the right to forgo therapies such as intravenous fluids, nasogastric feeding, supplemental oxygen, and others. Documentation of these choices is vital if the patient does not wish to undergo treatments and can be done on the MOLST form. Restricted intervention forms are also available in some states to augment the advance directives.

Pain and Symptom Relief

An important goal in palliative care is to keep patients as free of pain as is possible. Long-acting opioid preparations, when given in sufficient quantity in a regular dosing schedule with proportionate supplemental doses as needed, are effective in alleviating most chronic pain without significantly compromising quality of life (see Chapter 35). Knowing that they can control their own pain is reassuring to patients, especially those who have seen painful deaths. Unrealistic concerns about addiction or about respiratory depression from patients, families, and caregivers should be anticipated and addressed, as these worries often present a major obstacle to adequate pain relief. Withholding narcotics in the seriously ill because of unrealistic fears is unwarranted and cruel.

Delirium & Coma

Many patients die in profoundly altered states of sensorium. There is also an increasing number of patients with dementing illnesses in whom cognitive and affective life may have diminished significantly prior to the terminal episode. Terminally ill patients with delirium present the physician and the patient's family with a dilemma. Delirium may be due to reversible factors that, if treated, could extend life. The extent to which reversible causes of delirium are searched for and treated depends on the patient's current goals, previous directives, and concurrent discussions with the family in light of their underlying medical condition. The prior degree of suffering and the patient's wishes should largely determine what should be done.

 CASE ILLUSTRATION 6

Caleb, a 101-year-old rugged dairy farmer, has become partly deaf and then blind in the last 5 years of his life but remains alert and communicative. He develops a cough and fever, and despite treatment for pneumonia, becomes progressively more dyspneic. He tells his physician that he does not wish to be resuscitated. Because his elderly wife cannot care

for him at home, Caleb is hospitalized. He becomes progressively more confused and withdrawn, and his deafness and blindness further confound communication. He lies still in bed for long periods of time. Efforts by physicians and nurses to engage him in conversation are usually met with short responses such as yes, no, or okay. His physician asks him one morning what experiences he is having, and he replies that he is flying over fields of golden wheat on a sunny day. Then, in a voice of wonderment, he asks if he is still alive or if he has died. His physician replies that he is still alive. Caleb dies later that day.

The internal, subjective experience of a person dying with altered mental status may vary significantly from the outside perception. Patients who recover from delirium and coma sometimes report nightmarish, terrifying visions, out-of-body travel, or visions of light and angelic beings; others may not be able to remember anything about the experience. Occasionally, the disorientation becomes profound and the sense of the world is lost.

Patients who experience delirium at the end of life need supportive treatment. If not already done in advance by the patient, decisions about artificial hydration and feeding should be made and formalized through the designated health care agent. The agent or the family, taking into consideration the patient's condition and prognosis, must make a substituted judgment as to what the patient would want if they were able to understand the nuances of their condition. If this cannot be determined, the physician's decision should be based on a consensus among family and providers about what is in the best interest of the patient.

Providing nutrition and hydration through feeding tubes and intravenous lines when the dying patient can no longer eat or drink may appear compassionate, but such practices may inadvertently prolong dying and aggravate suffering. When a person with a terminal illness is actively dying, our acceptance of this fact should guide all treatments in the direction of decreasing the suffering, enhancing the quality of remaining time, and respecting the patient's dignity.

The Wish to Die

Sometimes, even with the best methods of palliative care, suffering cannot be alleviated to the patient's satisfaction. If this occurs, the patient may feel that dying is the only way out. The patient may no longer be able to tolerate the pain, humiliation, loss of control, increased dependency, or burden the illness places on the family. Such patients often actively begin to contemplate ending their life.

Table 40-2. Last resort interventions: definitions.

Term	Definition	Legal Status in the United States
Double effect	Administering drugs that are intended to relieve suffering but may unintentionally shorten life. The risk of shortening life must be proportionate to the degree of suffering. The clinician can foresee that life might be shortened, but it is not intended.	Legal
Withholding or withdrawing life-sustaining treatment	Withholding or withdrawing life-sustaining care that might result in the patient's death with the consent of the patient or surrogate. Justification based on the right to bodily integrity.	Legal with the proper consent
Palliative sedation to unconsciousness (also called terminal sedation)	With consent from the patient or surrogate, the patient is sedated to unconsciousness to relieve otherwise intractable suffering, and then food and fluids are withdrawn. Generally viewed as a combination of double effect and withdrawal of treatment, but not without moral controversy if viewed in aggregate.	Legal with the proper consent
Physician aid-in-dying (also called physician-assisted suicide)	Physician provides, at the patient's request, the means for the patient to end his or her own life. The patient then takes or does not take the overdose at a future time.	Illegal in most US states except for Oregon, Washington, Montana, and Vermont but difficult to prosecute
Active euthanasia	Physician administers an intentional lethal overdose of medication with the competent patient's informed consent. The physician is the direct agent causing death at the patient's request.	Illegal, and likely to be successfully prosecuted in the United States if discovered

CASE ILLUSTRATION 7

Marvin is 63 years old; he has amyotrophic lateral sclerosis and has been on a respirator at home for one year. He has lost the ability to use his arms and legs and requires total care. He increasingly resents his life on the respirator and finally requests that it be removed and he be permitted to die. He makes this request repeatedly over the course of a month. His primary care physician sees him several times on home visits and discusses the request with Marvin's family. They agree that the respirator should be stopped. A psychiatrist visits the patient and indicates that he finds Marvin competent, not depressed; he concurs with the patient, family, and primary care physician on removing the respirator. An attempt to remove the respirator without the sedative effects of morphine leads to air hunger and feelings of suffocation. A morphine drip is instituted and the respirator is turned off. The patient dies comfortably several minutes later, attended by his family and physician.

The ***double effect*** of providing medications intended to relieve suffering while taking the risk that they may unintentionally shorten the patient's life is an accepted part of medical practice and palliative care, provided the patient's suffering is proportionately severe. Withdrawing life-sustaining but burdensome treatments, even though the withdrawal leads to death, is also an accepted part of practice based on the patient's right to bodily integrity. These practices have widespread legal, ethical, and medical acceptance and should not be confused with the controversy surrounding assisted suicide and voluntary euthanasia. In this case, the patient's wish to die can be acceded to provided it is fully informed and not based on inadequate palliation. In such circumstances, treatments that are life-sustaining but very burdensome could be removed in conjunction with the provision of a high-dose narcotic that is intended to lessen suffering (Table 40-2).

Patients, however, may ask the clinician, sometimes in an off-hand way as if testing the water, about help in dying (either assisted suicide or euthanasia). This subject has both ethical and legal repercussions, and physicians are often as reluctant as their patients to discuss it.

If the patient has terrible suffering but does not have a life-sustaining treatment that can be withdrawn (e.g., respirator, dialysis, feeding tube) or the kind of pain that can justify high doses of narcotics, the request for help in dying would put the clinician in a more difficult position legally and ethically. **Voluntary active euthanasia** is the act of intentionally intervening to cause the patient's death, at the explicit request of, and with the full informed consent of, the competent patient. The physician administers a lethal agent, with the intent of both alleviating suffering and causing death. Although voluntary active euthanasia is legal is several western European countries, it is clearly illegal everywhere in the United States and would lead to prosecution if discovered. In **assisted suicide**, the physician provides the means (such as a prescription for barbiturates) at the request of the patient, but the patient must eventually take (or not take) the potentially lethal medication by his or her own hand. Assisted suicide is legal in Oregon, Washington, Montana, and Vermont, but it is illegal in most other states. There is an underground practice in these other states that is not actively prosecuted provided it is conducted in secret. There are now data about the legalized practice in Oregon and Washington which can allow for comparison of utilization patterns of assisted dying and other last-resort palliative care practices with other states.

CASE ILLUSTRATION 8

Sara, a bedridden 84-year-old woman with end-stage congestive heart failure, is seen on rounds. She is on multiple medications, including morphine, to relieve her dyspnea and pulmonary edema. Despite intensive treatment, even eating causes her to be dyspneic. She looks up from her bed and asks to be given a lethal dose of medicine so that she can die. When asked why she wants to die now, Sara replies that she has lived long enough—through the deaths of her husband, two of her children, three of her brothers, and both her sisters. Her one remaining son is dying of leukemia and has only weeks to live. She wants to die before him so that she will not have to grieve his death. Her request for lethal medication is not granted. Sara leaves the hospital with public health nurses and family to look after her. Her physician agrees to make home visits as Sara is too weak to travel to the office. A few days later, Sara is found dead in bed by the visiting nurse. The physician, called to the house to pronounce the patient dead, notices several empty pill bottles, including those from the morphine, at the bedside. The physician thinks that this may have been a suicide, but decides not to pursue it and simply completes the death certificate as for a natural death.

A patient's request to hasten death should be explored in detail. At first, it should be considered a cry for help. It may represent the wish to escape from depression, anxiety, uncontrolled physical pain, shame of dependency, and other psychosocial issues. Once the underlying reasons for the request are fully understood, the problem(s) can usually be ameliorated through appropriate techniques of palliative care, and the request is frequently withdrawn. If the request is ignored, minimized, or belittled, the patient is left to deal with these feelings alone, and may (as in case illustration 8) take an overdose because of suffering that might have been dealt with by other means.

There are times, as in our example, when protracted pain and other debilitating symptoms might make choosing death a plausible alternative to continued suffering. The relationship between the physician, patient, and family as well as the physician's own values determine the response to such requests. Clinicians who refuse to participate in assisted suicide because of their own moral positions should make this clear to the patient who inquires. In this event, they have an obligation to seek common ground with the patient and to continue to search for other avenues to relieve suffering. Usually such intractable suffering can be addressed with symptom management, withdrawal of potentially life-sustaining therapies, and terminal sedation as a last resort. In this particular case, if the patient's request was found to be rational and all reasonable alternatives had been explored, the patient could have stopped all of her heart failure medicines except for her morphine, which could have been titrated upward to control emerging shortness of breath. Those clinicians who are considering any last-resort options (legally permitted, and especially if legally prohibited) should fully explore the potential personal, professional, and legal consequences and get second opinions from experienced clinicians before proceeding. Guidelines for assisted suicide have been published, and clinicians confronted with a reasonable request to end life should refer to these, as well as to colleagues experienced in palliative care for help. In almost all cases, legally permissible and clinically preferable alternatives can be found.

ACCEPTANCE

Some patients are not afraid of dying and come to accept death as a natural step in completing the life cycle. Many such persons are able to die with grace and ease, demonstrating that death does not always have to be feared or denied. Furthermore, some patients experience profound personal growth in the process of dying. For some highly independent persons, this becomes a time to be more accepting and appreciative of the love and care of others.

CASE ILLUSTRATION 9

A 64-year-old veterinarian, Richard, develops headaches so severe that he can no longer carry on his surgical practice. Within 3 months, he is diagnosed with an inoperable brain tumor. Over the ensuing 6 months, he loses the ability to walk and swallow. Because of recurrent aspiration, he is placed on a home ventilator and fed through a gastrostomy tube. In the face of his overwhelming losses, he decides he wants relatives, friends, colleagues and members of his church to come to his home and tape a description of his life and journey to the point at which he is now. When this process is complete Richard says good-bye to his wife and family and requests that the respirator and fluids be withdrawn. With his physician's consent and instructions to family members, he is given regular doses of morphine and the respirator is turned off. He dies with his loved ones in attendance. His life and death leave a legacy of courage and an acquiescence to fate that touches the hearts of those he knew.

The search for love, a connection to others, and a sense of meaning is essential in helping patients through the dying process. The ability to experience love and meaning can ameliorate considerable suffering. If love and purpose can be found, then fears usually lessen, and dying may be accepted as an adventure and entry into the next phase of existence.

CARE OF THE FAMILY

Terminal illness can help resolve or intensify family conflict. Issues of power, money, allegiances, previous losses, and grief may surface along with unforeseen courage and the noblest sacrifices that family members may ever have made for each other. Paradoxical feelings of anger and love, fear and bravery, anxiety and compassion, depression and transcendence never seem to be far removed from dying patients and their caregivers.

The physician can be a healing presence in this volatile mix by including the patient's family and other caregivers as part of the treatment team. Such collaboration broadens the patient's network of support, enlisting new allies and more widely distributing the burden of care.

The clinician needs to communicate clearly with the family members regarding plans for care, prognosis, complications, and who will make decisions should the patient be unable. Establishing advance directives with the patient and the proxy is essential when it is likely the patient will lose capacity during the illness. The selection of a proxy forces the patient to choose among family members and may trigger old family wounds over who was favored and who has more power. The patient's wishes and choices should take precedence over what family members may want, although in actual practice this is sometimes difficult to achieve. When the patient loses mental capacity, the family becomes the focus of decision making, and processes are brought into play that may create conflict. Family pressures may even influence the decisions of a competent patient. The clinician may need to remind family members that whether the patient is competent or not,

the patient's values, beliefs, and preferences need to be honored.

When a family has many members, the clinician may want to meet regularly with a small group and at special times with more members. The family can be asked to designate representatives who can stay in close touch with the physician. If patients have lost the capacity to express their wishes and family members are in conflict about a certain plan, it is best to focus on what the patient would have wanted, applying the ethical principle of substituted judgment. If the patient's wishes are unknown, what is in the patient's best interest must be discussed. Views on what is truly in the patient's best interest may vary widely between family members and clinicians (see Chapter 11).

Unexpected Death

An unexpected death puts a particular strain on the family and the clinician. Sudden or traumatic death sends a shock through the family and, when it occurs in a medical facility, may elicit strong doubt about competence in clinicians. Meeting with the family, expressing sympathy, and answering questions in as straightforward a way as possible may be helpful. Family members should be allowed to view and stay with the deceased; when possible, the eyes and mouth should be closed and the limbs arranged peacefully. Strong emotional reactions should be anticipated and the tears of grief encouraged.

The clinician should recognize each family member present and solicit each person's reaction. Cultural norms may vary widely in the emotional behaviors displayed. The normal reactions to grief in some cultures (screaming, yelling, falling to the ground) may seem inappropriate or embarrassing to a clinician from another, less demonstrative background (see Chapter 15). Only through experience with various manifestations of grief can the clinician judge what "normal" grief should look like. Physicians and nurses may want to call in clergy and social workers; each may have something to offer a family that is trying to integrate the shock and loss.

When an unexpected death occurs in the context of ongoing medical care, the practitioner should critically examine what, if anything could have been done to prevent its occurrence. Self-recrimination and blame may initially be part of this process for the clinician, especially if a possible medical misjudgment was involved. Learning from the experience, discussing it with trusted colleagues, and disclosing it to the family are often appropriate. It is important that clinicians not bear the burdens of these experiences alone (see Chapter 37).

Unresolved Grief

Of all the causes of unremitting grief, one of the most overwhelmingly difficult for families and practitioners is the death of a child, especially when the death is unexpected. The parents' grief must be followed closely for signs of becoming pathological. The physician should not try to ameliorate the pain of the loss prematurely. Supportive listening, acknowledging and legitimizing the suffering, and expressing empathy may be the best initial approach. Follow-up visits to elicit stories and memories give the parents a chance to talk about the deceased if they choose. Discussing and expressing anger, guilt, and sadness can assist in the bereavement process. In many other cases, survivors are unable to deal with the loss of a parent, a sibling, a spouse or partner, or a long-time friend. Grief that is unresolved may lead to clinical depression, social isolation, and emotional numbing as well as multiple physical symptoms. Social problems such as drug abuse, marital and work conflicts, and feelings of hopelessness and abandonment may also appear. If the clinician cannot help the family resolve the grief, referral should be made to an appropriate support group or a therapist for counseling.

Under the Medicare Hospice Benefit, hospices provide bereavement support for at least a year to families of patients they have served. They also provide bereavement services to partners and close friends. Often, hospices provide this support to people in their community even if the death did not occur with hospice care.

SELF-CARE

How health care workers take care of themselves when involved in work related to death and dying has not received a great deal of attention. Burnout is common among physicians and nurses who work with patients who are suffering with a terminal illness. Having responsibility for dying patients' care and management in a society that denies death only exacerbates the problem. From the initial delivery of bad news about a new serious diagnosis, to discussions about disease recurrence, to the transition to hospice, to decisions about whether to attend the funeral, clinicians are confronted with thoughts and feelings that enmesh them with the patient and the family. How closely the patient's family resembles their own family dynamics or illness experience may determine how emotionally involved they become. The grief that follows the death of a close patient may be quite profound and requires time and reflection to heal. Unfortunately, most institutions do not have an organized way for caregivers to get and give support during these times. The feelings of loss need to be recognized and discussed. Support or bereavement groups may help in this process. Hospital morbidity and mortality committees review the decedent's medical care, but they rarely reflect on how caregivers felt about the death, or what effect it has on the staff. Setting aside time to review the death from this perspective is likely to be helpful for staff morale, cohesiveness, and healing (see Chapter 6).

Taking care of the dying patient enables clinicians to view death at very close range. Feelings of compassion and love as well as loneliness and vulnerability are frequently stirred up in providers. Healing responses may include turning to music, art, religion, literature, nature, humor, or psychotherapy for solace and understanding. Spiritual questions of purpose and meaning in life become more immediate in the face of impending death. Not only do workers in the realm of death and dying midwife patients through the dying process, but also the dying patient midwives us into a fuller experience of life.

Photo by Hank Christensen (www.hankchristensen. com)

SUGGESTED READINGS

Back AL, Arnold RM, Quill TE. Hope for the best, and prepare for the worst. *Ann Intern Med* 2003;138:439–443.

Block, SD. Psychological issues in end-of-life care. *J Palliat Med* 2006;9:751–772.

Casarett DJ, Quill TE. "I'm not ready for hospice": strategies for timely and effective hospice discussions. *Ann Intern Med* 2007;146:443–449.

Clinical Practice Guideline: Management of Cancer Pain. Agency for Health Care Policy and Research.Publication No. 94–0592. Available through the National Cancer Institute.

Meier DE, Back AL, Morrison RS. The inner life of physicians and the care of the seriously ill. *JAMA* 2001;286:3007–3014.

Quill TE. *Caring for Patients at the End of Life: Facing an Uncertain Future Together.* New York, NY: Oxford University Press, 2001.

Quill TE, Bower KA, Holloway R, et al. *Palliative Care Primer,* 6th ed. American Academy of Hospice and Palliative Medicine, Chicago, IL. 2014.

Quill TE, Lo B, Brock DW, Meisel A. Last resort options for palliative sedation. *Ann Intern Med* 2009;151:421–424.

Snyder L, Quill TE, eds.*Physician Guide to End-of-Life Care.* Philadelphia, PA: ACP-ASIM Publishing, 2001.

Sulmasy DP. Spiritual issues in the care of dying patients" ...*It's okay between me and God."JAMA* 2006;296:1385–1392.

WEB SITES

American Academy of Hospice and Palliative Medicine. www.aahpm.org. Accessed June 2013.

Center to Advance Palliative Care. www.capc.org. Accessed June 2013.

Compassion and Choices. www.compassionandchoices.org. Accessed June 2013.

Death with Dignity National Center. www.deathwithdignity.org. Accessed June 2013.

Education in Palliative and End-of-Life Care. www.epec.net. Accessed June 2013.

End of Life/Palliative Education Resource Center. www.eperc.mcw.edu. Accessed June 2013.

Hospice Foundation of America. http://www.hospicefoundation.org/ Accessed June2013.

National Consensus Project for Quality Palliative Care (2013). *Clinical Practice Guidelines for Quality Palliative Care, Third Edition.* http://www.nationalconsensusproject.org. Accessed June 2013.

National Hospice and Palliative Care Organization. www.nhpco.org. Accessed June 2013.

National Palliative Care Research Center. www.npcrc.org. Accessed June 2013.

Medical Orders for Life-Sustaining Treatment (MOLST). www.molst.org. Accessed June 2013.

Physician Orders for Life-Sustaining Treatment (POLST). http://www.polst.org/ Accessed June 2013.

SECTION VI
Teaching and Assessment

Competency-Based Education for Behavioral Medicine

41

Jason M. Satterfield, PhD & Eric Holmboe, MD

Wendy is a second year internal medicine resident currently struggling to feel "competent" as an outpatient primary care provider. Over the course of her internship year, her competence and confidence with inpatient care grew. However, her outpatient clinics were infrequent in comparison and she feels like she hasn't learned to be a "good primary care doctor." She shares her frustrations with her mentor—in part fueled by the breadth of skills required, the lack of benchmarks to measure her progress, and the lack of validated assessment tools. Her mentor attempts to help Wendy develop an individualized learning plan with formative assessments.

Medical education has recently undergone a transformation from process-oriented measures of success to more outcomes-oriented assessments that gauge what a learner can actually do and not only to what they have been exposed. Although the notion of competencies is not new, more recent conceptualizations move far beyond simple listings of skills and include multidimensional, dynamic, contextual, and developmental elements. This movement has been particularly transformative in the realm of graduate medical education (GME) with the advent of the Accreditation Council for Graduate Medical Education (ACGME) competencies and has become increasingly common as medical schools begin to embrace competency-based medical education (CBME) and translate the GME competencies for

medical students "further upstream." Learning objectives and related competencies are now more frequently articulated and tend to be more commonly linked to specific assessment tools that measure achievement of that specific competency. However, the practice of medicine is inherently complex and often requires subtle, nuanced skills that are both difficult to teach and challenging to quantify. In particular, competencies that fall within the realm of the Behavioral and Social Sciences (BSS) have proven particularly difficult to articulate, teach, and assess.

This chapter will first provide a brief overview of CBME that articulates common advantages and limitations of this approach. We then offer an update on the status of BSS curricular thinking within medical education, including the recent work of the Association of American Medical Colleges (AAMC) BSS Expert Panel, the BSS Curriculum Consortium (funded by National Institutes of Health [NIH]), and the behavioral science subcommittee of the MCAT 5th Revision (MR5) Committee (charged with creating the 5th version of the Medical College Admissions Test). This chapter presents a careful melding of the concepts and processes of CBME with the content of BSS by offering a synthesis of the innovative work emerging on both undergraduate medical education (UME) and GME levels. Specific assessment methods and evaluation tools for BSS competencies are described in Chapter 43.

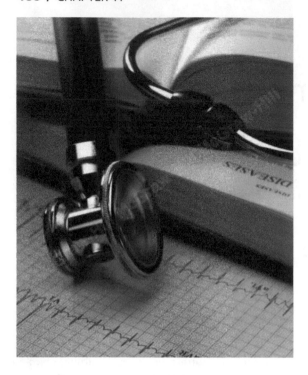

Pedagogical Building Blocks for CBME

The Royal College of Physicians and Surgeons of Canada define competency-based education and training (CBET) as "an outcomes-based approach to the design, implementation, assessment and evaluation of an education program using an organizing framework of competencies." CBET and CBME are intended to focus on outcomes, emphasize abilities, de-emphasize time-based training, and promote greater learner-centeredness. Epstein defines professional competence as "the habitual and judicious use of knowledge, technical skills, clinical reasoning, emotions, values, and reflection in daily practice for the benefit of the individual and community being served". More simply, Ten Cate defines competence as "the threshold level in the development of expertise that permits unsupervised practice".

A number of classical pedagogical and learning theories have helped medical education move from an expert-centric, apprenticeship model to a more evolved, evidence-based approach emphasizing adult learning and professional development. Medicine is perhaps unique in the number of disciplines, the quantity of knowledge, and the integrative capacity required to achieve even minimal competence. Miller's Pyramid offers a useful rubric in considering the progression of skill acquisition moving from Knows to Knows How to

Shows How to Does in a passing resemblance to the classic See One, Do One, Teach One. Dreyfus and Dreyfus present a continuum ranging from novice at one end, then progressing to advanced, competent, proficient, and expert. It is notable that in the Dreyfus model "competent" does not lie at the end of the continuum but precedes proficient and expert implying that competence is a stage, an important benchmark, on the way to becoming an expert.

In each of these important models and definitions it is clear that competence is thought to progress in a developmental fashion in response to direct (and indirect) intervention from the educational system and the learning environment. Recognizing this developmental aspect to competence, an international group developed a set of definitions to help clarify the confusion often engendered by the terms competencies, competence, and competent. Competencies are best viewed as "abilities." Competence and competent represent states of being that can be further subdivided into three categories:

- Competent: Possessing the required abilities in all domains at a specified stage of medical education or practice.
- Dyscompetent: Relatively lacking in one or more domains of required abilities at a specified stage of medical education or practice.
- Incompetent: Lacking the required abilities in all domains in a certain context at a defined state of medical education or practice.

Competence is acquired by the learner and not necessarily imparted by the faculty. Peers, patients, allied health professionals, the learner himself or herself, and others may be considered teachers capable of assisting a learner in acquiring competence. Once competent, learning and growth continue well into the professional years and perhaps for the rest of one's career. Competence is multidimensional and includes knowledge, procedural skills, metacognition, emotional management, social relationships, and communication. To best grasp how such breadth can be meaningfully captured and assessed to assist the faculty and learner in our opening vignette, it is helpful to review the history and evolution of CBME.

HISTORY OF CBET AND CBME

Competency-based medical education is not a new concept and represents an amalgam of educational theories, with origins in the work of Thorndike and Dewey. The earliest conception of competency-based training actually arose in the United States during the 1920s as educational reform became linked to industrial and business models of work that centered on clear specification of outcomes. However, the more recent conception of

Table 41-1. The Competency-based education and training (CBET).

CBET Principles	CBET Characteristics
1. Competencies are role derived, specified in behavioral terms, and made public	1. Learning is individualized
2. Assessment criteria are competency based and specify what constitutes mastery level of achievement	2. Feedback to the learner is critical
3. Assessment requires performance as the prime evidence but also takes knowledge into account	3. Emphasis is more on the exit criteria than on the admission criteria
4. Individual learners progress at rates dependent on demonstrated competency	4. CBET requires a systematic program (approach)
5. The instructional program facilitates development and evaluation of the specific competencies	5. Training is modularized
	6. Both the learner and the program have accountability

CBME had much of its genesis in the teacher education reform movement of the 1960s. This interest was spurred by a US Office of Education National Center for Education research grant program in 1968 to 10 universities to develop and implement new teacher training models that focused on student achievement (outcomes). Elam laid down a series of principles and characteristics of CBET in 1971 (see Table 41-1). In 2002, Carraccio and colleagues noted that some sectors in medical education explored competency-based models in the 1970s, but except for one study, no comparisons between competency-based and the traditional structure/process-based curricula were undertaken. The World Health Organization (WHO) commissioned a paper published in 1978 that strongly recommended the adoption of competency-based educational models for medical education, noting, *"The intended output of a competency-based programme is a health professional who can practise medicine at a defined level of proficiency, in accord with local conditions, to meet local needs."*

In the few studies within medical fields that have investigated competency-based models, there appear to be some benefits to trainees in the CBET model. For example, Johns Hopkins has employed competency-based approaches in its neurosurgery program, with success in accelerating competency in specific surgeries.

In 2002, the ACGME Outcome Project changed the accreditation focus from a program's process and structure (e.g., rotations, written curricula) to actual learner/program outcomes. Programs had to objectively document that their residents achieved competence in six general dimensions of practice—Medical Knowledge, Patient Care, Communication and Interpersonal Skills, Professionalism, Practice-Based Learning and Improvement, and Systems-Based Practice. In phase 1 of the Outcome Project, programs defined objectives to demonstrate learning in the competencies. In phase 2, they integrated the competencies into their curricula and expanded their evaluation systems to assess actual performance. In phase 3, programs are required to use aggregate performance data for curriculum reform—that is, examine important linkages between quality of patient care and education in the competencies. Phase 4 began in July 2011 and focuses on identification of benchmark programs and dissemination/adoption of emerging models of educational excellence. Each of the ACGME competencies are listed in Table 41-2 and paired with recommended assessment tools. Given the broad nature of these competencies, a substantial burden was placed on programs to define objectives and develop curricula.

In addition to the ACGME, a number of international competency frameworks have been developed to guide UME and GME curricula and assessment. Each provides a useful contrast to the ACGME approach, but like ACGME, is not specific to the social and behavioral sciences. Table 41-3 provides a side-by-side

Table 41-2. ACGME competencies and assessment tools.

ACGME Competency	Recommended Assessment Tools
Medical knowledge	MCQ exam, Oral exam
Patient care	Standardized patient, objective structured clinical examination (OSCE), patient survey, multi-source feedback (a.k.a. 360 degree assessment)
Communication and interpersonal skills	Standardized patient, OSCE, patient survey
Professionalism	OSCE, patient survey, multisource feedback
Practice-based learning and improvement	Portfolio, medical record review
Systems-based practice	MCQ exam, patient survey, multi-source feedback

Table 41-3. Medical competency frameworks.

ACGME (United States)	General Medical Council (Great Britain)	Scottish Doctor (Scotland)	CanMEDS Framework (Canada)
Six broad competency areas	Seven outcome categories for provisionally registered doctors	Twelve learning outcomes domains	Based on six physician roles and the integrative role of the medical expert
Medical knowledge	• Good clinical care	• Basic, social, and clinical sciences and underlying principles • Medical informatics	• Scholar
Patient care	• Good clinical care	• Clinical skills • Practical procedures • Patient investigation • Patient management • Decision making skills and clinical reasoning and judgment • Health promotion and disease prevention	• Health advocate • Medical expert
Interpersonal and communication skills	• Relationships with patients working with colleagues	• Clinical skills • Health promotion and disease prevention	• Communicator
Professionalism	• Health (self-care) • Probity (integrity)	• Attitudes, ethical understanding and legal responsibilities • Role of the doctor in the health service • Personal development	• Professional
Practice-based learning and improvement	• Maintaining good medical practice		• Manager
Systems-based practice	• Working with colleagues • Teaching and training, appraising and assessing	• Patient management • Role of the doctor in the health service	• Collaborator • Manager • Medical expert (integration of all roles)

comparison of these different competency frameworks. Competencies have been grouped by their approximate equivalence to the ACGME categories.

The American Board of Internal Medicine (ABIM) and the ACGME have sponsored the development of milestones for internal medicine residency training using the Dreyfus model of skill acquisition as the frame of reference for the milestones. They also have viewed competence as stage dependent to some degree. For example, what represents competence in interpersonal communication and skills changes as the resident progresses through the training program. The task force, therefore, used a hybrid of the Dreyfus and international group definition of competence to calibrate the milestones with the expectation that residents achieve, at a minimum, the defined level of competence before completion of residency training. The task force also included nonphysicians and trainees to ensure key developmental milestones were not missed and were stage appropriate. By the time a learner reaches competence, he or she has already progressed from simply applying rules to facts and features without context (novice) to considering the specific features of concrete situations (advanced beginner). The competent learner considers both context-free and situational elements but also hierarchically organizes and reduces them to a smaller set on which to base a decision. In addition, he or she becomes more intimately involved in the process and feels more responsible for the outcome. In the next stage, proficiency, learners solve problems with an intuition that usually derives from some time in independent practice. Thus, although it is expected that some residents will achieve proficiency in some competencies, the task force decided "proficiency" was the desired goal. They defined competence, however, in sufficiently robust terms that a resident deemed "competent" at graduation would be able to practice medicine effectively in an unsupervised clinical environment, a critical "entrustment" decision all training programs ultimately must make.

CBME has been embraced by UME as it moves away from the classic Flexner model of classroom-based basic science in years 1–2 with little clinical experience until year 3. Many medical schools have adopted the ACGME competency framework for both conceptual reasons and expediency. Presumably all graduating students will continue on to GME, and so will need to be familiar with the ACGME competencies. Conceptually, it is compelling to think of a full continuum of benchmarked competencies beginning with the first day of medical school and ending with achievement of competencies in residency. Of course, true CBME argues for a move away from time-based education, which could mean that some students (or residents) will achieve competence in less time whereas others may take longer. As with GME, UME BSS competencies are subsumed under the same rubric but perhaps less well articulated and more challenging to assess. Benchmarks for UME BSS competencies have not been developed, but helpful guidelines and tools have been provided by the Institute of Medicine (IOM) and AAMC (described below).

More recently, the concept of "entrustable professional activities" (EPA's) has emerged as a more practical and granular approach related to competency assessment. In medical training, a teacher essentially wants to train and "entrust" a learner to perform a particular activity such as performing a cardiac examination or diagnosing depression. Once "entrusted," the learner may continue to deepen that particular skill but can do so as a self-directed learner. Additional activities are added throughout training and potentially throughout an entire medical career. Although newer models of CBME have added contextual and multidimensional factors, the EPA approach does this in a more robust, holistic, systematic, and measurable way that yields practical outcomes.

Promises and Pitfalls of CBME

CBME represents a dramatic shift in the way we think about medical training and evaluation of medical learners at all levels. However, CBME is not without its critics. CBME, and particularly Milestones, struggle with the issue of granularity, or how atomistic one must be to reduce a complex skill into its constituent elements. Such reductions run the risk of becoming long, exhaustive lists of overlapping and sometimes redundant skills that still manage to be incomplete and may fail to capture the more subtle skills required in a complex interaction.

Particular "doctoring" skills, such as empathy or respect, and important skills like self-care or reflective capacity may prove particularly hard to benchmark and assess. Some have argued that the substantial assessment burden is amplified by the lack of psychometrically valid instruments and the lack of appropriately trained faculty evaluators. Beyond the obvious objections to the time, money, and resources required for CBME, some have argued that CBME focuses on the lowest common denominator rather than promoting learner excellence.

As the level of learner advances, competencies become more specialized, requiring ever greater levels of detail and specificity by program directors and evaluators. Proponents argue that despite these challenges, medicine has and always will be required to "entrust" its trainees to deliver medical care. Greater attention to specific, contextualized competencies makes this inevitable process more valid, reliable, and safe.

Creating a BSS Competency Framework

Despite the substantive struggles bound to arise from CBME, the challenge of articulating a particular skill set, describing its developmental progression, and developing assessment methodologies has important implications for the field. Recent educational research has supported the reduction of complex skill sets into constituent foundational skills, and CBME consensus conferences have affirmed the relative value of CBME in contrast to past guiding approaches. Moreover, CBME holds special promise for nonbiomedical disciplines often overlooked in medical curricula or thought to be too difficult to assess. BSS leaders have been required to articulate, operationalize, and justify BSS competencies thought essential to the practice of medicine. These initial efforts can be found in the work of the NIH BSS Curriculum Consortium, the IOM BSS Report Committee, and the AAMC BSS Expert Panel (see below).

Few would argue that BSS do not have a place within medical education and practice, but BSS is not always in sync with the culture of medicine which is still dominated by biomedicine. The BSS umbrella includes specific clinical content (medical knowledge) such as understanding the relationship between smoking and cardiovascular disease. However, BSS also includes methods of inquiry (qualitative or survey research) and introduces a philosophy of science and knowledge that includes the interdependence of variables, nonlinear causal models, tolerance of ambiguity, and social contextual factors. BSS includes meta-processes such as habits of mind, reflective capacity, self-regulation, professional identity development, and emotional management. And, finally, BSS speaks of the sociopolitical aspects of medicine, including medicine's "contract" with society, social justice, health care equality, ethics, and morality. In ACGME competency terms, BSS falls within all six competency domains but is most heavily represented in the Professionalism, Communication and Interpersonal Skills, and Systems-Based Practice categories.

Although lists of key BSS topics and more focused BSS competencies are available, they are not universally accepted and are paradoxically seen as both bloated and incomplete. Rather than focusing on the exclusion or inclusion of favored topics, these lists can serve as important starting points to develop and evaluate BSS curricula and competencies. To date, work to further define and list BSS topics and competencies has included the foundational work of the Association of Behavioral Science and Medical Education (ABSAME, the IOM BSS report (2004), the NIH BSS Curriculum Consortium, and more recently, the MR5 group and the AAMC BSS report (2011). Highlights from these seminal reports are presented below, and links to the full reports are provided at the end of the chapter.

ABSAME seeks to develop and promote the inclusion of the behavioral sciences in medical education. As part of that process, this AAMC-affiliated group developed one of the earliest and most comprehensive BSS content lists. Broad content categories included "Health, Illness, Sickness, and Disease," "Biological Components of Human Behavior," "Individual Behavior," "Interpersonal and Individual/Social Behavior," "Culture, Society, Institutions, and Organizations," "Epidemiology," "Clinical Reasoning," and "Psychopathology."

In 2004, the IOM released the report, *Social and Behavioral Sciences in Medical Education*. After a comprehensive review of BSS curricula across US medical schools, this report included five recommendations to move the field forward and presented a listing of six essential BSS content areas and 20 high-priority topics (see Table 41-4). These core content areas and topic listings have since been corroborated with a national faculty survey.

In response to one of the report recommendations, NIH funded nine medical schools to develop and evaluate BSS curricular innovations. Innovations have included greater explication of the IOM content areas, improved pedagogical methods, and more valid and reliable assessment tools for BSS competencies.

The MR5 Committee addressed the issue of BSS competencies even further upstream by specifying what BSS concepts, knowledge, and skills would be assessed for all medical school applicants taking the new MCAT starting in 2015. By setting the assessment standards, the MR5 committee essentially provided a road map to medical school advisors and applicants regarding what they should learn before applying to medical school. Table 41-5 lists the preliminary five core content areas and associated topics. As would be expected, these BSS areas represent the basic science of BSS, in contrast to the clinical applications of BSS described in the IOM report.

The report from the AAMC BSS Expert Panel, *Behavioral and Social Sciences Foundations for Future Physicians*, defines BSS within the context of medicine, illustrates the ways in which both BSS content and process influence teaching and clinical care, and provides a

Table 41-4. IOM content areas and high-priority topics.

Core Content Area	High-Priority Topics
1. Mind–body interactions in health and disease	• Biological mediators between psychological and social factors and health • Psychological, social, and behavioral factors in chronic disease • Psychological and social aspects of human development that influence disease and illness • Psychosocial aspects of pain
2. Patient behavior	• Health risk behaviors • Principles of behavior change • Impact of psychosocial stressors and psychiatric disorders on manifestations of other illnesses and on health behavior
3. Physician role and behavior	• Ethical guidelines for professional behavior • Personal values, attitudes, and biases as they influence patient care • Physician well-being • Social accountability and responsibility • Work in health care teams and organizations • Use of and linkage with community resources to enhance patient care
4. Physician–patient interactions	• Basic communication skills • Complex communication skills
5. Social and cultural issues in health care	• Impact of social inequalities in health care and the social factors that are determinants of health outcomes • Cultural competency
6. Health policy and economics	• Overview of the US health care system • Economic incentives affecting patients' health-related behaviors • Costs, cost-effectiveness, and physician responses to financial incentives

Table 41-5. MCAT BSS content.

Foundational Concept 1 (ways that individuals perceive, think about, and react to the world)	Foundational Concept 2 (factors that influence behavior and behavior change)	Foundational Concept 3 (factors that influence how we think about ourselves and others)	Foundational Concept 4 (ways in which cultural and social differences influence well-being)	Foundational Concept 5 (ways in which social stratification affects access to resources and well-being)
A: Sensing the environment 1) Sensory processing 2) Vision 3) Hearing 4) Other senses 5) Perception	A: Individual influences on behavior 1) Biological bases of behavior 2) Personality 3) Psychological disorders 4) Motivation 5) Attitudes	A: Self-identity 1) Self-concept and identity 2) Formation of identity	A: Understanding social structure 1) Components of social structure 2) Theoretical approaches 3) Specific social institutions 4) Culture	A: Social inequality 1) Spatial inequality 2) Social class 3) Health disparities 4) Healthcare disparities
B: Making sense of the environment 1) Attention 2) Cognition 3) Memory 4) Language	B: Social processes that influence human behavior 1) Socialization 2) How the presence of others affects individual behavior 3) Group processes 4) Culture	B: Social thinking 1) Attributing behavior to persons or situations 2) Prejudice and bias 3) Processes related to stereotypes	B: Demographic characteristics and process 1) Demographic shifts and social change 2) Demographic structure of society	
C: Responding to the world 1) Emotions 2) Stress	C: Attitude and Behavioral change 1) Associative learning 2) Observational learning 3) Attitude and Behavioral change	C: Social interactions 1) Self-presentation and interacting with others 2) Social behavior 3) Discrimination 4) Elements of social interaction		

short list of sample BSS competencies. More importantly, this report provides a robust curricular tool that guides educators and learners in identifying and elaborating BSS content that arises in any clinical case. This tool, the BSS Matrix, uses the IOM content areas (see Table 41-4) and the CanMEDS professional roles (see Table 41-6) as complementary rubrics to reduce complex clinical encounters into their foundational BSS competency units for further teaching and/or evaluation (see Figure 41-1).

Table 41-6. CanMEDS physician competency framework.

As *Professionals,* physicians are committed to the health and well-being of individuals and society through ethical practice, profession-led regulation, and high personal standards of behavior.

As *Communicators,* physicians effectively facilitate the doctor–patient relationship and the dynamic exchanges that occur before, during, and after the medical encounter.

As *Collaborators,* physicians effectively work within a health care team to achieve optimal patient care.

As *Managers,* physicians are integral participants in health care organizations, organizing sustainable practices, making decisions about allocating resources, and contributing to the effectiveness of the health care system.

As *Health Advocates,* physicians responsibly use their expertise and influence to advance the health and well-being of individual patients, communities, and populations.

As *Scholars,* physicians demonstrate a lifelong commitment to reflective learning, as well as the creation, dissemination, application, and translation of medical knowledge.

As *Medical Experts,* physicians integrate all of the CanMEDS Roles, applying medical knowledge, clinical skills, and professional attitudes in their provision of patient-centered care. Medical Expert is the central physician Role in the CanMEDS framework.

CanMEDS Physician Roles

	Professional	Communicator	Collaborator	Manager and Systems Thinker	Health Advocate	Scholar
Patient behavior		What are stages of change and how can I use motivational interviewing to help this patient?	How or when can I refer to a behavioral health counselor?	Are there quality indicators that track detection and intervention of binge drinking?		What are the evidence-based interventions for binge drinking?
Mind-body interaction						Is stress a causal factor for binge drinking?
Physician role & behavior	What are my ethical or legal responsibilities in this case?	What are my personal beliefs about binge drinking and do they influence my communication style?				
Doctor-patient interaction	How can I assess drinking and educate the pt about risks without sounding judgmental?	How can I build rapport and strengthen our connection?				Does research support particular communication strategies for educating pts about risk?
Health policy, economics and systems (including population health)			How can I communicate more effectively with ED docs?	Can I tap local resources to support behavioral change for this pt?	Could I promote better pt education programs in the ED?	
Social and cultural context	How can I be sensitive to his age, gender, culture, or socioeconomic status?					Is this problem more common in men?

IOM BSS Concepts & Evidence

Figure 41-1. The AAMC BSS matrix. Sample case: A 27-year-old man with atrial fibrillation following binge drinking episodes x2.

We resume our opening example to illustrate how the resident and preceptor could use the BSS Matrix to promote BSS competence.

Preceptor: Wendy, thank you for bringing this up. It might take a long time and a lot of patience before you can really start to feel competent as a primary care provider. There are a lot of skills involved and they are probably best taught while immersed in the context of caring for real patients. Do you have a case you can share with me? We'll use the AAMC BSS Matrix to identify some key learning issues for your development plan.

Resident: Well, my last patient was a 27-year-old man coming to see me after his second trip to the ED for a-fib following a night of heavy drinking. He was pretty shaken up by the experience and had no idea that binge drinking and atrial fibrillation could be related. He needed an INR check and warfarin adjustment but I wanted to counsel him about binge drinking. I'm not sure if I did a very good job of it.

Preceptor: Terrific case and lots of important behavioral and counseling issues we can discuss. Let's map it onto the BSS Matrix and see what roles and what content jump out at us. First, identify what roles you might be required to fill as his primary care provider. Next, think about the BSS core content you need to know and the competencies you need to possess. Let's fill in the cells with learning questions for this case together. (See Figure 41-1)

Preceptor: Great list! Now I'd like to ask you to circle the cell where you feel most competent already and the one to two cells where you feel least competent. Maybe we can start our conversation there and develop a learning approach to build your competence. [The conversation continues....]

As can be deduced from the above examples and the various BSS competency and content lists, the process of developing CBME for BSS requires a high level of faculty and learner engagement, time, resources, and, most importantly, an institutional or organizational culture that supports this material. However, it is important to remember that even if those necessary conditions are not present, organizational transformation does occur and can be stimulated from both the bottom-up and top-down. In Chapter 42, the authors carefully detail the necessary and sufficient conditions to support BSS education and the steps to promote cultural shifts that ensure both the quality and sustainability of the resulting product.

Although BSS competencies may "set the bar," it is the assessment toward achieving those competencies that allows us to "entrust" the learner with those clinical activities. Assessments may be formative (i.e., used to shape learning plans) or they may be summative (i.e., providing a grade or determining attainment of a particular skill level). Within the realm of CBME, most assessments measure skills or abilities rather than attitudes, since behavior and attitudes tend to be only weakly correlated. Direct observations of the learner are the most commonly used assessment methodology, but observations should occur frequently and require observer training and standardization. In Chapter 43, Carney and Milan describe a full menu of assessment and evaluation approaches, including the relative advantages and disadvantages of each approach. As they argue, regardless of the selected methodology, BSS competencies can and should be assessed frequently and in conjunction with other more biomedically based competencies.

Given the international convergence of competency-based models of medical education, ranging from medical school through medical residencies, it appears that CBME is here to stay for the foreseeable future. Although broad and including general "meta-skills" along with foundational scientific knowledge, the BSS fit within current CBME frameworks and can be measured with existing tools. As learners struggle to develop competence and teachers stretch to accommodate their needs, tools such as the AAMC BSS Matrix can identify the complex, interactive learning issues embedded in each case. Moreover, as the construct of EPAs further develops, perhaps BSS knowledge and skills can be seen as foundational to the practice of medicine in partnership with the biomedical sciences.

SUGGESTED READINGS

Carraccio C, Wolfsthal SD, Englander R, Ferentz K, Martin C. Shifting paradigms: From Flexner to competencies. *Acad Med* 2002;77:361–367.

Dreyfus SE, Dreyfus HL. *A Five-Stage Model of the Mental Activities Involved in Directed Skill Acquisition.* Washington, DC: Storming Media, 1980.

Epstein RM, Hundert EM. Defining and assessing professional competence. *JAMA* 2002;287:226–235.

Frank JR, Snell LS, Ten Cate O, et al. Competency-based medical education: theory to practice. *Med Teach* 2010;32:638–645.

Green ML, Aagaard EM, Caverzagie KJ, et al. Charting the road to competence: developmental milestones for internal medicine residency training. *J Grad Med Educ* 2009;1:5–20.

Long DM. Competency-based residency training: the next advance in graduate medical education. *Acad Med* 2000;75:1178–1183.

Satterfield J, Adler S, Chen CH, Hauer K, Saba G, Salazar R. Creating an ideal social and behavioral sciences curriculum for medical students. *Med Educ* 2010;44:1194–1202.

Swing SR. The ACGME outcome project: retrospective and prospective. *Med Teach* 2007;29:648–654.

Ten Cate O, Snell L, Carraccio C. Medical competence: the interplay between individual ability and the health care environment. *Med Teach* 2010;32:669–675.

WEB SITES

AAMC BSS Report (2011): https://www.aamc.org/publications. Accessed February 6 2014.

ABSAME: www.absame.org/dcms/curriculum. Accessed February 6 2014.

IOM BSS Report (2004): http://www.iom.edu/Reports/2004/Improving-Medical-Education-Enhancing-the-Behavioral-and-Social-Science-Content-of-Medical-School-Curricula.aspx. Last accessed 2/06/14.

MCAT (2011): https://www.aamc.org/students/download/266006/data/2015previewguide.pdf. Accessed February 6 2014.

NIH BSS Curriculum Consortium: http://obssr.od.nih.gov/training_and_education/bss_medical_school/index.aspx. Accessed February 6 2014.

Teaching Behavioral Medicine: Theory and Practice

42

Debra K. Litzelman MA, MD; Mark DiCorcia PhD; Ann Cottingham MAR, MA; & Thomas S. Inui ScM, MD

When one of my preceptors is running behind schedule during clinic hours he always pokes his head in the exam rooms of the patients who are waiting and apologizes for their wait. He also tells them that he hasn't forgotten about them and that he will be there to see them as soon as possible. I think that this is a great way to show respect for patients and their schedules and it helps prevent them from becoming angry and frustrated. This is a habit that I will definitely adopt when I am a physician.

Third-year medical student

One of my fellow students and I were on duty when there was a code called overhead. Everyone ran to assist in the code and the student was asked if she wanted to participate. This is something very neat for a third year because we never get to do that. However, the student spotted the wife of the coding patient at the end of the hall standing by herself with no one to comfort her. So instead of going to help in the code, the student went to talk to the patient's wife and explain to her what was going on. I thought that was very caring because no one else even noticed the wife standing there, and sometimes we get caught up in the chance to do something medical and forget about the families.

Third-year medical student

INTRODUCTION

Today it is widely recognized that high-quality patient care is built on a foundation of knowledge and abilities in the basic, clinical, and behavioral and social sciences. Social and behavioral factors are estimated to contribute to more than half of all causes of disease and death in the United States, including cancer, heart disease, chronic obstructive pulmonary disease, and type II diabetes. Growing knowledge of the complex behavioral, social, and psychological contributors to disease has important implications for clinical practice and physician education, both formal and informal. Physicians must understand these factors and their interrelationships, and be able to apply this knowledge in the care of patients to optimize health outcomes as well as to equip them with the skills that promote their own sense of

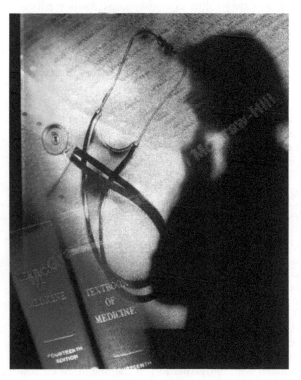

well-being, foster lifelong personal and professional growth, and decrease feelings of cynicism and burnout.

Whereas many health training programs have incorporated behavioral and social science content into their formal education, many curricula remain fragmented, incomplete, and marginalized. Emphasis on formal curricular development may also overlook the importance of the informal curriculum (or learning environment)— the physician and resident modeling of behaviors and attitudes that medical students experience every day. Therefore, educators must be attentive to both influences on student education. Using current theories of learning, this chapter illustrates innovative educational methods that integrate the formal and informal curricula to effectively teach social and behavioral science (SBS).

BACKGROUND

The IOM report, *Improving Medical Education: Enhancing the Behavioral and Social Science Content of Medical School Curricula*, identifies 26 topics in six SBS domains that are important to the education of future physicians (see Table 42-1). The demographic and social contexts contributing to the need for such training in the behavioral and social sciences have been well documented. Nevertheless, several decades of efforts to teach this content have resulted in mixed success. Medical education literature clearly identifies several types of difficulties specific to the teaching of SBS in the formal curriculum, including the marginalization of SBS content, lack of appropriately trained faculty, timing of teaching the SBS content, mismatch between teaching methods and context of use, and failure of social scientists and clinicians to work together to create effective learning experiences. It is not difficult to find examples. SBS content may be treated as an "add on" to the traditional basic science and clinical curricula. Medical training programs may lack support and incentives for faculty to include SBS content, and for career development programs in SBS. SBS topics may fit into available time slots rather than taught at the appropriate times in the trainees' development and in the appropriate depth. For example, topics such as death and dying are often covered in small-group discussions in the first or second year and not revisited in any formal way in the clerkship years, yet research on knowledge use and acquisition concludes that there is little immediate transfer of learning from one context of use to another. Thus, students who discuss death and dying only in the early year or two of training (academic context) will be challenged to exhibit professional and humanistic behavior in the presence of real patients (practice context) without further formal training in the clinical context.

There are also additional, well-documented structural impediments from a systems perspective to fully realizing the successful integration of SBS into the larger medical education curriculum. Medical education is by and large examination driven, quantitative in nature, and competition among and between students is based on these numerical rankings. This system continues to perpetuate the marginalization of SBS to a supporting or secondary role in the minds of faculty and students in favor of more influential "objective" measures. For example, on the national level, the Association of American Medical Colleges' Medical College Admission Test (MCAT) as well as other high-stakes examinations (e.g., USMLE Step 1) are not Pass/Fail despite sufficient evidence that once a learner achieves a particular threshold of success on the examination there is no difference in clinical performance based on achieving a greater numerical score. Yet, despite this evidence, many institutions continue to use the specific scores to screen applicants for entrance to US medical schools and residencies, and school administrators are under pressure, and in some cases even rewarded, for only recruiting and admitting those with the highest test scores instead of developing criteria that would focus on such areas as the 26 topics in the six SBS domains as the discriminating factors.

In response to similar concerns, Canada's McMaster University developed the Multiple Mini-Interview (MMI) for use in the admissions process. Resembling an objective structured clinical examination (OSCE) the MMI consists of short-interview stations that focus exclusively on noncognitive domains. The open-ended interviewer–applicant interactions instead revolve around areas such as the ability to collaborate, communication skills, and moral reasoning. By focusing on these noncognitive professional abilities the MMI has consistently demonstrated greater reliability (i.e., around 0.75) than standard interview methods to accurately assess for these qualities, which are grounded in SBS and valued in clinical practice. It has also been established that the MMI has a significant and moderately large positive correlation in predicting clinical clerkship performance as well as a statistically significant positive correlation for those subsections of national licensing examinations assessing professional quality domains.

On the local level, many courses in the basic sciences lend themselves to "multiple choice" measures making the evaluation of SBS content difficult to objectively evaluate given the time and resources SBS curriculum often requires in both teaching and evaluating. Therefore, even if SBS content is woven into the curriculum, it is often not as heavily weighted or given equal focus in course examinations. This not only perpetuates the idea that SBS content is not as important, but for the learner whose measure of success rests on quantitative

Table 42-1. SBS domains with priority topics and learning objectives.[*]

Domain: Mind–Body Interactions in Health & Disease
Biological Mediators Between Psychological and Social Factors and Health
Describe how behavioral and social factors and stress alter physiology to make disease more likely and the interconnectivity of homeostatic systems.   Explain the relationship between chronic stress, affective illness, social support, and health.
Psychological, Social, and Behavioral Factors in Chronic Illness
Understand the interrelationship between psychological, social, behavioral, and lifestyle factors and particular chronic medical conditions (e.g., diabetes, coronary artery disease [CAD], arthritis, cancer).   Understand and predict ongoing risky health behaviors.   Describe how to recognize stress in chronically ill patients.
Psychological and Social Aspects of Human Development That Influence Disease and Illness
Recognize the various life cycle theories (Freud, Piaget, Erikson, Bowlby) in normal development and the Epigenetic Principle of Life Cycle Theory.   Understand the interplay between stages of human development and disease states.
Psychological Aspects of Pain
Understand the wide range of psychosocial and cultural factors that influence the perception and expression of pain.   Be familiar with the classic gate control and contemporary theories of pain.   Perform a functional analysis of patients with chronic pain.   Describe the multimodal treatments for pain control.   Recognize the physician biases that influence the treatment of pain.
Psychological, Biological, and Management Issues in Somatization
Understand the definition, prevalence, common symptoms, and underlying affective illnesses associated with somatization.   List the diagnostic criteria for somatoform disorders.   Reflect on personal reactions to patients presenting with possible somatoform disorders.
Interactions Among Illness, Family Dynamics, and Culture
Understanding family and cultural influences on patient's interpretation of illness and treatment decisions and the importance of eliciting such Information.
Domain: Patient Behavior
Health Risk Behaviors
Understand the psychological factors associated with the development and maintenance of behaviors associated with major causes of morbidity and mortality.   Demonstrate the ability to assess patients for health risk behaviors.   Understand key strategies for prevention and cessation of these behaviors.   Reflect on the role of health care providers in instigating and maintaining changes in these behaviors.   Apply principles of motivational interviewing and counseling for behavioral change to the patient care situations.
Principles of Behavior Change
Demonstrate the ability to apply the various models (classical conditioning, cognitive social learning theory, health belief model, theory of reasoned action, stage-of-change model) available for guiding behavior change.   Understand how behaviors are acquired, maintained, and eliminated in the context of health risk.   Understand patient, family, and sociocultural variables that impact motivation to change behavior.
Impact of Psychosocial Stressors and Psychiatric Disorders on Manifestations of Other Illness on Health Behavior
Recognize the association between, and co-occurrence of, chronic medical illness and mental disorders.   Know and be able to discuss with patients the range of treatment options when medical and mental illness coexist.   Know the role of a primary care physician and specialist in the treatment when medical and mental illness coexist.   Demonstrate the ability to screen patients for depression.   Understand the pathogenetic relationships between depression and comorbid conditions.

(Continued)

Table 42-1. SBS domains with priority topics and learning objectives.* (Continued)

Domain: Physician Role and Behavior
Ethical Guidelines for Professional Behavior
Analyze ethical and professional dilemmas faced by health care professionals. Identify and apply guidelines of ethical decision making.
Personal Values, Attitudes, and Biases as They Influence Patient Care
Describe how the effect of family of origin, cultural background, gender, life experiences, and other personal factors may influ- ence your attitudes toward emotional reactions to patients. Identify methods for processing the highly emotional encounters that regularly occur in medical care.
Physician Well-Being
Recognize risk factors and warning signs for mental health issues in yourself. Develop personal wellness strategies.
Social Accountability and Responsibility
Engage in activities that foster the development of socially responsible leadership skills. Recognize the ever-changing health care needs of the community, region, and/or nation you serve.
Work in Health Care Teams and Organizations
Recognize the contribution that each member of the health care team has to offer. Identify ways to work effectively as a part of the team.
Use of and Linkage With Community Resources to Enhance Patient Care
Identify available community resources in the patient's community. Demonstrate a working knowledge of the types of interventions offered.
Domain: Physician–Patient Interactions
Basic Communication Skills
Demonstrate basic communication skills including, establishing rapport and building trust, eliciting adequate information to permit a robust differential diagnosis, understanding, and addressing patient. Understand how to engender (and potential barriers to development of) a therapeutic relationship. Demonstrate ability to express empathy, actively listen, elicit information about patients' lives and reasons for medical visit. Demonstrate motivational interviewing techniques and the 5 A's counseling skills.
Complex Communication Skills
Demonstrate ability to communicate effectively in contextual (cultural, translator, family) and developmental (pediatric, adoles- cent, geriatric) interview situations. Demonstrate ability to communicate effectively in assessment and counseling situations. Practice basic skills in communicating effectively in challenging situations using principles of patient-centered interviewing. Practice basic skills in communicating effectively with colleagues using principles of relationship-centered communication.
Context of a Patient's Social and Economic Situation, Capacity for Self-Care, and Ability to Participate in Shared Decision Making
Demonstrate an awareness of the patient's ability to participate in decision making. Identify necessary resources available to ensure access to care.
Management of Difficult or Problematic Physician–Patient Interactions
Describe approaches to working with patients in difficult situations. Identify taxonomy of difficult interviews (including personal or sexual history taking; abusive relationships; patients with HIV; breaking bad news). Identify key characteristics of difficult patient encounters, including personality types and stressful situations. Identify and use basic skills of patient-centered interviewing to ask sensitive questions and listen respectfully and nonjudgmentally.

(Continued)

Table 42-1. SBS domains with priority topics and learning objectives.* (Continued)

Domain: Social & Cultural Issues in Health Care
Impact of Social Inequalities in Health Care and the Social Factors That are Determinants of Health Outcomes
Analyze the intricate relationship that social factors (race, ethnicity, education, income, and occupation) have with patients' health.
Reflect on the impact your (students'/physicians') own social views can have on the delivery of effective health care.
Cultural Competency
Describe the impact the cultural context of illness can have on a successful patient–physician relationship.
Recognize ways that cultural competency encompasses language, customs, values, belief systems, and rituals.
Role of Complementary and Alternative Medicine
Describe complementary and alternative medicine treatments available in the local community and within local ethnic/cultural groups.
Recognize and apply required skills for eliciting information from patients seeking or using alternative treatment methods.
Describe to patients the efficacy and safety of alternative methods of treatment.
Domain: Health Policy & Economics
Overview of the US Health Care System
Appreciate the magnitude of the investment in health care services made by individuals and organizations in the United States, the impact of these expenditures on individuals and on organizations, and the limited "return on investment."
Explain why competition and other "market forces" may not work in health care.
Use state-of-the-art utilization controls within the TBL scenario in an attempt to allocate financial resources to critical sectors of care.
Economic Incentives Affecting Patients' Health-Related Behaviors
Appreciate how patients' values and life circumstances may affect their motivations for health-supporting behaviors, health care utilization, and preference for outcomes of health care.
Use this understanding to predict a patient's response to a complex and costly plan of care for several concomitant, chronic conditions, including the need to choose among therapeutic alternatives, adherence challenges, and patient-based assessments of risk.
Outline potential physician actions in this situation that might preserve the essential ingredients of effective care.
Costs, Cost-effectiveness, and Physician Responses to Financial Incentives
Appreciate how "delivery system" income is allocated to sectors of cost, using a microsystem model as an exemplar.
Apply this understanding, together with a statement of practice objectives, to develop the key elements of the practice in a financial context—staffing, services provided, in-office equipment, patients accepted, relationship to payers.
Variations in Care
Appreciate how large the variations in practice are, even in the presence of generally accepted evidence-based guidelines for care, and what some of the determinants of those variations might be.
Apply this knowledge to a specific case example, decide what "unwanted" variation means in this situation, and design a plan of action to eliminate this variation.

*Social and Behavioral Science Domains with Priority Topics are from a report issued by the Institute of Medicine (2004). Learning Objectives are used with permission from the Office of Medical Education and Curricular Affairs, Indiana University School of Medicine, (IUSM) Indianapolis, Indiana.

success (i.e., to get into medical school, a residency, or pass an examination), it creates a systems-induced survival strategy of "if it's not going to help me on the test then it's not important." This mentality or two-tiered system of valuing the objectively quantifiable over the more often subjectively qualitative SBS is as much a systems issue as it is those difficulties specific to the teaching of SBS in the curriculum noted above.

Finally, emphasis on discipline-based knowledge creates another barrier to integration of SBS content. True integration of SBS content requires disciplinary communities to work closely together to establish joint responsibility for knowledge creation, development and dissemination. With the exception of family medicine residency training programs, which have emphasized training in SBS, the same limitations and critiques directed toward undergraduate medical education hold true for graduate medical education as well.

Informal education in the SBS also has presented a challenge. Research indicates that it is the social environment of the medical school, the so-called "informal curriculum," that guides most aspects of a future physician's behavior. The role modeling that physicians and residents actually do, much more than what they say, powerfully influences the beliefs, values, and role expectations of physicians-in-training. Patient care and clerkship experiences—where physical, emotional, behavioral, social, and cultural issues become embodied for learners in their patients—have the potential to be particularly important behavioral and social science learning opportunities. Here attending and resident teaching could seamlessly integrate SBS education into daily clinical activities. Unfortunately, studies show that attributes such as social-mindedness and interest in the psychosocial issues embedded in all illness decline rather than improve during this time, and many students experience a diminishment, not enhancement, of their moral values base.

Work must be done to raise faculty and resident consciousness of the power that their words and actions have in shaping students' perceptions of patients, their specialty and medicine in general. Students and faculty benefit alike from the opportunity to process and learn from their own experiences, making each more conscious of the relationship between their values, actions, and behavior, and better prepared to model and teach the SBS aspects of patient care and the practice of medicine.

INTEGRATING THE FORMAL AND INFORMAL CURRICULA TO TEACH SOCIAL AND BEHAVIORAL SCIENCE

Educational Learning Theories Foundational to Creating Social and Behavioral Science Curriculum

As medical training programs seek to integrate their formal and informal curricula to improve SBS education, current learning theories provide a useful underlying framework. Understanding the various theoretical orientations will allow educators to address concerns raised in the IOM report about incorporating the most appropriate teaching methodologies when teaching SBS. The five learning theories described in the adult learning literature include behaviorist, humanist, social learning, cognitivist, and constructivist orientations. An overview of these orientations, associated educational methods, and theoretical principles are briefly summarized in Table 42-2.

Teaching Methods Foundational to Learning Social and Behavioral Sciences

The five Theoretical Orientations are presented as a frame for teaching SBS. A brief description of each of the suggested methods under each orientation is provided. Specific case illustrations applying the suggested methods in teaching and SBS are also included. In some cases, the

Table 42-2. Learning theories and orientations foundational to teaching and evaluating social and behavioral sciences.

Orientation	Educational Methods/Tools	SBS Abilities	Theoretical Principles
Behaviorist	Direct observation Standardized patients Checklists Rating forms	Clinical and psychomotor skills Other observable behaviors	Learning results from environmental factors and positive and negative reinforcement that shapes behavior
Humanist	Narrative reflection Problem-based learning	Self-awareness Autonomy Self-directedness	Learning results from the learners' desire to achieve their full potential
Social Learning	Role modeling Mentoring Collaborative/cooperative learning, for example, team-based learning	Social adaptability Teamwork	Learning results from the learners' interaction with and observation of others in a social context in which creative retrievable cognitive representations are used by learners when they are motivated to act
Cognitivist	Cognitive maps Reflective exercises	Insight Information processing	Learning results from relating new knowledge/experiences to existing knowledge/experiences
Constructivist	Reflective journaling Commitment to change statements Building portfolios	Ability to broaden one's perspective Critical reflection Ability to create meaning from experiences	Learning results from the learners' construction of meaning from experiences through critical reflection on their existing assumptions

examples provided by the authors could be categorized under more than one orientation. However, the main purpose of the illustrations is to provide a wide sampling of educational vignettes that integrate the formal and informal curricula as a foundation upon which to build an SBS curriculum for varying levels of medical trainees.

BEHAVIORAL ORIENTATION

The behavioral orientation is very useful for teaching technical, clinical, and psychomotor skills as well as other observable behaviors. Direct observation of trainees with real or standardized patients (SPs), particularly when trained observers utilize well-designed checklists and/or rating forms, provides valuable formative and summative assessment about trainees' social and behavior science competence.

Direct observation: Direct observation of trainees is an important way to foster medical trainees' basic clinical and communication skills as well as interpersonal and professional behavior; yet it is infrequently done. Here resident or student patient care competency, contextualized in the everyday interactions of the informal curriculum, or institutional culture, is brought into the formal curriculum for purposes of formative feedback.

Direct observation is itself a skill that requires faculty training and practice. Faculty training should focus on standardizing, to the extent possible, the behaviors of interest and how to accurately identify such behaviors in the trainees. This is especially important for high-inference behaviors, such as those provided below (see case illustration 1). For example, in the behaviorist approach, what does nonjudgmental communication about a sexually transmitted disease actually look like? Faculty should spend some time discussing these issues as part of the standardization and calibration process.

Standardized patients: In an effort to standardize training of doctor–patient communication, physical examination skills, and other areas, medical schools, residency training programs, and the National Board of Medical Examiners (NBME) have progressively moved toward using SPs. Simulations can be videotaped and used for self or group reflection. Paradigmatic examples could also be used for faculty development in recognizing and developing intercoder reliability on behavioral evaluations. From these examples, skills in providing feedback and creating learning opportunities could be developed.

HUMANISTIC ORIENTATION

The humanistic orientation promotes learning activities that are autonomous and self-directed for learners to develop a deeper understanding of the path needed to reach their full potential and, in return, recognize the humanness in themselves as well as their patients. Problem-based learning (PBL) and exercises that promote

self-assessment are educational tools for fostering humanistic-style learning.

Problem-based learning: Problem-Based Learning is a learner-centered method of small group learning usually built upon paper cases developed from real patient care vignettes. The case discussions generally evolve over several days or weeks with progressive disclosure of information to the students upon request or at critical times. Students identify their own learning issues and resources for finding solutions to their learning needs. A facilitator guides the process of the small group sessions but does not serve as a content expert for the learners. This process promotes autonomous, self-directed, lifelong learning skills and prompts learners to reflect on the cultural assumptions or observations that shape their list of learning issues and resources, providing an opportunity for integration of the informal curriculum.

 CASE ILLUSTRATION 1

As part of the first-year medical students' Concepts of Health and Disease PBL course, SBS objectives addressing principals of behavioral change have been woven into a case covering medical and genetic risk factors for cardiovascular disease (CVD). Students meet Monday, Wednesday, and Friday during 1 week to cover serial aspects of the case of: "Robert Richardson's Achilles Tendon."

Sample excerpts from the case:

Day 1:

Mr. Robert Richardson, a 44-year-old white male, visits his family physician, Dr. Roberts, for a follow-up of his myocardial infarct suffered several weeks ago. Mr. Richardson has been feeling well and continues his prescribed walking program. He is trying to follow his suggested diet and has begun a smoking cessation program. Mr. Richardson tells Dr. Roberts that he has been experiencing pain in his left Achilles tendon for the past several days. Mr. Richardson says that the pain had appeared several times during the past year. The pain usually resolved itself within several days without treatment.

Student instructions:

During the week the case is being presented, please make a commitment to change the following:

- *Engage in some form of aerobic exercise every day for at least 10 minutes.*
- *Take the provided pill twice a day. (Students are each given a packet of inert pills.)*
- *Diet—give up one thing that contributes to heart disease that you eat regularly.*

***Suggestions:** salt, red meat, butter, cheese, milk, eggs, fried foods.*

At the end of each day write a paragraph or two about the experience of complying with these activities. Did it all go as planned? Rate the amount of effort necessary to do these things, with 1 being the easiest and 10 being the hardest. What happened if things did not always go as planned? What did you struggle with? What were your successes?

Facilitator Notes:

The facilitator might consider doing these things as well to be able to aid in the discussion.

Guided self-assessment: Self-assessment exercises can be built into a variety of educational activities stimulated by prompting questions posed by medical educators. Creating a forum for students to safely discuss their personal reflections on journal entries or information collected as part of self- and peer-assessment programs can promote self awareness, personal growth, and professional development in one-on-one and group settings and is another example of formal/informal curricular integration. Students are asked in the formal curriculum to reflect upon and assess their abilities and performance in both the formal and informal curricula.

To be effective, self-assessment is not performed by the student in isolation. The impact of self-assessment is most valuable when performed with *guidance*, which we define as either externally provided data (e.g., peer assessment, etc.) or in conjunction with an advisor or mentor.

CASE ILLUSTRATION 1 (CONTD.): "ROBERT RICHARDSON'S ACHILLES TENDON" (PBL)

Sample excerpts from case:

Day 2:

Dr. Roberts reports that Mr. Richardson's lipid and enzyme values are improved, that he should continue to follow the prescribed treatment and that his prognosis will remain improved as long as he follows the diet, exercise, and medication program. He should have semi-annual checkups to follow his cholesterol and liver enzyme levels.

Facilitator Notes:

On the second and last day of the session, ask the following questions of the group.

Guided discussion of journals—prompting questions:

• *What was hardest?*
• *What was easiest?*
• *Any association with your lapses?*
• *How did you feel after you lapsed?*

How well did you comply with your journal writing?

Thinking about Mr. Richardson and what you learned with your own exercise, how could you help Mr. Richardson and his children to comply with these lifelong issues?

A sample of one student's self-assessment logged in her personal dietary/exercise/medicine adherence journal as part of the PBL exercise above:

Overall, this exercise has shown me that it is all too easy for a physician to become annoyed and frustrated with noncompliant patients, and write them off as not caring about their own well being or progress. Adherence with diet, exercise and medication is not as simple as it seems. I hope to remember those lessons in the coming years as I struggle with explaining to patients why it is so important, so they don't feel they are just doing something "because the doctor said to." First-year medical student

SOCIAL LEARNING ORIENTATION

According to the social learning orientation, learners assimilate new information and assume new roles through role modeling, behavioral rehearsal, and attending to observed behaviors. This orientation is central to the importance of the informal curriculum on shaping the professional development of trainees. Identifying ways to make stories about role models within an academic community more tangible and visible will inevitably lead to a heightened awareness about the importance of role modeling. Educational methods that promote collaborative, cooperative learning such as team-based learning (TBL) also highlight the complexities and value of collective problem solving and resourcefulness.

Role modeling: Role modeling shapes the professional culture or informal curriculum of an organization and substantially impacts the professional identity of trainees. The window into the impact of medical educators' role modeling can be seen in the trainees' stories about their learning environment. How the faculty conduct themselves and live their values through their actions can be influenced by integrating trainees' stories into the "formal" content of faculty development programs.

CASE ILLUSTRATION 2

Story of a negative role model from a student's professionalism journal maintained during her ambulatory block rotation.

During my second month I encountered a difficult patient that had chronic diarrhea as his primary diagnosis but also had a positive psychiatric history. During the course of his hospitalization the patient became very anxious and dramatic about every change that was being made to his care. We switched residents during this patient's hospitalization and our new resident was very aggressive. When we rounded together he hardly introduced himself to the patients before he asked direct and imposing questions or scolded them for behaviors like drinking if their diagnosis was pancreatitis. After seeing our difficult patient with diarrhea my resident pulled me aside and told me that he would give me some advice. He told me that I shouldn't be too nice to patients because it is not good to build a relationship. He said, "if you do this then it is very difficult to get them out of here." Considering this resident had been on service for only two days and barely knew any of the patients I felt his comment was offensive. I agree that there must be a line between being a patient's friend and a patient's doctor, but it is hard to imagine medicine without compassion and some empathy for those under your care. I understand hospitals are busy but because this resident didn't take the time to care I felt that our patients actually stayed longer because there was a lack of communication between our team and the patient about our goals and expectations. Third-year medical student

CASE ILLUSTRATION 3

Story of positive role modeling from a student's professional journal maintained during her medicine rotation.

One of the students on my team this month has had 3 patients back to back who have required palliative care. It had gotten to the point that several of us, including her, gently joked about her being a "bad omen" to the patients or a "black cloud." It was nothing mean or cruel, simply something to make her laugh or smile . . . something to keep her going and forget about the true impact of the situation. Her first two patients went home to die with their families. Her third patient presented with AMS and a terminal condition, and it was clear within hours of admission that the patient would die in the next few days. This student never spoke with the patient, as she was unresponsive, but she developed a relationship with the family. On the 3rd day, the student announced during rounds that the patient had passed away at 3:30 that morning. Her voice did not falter as she relayed the news, but we could all tell that it was difficult to get the words out. Our new attending, who

had only been with us for 1 ½ days and had only moments before asked to make presentations quick, stopped rounds, looked directly at the student, and simply asked "How are you feeling?" It surprised most of us at the table, and at first, the student didn't know what to say. Our attending continued to speak with her and discuss the impact of this loss. He encouraged her to stop and consider what she was feeling as the bond between a physician and patient is unique and special in its own way. He reassured her that it is okay to feel disappointed; it only means you truly gave yourself to that patient's care and invested an interest into their health. For the first time, the student admitted to the pain that she was feeling. I was really impressed with our attending's actions. As physicians, I feel as though most faculty are focused solely on the health of the patients and the information/aid that we can bring to the table. It was unique to see this physician take time to teach us a valuable lesson about personal care and coping. He even offered to speak with this student at any time if she wanted to talk. It was a great learning experience, and we felt as if he really cared about our education and growth as medical students. This whole time, the rest of us were trying to make her laugh to keep her going. It never crossed our minds that the best thing for her would be to stop for a moment and reflect. Third-year medical student

Team-based learning: Team-based learning has potential to be a major vehicle or education methodology for SBS. This methodology promotes active learning and effective team skills without requiring intensive faculty resources for tutoring sessions. TBL uses principles to develop small groups of students into effective learning teams who not only learn course content but also high-level content application, problem solving, and effective team interaction.

The three-part team learning instructional strategy puts these principles into action. Part I is the initial exposure to the concepts of an instructional unit through a Readiness Assurance Process. The Readiness Assurance Process begins with individual preclass work (through assigned readings, work on computer modules, and other modalities). It includes students completing an Individual Readiness Assurance Test (IRAT) during the first few minutes of class that covers the preassigned material. Immediately following the IRAT, the teams take the same test (a Group Readiness Assurance Test, or GRAT), which allows for peer discussion of important course content. The IRAT/GRAT tests are reviewed in class to ensure all students have thorough knowledge of foundational content. The instructor provides focused feedback and instruction on areas demonstrated to need additional clarification. Teams have the opportunity to appeal and defend any answers marked incorrect. This allows teams an opportunity to further review and discuss difficult concepts.

Upon completion of the Readiness Assurance Process, teams are ready to begin work on team application assignments (Part II). Team assignments allow students to increase their understanding of the main unit concepts by using them to solve a problem. Assignments generally ask team members to reach a decision (rather than write a report) and thus stimulate a high level of team interaction. At a given point, all teams simultaneously reveal their decisions and begin cross-team feedback and discussion. Team assignments for a given instructional unit usually progress from the simple to the more complex. Individual team members prepare for team assignments outside of class and then work together with their team members in class to reach a consensus conclusion. After sufficient team application practice, the instructor reviews the major course content and application learning points and students are formally assessed on an individual basis on their ability to solve a final application problem (Part III).

These team-learning experiences provide a perfect opportunity for learners to move from "stage-to-stage" as part of the process of professional development and role recognition. The experience of being a member of a TBL group also directly addresses key SBS learning objectives, including "*identify ways to work effectively as a part of a team*" and "*engage in activities that foster the development of socially responsible leadership skills*" (refer to Table 42-1 under the Physician Role and Behavior Domain). TBL also formally includes Peer Assessment in the sessions and can incorporate Self-Assessment as well.

Student narratives describing their experiences in the informal curriculum can provide opportunities for TBL groups to integrate multiple SBS competencies/domains into a discussion that addresses key learning objectives and exploration of the science supporting these objectives. Used in this way, narrative has the potential to utilize personal experiences of the informal curriculum to enhance the relevance and enrich the content related to formal curricular objectives.

COGNITIVIST ORIENTATION

The cognitivist orientation suggests that learners use cognitive tools such as insight, information processing, perceptions, and memory to facilitate learning by assigning meaning to events. Use of cognitive maps and reflection exercises are educational methods for promoting the cognitivist orientation.

Concept mapping: Concept mapping exercises provide trainees with a tool to graphically depict their understanding of complex problems or systems. Concept mapping offers a way for learners to incorporate new information into existing knowledge frameworks by associating relationships. Concept mapping can be used longitudinally to visually represent the progressively more complex neural connections in the developing mind. One can readily see the increasing complexity, hierarchical layers, and growing complexity of cross-linking between the pre- and postfigures (Figures 42-1 and 42-2) and when learners' cognitive development is tracked across time.

Analysis and reporting of developmental changes in concept mapping within individuals across time and between groups can be performed. Qualitative analysis of phrases and terms entered onto maps can be performed using software packages along with some quantitative or semiquantitative measures based on scoring schemes reported elsewhere.

 CASE ILLUSTRATION 4

Figure 42-1 **Concept maps:** Understanding factors influencing cardiovascular disease (CVD) risk.

CASE ILLUSTRATION 4 (CONTD.)

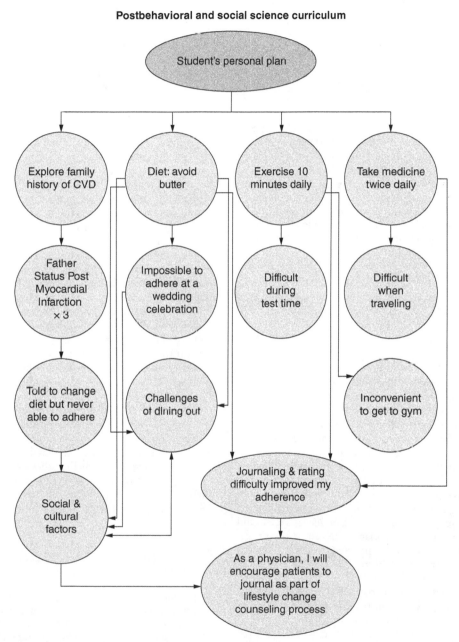

Figure 42-2. *Concept maps:* Understanding factors influencing CVD risk.

Reflective exercise: Medical training programs are increasingly incorporating 360-degree (multisource) evaluations for trainees. When accompanied by facilitated one-on-one reviews with mentors and advisors, these sessions offer the opportunity for learners to use a breadth of cognitive tools in an effort to assign meaning to these highly complex and personal data.

CASE ILLUSTRATION 5

A sample of one student's personal reflection stimulated by reviewing his self- and peer-assessment data during his annual meeting with his self-selected self- and peer-assessment advisor.

". . . the ideal professional physician must be respectful, tolerant, patient, and a good listener. From my peer assessment, I realize I don't need to be the first to speak when I think an underdog is being exploited . . . it is better to first listen to understand before making assumptions about whether a colleague is demonstrating tolerance . . . this will help me be a better doctor." Second-year medical student

CONSTRUCTIVIST ORIENTATION

The constructivist orientation supports the theory that knowledge is formed within the learner by integrating learning activities and experiences into knowledge and beliefs. The creation of meaning from these experiences emerges through critical reflection on existing beliefs and assumptions. Reflective journaling and active creation of learning or competency portfolios are examples of education methods used by educators to tap into constructivist learning styles.

Reflective journaling: Medical training institutions are including reflective journaling in their curricula. SBS constructs, such as identity, bias, privilege, social connections, and emotional management can be potent personal triggers requiring supported opportunities for reflection and growth. Reflection and reflective practice are essential habits of a good physician. (Although reflection is seen as a teachable skill with lifelong utility, it is especially important in the context of an intensive and challenging training environment.) Journaling exercises can range from brief informal invitations to write one's thoughts about a personal experience from the informal curriculum, to writing annual letters to one's self that are personally reviewed, to more extensive narrative writing exercises that are formally analyzed by faculty with expertise in "Narrative Medicine" (see Chapter 45). Reflective journaling can be solely for personal use and review, for one-on-one review with learner-selected and trusted mentors, for de-identified uses within small group seminars, or for required carefully evaluated narrative writing courses. Many guidelines for critical reflection exist. One example is the "LEAP" guidelines (LEAP = "**L**earning from your **E**xperiences as **A P**rofessional") that teach learners to write reflections similar to medical "SOAP" notes (i.e., the **s**ubjective experience, the **o**bjective data about the event, the learner's **a**ssessment of causes and **p**ossible learning points, and the learner's plan of what she/he will do next).

Reflective journaling serves to make more seamless the experience of the medical trainees regarding biomedical principles and social/behavioral principles in the context of patient care. Trainees' narratives can provide clear evidence of their ability to integrate these different dimensions of health and disease, in a more holistic manner than the knowledge measures or other quantitative measures of student performance. With permission, trainee's personal reflections (stories) can be used to generate new curricular materials linking informal and formal aspects of their training.

Commitment to change statements: Another approach to help learners integrate knowledge and experience is commitment to change (CtC) statements (see student journaling exercise on lifestyle change commitments above under case illustration 1). Research has shown the CtC method does enhance the probability of an individual making a change. At the end of an educational experience, the student is simply asked to write down a limited number of things they wish to change or accomplish as a result of the educational experience. In addition to writing what they would like to do differently, they can provide a rating on how motivated they are to make the change and how difficult they believe it will be to make the change. At a predetermined follow-up time, the student's CtC statements can be returned to them to reflect on whether they were successful in making the change and why. If they were not successful, they can also reflect on what the barriers were to making the change and lessons learned from the experience.

CASE ILLUSTRATION 6

Students select de-identified journal entries made by their cohort to discuss in small group, facilitated professionalism seminars during the medicine clerkship. In discussing their own narratives in a small group, the students are being professional as they talk and learn about professionalism. Reflection is stimulated by questions posed by the seminar facilitator such as: "What was it about this setting or these individuals that makes this possible?" As the students examine their experiences together, they are bringing their lived encounters—the informal curriculum—into the explicit, formal curriculum. Students report that the experience of being present to others' stories of professionalism helps them to feel less isolated and alone in their own experiences and also helps them to name professional issues that might otherwise go unacknowledged and unaddressed.

A sample from one student's professionalism journal entry made while on her third-year medicine rotation:

Today the fire alarms went off at the county hospital and all the elevators were stopped. I entered the stairwell on the 6th floor to go down stairs and encountered a hospital employee in a hair net coming up, four loaded food trays precariously stacked in her arms. Her breathing was loud and labored, and she implored Jesus with each exhalation. I ran down the few steps to her side and asked if she needed help. Between gasps and prayers she told me she was an asthmatic and really should not be climbing stairs, especially not six flights, and definitely not carrying four heavy trays. I relayed to her that a maintenance man told me it won't be long before the elevators are operating again, and maybe she could wait a few minutes. She replied, "we can't let the patients suffer just because the elevators are out and we've got a touch of asthma, now can we?" I was surprised by her dedication to her job and her care for the well-being of the patients. It reminded me how noble it is to be responsible at any level for the care of another human being, and how many important roles there are in providing that care to each patient. Third-year medical student

Portfolios: Learning portfolios aggregate learning products review and analysis by trainees and/or course and residency program directors. Portfolios have been found to be of high utility in documenting evidence of performance in SBS areas, such as self-awareness, professionalism, ethical judgment, and moral reasoning. Trainees can populate portfolios with documented experiences or activities from the formal or informal curricula. Given the sensitive nature of some materials entered into trainees' portfolios, several institutions have created ways to allow learners to self-populate both "personal" and "academic" versions of their portfolios. For ease of handling data, electronic portfolio tracking systems are increasingly available.

 CASE ILLUSTRATION 7

As part of an electronic portfolio pilot program, 16 first-year medical students from IUSM's Terre Haute campus were asked to self-populate fields built to document students' performance in each of the core competency areas. Four students chose to populate their academic portfolios with their reflective narratives written following their observations of an autopsy. One student mapped his narrative into the "Using Science to Guide Diagnosis, Management, Therapeutics and Prevention" competency, explaining that the experience helped him better understand the anatomy important for performing future procedures. One student added her story to the "Self-Awareness, Self-Care, and Personal Growth" competency stating, although she would never want to be a coroner, she now has a new appreciation for the important role these health care providers play as members of the larger health care team. Two students logged their entries into the "Moral Reasoning and Ethical Judgment" competency. One student reflected on the inappropriate behavior of the health care providers in handling human body remains of a deceased patient for whom some family members were likely still grieving. The second ethics entry included the student's reflection about how providers choose to deal with medical errors that resulted in a child's death. This demonstrates how a single curricular exercise can provide highly varied educational experiences for trainees uncovered through self-categorization based on the personal meaning these experiences had for the individual student. Portfolios can help document broad curricular exposure to all core competency areas as perceived by trainees.

Medical Education Methods Effective for Teaching Behavioral and Social Science

Educational methods found to improve student learning of traditional basic science or clinical content apply equally well to education in the SBS. Below are four examples.

ADULT LEARNING METHODS

The central tenet of teaching adult learners is recognizing and engaging their wealth of experience as an educational resource and creating "active" versus "passive" (e.g., lecture) learning activities. SBS lends itself to this approach because learners can often access the content through reflection on their own experience (e.g., racism, homophobia, caring for the elderly), in small group discussions or working together with peers on TBL cases. Students who participate in the learner-centered approach are more likely to go beyond passively absorbing the curriculum; they develop habits of inquiry, reflection, and teamwork as they move forward in the progressive development of a socially enlightened physician identity. In addition, activated learners participate in shaping the curriculum or delivering it to themselves and their peers. Further curricular enhancement can derive from interprofessional TBL experiences, as other disciplines such as nursing and social work have a long history of SBS-focused patient care and curriculum, which can increase its salience and influence on physician problem solving and worldview. These students may be especially motivated to develop and support SBS teaching not only in their practice but as models for future generations of physicians.

HIGHLIGHT CLINICAL RELEVANCE

An important mission of all medical schools is to graduate learners who are prepared for medical practice, and SBS curricula are central to this mission. Emphasizing clinical relevance for preclinical and clinical students can counter the perception that SBS lacks practical utility in patient care. Although there is no national consensus framework for presenting SBS material, existing guidelines may prove useful in determining how SBS content can best be implemented into clinical care. Early exposure to longitudinal patient care can provide students with a "lived" experience from the patient's perspective of interacting with a health care system that the students will soon be in a position to impact clinically, economically, and perhaps in policy. Although less factually based, a salient patient interview may prove far more memorable in illustrating the effects of poverty on health than a required journal article. Similarly, a well-crafted longitudinal patient care experience or PBL case that highlights issues such as substance abuse, social supports, and the value of the therapeutic relationships—while also integrating them with clinical and basic sciences—might more effectively convey those constructs compared to a didactic lecture.

INCLUDE A FOCUS ON QUALITY OF CARE:

An emphasis on quality of care further maximizes clinical relevance for students. Teaching students about the social and behavioral determinants of health, the major impact that SBS problems have on mortality, and methods of addressing these health risks moves the issue beyond a matter of political correctness or social trends. Teaching students how to ask about health-related behaviors and how to facilitate behavior change has direct benefits for quality of care. Teaching about health systems, health care teams, and ways to avoid medical errors clearly relates to quality improvement (QI). If SBS concepts are framed as practical tools to help students become better doctors, the perceived value increases. Furthermore, creating opportunities for students to be involved in actual, small-scale QI projects takes the process from passive knowledge attainment to actively acquiring the skills and efficacy to facilitate a measureable impact on both patients' and doctors' lives as well as the health care system as a whole.

CREATE A SPIRAL CURRICULUM

Given the vast amount of information to teach, many educators make the mistake of trying to teach too much at one time. Stand-alone behavioral science courses are so overfull that little time is left to promote clinical application and improve trainee retention. A developmentally appropriate "repetition and elaboration" approach should be created that first introduces the materials on a beginner's level, and then revisits those same constructs later with greater complexity and learner demand. However, in some instances these SBS linkages may already exist in the formal and informal curriculum, but they are poorly mapped and rarely if ever explicitly identified to the student in a purposeful way. This lack of purposefulness further perpetuates the belief that SBS concepts and curriculum are "just common sense" and do not require the same focus or prioritization as the biomedical sciences. Mapping would help identify areas where SBS concepts occur naturally in the curriculum, which in turn helps educators better identify and elaborate on them in a meaningful way. Mapping would also help curriculum designers identify specific lacunae where SBS needs to be addressed.

CREATING A COMMUNITY THAT MODELS AND SUPPORTS THE BEHAVIORAL AND SOCIAL SCIENCE KNOWLEDGE AND ABILITIES

The educational methods described above will be minimally effective unless grounded within a community that models and teaches these values, knowledge, and abilities. Serious attention to education in the behavioral and social sciences must, therefore, include attention to the informal curriculum of the institution that so strongly influences the developing professional identity and practice patterns of trainees. The educational methods described below are designed to foster the development of the medical training institution itself.

Promote Relational Practices across the Organization

Teaching behavioral and social sciences in the informal curriculum requires institutional and faculty/staff development that promotes key behavioral and social science-informed (relational) behaviors in the everyday environment. Practices that build relationships include faculty development that enhances both individual and group communication skills. New practices in meetings can enable participants to get to know the person, not just the position, sitting next to them. These include an invitation for participants to "check in" at the start of a meeting and share some small piece of personal or professional information ("My son won his bike race yesterday!" or "My clinical research project was funded!") that enables a deeper level of interaction. Collaboratively and transparently establishing the meeting agenda at the start of a meeting, ensuring that everyone has the opportunity to speak, and actively seeing and valuing a wide range of perspectives on any particular topic help to create an organizational culture that models the values and behaviors students are taught in their formal education.

Take Time to Examine and Publicize What Is Working Well

Traditional organizational development strategies often begin by identifying what is not working in the institution, the "problem," and focus on finding ways to avoid, decrease, or solve that problem. This deficit approach to change asks participants to address and study the question "what are we lacking?" In contrast, the organizational development method of Appreciate Inquiry (AI), grounded in positive psychology, challenges conventional approaches with the premise that people are more motivated to engage in change by finding what's working well and doing more of it. Described by its founder, David Cooperrider:

> Appreciative Inquiry is the cooperative search for the best in people, their organizations, and the world around them. It involves systematic discovery of what gives a system 'life' when it is most effective and capable in economic, ecological, and human terms. AI involves the art and practice of asking questions that strengthen a system's capacity to heighten positive potential. It mobilizes inquiry through crafting an "unconditional positive question".

AI seeks to discover what members of a community are already doing well, and to hold those achievements up as an attainable standard of success. It can be used by medical training institutions to identity existing strengths in key behavioral and social science domains, such as the ability to effectively address mind–body interactions in health and disease; understanding patient behavior and motivating behavioral change; exemplifying a professional physician role and behavior; demonstrating effective, compassionate physician–patient interactions; modeling facility in addressing social and cultural issues in health care; and demonstrating approaches to care that take into consideration health policy and economics. With its focus on the positive work that the institution is already modeling, AI inspires and motivates the community to reach its full potential.

Create a Reflective Community

Self-reflection is important not only for individuals but for institutions as well. It enables members to intentionally examine the professional and learning environments that they and their institution foster and promote. Institution-wide conversations about positive and challenging critical incidents—published in weekly newsletters or other public format—can promote open reflection about an institution's learning and professional environment, allow acknowledgment of error, promote discussion of values, and provide an opportunity for the members of an institution to thoughtfully consider the moral ethos of their culture.

SUMMARY

Medical training programs have employed a variety of organizational and theoretical frameworks as vehicles for increasing education in the SBS. These efforts, while important, are an incomplete solution. Attention to trainees' learning environment, and their experiential learning in the informal curriculum, are also critical. The authors suggest that educators consider including learning experiences that draw upon and integrate both formal and informal curricular content and experiences. They provide examples of educational activities within a range of theoretical orientations that accomplish this integration. Examples illustrate how narratives, generated by trainees and other members of the academic community about personal experiences and perceptions of the organization's professional culture, can be creatively integrated into the formal curriculum in a variety of contexts. This strategy promotes personal and organizational reflection and mindfulness, and reinforces the importance of lessons learned in the informal curriculum. This cyclical process promotes awareness of the individual community members' roles in the creation of a culture conducive to learning and caring for patients.

ACKNOWLEDGMENTS

The authors acknowledge Drs. J Satterfield, A. Schickedanz, R. Salazar, S. Adler, H. C. Chen, K. Hauer, D. Hughes, and G. Saba for providing contributions to the "Medical Education Methods Effective for Teaching Behavioral and Social Science" section. Funded in part by NIH Award R25AR060994.

SUGGESTED READINGS

Charon R, Holmboe E, Holmes J, et al. *Behavioral and Social Science Foundations for Future Physicians.* Report of the behavioral and social science expert panel. Association of American Medical College, Washington, D.C., 2011.

Cooperrider DL, Whitney D. "Appreciative inquiry: a positive revolution in change." In: Holman P, Devane T, eds, *The Change Handbook.* Berrett-Koehler Publishers, Inc., San Francisco, CA, 2005, pp. 245–263.

Frankel RM, Eddins-Folensbee F, Inui TS. Crossing the patient-centered divide: transforming healthcare quality through enhanced faculty development. *Acad Med* 2011;86:445–452.

Inui TS. *A Flag in the Wind: Education for Professionalism in Medicine.* Washington, DC: Association of American Medical Colleges, 2003.

Karnieli-Miller O, Vu TR, Frankel RM, et al. Which experiences in the hidden curriculum teach students about professionalism? *Acad Med* 2011;86:369–377.

Litzelman DK, Cottingham, AH. The new formal competency-based curriculum and informal curriculum at Indiana University School of Medicine: overview and five-year analysis. *Acad Med* 2007;82:410–421.

Reiter, HI, Eva KW, Rosenfeld J, Norman GR. Multiple mini-interviews predict clerkship and licensing examination performance. *Med Educ* 2007;41:378–384.

Satterfield JM, Adler SR, Chen HC, Hauer KE, Saba GW, Salazar R. Creating an ideal social and behavioral sciences curriculum for medical students. *Med Educ* 2010;44:1194–1202.

Suchman, AL, Sluyter, DJ, Williamson, PR. *Leading Change in Healthcare: Transforming Organizations Using Complexity, Positive Psychology and Relationship-Centered Care.* London: Radcliffe Publishing, 2011.

Suchman A, Williamson P, Litzelman D, et al. Toward an informal curriculum that teaches professionalism: transforming the social environment of a medical school. *JGIM* 2004;19: 501–504.

Torre DM, Daley BJ, Sebastion JL, Elnicki DM. Overview of current learning theories for medical educators. *Amer J Med* 2006;119:903–907.

WEB SITES

Improving Medical Education: Enhancing the Behavioral and Social Science Content of Medical School Curricula. http://www.iom.edu/CMS/3775/3891/19413.aspx. Accessed February 2014.

OSullivan P, Aronson L, Chittenden E, Niehaus B, Learman L. Reflective Ability Rubric and User Guide. MedEdPORTAL; 2010. Available from: www.mededportal.org/publication/8133. Accessed February 2014.

Team-Based Learning Collaborative: http://www.teambasedlearning.org/. Accessed February 2014.

Assessing Learners and Curricula in the Behavioral and Social Sciences

43

Patricia A. Carney, PhD; Felise Milan, MD; & Jason M. Satterfield, PhD

CASE ILLUSTRATION

In compliance with the recommendation for yearly alcohol screening for adults in primary care, a family medicine residency director wants to develop a curriculum to teach her residents how to use a validated alcohol-screening tool and provide brief alcohol counseling. Given competing educational demands, she wants this curriculum to be both efficient and effective. She plans to evaluate her residents and the curriculum....

INTRODUCTION

Medical training programs are increasingly focused on assessing clinical competencies that demonstrate a learner's readiness for (or progression toward) independent practice. Training programs must track a multitude of competencies or "entrustable professional activities" (EPA's) that often include both concrete observable procedures and more nuanced but essential doctoring skills, such as empathy and cultural sensitivity. Although the general principles of learner and curricular assessment hold equally true for the behavioral and social sciences (BSS), these content areas can be more difficult to operationalize and evaluate. Moreover, high-quality BSS teaching and assessment tools often require explicit, robust institutional support that relies on careful programmatic evaluations that compare institutional goals with curricular performance. Although evaluations assess a learner and/or program, the results should also iteratively drive curricular and institutional evolution.

This chapter provides guidance on designing evaluation strategies for assessing both medical learners and curricular programs with an eye toward continuous

improvement. In the section "Assessment and Evaluation Planning," we outline how to plan assessments including evaluation processes, methods, and tools for evaluation program design. In the section "Learner Assessment and Evaluation," we describe assessment methods and instrumentation that can ensure learners have the skills needed to address behavioral and social issues that influence health. In the section "Program Evaluation," we address how measurements can be used to assess curricular and program performance. Lastly, in the section "Educational Research and Scholarship," we underscore the importance of educational scholarship and research as a means to move the science of educational evaluation forward.

Fundamental principles have influenced the content of each section. First, evaluation is as important as the training curricula delivered. Evaluations should not be an afterthought after the curriculum has already been delivered. Second, just as we urge our learners to practice evidence-based medicine, we urge educators to practice evidence-guided teaching. Although educational science is young, there is a growing body of research to guide selection of teaching interventions, curricular timing and "dose," and the choice of valid and reliable assessment tools. Educational tradition and convenience are simply not sufficient to guide efficient and effective uses of precious training hours. Finally, we assert that rigorously developed, delivered, and evaluated curricula should be published and shared as scholarly peer-reviewed works to advance educators' skills and the field.

ASSESSMENT AND EVALUATION PLANNING

Evaluation designs are critical for determining the impact of curriculum or teaching approaches on learners' knowledge, attitudes/values, and skills. Evaluation design selection might also consider cost effectiveness, systems change, or impact on patient or clinical outcomes. Implementing a design to test established or new curricular strategies takes careful planning and measurement considerations. The best approach for evaluation design is to develop the assessment(s) *as the curriculum or educational program is being developed,* rather than after. Too often, evaluations are planned at the end when opportunities to revise for meaningful assessment of learner and program outcomes have passed. Early evaluation planning will ensure that programmatic goals have been articulated, learning objectives are measurable, best approaches for evaluation have been identified, and the processes for evaluation are timed for best results. Although the planning process will vary based on resources, expertise, and other contextual factors, the following four questions highlight common issues to be considered during evaluation planning.

1. What is the goal of the evaluation? All educators assume their training program "works" but the specific purpose of the education may vary. For example, does the intervention target changes in attitudes, knowledge, or skills? Does the program intend to demonstrate minimally sufficient competence or extraordinary talent and achievement? Will the results be formative or summative? Will the data be used to influence institutional policy or to identify strengths or weaknesses of the program?

2. Which theoretical models will best guide evaluation designs and specific curricular content? For example, an educator interested in determining "competence" could use the Dreyfus model of skill acquisition that starts at novice, and progresses to advanced beginner, competent, proficient, and expert. In this case, assessment tools that target a determined threshold for "competence" and benchmarked steps leading to competence would be needed. Other models that guide evaluation development include Miller's pyramid (knows, knows how, shows how, does), Kirkpatrick's hierarchy of evaluation (assesses level of impact of the curriculum ranging from learner satisfaction to changes in clinical outcomes), or Bloom's taxonomy.

Models that guide educational content might include the Transtheoretical (Stages of Change) Model and motivational interviewing that matches behavioral counseling to patients' readiness to change (see Chapter 19). A demonstration of "competence" would require the use of the general Dreyfus model with specific assessment items relevant to motivational interviewing.

3. What are the available evaluation resources? Resources include time (for faculty and/or learners), money, faculty/evaluator skills, and buy-in from program leaders and learners. Assessments may range from time, cost, and labor-intensive standardized patient (SP) assessments to quicker and cheaper peer–peer observations. Careful attention must be given to the test characteristics of the assessment tools chosen and whether feasibility compromises the utility of the results.

4. What are the key methodological considerations? Even with clear goals and sufficient resources, critical decisions must be made that can affect the value of evaluations. As discussed below, psychometric properties such as reliability, validity, and fidelity of instruments must be considered. Standard setting, benchmarking, scoring, and remediation should also be determined. All four key considerations are applied to the opening Case Illustration in Table 43-1.

Creating Reliable and Valid Instruments

Concepts of reliability and validity are central to designing and implementing high stakes assessments. The higher the stakes associated with the assessment (e.g., pass or fail a course/clerkship), the greater the need for the assessment to be valid and reliable. In very simple terms, validity refers to whether the assessment measures what it intends to measure. A common misconception is that assessment instruments can be considered universally valid, when, in fact, validity can only be shown for a given population and context. Validating an assessment consists of evaluating potential threats to validity to ensure that the assessment actually

Table 43-1. Developing assessments for an alcohol counseling curriculum.

1. Goals of the Curriculum	2. Theoretical Model(s)	3. Resource Considerations	4. Methods: Tools	Methods: Timing
To produce lasting changes in resident knowledge and skills regarding alcohol screening and brief intervention.	- Miller's pyramid - National Institute on Alcohol Abuse and Alcoholism (NIAAA) clinician's guide to patients who drink to excess - Stages of change and motivational interviewing	- 3 hours of large group didactic time - 4 hours of small group discussion or role play - Use of three SP cases about alcohol use	- SP examinations - Written test - Survey - Focus groups	- Pre knowledge test - Post-SP examination - Post-written examination - Post-survey and focus group

represents the intended construct as applied in the intended setting. Common threats to validity include construct underrepresentation (e.g., too few items or cases) and construct-irrelevant variance (e.g., flawed rating scales, poorly trained SPs).

Reliability in educational assessment is a measure of reproducibility. Statistical methods of measuring reliability determine the difference between the "true score" and the "observed score" or the amount of error in the observed score. The greater the measurement error, the less reproducible the assessment becomes. There are three different questions to be asked about the reproducibility of a given test score if it were given to the same group of students more than once: (1) Would the same students pass or fail? (2) Would the rank order from best to worst score be the same? (3) Would all the students receive the same scores? Three different theories can be used statistically to assess reliability, including classical test theory (using Cronbach's alpha), generalizability theory, and item response theory. A psychometrics consultation can often answer these and many key evaluation development questions.

Standard Setting and Grading

Standard setting refers to the process of determining a cut score or passing score. For traditional assessments, such as multiple-choice examinations, standard setting techniques are well developed. For any performance-based assessments to be effectively used for summative decisions, setting defensible standards is necessary. Although standard setting may require attention to psychometrics, ultimately it incorporates consideration of institutional culture, policy, and resources.

Determining the passing score means determining how many students are going to fail. The "stakes" or ramifications of failing an assessment (e.g., repeating a course, need for remediation, ability to graduate) will play the largest role in determining how to set the passing score. Two broad categories of standard setting are normative (grading on a curve) and absolute or criterion referenced. Normative grading involves determining how a cohort of learners performed and then setting a cut-point as a multiple of standard deviations below the mean. Criterion-referenced standard setting is more work intensive but usually favored for performance-based assessment, as it is based on how each learner performs against a determined competency standard. Grading can be compensatory, allowing a learner to compensate for a low performance in one domain or case with higher performance on another, or noncompensatory. Noncompensatory grading will result in a greater number of students failing the assessment. For example, if students need to pass a certain number of cases to pass an Observed Standardized Clinical Examination (OSCE), they can compensate for poor history taking with outstanding interpersonal skills. If students must pass the history and interpersonal aspects of each case to pass an examination, passing will be more difficult.

LEARNER ASSESSMENT AND EVALUATION

Ideally, learners (and programs) will be assessed at multiple points with performance data being used to iteratively drive improvements. In a competency-based model, a threshold is set that all learners must achieve; however, benchmark or milestones on the path toward competence can be used to track learner progression toward more advanced skills over time. Programs should articulate skill development pathways that repeatedly assess learners and offer remediation, as needed.

A number of validated assessment tools are available for the BSS (see Suggested Readings and resource links). Table 43-2 provides examples of specific tools that assess core BSS areas such as social attitudes and behavior change counseling. Evaluators may select validated tools or develop their own based on the specific assessment needs. Remember that assessment instruments are not universally valid or reliable. Although it is helpful to review the psychometric properties of tools as they have been previously studied, it will still be necessary to evaluate any tool's performance when used with learners in the context of your assessment. Assessment goals (e.g., changing attitudes, knowledge, or skills), available resources, and preferred methodologies all inform the selection of measurement tools.

Assessing Attitudes

Educational programs seek to instill particular values or attitudes in their learners (e.g., empathy, respect, nonjudgment, egalitarianism). Educational activities are often indirect or occur on an experiential level and can be highly influenced by institutional culture and the "hidden curriculum" (see Chapter 46). Attitudes are most commonly assessed with self-report surveys that are highly efficient but have fairly obvious demand characteristics. Respondents may know the socially desirable answer and may not answer honestly. Indirect testing measures, such as the Implicit Associations Test (IAT), attempt to tap unconscious bias by tracking milliseconds of reaction time to words paired with race, gender, or other demographic identifiers. Multisource feedback (also known as "360-degree evaluations") involve eliciting learner evaluations from peers, allied health professionals, patients, and others with first-hand knowledge of the learner's tone, emotion, and behaviors—all of which infer attitudes.

Table 43-2. Examples of BSS assessment tools for learners.

Assessment Tool	Description	Where to Find It
1. Attitudes Toward Social Issues in Medicine	A 63-item Likert-type attitude survey with seven subscales including social factors, interprofessionalism, and prevention.	Parlow & Rothman. J Med Educ 1974;49:385–387.
2. Video Assessment of Simulated Encounters (VASE-R)	Three video-based case vignettes are used to assess learner skills in motivational interviewing.	John S. Baer, PhD VA Puget Sound Healthcare System-Seattle jsbaer@u.washington.edu http://adai.washington.edu/instruments/VASE-R.htm
3. Cognitive Behavior Survey	A seven-scale, 120-item questionnaire that profiles cognitive, meta-cognitive, and experiential aspect of learning for residents or students.	Dr. Rudolph Mitchell, Massachusetts Institute of Technology, (rudy@mit.edu). See *Acad Med* 2009;84:918–926.
4. Brief Negotiated Interview (BNI)	A 21-item checklist used to evaluate the quality of a brief negotiated interview for problematic substance use.	http://www.ihs.gov/nc4/documents/appendix_a_yale_bni_manual.pdf

Assessing Knowledge

Educational or learning objectives are critical for both curriculum development and evaluation. Objectives should specify observable and measurable changes brought about as a consequence of curricular exposure. Even for objectives limited only to medical knowledge, the levels or content of knowledge expected can vary, ranging from simple recall to complex synthesis using foundational knowledge and principles (see Bloom's Taxonomy). Written tests are commonly used to assess medical knowledge, but their content and format should be determined by knowledge level expected. Because learning can occur at many levels, from simple recall to problem solving, multiple-choice questions (MCQs) should target the level of learning appropriate to the content taught. Characteristics of effective MCQs are related to the item, the question stem, and answer options. Poorly constructed MCQs will not produce accurate or meaningful test scores and could negatively affect learner pass rates. Tips for developing MCQs can be found on The National Board of Medical Examiners web site.

Although MCQs can be problematic in nearly any content area, they are especially difficult to develop for BSS content. MCQ's commonly test recognition (choosing an answer) rather than recall (constructing an answer), allow guessing, and are time-consuming to construct with choices that are neither intuitive nor unequivocally correct. Thus, case write-ups, critical essays, or innovative tools like concept mapping might better assess a learner's mastery of BSS content. For example, in the UCSF School of Medicine, medical students keep a "sociocultural skills tracker" that includes a longitudinal series of patient-based assignments to demonstrate progress toward competence working with patients of diverse backgrounds.

"Tracker" entries are used to provide feedback and shape subsequent exercises.

Assessing Skills

Achieving behavioral science competency includes mastery of broad content as well as communication and interpersonal skills. Although relatively little has been studied about assessing students' behavioral science knowledge, a rich literature exists on performance-based testing to assess communication skills. Most of this work assesses learners at the "shows how" level of Miller's pyramid (know, knows how, shows how, does) and are stronger predictors of whether learners will demonstrate these skills in the clinical setting than written examinations. Using unannounced SPs in the clinical setting is an example of a performance-based assessment that evaluates learners at the "does" level of the pyramid, assuming they are unaware they are being assessed.

In the following section, we discuss several methods of performance-based assessments to evaluate communication and interpersonal skills. Many of these performance-based assessment methods can also be used to directly measure knowledge and indirectly measure attitudes.

Direct Observation

Direct observation of learners in medical education is essential but underutilized, especially in clinical settings. Both the Liaison Committee on Medical Education (LCME) and Accreditation Council for Graduate Medical Education (ACGME) require ongoing assessment of trainees that includes direct observation of clinical skills. The Mini-Clinical Evaluation Exercise (mini-CEX) is the most studied format for performance evaluation using direct observation. Less formal observations are also commonly done using behavioral checklists, global rating scales, or other observational tools.

INTER-RATER RELIABILITY

Several factors are important to consider when evaluating the quality and accuracy of assessments using direct observation. Overall assessments based on clinical observation generally have poor reliability. Variability in rater assessments has been attributed to measurement errors of leniency, bias, and poor performance discrimination. Whereas case specificity is typically unavoidable and affects reliability, rater variability also plays a role in accuracy. Judgments made by raters can be extremely subjective, influenced by raters' moods and likely to be idiosyncratic.

Using interviews of faculty raters, Kogan and colleagues identified four themes that provide insight into how ratings form: (1) faculty rely on variable frames of reference during observations including their own performance, performance by others known to them at different levels of training, standards of performance considered necessary for patient care, and patient outcomes; (2) inference often plays a key role, including assumptions about learner motivations and attitudes; (3) faculty use variable approaches to synthesizing judgments into numerical ratings across or within different observations; and (4) contextual factors (complexity of the encounter, learners' level of experience, the faculty–resident relationships), and residents' responses to feedback play a role in faculty judgments. Thus, raters need both tools and training to improve reliability.

OBSERVATION TOOLS

Tools to guide observations and structure assessments come in different forms. Kogan and colleagues published a systematic review of tools for direct observations with students, residents, and fellows in clinical settings. Another review of tools to assess communication skills evaluated 15 instruments based on criteria from the Kalamazoo Consensus Statement. Global rating scales have been found to be the more efficient of these tools, and are as reliable as checklists when completed by expert faculty. Checklists have advantages for lesser-experienced raters such as students or SPs.

Both checklists and rating scales vary greatly in length and format based on the objective of the assessment, the aspects of performance being assessed, and who is doing the rating. Checklists typically measure a list of behaviors observed that can be scored dichotomously as "done" or "not done." This approach is not ideal for assessments of complex and nuanced behaviors such as empathy or respect. In general, rating scales measure implicit processes and offer a range of responses usually on either a numerical or Likert-type scale or a behaviorally anchored rating scale (BARS). BARS specifically list the learner behaviors that must be observed to achieve a particular score. For example, for the item, "*Allows the patient to tell their story,*" the behavioral anchors can range from the lowest level

"*fails to let patient tell story or sets pace with closed Q&A style, not conversational*" to the highest level of "*encourages and lets patient tell story with open-ended questions and doesn't interrupt patient.*" Behavioral anchors can improve inter-rater reliability as they provide a more explicit definition of each level of performance. Global rating scales use fewer items but assess larger domains that may be difficult to reduce to a micro-skill set (e.g., empathy, cultural sensitivity). Global rating scales have been shown to be reliable when used by expert faculty or well-trained raters.

OBSERVER TRAINING

Despite the difficulties inherent in faculty raters, their assessments of learners' performance are essential for any educational program. Faculty training can improve their observation skills, which is far more important than choosing the "perfect" rating instrument.

Behavioral Observation Training (BOT) focuses on improving the ability of the observer to detect, perceive, and remember performance of learners. Strategies include practice by increasing the number of observations done, using a tool to record observations, establishing the learning objectives, and considering encounter logistics. Performance Dimension Training (PDT) is designed to familiarize faculty with the definitions and criteria for the competencies being observed. When faculty understand performance dimensions as a group, it is easier to achieve consensus on behaviors that constitute a superior versus inferior performance. Frame of Reference Training is an extension of PDT. It encourages faculty consensus and distinguishing minimum criteria for performance levels. Training includes several exercises where faculty work together to set criteria for satisfactory performance and create a BARS. Vignettes are viewed and rated using the scale, followed by feedback from the session trainer on the "true" ratings with explanations. Finally, Direct Observation of Competence training (developed by Holmboe and colleagues) incorporates elements of all the above rater training methods and adds relevant, practical exercises in direct observation. These exercises can be done in faculty development sessions and have been shown to lead to meaningful improvements.

Clinical Simulations

OSCE/CLINICAL SKILLS EXAMINATIONS

Since direct observation by faculty in clinical settings does not have the reliability necessary for high stakes assessments, most institutions now rely on structured performance testing. Clinical skills examinations, such as OSCEs or Clinical Performance Examinations (CPEs), are used by many programs to assess progression of learners to the next level of training. The United States and Canada both include a Clinical Skills Examination as part of their medical licensure requirements. These examinations often include a series of encounters with SPs who have been trained to portray patients with specific medical needs. By holding variables in the encounter constant, the reliability of these examinations is greater than observations with real patients. However, artificially creating and standardizing patient encounters does not fully eliminate threats to validity.

Standardized clinical examinations measure a learner's skills at the "show's how" level of Miller's pyramid; however, this occurs in an artificial situation. The key question for Clinical Skills Examinations is how well its scores predict learner performance in actual clinical settings (e.g., the "does" level of Miller's pyramid). Several studies support the predictive validity of CPE communication scores showing strong correlations between medical student CPE scores and later performance as residents. Although evidence supports the validity of CPE to assess communication, there are many aspects of communication in real clinical settings that are unmeasured, such as team communication and adaptability of communication styles in various clinical settings.

Contextual fidelity, or the extent to which the CPE can be affected by the learner, environment, task, or technical system, can threaten the validity of communication skills assessment. Also, the artificial context of the CPE may deprive the learner of contextual cues found in a real clinical environment and, therefore, stymie the learner's ability to communicate empathically. To consider these challenges to validity, some experts recommend the use of reflective practice, challenging cases, and rater training on how to give feedback to enrich the SP simulations in evaluating empathy. When the artificiality of the testing environment is further increased by "over standardization" in SP training, this can lead to encounters that lack fidelity and validity.

There is some debate about whether BSS skills can be reliably assessed using clinical cases or whether they are more accurately assessed when the explicit goal of the case is BSS focused, such as smoking cessation counseling. Some have also questioned whether general assessment of a learner's BSS skills can be measured across several cases or requires case specificity. Generally, each clinical case in a CPE has a separate and relevant content checklist for history and physical examination items, but the CPE may have only one global checklist (global rating scale) to evaluate the BSS skills across all cases. A study by Guiton of fourth-year medical students found high generalizability for seven communication skills across seven OSCE cases, supporting the ability to identify a set of generic communication skills across cases. However, they also found significant case-student variability in communication scores. This suggests that even though one communication skills checklist can be used across several cases, in any performance assessment of communication skills, several cases providing a variety of communication (or BSS) challenges should be used to achieve adequate reliability.

Although inter-rater reliability is generally greater in CPEs than in directly observed encounters with real patients, it is important to address this form of reliability when assessing BSS skills. There are inconsistent findings in the literature as to whether faculty and SP ratings correlate or if faculty are rating something different than SPs in assessments of communication and other BSS skills. Faculty are often looking for communication behaviors or skills that are known to be effective with patients, and SPs are reporting their experience from inside the interaction on the effectiveness of the skills observed. Some differences between expert faculty and SP raters have been found when global ratings are used in lieu of checklists. Training raters and using standardized tools (e.g., checklists) can reduce the number of raters needed for reliability and can increase inter-rater reliability.

HIGH TECH SIMULATION

Technically sophisticated mannequins and task trainers have been increasingly integrated into medical education for both teaching and assessment of clinical skills. A growing literature demonstrates that the practice of high-risk procedures on computerized, highly technical mannequins that appear to blink, sweat, and breathe create enough realism or fidelity that the skills demonstrated in these scenarios carry over to real clinical situations. Psychological fidelity—or how "real" the situation feels—and whether it requires the same cognitive and emotional skill set as a real situation must also be considered. Although medical procedures are well suited for high-simulation mannequin assessments, they can also be used to test teamwork skills, clinical reasoning, and emotion/stress-management.

Patient-focused simulation training involves a combination of mannequins and real people within a simulated scenario to provide psychological and functional fidelity. These simulations allow learners to tap into conscious and unconscious responses that can provide opportunities to assess skills of delivering bad news, communication of medical errors, ethical decision making, and end-of-life care, to name a few.

Computer-based virtual patients are another emerging technology for BSS assessment. More can be learned about the use and development of virtual patients on the MedBiquitous web site (see resource links).

PERFORMANCE PORTFOLIOS

Assessment of learner attitudes, knowledge, and skills is complex and requires a robust toolbox of assessment instruments. For BSS skills the most valid evaluations use planned overlaps among SPs, case assignments, faculty observations, and other "real-world" tools such as multisource feedback or chart review. These diverse data elements are often integrated into "performance portfolios" where learners and mentors are given some latitude in selecting artifacts that demonstrate progression toward or achievement of competence. By drawing from a pool of validated assessment instruments and evaluation data (e.g., CPE, OSCE), portfolios ensure some level of standardization while still allowing sufficient flexibility for learners with different strengths and needs. Ideally, portfolios serve both summative and formative purposes.

PROGRAM EVALUATION

Accumulated learner assessment data inform how well a program is operating to develop knowledge, behaviors/attitudes, and skills of its graduates. However, program evaluations might also include institutional impact, cost, conformity with program objectives or goals, and unplanned impacts on other programs or schools. As with learner assessments, program evaluation should be designed concurrently with the program itself and not added on after program completion. Moreover, program evaluation data hold great value as a summative process that drives curricular change. A simple program evaluation cycle is commonly used that begins with curricular planning and preparation then moves to teaching, data collection, reflection, analysis, and revision.

Kirkpatrick's hierarchy of evaluation is shown in Figure 43-1. Satisfaction surveys (the lowest Kirkpatrick level) are most commonly used but do not assess a program's success in impacting knowledge or skills. Ideally, medical educators could show that their training interventions affect learner behavior in the real world and ultimately influence patient outcomes.

The chosen Kirkpatrick level and matched assessment tools will depend on a variety of factors including programmatic goals, resources, feasibility, audience, and preferred methodologies. In addition to the evaluation tools described under learner evaluations (e.g., CPE, MCQs), sources of evidence for program evaluation might include satisfaction surveys, graduation or exit interviews, focus groups, and ratings from expert/outside observers. Table 43-3 provides examples of BSS program assessment tools.

CASE ILLUSTRATION (CONTD.)

After collecting learner data from SP (CPE) examinations around alcohol screening and brief interventions, a satisfaction survey and focus group are administered as a final program evaluation tool. The family medicine residency director reviews the data to evaluate and improve the alcohol counseling curriculum. She first turns to mean composite scores for residents completing the CPE.

The CPE composite data presented in Figure 43-2 show that Relationship Development and Physical Examination skills are better developed in this class of family medicine residents than their history taking. It also shows that scores on alcohol screening and counseling (a more specialized skill set) are about the same as general history taking. These mean scores from all learners reflect how well the program is performing in teaching these skills. Typically, a benchmark above 85–95% demonstrates that the examination is developmentally appropriate for residents. With a benchmark score below 85–95%, the examination may not be not performing well, either because it is too hard, not well designed, or the curriculum was not effectively taught. Because history taking and alcohol counseling scores in this figure are lowest and the benchmark is low at 80%, both this portion of the examination and the curriculum addressing these skills should be reviewed. In Kirkpatrick terms, this CPE assesses changes in learner skills but is not able to address changes in actual clinical practice or changes in patient outcomes.

Resident satisfaction surveys and focus groups addressed the lowest Kirkpatrick level of learner reaction but still provided important formative feedback to shape future curricular iterations. Learners were generally satisfied with the curriculum and would recommend it to their peers. However, residents requested more training in learning how to access community alcohol treatment resources and more direct observations of their counseling skills with real clinic patients. Interestingly, residents also noted there was great preceptor variability in alcohol screening and counseling skills and suggested the inclusion of faculty preceptor training.

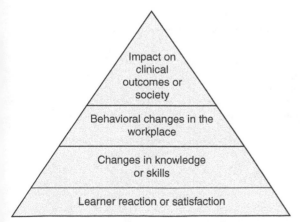

Figure 43-1. Kirkpatrick's hierarchy of evaluation.

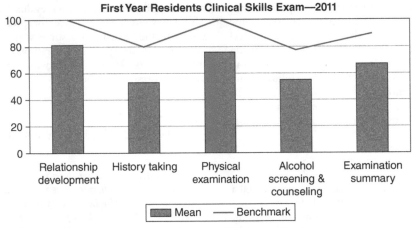

Figure 43-2. Mean composite scores for the resident Clinical Performance Exam.

The above case illustrates how data generated from learner evaluation can then be used to improve both the curricular program and the faculty teaching in it. This comprehensive evaluative approach should be routinely used to make the most of the evaluation data collected.

EDUCATIONAL RESEARCH AND SCHOLARSHIP

Research into the development and delivery of valid and reliable tools is a high priority and should be considered on par with other more traditional academic research pathways. It is the responsibility of deans, curriculum leaders, and educators to rigorously design and study their curricular innovations and to submit them to peer-reviewed journals for appropriate critique and dissemination.

Although educational funding streams pale in comparison to clinical research, organizations such as Agency for Healthcare Research and Quality (AHRQ) or Health Resources and Services Administration (HRSA) and foundations such as FIPSE, Harvard-Macy, and Stemmler regularly support educational research projects. Innovative programs to support faculty development in educational research skills are increasingly common as are Master's programs in education. As with any scholarly endeavor, adherence to ethical and practical guidelines regarding subject recruitment, data collection methods, and authorship is expected. In the end, "raising the bar" in BSS assessment and evaluation presents a "win-win-win" situation—learners receive higher quality feedback, programs and curricula constructively evolve, and contributions to educational science are recognized for academic advancement.

Table 43-3. Examples of BSS assessment tools for programs.

Assessment Tool	Description	Where to Find It
1. Tool to Assess Cultural Competence Training	A self-administered curriculum assessment tool used to identify gaps and redundancies in cultural competence curricula.	https://www.aamc.org/initiatives/tacct/
2. Communication, Curriculum, and Culture Instrument (C-3)	A 29-item tool used to assess the "hidden curriculum" of an institution.	Haidet P, et al. Characterizing the patient-centeredness of hidden curricula in medical schools: development and validation of a new measure. *Acad Med* 2005;80:44–50.
3. Association of American Medical Colleges (AAMC) Graduation Questionnaire (GQ)	An AAMC web-based survey administered to all graduating medical students including 24 potential BSS variables.	Carney PA, et al. Utility of the AAMC's Graduation Questionnaire to study behavioral and social sciences domains in undergraduate medical education. *Acad Med* 2010;89:165–176. www.aamc.org.

SUGGESTED READINGS

AAMC. Medical Simulation in Medical Education: Results of an AAMC Survey.https://www.aamc.org/download/259760/data/medicalsimulationinmedicaleducationanaamcsurvey.pdf. Accessed February 2014.

Cook DA, Beckman TJ, Bordage G. Quality of reporting of experimental studies in medical education: a systematic review. Med Educ 2007;41:737–745.

Corbett E, Jr., Berkow R, Bernstein L, et al. *Recommendations for Clinical Skills Undergraduate Medical Education.* Association of American Medical Colleges, Washington, D.C., 2008. Available at: https://www.aamc.org/download/163788/data/recommendations_for_preclerkship_skills_education_for_ugme.pdf. Accessed February 2014.

Downing S, Yudkowsky R. *Assessment in Health Professions Educations.* New York, NY: Routledge, 2009.

Duffy D, Gordon G, Whelan G, Cole-Kelly K, Frankel R, & All Participants in the American Academy on Physician and Patient's Conference on Education and Evaluation of Competence in Communication and Interpersonal Skills. Assessing competence in communication and interpersonal skills: the Kalamazoo II report. *Acad Med* 2004;79:495–507.

Epstein RM. Assessment in medical education. *N Engl J Med* 2007;356:387–396.

Epstein RM, Hundert EM. Defining and assessing professional-competence. *JAMA* 2002;287:226–235.

Haidet P, et al. Characterizing the patient centeredness of hidden curricula in medical schools: development and validation of a new measure. *Acad Med* 2005;80:44–50.

Kneebone R, Nestel D, Wetzel C, et al. The human face of simulation: patient-focused simulation training. *Acad Med* 2006;81: 919–924.

Kogan J, Holmboe E, Hauer K. Tools for direct observation and assessment of clinical skills in medical trainees: a systematic review. *J Am Med Assoc* 2009;302:1316–1326.

Schirmer J, Mauksch L, Lang F, et al. Assessing communication competence: a review of current tools. *Med Stud Educ* 2005; 37:184–192.

Schuwirth L, Van Der Vleuten C. General overview of the theories used in assessment: AMEE Guide no.57. 2011;33:783–797.

WEB SITES

MedBiquitous. http://www.medbiq.org. Accessed February 2014.

American Board of Internal Medicine Mini-CEX. http://www.abim.org/program-directors-administrators/assessment-tools/mini-cex.aspx. Accessed February 2014.

NBME MCQ Guide: http://www.nbme.org/publications/item-writing-manual.html. Accessed February 2014.

AAMC Tool to Assess Cultural Competence Training: https://www.aamc.org/initiatives/tacct/. Accessed February 2014.

Brief Negotiated Interview: http://www.ihs.gov/nc4/documents/appendix_a_yale_bni_manual.pdf. Accessed February 2014.

VASE-R: http://adai.washington.edu/instruments/VASE-R.htm. Accessed February 2014.

Evidence-Based Behavioral Practice

44

Bonnie Spring, PhD, ABPP & Stephen D. Persell, MD, MPH

RELEVANCE OF BEHAVIOR TO MEDICAL PRACTICE

Human behavior has a major impact on health and well-being. The patients that you see in medical practice are likely to have behaviors (e.g., smoking, drinking, and eating habits) that place them at risk of developing chronic disease. Equally likely, they may have psychological problems (e.g., depression) that impair their quality of life and undermine their motivation to follow your treatment recommendations. Moreover, if you treat families and see the same patients over many years, you may observe unhealthy behaviors long before you see the emergence of biological risk factors like hypertension, hypercholesterolemia, or hyperglycemia. By helping your patients to address unhealthy behaviors, you have the opportunity to help them prevent the onset or worsening of chronic diseases. Just as in evidence-based medicine, you should know how to find and appraise the evidence base for behavioral (nondrug, nonsurgical) treatments, so you can help your patients with the most appropriate behavioral treatment option. Below is a case you might encounter in the primary care clinic.

CASE ILLUSTRATION 1

A 43-year-old man presents for a preventive care visit. He has not had any preventive care in over 5 years but at an urgent care visit 4 months ago he was told he had high blood pressure. His past medical history is remarkable only for mild eczema. He is married, has two children, and works as an attorney. He says his work is sometimes stressful but denies a depressed mood or loss of interest in leisure activities. He has no difficulty sleeping. He recently cut back to about five cigarettes per day and has three to four alcoholic drinks almost every night. He does not exercise regularly, but walks about 5 minutes twice a day to the train. He does not follow any particular diet: breakfast is usually coffee and toast; lunch is fast food or a deli sandwich; he snacks on cookies or pastries at work. His wife cooks "healthy food" sometimes and they order from restaurants frequently. On physical examination his weight is 207 lbs with a body mass index of 29.7 kg/m². An average of three office blood pressures is 139/88 mm Hg. The rest of the examination is normal except for an eczematous rash on his arms. As you prescribe triamcinolone cream for his rash, you consider how best to counsel him about behavior change. The list of changes you think would be beneficial include: (1) stopping smoking; (2) reducing total calories; (3) following a diet low in sodium and high in vegetables, fruits, whole grains, and nonfat dairy products; (4) reducing saturated fat in his diet; (5) reducing alcohol use to no more than two drinks per day; and (6) increasing the amount of moderate-intensity physical activity he does by an additional 90–120 minutes each week.

APPLYING EVIDENCE-BASED PRACTICE IN PRIMARY CARE

This patient has several risk factors and behaviors that put his health at risk and that are potential targets for behavior change interventions. You are probably familiar with how to practice evidence-based care when making medical decisions about the use of medications or procedures. There is also a scientific evidence base about how to treat most unhealthy behaviors. For the purposes of this chapter, we use the broader term "evidence-based practice" (EBP) that includes both traditional evidence-based medicine and evidence-based behavioral practice.

EBP 5A's: Ask Questions

A practical way to approach EBP is by using a 5-step process better known as the "5A's,": Ask, Acquire, Appraise, Apply, and Analyze & adjust (see Figure 44-1).

Figure 44-1. Five steps of evidence-based practice. Source: www.ebbp.org.

reversing disease risk factors and promoting health protection.

Early in their careers, most physicians become familiar with the evidence base that evaluates which biomarkers warrant consistent clinical attention because they are risk factors for the development of chronic disease. They also learn to monitor and treat elevated cholesterol, blood pressure, and glucose to slow the patient's progression toward clinical disease. For disease prevention to be effective, it is important for physicians to recall that many unhealthy behaviors (e.g., substance use, physical inactivity, overeating) warrant as urgent attention as risk biomarkers. By asking prognostic questions and consulting the scientific literature, you can master the knowledge base that supports the contention that lifestyle behaviors are just as strongly associated as risk biomarkers with the onset of disease. With that awareness, you can then inquire about the best ways to treat unhealthy lifestyle behaviors.

EBP 5A's: Acquire and Appraise

Next steps in the EBP process are to acquire the evidence and critically appraise it for its quality and relevance to your patient. As a health care practitioner, you are a consumer of research; sometimes you will look for primary research evidence such as individual research studies, including clinical trials. More often you will turn to a secondary, synthesized evidence base that has been assembled in the form of systematic reviews.

The first step is to ask focused questions that can be answered through review of the scientific literature. Two kinds of questions connect health care providers with the knowledge base needed to offer best preventive care. The first (prognostic questions), asks which factors (i.e., biomarkers, behaviors, environmental conditions) convey risk or protection with respect to the likelihood of developing a chronic disease. The second (treatment questions) asks which treatments are most effective at

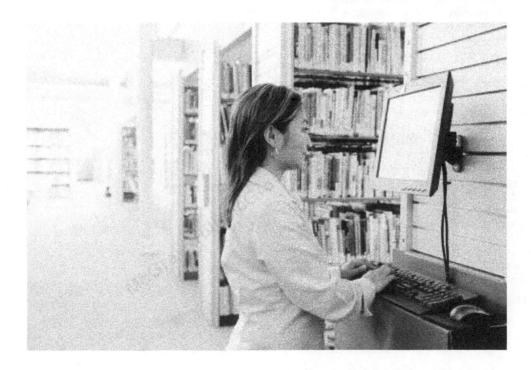

Much research exists about the lifestyle risk behaviors and treatment options for the patient described in the case. This evidence has often undergone systematic reviews to develop evidence-based treatment guidelines. For example, the *Guide to Clinical Preventive Services,* prepared by the US Preventive Services Task Force (USP-STF), rigorously evaluates and makes recommendations about the merits of preventive measures, including screening tests, counseling, and preventive medications. Another guideline, *Treating Tobacco Use and Dependence,* prepared by the US Public Health Services (USPHS), evaluates and makes recommendations about treating tobacco use. The National Heart, Lung, and Blood Institute has systematic reviews and guidelines about obesity treatment and about lifestyle interventions to reduce the risk of cardiovascular disease. Each review grounds interpretation of the evidence in an analytic framework that summarizes observational epidemiologic studies showing evidence of harms from the unhealthy behavior, as well as evidence of reduction in these harms when the behavior is stopped. These guidelines offer many recommendations relevant to your patient's smoking, unhealthy use of alcohol, obesity, and sedentary lifestyle.

BRIEF VERSUS INTENSIVE BEHAVIORAL INTERVENTIONS

The act of having a healthcare professional identify an unhealthy behavior, provide brief counseling to promote change, and follow up produces measureable improvement in several risk behaviors, including cigarette smoking. Usually, however, behavior changes are small and most patients do not respond. It is very important that the physician not interpret this experience to mean that behavior cannot be changed. After all, most unhealthy habits were acquired over a period of many years and have become deeply ingrained. More intensive treatments (that involve more and longer counseling sessions with specially trained providers) produce larger behavioral improvements in a greater proportion of those treated. For example, the Diabetes Prevention Program and Look AHEAD established that multiple sessions of diet, exercise, and behavior change counseling could produce a 7–8% weight loss, improved glycemic control, delayed progression of diabetes, and improved cardiovascular risk factors. Similarly, many studies synthesized to develop the USPHS Tobacco Guideline show that providing a greater number of counseling sessions or offering counseling combined with quit smoking medications substantially improves the patient's odds of becoming smoke free for the long term.

MULTIPLE UNHEALTHY BEHAVIORS

While the evidence supporting the effectiveness of intensive health behavior change treatments is strong, derived from well-executed multisite randomized

controlled trials, the research on health behavior change is particularly sparse in terms of indicating how to treat multiple co-occurring unhealthy behaviors. A majority of treatments directed at health behavior change address a single behavior, for example, excess alcohol intake, obesity, or risky sexual behavior. It has not been well studied how many behaviors are feasible to change at once, whether attempts to change multiple behaviors should be made simultaneously or sequentially, how to prioritize which behavior(s) to tackle first, or whether it is more effective to encourage patients to increase healthy behaviors or decrease unhealthy ones. If several behaviors in sequence will be changed, there is little research to guide the practitioner about how long to wait before tackling a new behavior and what sequence of behaviors will maximize the chances of success. These are important gaps in knowledge that clinicians and patients need researchers to fill.

EBP 5A's: Apply

Having asked key questions about the patient's health risks and treatment options, and having acquired and appraised the evidence, you have now reached the *apply* step in the EBP process. Deciding how to apply the evidence is the heart of how clinicians translate research into practice. As Figure 44-2 illustrates, making decisions about how to apply evidence requires integrating data from each of the three circles: best available research, patient characteristics (including preferences and values), and resource considerations (including practitioner expertise or skills).

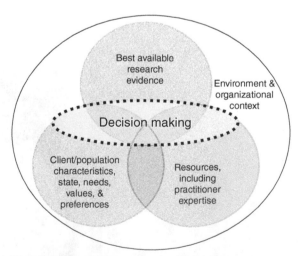

Figure 44-2. Elements that need integration in evidence-based practice. Source: Spring B, Hitchcock K. Evidence-based practice in psychology. In: Weiner IB, Craighead WE, eds. *Corsini's Encyclopedia of Psychology,* 4th ed. Wiley, 2009, pp. 603–607.

For this patient, there are a number of effective interventions, some brief and some intensive, to address his risk behaviors. With so many unhealthy behaviors, the real challenge is to know where to begin. To prioritize which behaviors to treat, you will want to consider all three circles. An important first step is to evaluate the magnitude and immediacy of risks associated with each of the patient's health behaviors. Research evidence informs you that, ordinarily, smoking and obesity top the list of risk factors that have the greatest harmful impact. For this patient, though, his alcohol use could pose a greater immediate risk of harm. You might also want to evaluate whether a coexisting mental health disorder like depression or anxiety is present that warrants treatment in its own right and that could complicate efforts at behavior change.

To address the patient's risk of drinking, you will probably want to start off with a procedure called SBIRT (Screening, Brief Intervention, and Referral for Treatment). Based on the patient's responses to a screening questionnaire, you would inform him about how his amount of drinking corresponds to a level of intake that is considered low risk. You would then assess his motivation or level of readiness to change. Depending on his readiness, you and the patient might collaboratively set a goal that falls somewhere between touching base about drinking at the next medical appointment, to reducing his number of drinks per week, to beginning intensive treatment with a substance abuse counselor. Alternatively, the patient may not be interested in changing his drinking, but motivated to become more physically active. The more the patient can be engaged in collaborating to formulate a behavior change goal, the greater the likelihood that he will follow through, thereby growing more confident and motivated to attempt new healthy changes (see Chapter 19).

Another key consideration arises from the third circle: resources. What assets are available to support your patient's behavior change? Financial resources will probably factor in, as may your team's time and professional skills. As practitioners acquire knowledge of evidence-based interventions to change behavior, they need to maintain self-awareness of their own skills, time, and resources. They need to be aware of their own limitations and understand when the evidence suggests that a behavior change intervention that they cannot provide is likely to be more effective than what they can offer. If they are unable to develop those services in their practice, they should refer patients to practitioners and programs in their community that can provide them. To adequately support health promotion, the physician needs to cultivate a professional referral network that includes experts in behavior change (psychologists), nutrition (dieticians), and exercise (kinesiologists, exercise physiologists). To serve those without resources to pay for intensive behavioral treatments, the doctor will also want to keep on hand a roster of no- or low-cost resources, including free telephone counseling services (e.g., smoking quit line), community programs (e.g., training clinics that offer free or sliding scale billing, church-based programs, YMCA), Internet or mobile treatment programs, and books.

EBP 5A's: Analyze and Adjust

At the end of the day, the best intervention is not necessarily the one supported by the highest quality clinical trial evidence, but rather the one that works for the particular patient. The treatment supported by the best available evidence is the best initial treatment to try, but decision making about intervention begins rather than ends when an initial treatment is selected and delivered. The important rest of the story unfolds by measuring and analyzing what benefits (positive behavior changes) and harms (side effects, distress, worsening of other health behaviors) accrue to the patient as a result of receiving the chosen treatment. If the balance of benefits and harms continues in an unfavorable direction, the provider will want to consider adjusting the type, dose, or administrator of the treatment.

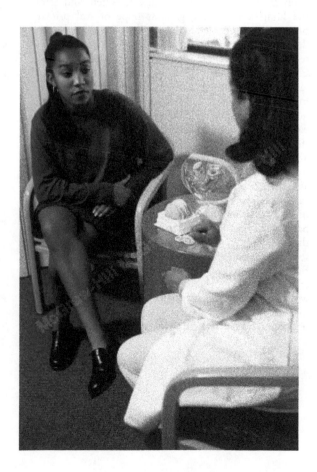

Physicians should not be surprised if the benefits they observe from any treatment in actual clinical practice are smaller than those seen in research studies. There are many reasons for this discrepancy. Clinicians who provide an intervention in actual practice may be less well-trained, exert fewer checks on the quality of treatment delivery, and provide less intensive care because they have competing priorities. Cost may also be a barrier that constrains patients' full engagement in treatment; behavioral interventions may be expensive, and third-party coverage may be less generous or nonexistent for these services. Out-of-pocket costs to the patient can pose a real obstacle to full engagement with treatment.

SETTING UP A PRACTICE TO SUPPORT EVIDENCE-BASED BEHAVIORAL PRACTICE

Prospects for preventive medicine hinge upon making evidence-based behavioral practice a reality. Because lifestyle behaviors constitute the major preventable causes of chronic disease, monitoring and treating them effectively through the entire health care system and across the lifespan offers the greatest hope of real primary prevention. Useful tools that fit into the clinical workflow can help make it easier for clinical practices to systematically complete screenings for risky behaviors. Changing the roles played by care team members can take some of the burden off the physician and may make the delivery system more reliable. Electronic health record tools like clinical reminders can encourage completion of standardized health behavior assessments that serve as screeners or that track progress over time. Tools like Internet portals connected to patients' electronic health records can allow patients to complete assessments prior to a medical visit so that the patient can self-monitor personal progress over time. Mechanisms that simplify and expedite the process of referring patients to expert interventionists are also needed so that the barriers to referral are reduced when patients require more than just brief behavioral treatment. Because we cannot manage what we do not measure, effective health promotion through lifestyle intervention would be enhanced by increased use of performance measures that assess screening for and treatment of risk behaviors. Some of these exist (such as those developed by the Physicians Consortium for Performance Improvement convened by the American Medical Association) and are used to varying degrees. Assessing and intervening with risk behaviors in a manner that integrates best available research, patient characteristics and resources is the pathway to integrative care that prevents illness in addition to managing disease.

SUGGESTED READINGS

Fiore MC, Jaen CR, Baker TB, et al. *Treating Tobacco Use and Dependence: 2008 Update.* Clinical Practice Guideline. Rockville, MD: U.S. Department of Health and Human Services. Public Health Service, May 2008.

Folsom AR, Yatsuya H, Nettleton JA, Lutsey PL, Cushman M, Rosamond WD. Community prevalence of ideal cardiovascular health by the American Heart Association definition, and relationship with cardiovascular disease incidence. *J Am Coll Cardiol* 2011;57:1690–1696.

Guyatt G, Rennie D, Meade MO, Cook DJ. *Users' Guides to the Medical Literature: A Manual for Evidence-Based Clinical Practice,* 2nd ed. New York: McGraw Hill Publishers, 2008.

Satterfield J, Spring B, Newhouse R, et al. Toward a transdisciplinary model of evidence-based practice. *Milbank Quarterly* 2009;87:368–390.

Spring B, Hitchcock K. Evidence-based practice in psychology. In: Weiner IB, Craighead WE, eds. *Corsini's Encyclopedia of Psychology,* 4th ed. Hoboken, New Jersey, 2010, pp. 603–607.

Stead LF, Bergson G, Lancaster T. Physician advice for smoking cessation. *Cochrane Database Syst Rev* 2008;(2):CD000165.

U.S. Preventive Services TaskForce. *Guide to Clinical Preventive Services,* 2010–2011. AHRQ Publication No. 10-05145, September 2010. Rockville, MD: Agency for Healthcare Research and Quality, 2010.

Wing RR; Look AHEAD Research Group. Long-term effects of a lifestyle intervention on weight and cardiovascular risk factors in individuals with type 2 diabetes mellitus: four-year results of the Look AHEAD trial. *Arch Intern Med* 2010;170:1566–1575.

WEB SITES

Evidence-based behavioral practice. www.ebbp.org. Free online modules that illustrate the EBBP process for both individual and public health. Accessed February 2014.

Duke and UNC Chapel Hill online EBP module. http://www.hsl.unc.edu/services/tutorials/EBM/index.htm. Accessed February 2014.

Physicians Consortium for Performance Improvement. http://www.ama-assn.org/apps/listserv/x-check/qmeasure.cgi?submit=PCPI. Accessed February 2014.

Narrative Medicine

Jonathan Amiel, MD; Anne Armstrong-Coben, MD; Melanie Bernitz, MD, MPH;
Julie Glickstein, MD; Deepthiman Gowda, MD, MPH; Gillian Graham, MS;
Nellie Hermann, MFA; Constance Molino Park, MD, PhD; Delphine Taylor, MD;
& Rita Charon, MD, PhD

A group of physicians, writers, and educators sits around a conference table in a busy medical school, eating hurried lunches, coordinating course materials for medical students, reviewing with excitement or concern what just happened in their first-year medical interviewing courses. More people gather, and the room quiets. Today, the novelist on the faculty reminds them, they are reading "Aquarium," a personal essay written by writer Aleksandar Hemon who has lost his baby daughter to brain cancer. The mood in the room shifts from light camaraderie to an attentive sense of purpose. "I had such a hard time reading this," a seasoned family physician sighs. "It made me want to run home and pick up my baby," offers the hospitalist.

As the conversation develops, the novelist draws the group's attention to the essay's title and its governing image, an important metaphor for his experience with illness and loss. "The whole thing is about an aquarium," an internist and literary scholar offers. "You feel very much like an outsider reading this," admits a pediatrician.

After some discussion, the novelist offers a writing prompt: *Describe an aquarium that you yourself have been in.* The group members take out pen and paper and, heads bowed, write intently for 4 minutes. When the time is up, many offer to read their work. Some read aloud descriptions of experiences with literal aquariums, marveling at the foreignness of aquatic life. A psychiatrist and a general internist each read aloud what they wrote about-times when they felt isolated in family or work and unable to truly communicate with those around them. Some wrote about feeling that, as doctors, they are inside an aquarium; others wrote about the experience of being on the outside. "The whole patient experience is like being in a fishbowl," reflects a pediatrician, "and in the story, the doctors are in a fishbowl too." The internist and literary scholar replies, "But this story is like instructions about how not to be marooned. It gives a glimpse into that fishbowl, but also says *and*

then you can write. It opens up a way to talk about and then use the imagination and the power of words."

WHAT IS NARRATIVE MEDICINE?

This session is a typical example of the kind of work this group does every week. They are medical educators, the faculty of Foundations of Clinical Medicine (Columbia's "doctoring" course) who employ the techniques of narrative medicine to sharpen their clinical skills, deepen their teaching, and reflect on their work. Narrative medicine developed out of the integration of medicine and literary studies to fortify clinical practice with the narrative competence to recognize, absorb, metabolize, interpret, and be moved by the stories of illness. Its unifying tenet is that the giving and receiving of accounts of self are the central events in health care—whether the account is given by a patient, family member, student, clinician, or members of the lay public and whether it is received by a doctor in the office, a circle of peers in a teaching session, a multidisciplinary team meeting in a clinic, or a Congressional hearing about health reform. Although arising only in 2000 from earlier efforts in humanities and medicine and primary care medicine, narrative medicine has spread quickly first at its home at Columbia University and then throughout the United States and abroad. Synthesizing theories and methods from the humanities, the social sciences, and the behavioral sciences, narrative medicine models a bridge among disciplines and, more importantly, supports the interior integration of cognitive, behavioral, imaginative, aesthetic, and affective states to which the effective clinician aspires.

Narrative medicine unfolds in three broad and simultaneous movements—**attention, representation, and affiliation**. These movements conceptualize and then guide a clinical and teaching practice that can establish contact with self, patients, students, colleagues, and the public that medicine serves. We will first define these movements and then follow with real-life examples.

Attention is that state of receptivity whereby a listener or witness or reader can receive the account given by another. To attain the state of attention, the receiver focuses closely and deeply on the person giving an account, whether that person is a patient, a student, a novelist, a poet, or even a painter or a composer. The receiver does not efface himself or herself but rather offers the contours of the self as a container for what is given by the other. Combining mindfulness with curiosity, the receiver captures all that the other transmits, squandering no word or silence or gesture or mood from the evidence that emerges from the encounter.

Representation includes the means by which any attentive witness confers form on what is received. Typically this is done with language as one writes a story or a vignette or a progress note to capture that which has been received from the other. (Although visual representations can also be made, we restrict ourselves here to written representations.) What is represented can be read—by the writer, by the subject of the representation, or by others involved in the clinical process. Because, as psychotherapist Hans Loewald suggests, writing is a sensorimotor act that transforms the immaterial into the material, it allows the writer to communicate what was not known until the writing to self and then to others.

Affiliation is the ultimate goal of any clinical act—affiliation between patient and clinician, between clinician and colleagues, between clinician-teacher and student, and between health care professionals and the public we serve. Robust affiliation provides the grounds for any event of healing.

These movements intensify one another, attention fueling the capacity to represent, representation fortifying the capacity to attend, and both of them spiraling toward affiliation. Doctor and patient write their way through clinical events. Medical students write reflective essays about early clinical experience, and their teachers receive them with newly developed skills in close reading. Patients and clinicians share writing groups to write about their lived experiences with illness. Multidisciplinary teams meet on the wards or the clinics to develop their own capacity to collaborate and unite. These methods permit us to get under the distinctions that typically isolate us from one another and bring us, in common, onto the grounds of human suffering and the desire to lessen that suffering.

NARRATIVE MEDICINE IN CLINICAL PRACTICE

Querying all faculty of Columbia's Foundations of Clinical Medicine course, we compiled a table of goals that have been accomplished in clinical practice

Table 45-1. The movements of narrative medicine.

Attention
Self-awareness and self-care
Recognition of the patient
Recognition of colleagues
Representation
Writing as discovery
Writing in the shadow of texts
Writing with patients
Affiliation
With patients
Among colleagues
Among human beings

through the use of narrative methods (see Table 45-1). Selections from our respondents' accounts of accomplishing some of these goals in practice thicken the descriptions of our listed goals. We categorize these goals according to the three movements of narrative medicine, although it is easily seen how these movements converge and occur simultaneously.

Attention

CASE ILLUSTRATION 1: SELF-AWARENESS AND SELF-CARE

Several years ago, I cared for a retired health care professional whom I found to be enormously difficult to care for. . . . I was unsuccessful at bringing her attention to the likely undercurrent to her various somatic complaints—a long-standing and untreated depression and anxiety disorder. . . . [S]he expressed to me that she felt I was not providing adequate care. Ultimately, I felt frustrated and powerless, and in light of her impression about my care, I suggested that she switch to another physician. Soon after this clinical relationship ended, I reflected and wrote about this patient in our Narrative Medicine group and shared my writing with the others. Through the writing, I clarified the events that led to certain outcomes and I understood more deeply what I felt was at stake for me. As a clinician, I felt as though I had failed and had abandoned the patient. As an educator, I felt particular shame, given that I had unsuccessfully managed this clinical relationship, yet teach students how to navigate communication with "difficult patients." In the writing and telling, others were able to relate to my experience and normalize what was going on. I was able to forgive myself, and I reframed what had become an overly harsh self-judgment. I recognized my own humanity In the enterprise.

(Written by a general internist)

CASE ILLUSTRATION 2: RECOGNITION OF THE PATIENT

I had just spent some time doing intense narrative medicine work. . . . When I walked into my practice I felt more excitement than stress when I saw the box of charts. I looked upon this as opportunity to hear patient stories rather than feeling burdened by the workload. I saw a mother and son that afternoon. The child had a superficial cut that required little medical care. My "former self" (and the fact that there were numerous patients waiting) would have likely left it at that. . . . Superficial cut, antibiotic ointment, anticipatory guidance about keeping him away from scissors. However, my head began to ask more questions and my eyes were more in tune to the Mom. I realized I had not heard the whole story. I probed more, listened more intently, and discovered why she was really there. The mother had taken boarders in to her apartment who were HIV positive. These individuals had had a number of violent fights, which included cutting with scissors. She had asked them to move out. During the move, her son had found the scissors and cut his hand. This was her true fear. Using narrative attention, the desire to hear the story, enabled me to address what was really needed that day.

(Written by a general pediatrician.)

Representation

CASE ILLUSTRATION 3: WRITING AS DISCOVERY

We were asked to identify a difficult patient and write about them. I had never previously written about a patient in this manner, and never really taken the time to consider why I reacted in such a way to certain patients. It is always easy to identify the "heart sink" patients, the ones whose names you see on your schedule and who you hope will not come in that day. The patient I chose to write about on that day was one [with] few "real" medical issues, but [who] always tried to cloak her reason for the visit with a physical complaint. . . . When writing about her, I realized that I actually really did like her. . . . Subsequent to writing about her, I felt a lot less frustrated about the situation. I actually welcomed seeing her on my schedule. I felt empowered to know what my role was and what my duty was towards her. I felt like I did have something to offer, I realized that there was a reason why she chose to come back and see me again and again. I felt honored. And now that she has moved on and is no longer my patient, I actually miss her. . . . [M]y resentment turned to gratitude. Through writing that first time about a patient I have started on my own journey towards understanding the power of narrative on my own personal journey as a physician.

(Written by a family physician who practices in Student Health.)

CASE ILLUSTRATION 4: WRITING WITH PATIENTS

A 53-year-old business executive, for whom I'd served as internist/endocrinologist for 10 years, suddenly and almost parenthetically said she sometimes thought of her long deceased sister when she came to my office. . . . I silently wondered if the stressful time of menopause with possible thoughts of mortality had reawakened feelings of loss, especially of an older sister, and I suggested that perhaps she'd benefit from writing about why she might associate our visits with thoughts of her sister's death. A month later the patient returned having written on the topic and wanting to share thoughts and memories. She vividly recalled that ten years ago I'd been the first physician to have paused during the routine family history after she'd impassively recited yet again that her older sister had committed suicide when they were both teenagers 30 years earlier. She had even on occasion thought vaguely of exploring memories of her sister's early death with me and then perhaps a psychiatrist but only now, after writing about her sister and her own concerns about mood, did she have the courage to begin this.

(Written by an internist/endocrinologist
in private practice.)

Affiliation

CASE ILLUSTRATION 5:
AFFILIATION WITH PATIENTS

I run a narrative medicine seminar for a group of health care professionals at the hospital. It happens that three of the persons who attend the group are also my internal medicine patients. Every month, we gather to read together and then to write in the shadow of what we have read. Once, I chose a poem by Rachel Hadas, "Tenor and Vehicle," as the text. In it, the poet conveys the close relationship between ivy and the wall on which it climbs—both of them dependent on the other for existence and supportive of one another's thriving. Some of the writers wrote about their own practice in the hospital, caring for very dependent and needy patients. One of my patients, who was undergoing an incredibly challenging health situation and finding great resilience and courage in the face of it, wrote of how this poem seemed to her to be her own vows for her up-coming marriage. It was a stunning expressive act not only for the writer vis-à-vis her love relationship but also for all the other members of the group, able to see how vast was the reach of this short poem.

(Written by an internist who practices
in the medicine clinic.)

CASE ILLUSTRATION 6:
AFFILIATION WITH PATIENTS AND FAMILIES

The ultimate goal for the fetal cardiologist is to facilitate the best possible outcome for the fetus and the family. . . . During the patient encounter, the physician changes narrative perspective from the interpreter of the medical images and data, to the narrator of the diagnosis and prognosis for the baby, to the listener while the parents serve as narrator of their lived experience and support milieu, to a participant in the integration of all the above information in guiding the parents towards a final decision. During each process, the narrative techniques of empathy, imagination, and of entering the patient's presence with attuned concentration and observation allow the physician to adapt himself or herself to the individual needs of each patient and to form an individual bond that will be the foundation for the stressful journey upon which he or she is to embark with the parents.

(Written by a fetal cardiologist who practices in
the fetal echocardiography unit.)

WHY WE READ AND WRITE

These examples demonstrate some of the guiding goals and powers of narrative medicine. As a discipline based in textual practices, narrative medicine can train its students to do what close readers and writers do—enter alien narrative worlds, comprehend those worlds from others' points of view, co-create with the inhabitant of these worlds the substrate for meaning, and be nourished by the process. Adopting the policy that every word counts, close readers learn to take account of the formal features of a text—its genre, diction, temporal structure, metaphors, narrative strategies—so as to receive the full "message" of what is written. Whether reading Aleksandar Hemon's "The Aquarium" or a Stephen King thriller, the reader surrenders to the demands of the text, wondering why the story is told the way it is told or why it triggers particular moods or thoughts. Perhaps one reason that serious readers seek out opportunities to read with others or to read what others have written about a text is to learn how infinite are the potential interpretations of any stretch of text. Readers learn to honor the text as an entity unto itself as well as a powerful mirror for the self of the reader. When in the clinical setting, these readerly skills get transposed to powerful skills of attentive listening to patients' words and silences and bodies. The reader/listener enters the patient's world with openness and curiosity, able more effectively to imagine the whole, to raise consequential hypotheses about what goes on, to accept the strangeness of any alien world as plausible if not necessary and ultimately to make contact with the patient. The reader/listener seeks out groups of peers to work with, realizing how enriched is one person's interpretation by congress with others.

As is demonstrated in our clinicians' responses to our query, narrative medicine has developed many forms of writing in its practice. In all cases, the writer needs a reader. The faculty-participants in this project were trained in close reading as they wrote in concert with their peers. Always, what any of us wrote was read or listened to closely and skillfully by our peers. By developing the reading capacities of our faculty, we could assure that when students are asked to write about their experiences, they will obtain close and skilled reading of their texts. We furnish faculty members with "readers' guides" instead of rating scales so that they can attend to what their students express, not to judge and rate the levels of reflection achieved but rather to read the text closely enough to be able to say what is seen.

Some reflective writing practices are practical means to concentrate attention on a particular clinical situation—write about a challenging patient; write about a patient you brood about; write about a patient you love. Other practices that engage clinicians and patients in writing seem farther afield from clinical practice, although these too circle back very directly to the writer's capacity to offer or receive health care. Often, the writing is encouraged by first reading a literary text with a group—a poem, a paragraph of a novel, a short story, an intern's progress note, a prayer. A narrative medicine group adopts close reading techniques in which one inspects the form, the tempo, the mood, and the movements of the text. You might feel like you were in English class for this part of the narrative medicine seminar. But unlike the English teacher, the narrative medicine teacher will offer a writing prompt that invites you to consider some aspect of your own experience. Creating the writing prompt is the hardest part of teaching narrative medicine, for it has to be an economical and compelling invitation to expand the mind of the learner toward both the "business" of the text and the interiority of the reader.

Here are a couple of examples.

the death of fred clifton
11/10/84, age 49

i seemed to be drawn
to the center of myself
leaving the edges of me
in the hands of my wife

and i saw with the most amazing
clarity
so that i had not eyes but
sight,
and, rising and turning,
through my skin,
there was all around not the
shapes of things
but oh, at last, the things
themselves.
(Clifton, 51)

The prompt used sometimes in teaching this poem is, "Write about the things themselves." One of us recently taught this poem using this prompt to a group of palliative care fellows. No matter how many deaths these doctors had accompanied, they wrote about "the things themselves" in their own lives. One intensivist wrote four words: "Love, Family, Work, Joy." Those of us hearing these words told him he had just written the words on his own family crest. It was as if he had found a direct line to those essentials within the edges of self, thereby bringing into immediate contact the dilemmas of his dying patients with his own search for meaning in his life.

A paragraph from a book on illness narratives offers the following story written by Eduardo Galeano that, Arthur Frank heard years ago and finds himself still brooding about and sharing with others:

> Fernando Silva ran the children's hospital in Managua. On Christmas Eve, he worked late into the night. Firecrackers were exploding and fireworks lit up the sky when Fernando decided it was time to leave. They were expecting him at home to celebrate the holiday.
>
> He took one last look around, checking to see that everything was in order, when he heard cottony footsteps behind him. He turned to find one of the sick children walking after him. In the half light he recognized the lonely, doomed child. Fernando recognized the face already lined with death and those eyes asking for forgiveness, or perhaps permission.
>
> Fernando walked over to him and the boy gave him his hand.
>
> "Tell someone . . ." the child whispered. "Tell someone I'm here." (Frank, 4)

The prompt we have used with this paragraph, taken from Art Frank's explanation of what stories can do to their readers is, "Write about a story that is working on you." This prompt can be met either with a clinical story still gripping the writer or, as likely, an event from childhood, a fairy tale, or a parable from a Gospel.

These examples of writing prompts suggest, we hope, the function of the writing of narrative medicine. The learner is not asked to write "about" the text but, rather, from within the mood and train of thought of the text and the conversation the group has experienced about it. Writing in the shadow of the text suggests that powerful states of contemplation and reflection can be entered—oftentimes very quickly—by paying serious attention to well-written texts. Close reading might be a form of meditation, in which the reader concentrates on the text in its entirety—not only its linguistic freight but its music, its echoes to other texts, its balance, its jar, its form. Captivated, the reader can then be taken to places, in his or her writing, that might have been hard to achieve without first reading. Another way to say this is that the reader is quickly made permeable to the text, first, and then that permeability is extended to self. Such states, we know, are achieved when beholding great works of art or hearing great musical compositions. These findings fuel the recent trend in bringing medical students to art museums or symphony halls, not to civilize them but to confront them with the otherness of great beauty, a confrontation that invariably brings them closer to their selves.

These examples from narrative medicine practice hint at the pleasure and freedom available in simple reading and writing exercises. When a writer reads aloud to a group what he or she has written in the shadow of a text, the group members expand *their* minds toward the text as well as toward the writer. Writing as discovery, as Loewald describes it, these learners gain access to what they know but might not realize they know. They then accept the risks of exposing this "newly known" to self and listener, thereby intensifying both self-awareness and contact with peers. Even when a narrative medicine group is composed of persons unlike one another—nurses, social workers, patients, doctors, administrators might be in the same group—the reading and writing actions release them from the distinctions that typically separate them. They are equals in the reading and writing if not in the hierarchical structures that contain them.

NARRATIVE MEDICINE IN TEACHING

Armed with an understanding of the important clinical goals reachable through the use of narrative methods, we turn to ways in which we have used narrative medicine methods in our teaching practice. The educational goals parallel the clinical goals. Here, we display the educational experiences in a developmental sequence, starting with the premedical student and ending with the senior resident, suggesting which movements and specific goals have been reached in each example.

CASE ILLUSTRATION 7: PRE-MEDICAL STUDENT— REPRESENTATION (WRITING AS DISCOVERY)

A premed student was asked to witness my office. She had been an art history major who was embarking on a Master's degree in international health. She wrote witness notes (similar to field notes an anthropologist might write) after observing in clinic, and I could see that she was "getting" what was going on between my patients and me, attentive to aspects of the encounters that I had not noticed myself. Her first personal statement for medical school applications was a smart crisp statement about international health movements and health care reform. Then, after her month of writing about what she witnessed in the office, she totally revised her statement. Her exposure to what patients said about themselves and the narrative routines in my practice transformed her view of what sick people really need and what doctors can to do help them.

CASE ILLUSTRATION 8: FIRST-YEAR STUDENT— ATTENTION (SELF AWARENESS)

A student told a story [in class] last week about the experience of seeing a patient interviewed in front of the whole class. It sounded like an old-time "demonstrate the pathology" session, with the patient passive and seemingly clueless and the doctor all-powerful. The student cried when she related the story and the whole group resonated. When I ran into her on the subway yesterday, she told me she hadn't realized how upset she was. But articulating the experience helped her to realize and think about why this was so disturbing.

CASE ILLUSTRATION 9: FIRST-YEAR STUDENT—AFFILIATION (WITH PEERS)

[A first year medical student] came into the standardized patient encounter eager and animated. She began well, introducing herself and setting the tone. The patient was quiet and depressed, yet the student was unable to change her tone to respond

to the patient's cues. She continued the interview, but her enthusiasm and energy pushed the patient further and further away.

The semester continued and her enthusiasm did not wane. She continues to grapple with managing her perky manner while interviewing with a patient who was quieter, depressed, or troubled. She told me that her outward demeanor was actually covering up extreme anxiety about the patient interaction, and that her often almost manic interviewing skills were a result of her protecting herself from falling apart during patient interviews.

She wrote about her patient encounters, and often shared to the class what she wrote. She wrote about accepting the anxiety, and learning to read the physical manifestations, the clammy palms, the racing heart. She wrote that she has learned to just feel these sensations and not let them overshadow what she needs to say to the patient or do for the patient. She wrote that she has learned to let go of the anxiety surrounding the patient interview and instead feel the excitement of caring for the patient.

Although she has been writing about how it feels to interview, her objective ability to interview a patient, in a more controlled, dignified, professional way, has improved dramatically. The enthusiasm is still palpable, yet the energy is more controlled. I believe her ability to use narrative writing to express her feelings regarding the interview has allowed her to see herself in a way that she never would have, even with her preceptor or her peers commenting on her interview skills numerous time. The self-reflection that came from the narrative allowed her to undergo a truly transformative experience that will benefit her future career as a doctor.

CASE ILLUSTRATION 10: SECOND-YEAR STUDENT — REPRESENTATION (WRITING AS DISCOVERY); ATTENTION (SELF-AWARENESS AND SELF-CARE)

After reading the paragraph from Art Frank's book about the dying child, I invited my students to write about a story that is working on them. One student had not disclosed in the context of our seminar complex events of her childhood related to the serious illness and death of a sibling. Until given this opportunity to write, the student had not disclosed the challenging role she herself had been asked to play in obtaining health care for her family. How did she benefit from writing about this? The permission to write let her acknowledge that these events, and her role in

this story, had created who she is, and are part of the reason she is in medicine in the first place.

CASE ILLUSTRATION 11: THIRD-YEAR STUDENT—ATTENTION (SELF-AWARENESS); AFFILIATION (WITH PEERS)

While precepting third-year students on their internal medicine rotation, I devote one session a week to writing in the Parallel Chart, where I invite students to write about aspects of their patients that are critical to their care but that do not belong in the hospital chart. One student bristled at the idea of writing as discovery, saying she hated to write and, instead, just took long runs and did her contemplation and self-examination in that way. I invited her simply to bring in to class lists of things that went through her mind as she ran across the George Washington Bridge. She did so, and she created luminous texts filled with fragments of images that cohered into fragile meaning. I told her she was writing poems. She started bringing poems into our sessions. When she brought Dylan Thomas's "Do Not Go Gentle into That Good Night" and read it with her classmates, she made a breakthrough in the care of a dying patient in her care, able for the first time to leave her own perspective on his care and to comprehend his and his family's continuing wish for aggressive care.

CASE ILLUSTRATION 12: FOURTH-YEAR STUDENT—ATTENTION (SELF-AWARENESS); AFFILIATION (WITH PATIENTS)

[During a fiction-writing workshop, I gave medical students a prompt to write of a complicated situation from a point of view other than their own.] One student said that imagining her patient as if she were he changed everything for her. He had made her cry, she said, this was years before, and she hadn't been able to forget him and his hostility. But when she wrote from his point of view, suddenly she felt she could understand him—understand why he was rude to her—even if it were only her imagination of why. It was enough. She felt better. It wasn't about her after all.

Manet/The Old Musician. Open access image download. Please visit images.nga.gov for more information. A13252.jpg. Edouard Manet, French, 1832-1883, The Old Musician, 1862, oil on canvas.

CASE ILLUSTRATION 13: HOUSE OFFICER—ATTENTION (TOWARD PATIENT, SELF-AWARENESS)

I try not to interrupt the harried resident who is getting paged back on the floor, who has papers to be signed, and whose patient just wants to see the GI doctor, no matter that she had a normal colonoscopy last year in the Dominican Republic. "Strange," I say, after consciously not asking for clarifying details or asking for a differential diagnosis. "What do you think is going on here? Why is this 38-year-old woman so adamant about a referral?" The resident looks at me, lists the possibilities, appropriately including a concern for domestic violence or nonconsensual sex, and then stops and stares. "Why don't you ask her what she is concerned about?" With a shrug, she gets up and returns a few minutes later, now glowing: "Aha! Her mother-in-law—mother-in-law had colon cancer, and she's worried she could have it!" This patient-narrative approach does not discredit the physiologic or epidemiologic approach to diagnostic reasoning. It simply contextualizes it, and, I believe, saves a great deal of time and money. As a supervisor and teacher, if I use the same stance toward my learner, who indeed is telling me a story, allowing myself to be the receiver at first, not yet the coach, then perhaps I am modeling behavior I would hope they would adopt in their own clinical work.

We see a developmental sequence unfolding for learners in our school and teaching hospital. Since narrative work has been adopted as one of our teaching and practice methods, the students are exposed to it longitudinally while their own skills deepen and complicate. From the premedical and first-year students' early experiences of "seeing" what goes on either in office hours or in some lecture in the amphitheater, the students progress to more consequential telling of the self and claiming for oneself the formative force of autobiographical truths. They discover their peers to be valuable witnesses and confirmers of their own experiences. Their skills as readers of texts and spoken language come to represent valuable resources for their lives as doctors and as persons. More seasoned students write their ways through the inevitable assaults and sadnesses of ward medicine. By turning their developing writing powers to face actual conflicts or dilemmas with patients, they start to use these techniques to establish genuine contact with patients and then to solve clinical problems.

What Is Narrative Medicine *For?*

A short poem by Philip Larkin gives us courage to ask, "What is narrative medicine *for?*"

> Days
> *What are days for?*
> *Days are where we live.*
> *They come, they wake us*
> *Time and time over.*
> *They are to be happy in:*
> *Where can we live but days?*
>
> *Ah, solving that question*
> *Brings the priest and the doctor*
> *In their long coats*
> *Running over the fields.*
> (Larkin, 98)

These examples, whether from clinical practice or in classroom or ward teaching, demonstrate the utility and gifts of narrative routines in health care. We hope you can trace the similarity of our work with patients and peers and our work with students. We fuel our own teaching of these skills with the benefits that these skills have given to us in practice. Our own clinical-narrative experience gives us a place from which to continue to develop these skills, to research their outcomes for other groups, and to convey them to learners who have entrusted us with their educations.

Narrative medicine methods donate methods of teaching, methods of doing, and methods of studying what might have been accomplished. As this young field develops, a robust outcomes research agenda is unfolding. Using various methodological approaches, researchers are measuring and articulating the consequences for clinicians, students, and patients of rigorous narrative work in clinical settings. Already, researchers in narrative medicine have documented improvements in team cohesion, deepening of cultural sensitivity, improvements in individual practitioners' ability to adopt patients' perspectives, improvements in medical interviewing and relationship-building skills, decreases in burnout, and decreases in compassion fatigue.

The field of narrative medicine is continuing its search for insight, for contact, for affiliation. In days of health care reform, of now drastic movement toward accountable care organizations and medical homes, where the care will be delivered and funded on the basis of not just cost effectiveness but continuity, the health of teams and the inner health of individual practitioners will be critical. We think that narrative training will equip both seasoned and emerging clinicians with the wherewithal to come to know the self, to be permeable to peers and patients, to make that healing contact with patients and peers now so dangerously lacking in the care we give to our sick. We close with Henry James's description of what the reader does:

> To lend himself, to project himself and steep himself, to feel and feel till he understands and to understand so well that he can say, to have perception at the pitch of passion and expression as embracing as the air, to be infinitely curious and incorrigibly patient, and yet plastic and inflammable and determinable. . . . [T]hese are the fine chances for an active mind, chances to add the idea of independent beauty to the conception of success.

ACKNOWLEDGMENTS

We acknowledge our faculty colleagues in the K07 seminar and the students in the Foundations of Clinical Medicine course at the College of Physicians and Surgeons of Columbia University. This work is supported by NIH NHLBI R25 HL108014, "Enacting the Behavioral and Social Sciences in the Clinical Setting: Institution-Wide Teaching of Effective Team-Based Patient Care."

SUGGESTED READINGS

Charon R. *Narrative Medicine: Honoring the Stories of Illness.* New York: Oxford University Press, 2006.

Charon R. At the membranes of care: stories in narrative medicine. *Acad Med* 2012;87:342–347. doi: 10.1097/ACM .0b013e3182446fbb.

Clifton L. *Blessing the Boats: New and Selected Poems 1988-2000.* Rochester, NY: BOA Editions, Ltd. 2000.

Engel JD, Zarconi J, Pethel LL, Missima SA. *Narratives in Health Care: Healing Patients, Practitioners, Profession, and Community.* Oxford UK: Radcliffe, 2008.

Frank AW. *Letting Stories Breathe: A Socio-Narratology,* Chicago: University of Chicago Press, 2010, p. 4.

Hemon A. The aquarium: a child's isolating illness. *The New Yorker,* June13 & 20,2011, pp. 50–62 .

James H. Criticism. In: Shapira M, ed. *Selected Literary Criticism.* Cambridge, UK: Cambridge University Press, 1974.

Larkin P. Days. In: Thwaite A, ed. *Collected Poems.* London: Farrar Straus Giroux and the Marvell Press, 1989.

Loewald H. *Sublimation: Inquiries into Theoretical Psychoanalysis.* New Haven: Yale University Press, 1988, p. 47.

WEB SITES

Program in Narrative Medicine web site with events, resources, seminars. http://www.narrativemedicine.org/. Accessed February 2014.

Master of Science in Narrative Medicine, Columbia University. http://ce.columbia.edu/Narrative-Medicine. Accessed February 2014.

Online bibliography on Literature, Medicine, and the Arts from NYU. litmed.med.nyu.edu/. Accessed February 2014.

Educating for Professionalism

46

Richard M. Frankel, PhD & Frederic W. Hafferty, PhD

KEY CHALLENGES IN EDUCATING FOR PROFESSIONALISM

Concerns about medicine's status as a profession have been growing for the past 80 years. By the late 1990s, many experts felt that medicine had become self-serving and insular, had violated its social trust, and was in danger of losing its vaunted professional status. The slowness of medicine's awakenings notwithstanding, the inaugural decade of the twenty-first century was marked by a flurry of actions deigned to define, assess, and institutionalize professionalism within the classrooms of medical education and hallways of clinical practice. By 2000, for example, virtually every medical school and residency program had implemented some type of formal professionalism curriculum.

Medical professionalism faces a number of challenges. Perhaps the most important is the need to reconcile professionalism being taught in the "classroom" (which includes the professionalism embedded in the codes, charters, competencies, and curricula) with professionalism being observed by learners in the clinical settings modeled on a day-to-day basis by more senior clinicians and faculty. At root is a classic hidden curriculum problem of the gap between efforts to formalize professionalism instruction and the day-to-day or moment-to-moment lived experience of trainees. In some cases, the gap has been great enough to cause some trainees to "push back" against and disavow the formal professionalism curriculum. Successfully developing and implementing approaches to teaching professionalism that integrate elements of the formal and informal or hidden curriculum remain elusive.

Competency-based medical education has further defined, benchmarked, and assessed professionalism. The Accreditation Council for Graduate Medical Education (ACGME) professionalism competency emphasizes the development of professional character, high standards of accountability, humanism in all dealings with others, and altruism—putting the interests of the patient before self-interest. There are now a large number of readily available formal professionalism curricula, assessment tools, and literature (see web links and Suggested Readings). Although the challenge of formal versus informal curricula remain, these resources identify important aspects of professionalism and point to areas for further curricular development.

Professionalism requires attention to several domains of physician behavior, including truth-telling, confidentiality, disruptive behavior, assuming responsibility, respectful communication with patients and colleagues, giving and receiving feedback, bullying, sexual harassment, personal appearance and attire, and others. In this chapter, we focus on three major professionalism issues: inappropriate use of social media, plagiarism, and boundary violations. We first define each challenge, then illustrate each with one or more cases. We end the discussion of each challenge with commentary regarding educational and institutional implications in four areas: (1) formal/informal curriculum; (2) faculty development; (3) institutional response; and (4) remediation.

Social Media

The explosive growth in information technology, especially the adoption of social media, presents a new challenge to professionalism. Concerns about sharing confidential patient information on public social media web sites, posting of inappropriate personal information, using social media at inappropriate times such as on rounds or during lectures and other educational activities, and failure to maintain good professional boundaries by, for example, "friending" patients on social media sites are among the problematic behaviors that have been noted among recent cohorts of medical students and residents. "Millennials," or Generation Y (those born between 1980 and 1994), which includes medical students, residents, and to some degree fellows and junior faculty are almost constantly engaged in using social media. It is estimated that in the United States alone there are over 120 million users of Facebook, and that number is growing rapidly. This method of communication has supplanted other forms of interaction, including the telephone and even e-mail, which is more commonly used by older faculty. In the area of social media, faculty are what Prensky has termed "digital immigrants," whereas their younger charges who grew up with digital technology are "digital natives." Capitalizing on the benefits and understanding the risks inherent in social media remains a challenge for undergraduate and graduate training programs.

CASE ILLUSTRATION 1: "A CLICK IS ALL IT TAKES"

A Student Reports: I recently posted an offensive and tasteless "doctor joke" for my friends to see on Facebook. Another medical student who viewed it thought the posting was highly unprofessional and put the school in a potentially negative light so brought it to the attention of school administrators. As a result of my actions I was required to make an appearance before the student promotions committee and face the possibility of dismissal for behavior unbecoming a medical student.

As a result of this experience I have become acutely aware of the attractions and dangers of social networking and its potential to do harm. Since a case in which a student at Rutgers committed suicide after compromising information about him was circulated on social networking sites, I have come to realize that I have a responsibility to recognize that one click of the mouse is all it took to jeopardize my entire future as a physician. (MS II)

The essay above, written by a second-year medical student and president of his class was published in SCOPE, Indiana University School of Medicine's weekly electronic newsletter that is distributed to the entire medical staff of some 2500 people on nine different campuses. It was written after the student had been cited for unprofessional behavior and only was permitted to stay in school contingent upon successful remediation with the school's competency director. The essay was voluntary, the result of a conversation between the student and two faculty members about alerting other students to the risks of posting information on social networking sites.

The student volunteered to give a presentation based on his case to the entering freshman class.

Educational and Institutional Implications

1. Formal/Informal Curriculum
   • Many students and residents are unaware of the risks of using social media. For example, a study of online posting by medical students and residents found that only 37.5% made their Facebook pages private.
     • Education can be effective. One school that developed an educational intervention around Internet privacy saw an 85% drop in publicly available Facebook pages.
   • Modeling professional behavior in the informal curriculum
     • Engaging students in respectful dialogue and discovery about how and why they use social media can be helpful in bringing about behavior and culture change.
     • Enlisting student leaders who may have had experiences with professionalism issues relating to Internet usage may also help students recognize that the issue is serious and affects their peers and colleagues.

2. Faculty Development
   • Inappropriate use of social media among faculty has increased as evidenced by a recent flurry of articles in the popular press and a study of the actions of state medical boards dealing with this issue.
     • Faculty development programs focusing on the use and abuse of social media by students and colleagues can be helpful in raising awareness of the risks involved.
     • Encouraging faculty to lead by example in the use of smart phones and other handheld devices can also be effective in addressing inappropriate usage.

3. Institutional Response
   • The use of social media by medical trainees is growing.
     • Surveys by school administrators to determine the extent of social media use and its appropriateness/inappropriateness can help give the school a sense of the extent of social media practices among students, residents, and faculty, and help shape institutional policy.
   • Few schools have written policies that specifically deal with social networking, but schools with any written policies about unprofessional behavior are better able to handle violations than schools without written policies.

- Developing written policies that take into account school size and the range of problem behaviors can be helpful in crafting institutional responses that are targeted and appropriate.
- Collaborative engagement of students, residents, and junior faculty in policy development facilitates implementation of the policies in question.

4. Remediation
- There are currently no national standards for remediation of unprofessional behavior involving social media among medical students and residents. It falls to individual deans, course and clerkship directors, and faculty to come up with remediation procedures that are fair and fit the questionable behavior.
  - Apart from dismissal from school, remediation is best accomplished in the spirit of improvement and increased awareness of the risks associated with social media use. Personal research by students who have violated social media standards into what is known about millennials and their status as "digital natives" along with journaling and reflection are often useful.
  - Recruitment of student leaders who have had professionalism lapses and who share messages about the risks of inappropriate use of social media can be an effective method of "spreading the word" about expectations and appropriate behaviors.

Plagiarism

Another challenge in educating for professionalism is plagiarism. This problem may, in part, derive from the "digital divide" between generations and their knowledge and understanding of the rules that govern electronic, print, and written media. For example, evidence of plagiarism was found in 5.2% of the personal statements of residency applicants to a single institution by comparing them with readily available Internet sources. Likewise, in their undergraduate coursework some medical students believe that citing Internet sources such as Wikipedia or other websites is unnecessary because of the "open source" nature of these sites. Equally concerning is the trend among some faculty and trainees to "cut and paste" medical records in clinical care. Residents may observe their attending physicians engaging in this practice or get the message that it is okay to "cut and paste" a patient's history from day to day or from previous hospital admissions. Medical students, for whom there is typically no formal instruction in this area, learn to follow suit. The result is an "epidemic" of behavior that is a threat to both professionalism and quality of care.

CASE ILLUSTRATION 2: PLAGIARISM

A. Residency Application	B. Internet Match http://csa-notes.com
"I am accustomed to working for long hours, making decisions under pressure and performing multiple tasks simultaneously. I possess a sound medical knowledge base and aspire to further my education. I am a team player who enjoys collaborating with others and can assume leadership when appropriate."	"I am accustomed to working for long hours, making decisions under pressure and performing multiple tasks simultaneously *and working independently*. I possess a sound medical knowledge base and aspire to further my education. I am a team player who enjoys collaborating with others and I can *communicate clearly* and assume leadership when appropriate."

The Oxford English Dictionary defines plagiarism as "the wrongful appropriation or purloining and publication as one's own, of the ideas, or the expression of the ideas … of another." The two samples above come from the personal statement of an application for residency at Harvard Medical School (Column A) and a popular web site with examples of application essays (Column B). With the exception of two phrases deleted by the applicant and highlighted in italics, they are identical. Applicants must certify in writing that their essays are accurate and original. In the case of a residency application, the response to plagiarism is straightforward and involves rejecting the application and the applicant. With increasingly sophisticated tools available to prospective applicants as well as to faculty and administrators, the challenges of educating about, and monitoring for, plagiarism have become more pressing.

Educational and Institutional Implications

1. Formal/Informal Curriculum
- Plagiarism may occur in many forms in preclinical and clinical contexts.
  - It is not safe to assume that students and residents would have learned about plagiarism in college. Consequently, formal instruction on the various types of plagiarism in medicine can help trainees be aware of what is and what is not considered plagiarism.
  - Certification may be another alternative for teaching about plagiarism. In the same way that researchers must obtain human subjects certification to do their work, trainees would have to

complete one or more modules on plagiarism and become "certified." This would ensure that subsequent plagiarism breaches could not be attributed to sheer lack of knowledge and would make clearer to students the consequences of such actions.

- Use of informal channels such as reviewing articles in a journal club format, brown bag discussions, or "Ethics at Lunch," led by students with input from faculty advisors, can be a useful avenue for raising awareness about falsification and plagiarism.

2. Faculty Development

- Many faculty members who suspect plagiarism in written reports are hesitant to invest the time and energy to prevent or "prove" these occurrences. Several automated programs are available to check for plagiarism (e.g., www.duplichecker.com, www.scanmyessay.com, and www.turnitin.com for admissions essays). In addition, faculty may not readily make the connection between activities like cutting and pasting of notes in the electronic medical record and plagiarism.
  - Faculty development seminars on how to detect and respond to instances of plagiarism can be quite useful in addressing the problem.
  - Raising awareness of faculty about the risks (malpractice and otherwise) of cutting and pasting their own hospital notes and the fact that residents and students will do as they see their role models doing may help address this problem.

3. Institutional Response

- Clearly stated institutional policies, procedures, and consequences regarding plagiarism in the preclinical and clinical years are essential for students and residents to understand the risks involved in copying one's own or another person's words and ideas or falsifying records.
  - Academic policies as well as student promotions committees can be helpful in setting standards. Working together with student leaders to develop standards can facilitate their acceptance by the student body.
  - Using the honor code, if one exists, to clearly define the role of plagiarism can help students understand what is expected of them in this domain.

4. Remediation

- Remediation depends in large measure on the type of plagiarism that has occurred. Serious cases involving the scientific integrity of a piece of work by stealing another's ideas and representing them as one's own should be dealt with by considering failure in a course, clinical rotation and in some cases, dismissal from school.

- Plagiarism of any sort is a serious offense, whether premeditated or inadvertent. Remediation is often more successful if the trainee has a clear sense of what rule or norm has been violated and what its present and future impact may be. Using literary examples like the historian Stephen Ambrose whose otherwise unblemished career was sullied when it was discovered that he had plagiarized his own and others' works in his books are useful in bringing plagiarism issues to the forefront.

- It may also be useful to bring attention to the link between unprofessional behavior of undergraduate medical students, including plagiarism, and risk of subsequent censure by state boards of medical practice.

Boundary Management

Another challenge for professionalism training is boundary management. Although there are dimensions of boundary management that touch upon the use of social media, for example, whether it is appropriate for physicians to be "friends" with their patients on Facebook, or First Amendment issues of whether schools or residency programs have the right or obligation to monitor their trainees' individual postings, students and residents also confront a range of boundary issues in their day-to-day work and roles. Little attention is paid to these issues in the formal professionalism curriculum, because the issues are not recognized or do not fit well into the global categories of professionalism such as altruism, beneficence, or humanism. In addition, abstract discussions of professionalism often exclude issues of power and hierarchy which dominate many students' thinking and experience. A particular challenge in this regard is the transition from classroom learning, which typically takes place in the first and second year of medical school, to clinical rotations where classroom learning is disregarded or derided. Students are often left on their own to piece together the appropriate boundaries of their professional role in regard to patients, peers, allied health professionals, and teachers while realizing that they are often at the lower rungs of power and potentially vulnerable to negative evaluations should they incorrectly define their professional role.

CASE ILLUSTRATION 3: MANAGING PROFESSIONAL AND PERSONAL BOUNDARIES

Scenario 1

An intern went out of his way to 'warn' the members of our team that a particular. . . [professional] working with us was 'an idiot' . . . I thought this was extremely disrespectful to the [professional], who was unaware of any of this . . . I wanted to say something but I wasn't sure if that was my place. I had no idea how to handle the situation. (Narrative written by a third year medical student.)

Medical students frequently struggle with the concept of professional boundaries, especially as it relates to their role in hierarchical situations. On their clinical rotations, and in their role primarily as observers, students often witness behaviors in others which they perceive to be unprofessional but feel powerless to address. Fear of reprisal, loss of face among peers, and being labeled a "whistleblower" or a troublemaker are frequent reasons given by medical students for failing to act in the face of behavior perceived to be unprofessional. In these cases, as illustrated above, boundaries defined by power differentials may be particularly difficult for students to navigate. Especially troubling to medical students are situations that involve disrespect. Boundaries are not specifically included in the Association of American Medical Colleges (AAMC) professionalism categories, but can be considered proxy measures for concerns about personal and professional conduct.

CASE ILLUSTRATION 3 (CONTD.)

Scenario 2

I was sitting in the conference room when the assistant came in and said, 'You have a patient in the exam room who is going to make your day.' I walked in and this woman is dressed in like a wet tee-shirt, no bra, very good looking and shapely. I started talking to her and she was giggling every other word and acting more inappropriately than I'm used to . . . And it was very uncomfortable because I was sitting in that room looking at her and I couldn't divert my attention from looking at her breasts. I tried to spend a lot of time looking down at her chart, but every time I looked up my eyes zoomed in on her breasts. She was controlling my eyes ... jiggling those things around so that her already prominent breasts were more prominent...She was just too flirtatious for me. I was really uncomfortable. (Third-year resident)

Sexuality and sexual feelings are a normal part of being human. Sexual feelings between a doctor and patient are not abnormal, but they can sometimes be confusing and troublesome. When acted upon, they can be dangerous to the relationship and potentially exploitative. In previous research based on the narratives of students, residents, and practicing physicians,

we found that the majority of situations in which providers' sexual feelings came into play involved boundary confusion on the physician's part. These situations typically involved their recognition of a sexual attraction or the potential for becoming aroused during the medical visit. Very infrequently, the feelings led to a boundary crossing where physician and patient mutually disclosed their feelings of attraction to one another. Much more frequently, the physician took steps to avoid the feelings by fleeing the encounter or skipping portions of the physical examination. Both male and female physicians described failing to do rectal, genitourinary (GU), and breast examinations to avoid boundary confusion. The above narrative from a third-year resident in internal medicine graphically illustrates the effect sexual feelings and assumptions about others' behavior can have on the medical encounter.

It is clear from this narrative that the patient's appearance and manner of interacting (inappropriately described by the assistant as "a patient who's going to make your day") led the resident to "sexualize" the situation and make some assumptions about the patient, her behavior, and her intentions. He then became caught and confused between the nature and boundaries of the doctor–patient interaction, and those of an encounter between himself as a sexually interested man and an attractive woman. It is interesting to note that the resident did not recognize his own role in nonverbally encouraging the very behavior that made him so uncomfortable. He reported that each time he looked up, his eyes zoomed in on her breasts, the result of which he felt was to make her display them even more prominently. The resident was clearly stuck, attracted to his patient, and at the same time struggling to distance himself sufficiently to maintain an appropriate professional boundary. He knew something was wrong, but was not sure what it was, or what to do about it. This sense of helplessness and lack of clarity is typical of confusing boundary situations.

As it happens, our resident is not alone in feeling a confusing attraction to his patient. Prior research among psychiatry residents has found that most men and about half of the women reported sexual attraction to one or more patients, and 1% acknowledged sexual contact with patients. Another study found that 57% of medical students had sexual feelings about patients, and that males had them more frequently than female students. Twenty-one percent of the students surveyed thought it was okay to have sex with patients. The same study reported that there was no teaching in the undergraduate curriculum about sexual boundaries in medical care.

Educational and Institutional Implications

1. Formal/Informal Curriculum
   - Both students and residents find it difficult to act in the face of witnessing unprofessional behavior

or experiencing sexual feelings that could threaten or cross boundaries.

- Curriculum offerings that focus on duty, responsibility, and accountability can help trainees define boundaries so that they have a clear understanding of the issues involved.
- Curricula should discuss physical and sexual boundaries with patients, peers, and faculty. Role-plays could address ways to respond to sexual confusion or boundary transgressions. Clear legal and ethical ramifications should be discussed.
- Communication skills for dealing with conflict, especially where there is an authority gradient, can be helpful in giving students and residents the requisite skill set to successfully address boundary crossings and violations.
- Curriculum content that reinforces the consequences of boundary confusion, crossing, or violations for patient safety and quality can help raise awareness of the larger issues that underlie professionalism. For example, using evidence to show that disruptive surgeons have worse complication rates and are more likely to be sued frames unprofessional behavior as a risk rather than a personality trait.
- Looking for positive examples of maintaining healthy sexual and other boundaries among students, residents, and faculty can also be helpful in terms of reinforcing desired norms in the informal curriculum.

2. Faculty Development
- Faculty members are often unaware of how their behavior affects students and residents. Strong emotions such as frustration, anger, and contempt are amplified among students and residents who view themselves in a "one down" position. Relational coordination and safety in the learning environment suffer when students feel intimidated or humiliated.
  - Faculty development programs that emphasize new rules and regulations with zero tolerance for disruptive behavior, mistreatment of trainees, or sexual boundary violations can help inform faculty members and raise awareness.
  - Opportunities to practice skills of maintaining healthy boundaries with peers can help surface personal and professional boundary issues that were never taught in medical school or residency. Working through cases with peers helps to create a culture of respect among faculty with a "trickle down" effect on residents and students.
  - Faculty development courses such as the ones put on by the American Academy on Communication in Healthcare use skill development

and personal awareness together to teach faculty how to create a safe, satisfying learning environment for trainees and how to recognize and deal effectively with sexual and other boundary issues.

3. Institutional Response
- Clear institutional policies for dealing with boundary concerns and violations are critical to creating safe, supportive work environments.
  - Having personnel and procedures in place for faculty and trainees to present their concerns, have them investigated and hopefully resolved in a nonjudgmental way can help reinforce both the informal and formal curriculum.
  - Orientation programs for entering medical students, residents, and fellows with opportunities for small group discussion and role play can be helpful in putting the issues of healthy boundaries in a positive, constructive light. Similar programs are useful in orienting new faculty and staff.

4. Remediation
- Remediation for students who have engaged in unprofessional behavior that threatens or crosses personal or professional boundaries should be handled on a case-by-case basis. Obviously, remediation will depend on the seriousness of the boundary issue in question. Consequences, too, will vary from dismissal from medical school to learning about the risks of boundary confusion, boundary crossings, and boundary violations.
  - If it is determined that the boundary issue is one in which there is a deficit in performance, suitable remediation might include activities such as: coaching and role play; research on the causes and consequences of boundary issues in medical students and residents; developing and presenting a teaching module to peers on professional boundaries; counseling and psychotherapy; and close supervision by faculty during clinical rotations.
  - If it is determined that the boundary issue is due to an impairment, steps should be taken to alert institutional representatives who are prepared to deal with such issues.

SUMMARY AND CONCLUSION

In this chapter, we have tried to bring to light some of the most pressing professionalism issues that trainees encounter. Although global concepts like altruism, respect, and equity are enormously helpful in setting community or disciplinary standards of behavior, the lived experience of medical students and residents is much more tightly bound to the local cultures and contexts in which they live and work. One of the most important aspects of educating for professionalism is to build bridges between students' experiences in the informal curriculum and the global concepts they represent.

One pedagogical and practical challenge is to remain nonjudgmental about the behaviors observed in, or reported by, students and residents. It is very easy to slip into the role of moral arbiter in situations in which unprofessional behavior is being discussed. The surgeon who yelled at a student or the attending who admonished a patient to lose weight may have had good reasons for doing so (e.g., the student was about to break the sterile field, and the patient had dangerously high blood pressure and was at imminent risk of a heart attack). Rather than acting on the student's or resident's behalf in the face of a reported boundary issue, helping trainees to develop their own skill set for dealing with the behavior, and closely monitoring their progress can be very fruitful. Obviously, if there is suspicion that the issue represents a boundary violation with potential for harm to the trainee, immediate action and fact finding may be required.

At the student level, professionalism challenges tend to be recurrent; caring, compassion and communication (especially across an authority gradient), respect, and teamwork tend to dominate the concerns. For residents, autonomy, conflicts of interest, and mistakes take on special importance. For both students and residents, boundary issues, albeit different for each group, tend to occur with great frequency in professionalism discussions.

Pedagogically it is helpful to start with trainees' lived experiences of professionalism and deepen reflection on them through small group discussion, use of student narratives, and facilitated faculty discussion. This approach optimizes the likelihood of making professionalism education salient and engaging for both students and faculty. Discussions of topics like medical mistakes, boundary issues, sexuality and professionalism, impaired physicians, quality and safety, and conflicts of interest can help highlight and deepen trainees' understanding of their own and others' behavior and reinforce the value of professionalism to the individual, community, and society. From a practical point of view, focusing on professionalism as a way of being rather than an abstract set of concepts helps trainees make connections between their existence in the real time environments in which they are training and their hopes, dreams, and aspirations for their lives in the profession of medicine.

SUGGESTED READINGS

Ginsburg S, Regehr G, Lingard L. The disavowed curriculum: understanding students' reasoning in professionally challenging situations. *J Gen Intern Med* 2003;18:1015–1022.

Greysen SR, et al. Physician violations of online professionalism and disciplinary actions: a national survey of state medical-boards. *JAMA* 2012;307:1141–1142.

Hafferty FW, Levinson D. Moving beyond nostalgia and motives: towards a complexity science view of medical professionalism. *Perspect Biol Med* 2008;51:599–615.

Karnieli-Miller O, et al. Exploring the meaning of respect in medical student education: an analysis of student narratives. *J Gen Intern Med* 2010;25:1309–1314.

Papadakis MA, et al. Disciplinary action by medical boards and prior behavior in medical school. *N Engl J Med* 2005;353:2673–2682.

Passi V, Doug M, Peile E, Thistlethwaite J, Johnson, N. Developing medical professionalism in future doctors: a systematic review. *Int J Med Educ* 2010;1:19–29.

WEB SITES FOR FURTHER LEARNING

American Academy on Communication in Healthcare. http://www.aachonline.org/. Accessed February 2014.

ABIM Project Professionalism. http://www.abimfoundation.org/en/Resource%20Center/Bibliography/~/media/Files/Resource%20Center/Project%20professionalism.ashx. Accessed February 2014.

AMA Position Statement on Medical Professionalism. http://ama.com.au/node/5449. Accessed February 2014.

Annals of Internal Medicine Physician Charter on medical professionalism. http://annals.org/article.aspx?volume=136&issue=3&page=243. Accessed February 2014.

American College of Physicians: Medical Ethics and Professionalism Cases. http://www.acponline.org/running_practice/ethics/. Accessed February 2014.

Trainee Well-Being

John F. Christensen, PhD & Mitchell D. Feldman, MD, MPhil

Becoming a health professional is a challenging and complex process. Trainees frequently experience stressors that exceed their previous life experience and coping skills. These demands are proportionate to the responsibility and complexity of caring for patients in all their variability and vulnerability. These demands of professional training are enormous, and trainees often neglect their own physical, emotional, relational, and spiritual health; however, a central component of professionalism is awareness of one's own limits, and mindfulness about the wise allocation of one's energy in providing quality patient care (see Chapters 6 and 7). Neglect of this awareness may sow the seeds of burnout and lead to poor quality care and medical error (see Chapter 37). Close attention to maintaining well-being, however, can enhance satisfaction with medicine as a career and optimize the clinician–patient relationship. Given that trainees are vulnerable to pressures to postpone their own well-being until training is completed, it is paramount to include promotion of self-care in the formation of health professionals.

 CASE ILLUSTRATION 1

Jill Rayburn had not slept in 30 hours. She had been studying for her pathophysiology examination for a week, and still she felt ill prepared. As a second-year medical student she was beginning to wonder whether she was cut out for medicine, in spite of the fact that she was in the upper 20% of her class. Many of her classmates seemed to be on top of the material to be mastered for this examination. Some of them had even gone for a hike yesterday afternoon. Last night she declined an invitation to play indoor soccer. It was mid-January and cold outside, and she was tired of being stuck in the library. She was beginning to resent the professor who invited her to coauthor a paper, even though at the time she felt flattered that he had singled her out for this honor. Now she did not feel up to the task, and she wished she had started preparing for this examination earlier rather than working on the paper. She looked back to her days of high school and college, when she was consistently at the top of her class, and remembered many carefree days. She wondered what had happened to that teenager with the sense of humor and the time to hang out with friends. Now as she looked ahead to the remainder of the winter, all she saw were more deadlines and isolated days in the library without respite. She wondered if she would ever have fun again.

A common trait of physicians is compulsivity. Although many attributes of compulsivity—thoroughness, accuracy, second guessing, monitoring changes—are beneficial to patient care and success in medical training, this trait may also erode the personal health, satisfaction, and well-being of the physician. Early in her training, Jill is manifesting many of the associated characteristics of compulsivity that if unchecked by reflection can lead to cynicism and burnout by the time she is a resident. She is beginning to question her competence, in spite of the fact that she is in the top fifth of her class. Ultimately, she is at risk of developing what has been labeled the "imposter syndrome," in which the individual feels that she has fooled others into thinking she is competent, but the threat of being unmasked lurks at every turn. Jill is also feeling guilt about not having been wiser in her allocation of time. No matter how hard she has worked, it does not seem to be enough. In addition to self-doubt and guilt, Jill is also carrying a burden of responsibility for meeting all her obligations, and she feels alone with that burden. She thinks about her peers enjoying an outing together and envisions continued isolation for herself in the library. This triad of doubt, guilt, and an exaggerated sense of responsibility has been described by Gabbard as constituents of the compulsivity that is a "normal" trait in most physicians.

Jill's discontent has its roots in the early conditioning of many bright young people in American society that implies that our value or worth as persons is linked to academic success or outward performance. Most of us have an inherent need for love and acceptance, and when children are repeatedly told that they are special and valued only when they are "exceptional," that is, at the top of their class in grades and stars in various performance endeavors, they begin to link their personal worth to meeting these standards of excellence. This high need for achievement collides with the reality that many of one's peers in medical school also came from the top of their class and consequently being smart and performing well are not so exceptional. They must work harder to stand out. Being less than outstanding is construed as having failed to meet an essential marker of their worth and value as a person. They are left with the dilemma of backing off from overwork and consequently carrying the self-stigma of being "second best," "ordinary," "mediocre," and unconsciously feeling less lovable; or of working harder to stand out. Paradoxically these efforts to excel and "stand out" can lead to the very isolation and loneliness from which they are trying to escape.

Some trainees may have the nagging thought that overwork is not good for them, that taking care of themselves by getting enough sleep, exercise, eating well, having fun, and spending time with friends are all important; but in the "psychology of postponement" they think, "As soon as this exam is over, then I can unwind." In addition, their elevated expectation of themselves multiplies this self-bargaining: "As soon as I get into the residency I want, then I can relax;" "as soon as I get accepted for a fellowship, then I can start working out;" "as soon as I start my first real job, then I can have a life." Thus, early in professional training a habit of postponement can develop that if unchecked can lead to neglecting many of one's most valued relationships and activities throughout one's career. Sir William Osler in a commencement address to graduating medical students in 1889 had these words to say about postponement:

> Engrossed late and soon in professional cares . . . you may so lay waste that you may find, too late, with hearts given way, that there is no place in your habit-stricken souls for those gentler influences which make life worth living.

Jill's story also illustrates the insidious manner in which the system of medical education with its overt and covert rewards and punishments can reinforce the student's inherent compulsivity. Her exceptional performance has been noticed by one of her professors, who asks her to work with him as coauthor on a paper for publication. It is natural for teachers to ask top performers to do more, yet neither the teacher nor the student pauses to reflect on the potential toxicity of rewarding overwork. Medical school traditionally is better at channeling students into ever-refined strata of academic and professional success than at mentoring them into building a career in which their professional endeavors unfold within a context of a healthy life well lived. Unless Jill were to encounter a mentor who has this broader grasp of personal and professional well-being, her role models and professors will continue unwittingly to provide a "hidden curriculum," in which being a successful physician entails putting one's own life on hold.

 ## CASE ILLUSTRATION 1 (CONTD.)

Jill was walking across the quadrangle after her pathophysiology examination and failed to notice Dr. Ann Bennington, her teacher from the previous term in a class on the medical interview. Dr. Bennington noticed Jill's hunched over posture and drawn facial expression. "Jill, you look like you have the weight of the world on your shoulders and haven't slept in days. How are you doing?" Jill managed a smile and protested, "I'm fine. I just finished the pathophys exam." Ann confronted her mildly, "Well you look exhausted. When's the last time you had an evening off?"

When she noticed a tear forming in Jill's eyes, Ann replied, "Jill, I suspect you're carrying more of a burden than you let on to others. I'd really like to talk with you more about this." She then suggested they meet later that afternoon in her office. At the meeting later in Dr. Bennington's office, after some initial hesitation Jill opened up with the self-doubt, emptiness, fatigue, and isolation she had been feeling the last few weeks. After a pause, Ann replied, "You know, Jill, you remind me of myself when I was a medical student." Noticing Jill's tears, she continued, "The fact that you are one of the brightest people in your class doesn't seem to matter to you now, and I think I know why. Like me you are perfectionistic, and there are reasons too numerous for us to go into now why we are that way. But one of the effects of that perfectionism is that we never feel we can get enough praise or external validation for our worth. That's because we weren't taught to value ourselves from within, that we are lovable and have immense worth before we ever set out to do great things." She paused to observe Jill's response. Since she was breathing more freely and seemed curious, Ann continued: "There's nothing wrong in striving for excellence. In fact that's desirable. But what we mean by 'excellence' needs to be challenged. Your work as a physician, like your work as a student, will always occur within a real world context of the various values you hold and commitments you have made, as well as the limitations of time, personal energy, and competing tasks. Bumping up against these limits can be humbling, but ultimately accepting those limits and allowing your excellence to be contextualized into your life will give you wisdom. Your body, mind, and spirit are giving you feedback that you ignore only at your peril. Rather than anesthetizing yourself to this pain, let it teach you more about yourself and the full context of joy of which you are capable. To the extent you can let your awareness of the origin of this pain lead you to greater self-acceptance, you will be an excellent physician and a healing presence for others."

Jill's chance encounter with Dr. Bennington, along with Ann's willingness to mentor Jill about the importance of honoring life values in becoming a doctor, shows the powerful influence of senior physicians who have struggled themselves to attain life wisdom in revising the "hidden curriculum" of medical training. In choosing mentors, students would do well to seek out physicians who tolerate the tension of keeping their personal and professional lives in balance and who explicitly honor a variety of values beyond their professional lives, including family relationships, friendships, recreational pursuits, hobbies, and personal self-care. Having a mentor is a critical component of career satisfaction and success in medicine. The mentoring relationship has been described as one of the most complex and developmentally important in a person's life. Mentors act as teachers, exemplars, and guides for their mentees. On a practical level, medical students and residents who have a mentor report better career preparation than do those without a mentor. Ideally, the mentoring relationship provides some benefits to both mentor and mentee, such as opportunities for collaboration, mutual teaching and learning, and the promotion of self reflection as illustrated by the above vignette.

Among the perspectives worth cultivating is the awareness that becoming a health professional is a process that occurs over several years and that self-perceived imperfection is an inherent part of that process. It is helpful to think of ourselves as "becoming" rather than insisting on holding an image of what we have not yet become, then unfavorably comparing ourselves with that image. Given the continual pressures inherent in medical training to judge our own competence, it is important to cultivate the equally important capacity for "self-appreciation." When we respond to a sunset, to the first flower blooming in the garden in spring, or to the final movement of Beethoven's *9th Symphony*, this is typically not an act of judgment, but one of appreciation. It is impossible to engage the "judgment" and "appreciation" centers of our minds at the same time.

The exaggerated sense of personal responsibility that is part of the compulsive triad is often reinforced by the competitive climate of getting into medical school and advancing through training. This attitude is frequently carried into residency training and subsequent practice, in which the illusion is maintained that one is a self-sufficient professional, that asking for help is a sign of weakness, and that competency is distinguished by the ability to "go it alone." Nothing could be further from the way health care is actually delivered, in which systematic attempts to improve quality and reduce error now demand that teams of professionals from various disciplines work cooperatively to provide patient care and promote the health of the community. The best medical schools are beginning to train for this, and the Accreditation Council of Graduate Medical Education (ACGME) states that "systems-based practice," which largely involves working as part of a team, is one of the core competencies to be mastered during residency (see Chapter 41). Whether or not teamwork is reinforced by one's medical school or residency, cultivating the practice of working cooperatively with others and committing oneself to helping colleagues succeed can contribute enormously to one's personal and professional satisfaction.

 CASE ILLUSTRATION 1 (CONTD.)

In April of her fourth year of medical school Jill dropped by Dr. Bennington's office to let her know she would be going to a family medicine residency in the South. "How are you feeling about the match?" Ann asked. "Well, to tell you the truth," Jill replied, "my first choice was another program where I could have pursued some work in epidemiology based on that paper I co-authored a couple of years ago. Since the match, however, I've thought more about the program I'm going to, and especially about one physician on the faculty there who interviewed me. I was struck by the pictures he had on his wall of his wife and children, his children's poems and drawings, and what he shared with me about how much their training program valued both professionalism and the personal growth and life satisfaction of their residents." Ann smiled and nodded. Jill went on, "I have you to thank for reaching out to me at a critical moment a couple of years ago and helping me realize there was more to me than trying to be a star. You helped me realize the value of humility, which includes appreciation of my gifts as well as acceptance of my limitations. You also gave me the greatest gift, which was affirming my own capacity for appreciating my life and for letting that be the ground from which to appreciate others." In June, after her white coat ceremony Jill

opened a card from Dr. Bennington, which contained this poem by Derek Walcott:

Love After Love
The time will come
when, with elation
you will greet yourself arriving
at your own door, in your own mirror,
and each will smile at the other's welcome,
and say, sit here. Eat.
You will love again
the stranger who was yourself.

Give wine. Give bread. Give back your heart
to itself, to the stranger who has loved you
all your life, whom you ignored
for another, who knows you by heart.
Take down the love letters from the bookshelf,
the photographs, the desperate notes,
peel your own image from the mirror.
Sit. Feast on your life.

 ## CASE ILLUSTRATION 2

Bill Trimmell was shaking as he sat in the resident's room wondering why he had yelled at the patient he had just admitted to the hospital, scolding her about not doing enough to monitor her blood sugars, and therefore contributing to her hyperglycemia and subsequent infection. As he reflected on the unpleasant conversation with her, he suddenly asked himself, "What am I doing?" This was only the second admission of the day, and already he could not wait to go home. He had had a busy morning caring for a patient he had admitted to the Intensive Care Unit, leaving him only 10 minutes over the noon hour to eat a stale bagel left over from the morning conference. Bill was only a third of the way through his second year of internal medicine residency, and he found himself more often than not resenting many of his patients and wondering what had happened to the altruistic dream of helping people that had led him into medical school. Why did he feel like he no longer cared?

Bill is showing the classic signs and symptoms of *burnout*, which consists of emotional exhaustion (including compassion fatigue and dissociation from feelings in general), depersonalization in relationships (treating oneself, patients, coworkers, and family members as objects), and a perceived clinical ineffectiveness. Burnout has been described as "an erosion of the soul," and it spreads gradually and continually over time, sending people into a downward spiral in which it is difficult to recover if one remains in the circumstances that generated it. Burnout has been associated with impaired job performance and poor health, including headaches, sleep disturbance, irritability, relationship difficulties, fatigue, hypertension, anxiety, depression, myocardial infarction, and chemical dependency. Cognitive performance as well can be compromised by burnout. A national US study of internal medicine residents found that symptoms of burnout, which were associated with higher medical school debt, were also associated with lower In-Training Examination scores. For physicians the seeds of burnout may be sown in medical school and residency training, where fatigue and emotional exhaustion are often the norm. By mid-career, the momentum of this condition is maintained by the subtle reinforcements in the work setting for being a hard worker and placing service to others before self-care.

All too often residents are confronted with the reality of patients who for one reason or another are nonadherent to medical regimens, or who have chronic health problems that are refractory to interventions (see Chapters 4 and 20). Unremitting exposure to cases in which one's own efforts appear futile can engender frustration and cynicism. Without the opportunity to discuss these common experiences with their peers and faculty, trainees may begin to experience the early symptoms of burnout.

Ward residents like Bill may begin to view their work in terms of the tasks involved in admitting and discharging patients, rather than in terms of the patient's experience of illness. Terry Mizrahi, a medical anthropologist, spent several months observing teams of ward residents in one training hospital, and through observation of what they did and what they communicated among themselves she concluded that the job of the ward resident is "getting rid of patients."

Frequently, underlying this detached attitude is "compassion fatigue," in which an overload of suffering threatens to run our emotional tank dry and lead to *dissociation*, characterized by a withdrawal of attention from emotions and somatic sensations as we focus cognitively and visually on complex patient care problems or get absorbed in our "to do" list. We become anesthetized to feelings and cannot relate to family and friends once we leave work. The cognitive correlate of dissociation is *decontextualization*. This involves a habit of thinking of others (and even ourselves) in a utilitarian way that abstracts and constructs persons into categories that have usefulness for our jobs and getting our tasks done in a timely way. This habit of thinking ignores the full life context in which others (and we ourselves) are embedded. Thus, we relate to patients as diagnoses or appointments on the schedule, to coworkers as facilitating or impeding our work, to family and friends as intruding or placing unrealistic demands on our time, and to ourselves as task-processing machines.

Bill understandably feels a disconnect between the sense of vocation he once felt about medicine and the sense of futility about how he spends his working hours. In the absence of time to reflect on what is happening or discuss it with others, he finds himself slipping into disillusionment and cynicism. His job as a resident has begun to feel meaningless.

CASE ILLUSTRATION 2 (CONTD.)

In January of his second year, Bill attended a resident well-being retreat offered three times a year to all residents in his program. This particular retreat was focused on finding personal renewal in the work of caring for patients. During a small group discussion, one of the senior residents shared that she had felt burned out and uncaring by the middle of her second year. This led to a discussion about burnout and the vulnerability most residents have to this phenomenon. Another resident stated that what had helped him was observing an attending at the bedside of a dying patient showing considerable patience and compassion and asking him how he did that. This attending had replied that he kept a journal of memorable events from the day that gave him an opportunity for reflection. As the group talked, it became clear to Bill that he was not alone with this erosion of meaning and that there were personal and group strategies for renewing his enthusiasm for medicine.

Carl Rogers once said that "what is most personal is most universal." Nothing can be so personally isolating as the perception that one has lost one's way professionally. It is reminiscent of the poignant lament of Dante at the opening of the *Divina Comedia*:

> In the middle of the road of my life I awoke in a dark wood where the true way was wholly lost.

Nothing can be so healing and reassuring as to know that others have traveled the same road and have emerged as colleagues to admire and emulate. The value of retreats, support groups, or even impromptu discussions during lulls in the pace of work to share common experiences and struggles is to remind trainees that they are part of the human community and that they have the capacity for renewal and change.

Support groups are an especially valuable learning format in residency training programs to help residents navigate personal and professional developmental tasks, learn self-management and emotion management skills, build authentic community with their peers, and promote their well-being. Developmental challenges common to residents include establishing one's professional identity, developing professional confidence, coping with patient deaths, erosion of an idealized view of medicine, cognitive and behavioral management of stress, assuming the responsibility of a team leader, developing a reflective capacity for self-awareness, finding a career path, and learning self-acceptance and the limitations of personal control. Having a safe and confidential format for sharing these issues with one's peers is vital to a resident's professional development, and training programs would be wise to incorporate this into their curricula.

Emotional Intelligence

Among the strategies that trainees can use for restoring a capacity for compassion and enjoyment of work is the cultivation of "emotional intelligence." Developing self-awareness is essential to emotional intelligence. This is a challenge for clinicians who have been trained to dissociate from their feelings as a way of being "objective" in their professional role with patients. Since the quality of clinicians' relationships with their patients is a major component of the therapeutic process as well as a major contributor to their own well-being, developing self-awareness to maximize this process is essential (see Chapter 7). Emotional intelligence includes developing a language for one's emotions and a capacity of self-disclosure to others. The mirror of this process of self-awareness and self-expression is the capacity to recognize emotions in others. We can use our own emotions to develop hypotheses about what the other is feeling. We can learn to check out feelings with others, reflect feelings, comment on what we are observing, and receive the emotional disclosure of others without judgment. It can be helpful to regard emotions as value-neutral information that is passing through our awareness like weather systems, which in themselves are neither right nor wrong. Thus we can think of attending to the patient's feelings as getting a "weather report" and awareness of our own feelings as "checking the weather." Accepting our own emotions and those of others can be liberating and allow us to be fully present to others and ourselves (see Chapters 2 and 7).

Other components of emotional intelligence include controlling impulses, especially by delaying our response in conflict situations, delaying gratification for the sake of achieving goals, and using cognitive reframing and self-instructional statements to regulate our moods. We can enhance our emotional intelligence by naming internally what we are feeling at the moment, keeping a journal that captures the predominant feelings we have experienced on a given day, practicing using emotional words with friends and intimate partners, reflecting the feelings that others disclose to us, and in some cases by engaging in psychotherapy to enhance our emotional literacy.

Self-regulation of anxiety and situational stress is a skill that can be learned in the context of training. It is an essential prerequisite for the accurate perception of patients' distress, which facilitates the use of empathy skills (see Chapter 2). A Belgian study of resident physicians on an inpatient rotation found that their self-reported anxiety and physiologic measures of sympathetic nervous system arousal were inversely related to their ability to detect patients' distress.

Bill's feeling of futility in caring for patients who did not get better in spite of his best efforts emanated from his own beliefs and expectations about control. Gaining clarity about the extent to which control is possible in the events of our lives, and in the profession of medicine in particular, is essential to satisfaction with the work of being a doctor. Although people tend to be more satisfied when they perceive a greater control over the events that impact them, most of the outcomes of patient care are multidetermined and to a large extent dependent on many forces beyond the physician's control, including patient choices as well as genetic and environmental variables. Thinking in terms of "influence" rather than "control" may be more realistic. Within the large array of factors that contribute to illness and health, physicians can have enormous influence, but medical care is only one of several events that contribute to the eventual outcome. Assuming a Zen approach of focusing on "right action" in the moment—whether it is the exercise of empathy, conducting a careful physical examination, engaging clinical reasoning, or performing a procedure—and releasing the need to have the outcome be a marker of one's competence, can provide a helpful cognitive framework for self-assessment. Other strategies for inoculating ourselves against futility may include finding meaning in small victories, such as preventing a hospitalization for a patient with chronic emphysema; using a recurrent worsening of a condition, such as a patient repeatedly admitted for diabetic ketoacidosis, as an opportunity to learn more about clinical medicine; regarding "difficult patients" as visiting professors because of the learning they can provide about how to manage such patients; focusing on the quality of the relationship with the patient whose condition is worsening; and spending some reflective time recalling the positive connections with patients who appreciate the work we do.

Common to several of the unhealthy habits described above (compulsiveness, the psychology of postponement, dissociation from feelings, and tolerating conditions of burnout) is the notion of work as *energy depletion*. Hence many physicians, nurses, administrators and others view weekends, vacations, and time with family as the opportunity to recharge and recapture a more expansive awareness. Some seek to expand the time available for recharging by working parttime. The converse of protected "personal time" is the intense compression of "work time" and the density of tasks to be processed in a given day. During this surreal pursuit of the processing of tasks in which "productivity" is equated with "being good," an altered state of consciousness emerges (see Chapter 5). This is a trance that one enters in the presence of certain ritualistic cues (the door to the office, turning on the computer, checking the schedule, retrieving voice mails) and may include running an incessant "to do" list, looking for brief tasks to process in an illusory pursuit of "closure," a shortened attention span, irritability in the presence of lengthy or labored conversations, a habit of checking and rechecking one's work, stewing about difficult interactions in the past, and worrying about future events.

Renewal, Reflection, and Mindfulness

Steve McPhee, a professor of medicine at UCSF, has used the metaphor of solar-powered versus gasoline-powered automobiles to contrast different approaches to human energy in our daily lives. The notion of work as a locus of energy depletion (requiring a leaving of work to find energy renewal) is similar to the nonrenewable dependence of industrial societies on fossil fuels. In the long run, such a view of one's own energy is unsustainable. An alternative perspective is that *energy renewal* is continually available as one moves through the day, whether at work or away from work. This is analogous to the solar-powered car, which requires the opening of panels to draw on the renewable energy from the sun. Such a fundamental shift in our thinking about energy may entail reevaluating our notion of who we are. The fossil fuel model represents a view of oneself as an individual source of productivity and accomplishment, acting with agency upon the material world and upon people's lives to achieve outcomes. The solar panel model suggests a view of oneself as a medium of energy exchange, a self-organizing system much like a candle flame that gives off light in the process of continuous transformation, a system that is embedded within, and a part of, larger self-organizing systems such as a doctor–patient relationship, a health care system, a society, a the earth itself.

Trainees should ask themselves: How can we open ourselves to renewal as we move through our days, both at work and at home? What is the psychological equivalent of "opening our solar panels?" One approach is the cultivation of *mindfulness*, which is the practice of being present to where we are and what we are doing. It is the discipline of living an intentional, conscious life (see Chapter 7). Our stream of consciousness often includes thoughts about the past, sometimes accompanied by regret or resentment, and thoughts and images of the future, sometimes threatening, sometimes escapist. Mindfulness is a counterweight to this enchantment with the "there and then" by increasing our skill at being present in the "here and now." Mindfulness involves nonjudgmental attention to our emotional and mental states as they pass through awareness. We learn to see ourselves as vessels through which the various feelings of joy, sorrow, anger, affection, peace, and agitation flow without defining who we are in any moment of intensity. Twenty minutes a day practicing mindfulness meditation can enhance our capacity for mindful attention. This practice can help physicians be present to patients without interference from what happens before or after that encounter. Mindfulness is also the gateway to accessing opportunities for personal renewal in the midst of work, where in addition to expending energy, we are also receiving energy from personal interactions or the satisfaction of work well done.

The process of approaching each day with mindfulness and openness to the uncertainty of who will walk in the door next, and nonjudgmental attention to the "weather" of our own emotions and those of others, is captured in this poem by Rumi, the thirteenth-century Sufi mystic whose verses reach across the centuries and cultures to speak to our own experience:

The Guest House
This being human is a guest house.
Every morning a new arrival.

A joy, a depression, a meanness,
some momentary awareness comes
as an unexpected visitor.

Welcome and entertain them all!
Even if they're a crowd of sorrows,
who violently sweep your house
empty of its furniture,
still, treat each guest honorably.
He may be clearing you out
for some new delight.

The dark thought, the shame, the malice,
meet them at the door laughing,
and invite them in.

Be grateful for whoever comes,
because each has been sent
as a guide from beyond.

Incorporating a brief period of reflection at the end of each day is one way of conditioning ourselves to perceive the opportunities for personal renewal and meaning contained in various encounters of the day. Using a journal or simply reflecting back for a few minutes on the events of the day can offer a transitional time to let go of the day and absorb the gifts that came our way. Angeles Arrien suggests that we ask ourselves three simple questions: "What surprised me today? What moved me today? What inspired me today?" Sometimes we may find that there has been great meaning in our encounters with the full panoply of human experience, including suffering. A related practice is that of keeping a "gratitude journal," which can be done at the end of the week. This involves writing down a few things from the week for which one is thankful, from simple events like watching a particularly beautiful sunrise to more profound ones like a satisfying encounter with a patient with whom one had a previously troubling relationship.

 CASE ILLUSTRATION 2 (CONTD.)

In the weeks following the resident retreat, Bill experimented with keeping a journal.. Gradually he found himself noticing sources of energy boost during his day—a joke shared with the nursing staff, the satisfaction of having been present to a patient's distress with compassion, learning a new way of working up patients for certain illnesses, being able to guide an intern in managing a difficult admission, observing a faculty preceptor facilitate a difficult family meeting about end-of-life care. He read a little each day in an introductory book on mindfulness meditation and on some days was able to take 5 minutes to practice meditation before his day began. Some days were incredibly busy, and he was still confronted with uncertain medical dilemmas and difficult patients, but he seemed to take it more in stride. He found himself more frequently centering himself before walking into the next patient's room by taking a couple of breaths and letting go of what went before, while embracing the unknown of the encounter awaiting him. Most helpful to him were some discussions with fellow residents in which he found himself more willing to share the stresses and uncertainties of his work and to enjoy the comradeship of knowing he was not alone.

Intimacy and Value Clarification

If our relationship commitments are consistently subordinated to work demands, a review and clarification of our values is in order. Although humbling, we can get a glimpse into our value hierarchy by examining how we actually spend our time and energy in any given week. We may find that what our practice reveals is at variance with what we tell ourselves and others about our deepest values. We also may find that much of the way we spend our time is in response to urgent demands that are not that important in the long run.

In addition to the challenge of nurturing our relationships with family and friends when constrained by professional demands, another barrier is posed by a fear of intimacy or the lack of skill in sharing our inner selves with others. Since clinicians spend much of their time on the receiving end of others' confidences and disclosures, they may have less practice in self-disclosure. It is in relationship with others, however, that we deepen our identity and sense of who we are as persons. This requires not only the presence of close relationships, in and out of medicine, but also time spent with them and the capacity for self-disclosure and intimacy.

- *Friends.* Given the general erosion of community in American life, we must actively seek connections with others. Sometimes opportunities for forming friendships will arise in the work setting, and there it depends on our willingness to take the initiative. We also can develop hobbies and interests outside of medicine that form natural settings for people with similar interests coming together, whether it is through the arts, volunteer work, political action, a faith community, sports, or engaging in outdoor activities. It is not sufficient to have a network of friends without developing our capacity for self-disclosure. Learning to confide in trusted friends is an essential counterbalance to long hours of receiving the confidences of patients in our professional roles.

- *Intimate partners.* A love relationship sustained over time can be one of the great spiritual paths to our growth and development as persons. A long-term and even life-long journey with an intimate partner is a cauldron which both tests our identity and expands our capacity to embrace life and endure its stresses and challenges. It is in such a relationship that we can learn acceptance of ourselves with all our flaws and virtues. We also can learn the art of compassion through nurturing our beloved and seeking their well-being. Building and maintaining a successful partnership requires scheduled time. Enhancing our interpersonal communication skills—especially the art of active listening, disclosure of feelings, and negotiating respectfully when there are differences and conflict—is central to an enduring relationship. Other vital intimacy skills include awareness of our family of origin influences on couple communication and expectations; learning to tolerate differences in tastes and preferences; clarifying mutual values as a couple; and negotiating time, sex, money, space, division of labor, and whether and how to raise children. Romance and sex may occur spontaneously in the early stages of a relationship, but over time require our intentional planning to create the time and conditions for this vital component of a relationship to be a lasting source of mutual renewal. Sometimes couples get stuck in stagnating patterns or impasses in their communication, and at such times couple counseling can be a valuable resource.

One constraint to giving ourselves the needed time to honor personal values and relationships may be concern about money. Many physicians at the beginning of their career are understandably worried about paying off medical school debt. This may lead to working longer hours in the earlier years, or even moonlighting, which diminishes time and energy for family, friends, and hobbies. Sometimes material aspirations and the consumer mentality of our culture lead us to encumber more debt than is necessary, and we end up trading valuable time for more money to service those debts. The way money flows through our lives and whether it is a burden or a useful tool will depend on our core philosophy about wealth. Engaging in a process of clarifying our life values and financial goals, either through consultation with a financial planner or reading financial self-help literature, can provide a framework for making wise decisions about what we need to sustain our lives and how much time and energy we will expend in generating an income to support those needs. One physician couple reported a process of reflection they used when they realized they were "sacrificing precious time and earning money to support a lifestyle not worth living." They engaged in a process of value clarification and financial assessment that eventually led to downsizing their material possessions, eliminating debt, and embracing a path of "voluntary simplicity." They traded financial wealth for the time to travel, spend more time with their families, and pursue other interests.

Organizations and Trainee Well-Being

Although it is essential to engage in self-reflection, value clarification, and behavior change to move our own lives toward renewal and sustainability, viewing this solely as a personal project will not be sufficient to make meaningful changes. Well-being is not only an individual process, but a political process as well. With the best of intentions we may begin a practice of mindfulness, enhancement of our intimate relationships, and caring for ourselves physically—only to have those intentions evaporate at the next attending rounds or faculty meeting where overwork is reinforced and rewarded with admiration, the esteem of colleagues, and the imperatives of meeting productivity expectations. For the well-being of trainees to thrive, the organizations in which they are trained and work (hospital systems, group practices, academic medical centers, and government institutions) must be sustainable enterprises that value the health and well-being of all their workers. Each of us has a responsibility not only to ourselves but to our colleagues and our profession to engage in the difficult work of changing our organizations—medical schools, residencies, health care systems, and practice settings—so that they allow time and energy for "those gentler influences which make life worth living."

CONCLUSIONS

The woodblock print seen below, *The Great Wave off Kanagawa*, by the artist Katsushika Hokusai, is from a series entitled "36 Views of Mt. Fuji." It captures several of the elements of personal and organizational well-being we have discussed above. The first and most obvious element is the waves, which are relentlessly chaotic and threaten to capsize the boats. The waves call to mind the ongoing challenges and uncertainty of clinical training and practice. The second element is the people in the boats, who require cohesion, teamwork, and ongoing communication to keep the boats headed into the waves and moving successfully forward on their journey. Our colleagues and team working alongside us are a vital resource for navigating each day of patient care and the developmental hurdles of professional formation. A healthy organization provides such a disciplined collaboration for its members, so that no one person bears the sole burden of responsibility. The third element is Mt. Fuji, at first indistinguishable from the waves, which in its deeply grounded stability provides the still point in the center of this painting around which the chaos revolves.

Mindfulness and self-awareness can provide such an inner stillness allowing us to rest at the deepest center of ourselves as we continually adjust our balance to catch the next wave.

Training health professionals in this complex, information-rich and choice-rich era of human history requires new skills that were not required of previous generations. At the same time, doing so in a way that sustains both educators and trainees as persons requires drawing upon the "practical wisdom" of previous generations. This practical wisdom, what Aristotle called *phronesis*, incorporates the cognitive, emotional, behavioral, and interpersonal skills to expand our capacity as persons and reduce or eliminate the nonimportant and unnecessary loads that erode our spirits. We also need to develop a practical wisdom of working within health care systems that is mindful of the factors that promote sustainability, such as expanding our capacity for service through teamwork, clarifying the organization's values, and establishing structures and processes that promote the well-being of health care workers. This perspective is the responsibility of trainees and faculty alike. Developing the practical wisdom to engage in this work in a sustainable way is our personal and collective challenge.

The Great Wave off Kanagawa, Katsushika Hokusai, c. 1830

SUGGESTED READINGS

Barks C, trans.. *The Essential Rumi*. Edison, N.J.: Castle Books, 1997.

Christensen JF, Feldman MD, eds. Recapturing the spirit of medicine (Special issue on physician well-being). *Western J Med* 2001; 174:1–80.http://www.ncbi.nlm.nih.gov/pmc/issues/116276/. Accessed February 2014.

Elgin D. *Voluntary Simplicity: Toward a Way of Life that is Outwardly Simple, Inwardly Rich*. New York: William Morrow, 1993.

Gabbard GO. The role of compulsiveness in the normal physician. *JAMA* 1985;254:2926–2929.

Gabbard GO, Menninger RW. The psychology of postponement in the medical marriage. *JAMA* 1989;261:2378–2381.

Kabat-Zinn J. *Wherever You Go There You Are: Mindfulness Meditation in Everyday Life.* New York: Hyperion, 1994.

Kinder G. *Seven Stages of Money Maturity.* New York: Dell, 1999.

McPhee SJ. Letter from the abbey. *Western J Med* 2001;174:73–75.

Meunier J, Libert Y, Merckaert I, et al. How much is residents' distress detection performance during a clinical round related to their characteristics? Patient Educ Counsel 2011;85:1880–1187.

Mizrahi T. *Getting Rid of Patients.* New Brunswick, N.J.: Rutgers University Press, 1986.

Osler W. Address to students of the Albany Medical College, February 1, 1899. *Albany Med Ann* 1899;261:307–309.

Ratanawongsa N, et al. Well-being in residency: a time for temporary imbalance? *Med Educ* 2007;41:237–280.

Satterfield JM, Becerra C. Developmental challenges, stressors, and coping strategies in medical residents: a qualitative analysis of support groups. *Med Educ* 2010;44:908–916.

Spickard A, Gabbe SG, Christensen JF . Mid-career burnout in generalist and specialist physicians. *JAMA* 2002;288:1447–1450.

Thich Nhat Hanh. *The Miracle of Mindfulness: A Manual on Meditation.* Boston: Beacon Press, 1987.

Walcott D. *Collected Poems 1948-1984.* New York: Farrar Strauss & Giroux, 1987.

West CP, et al. Quality of life, burnout, educational debt, and medical knowledge among internal medicine residents. *JAMA* 2011;306:952–960.

OTHER RESOURCE

Christensen JF. Balance and Self-Care. *Web-based learning module in Doc.com: An Interactive Learning Resource for Healthcare Communication.* American Academy on Communication in Healthcare. www.aachonline.org. Accessed February 2014.

WEB SITES

American Medical Student Association. Resources on medical student well-being. http://www.amsa.org/well/. Accessed February 2014.

The Foundation for Medical Excellence (Annual conference on physician well-being). http://www.tfme.org. Accessed February 2014.

Financial Integrity (Transforming our relationship with money). http://www.financialintegrity.org/index.php?title=Main_Page. Accessed February 2014.

Seligman M, et al. Positive Psychology Annotated Bibliography. Center for Positive Psychology, University of Pennsylvania. http://www.ppc.sas.upenn.edu/ppappend.htm. Accessed February 2014.

Index

Note: Page numbers followed by *t* indicate tables; those followed by *f* indicate figures.

CPSIA information can be obtained
at www.ICGtesting.com
Printed in the USA
BVHW01s0816160818
524651BV00005B/31/P

5539 014

9 780071 767705